Equine Breeding Management and Artificial Insemination

Equine Breeding Management and Artificial Insemination

SECOND EDITION

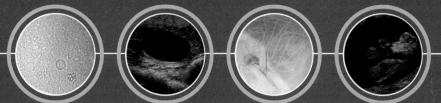

Juan C. Samper, DVM, MSc, PhD,
   Diplomate American College of Theriogenologists
Veterinary Reproductive Services
Langley, British Columbia, Canada

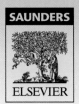

SAUNDERS

ELSEVIER

636.1
E648e

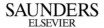

11830 Westline Industrial Drive
St. Louis, Missouri 63146

EQUINE BREEDING MANAGEMENT AND ARTIFICIAL INSEMINATION, SECOND EDITION   ISBN: 978-1-4160-5234-0
Copyright © 2009, 2000 by Saunders, an imprint of Elsevier Inc.

Notice

Knowledge and best practice in this field are constantly changing. As new research and experience broaden our knowledge, changes in practice, treatment and drug therapy may become necessary or appropriate. Readers are advised to check the most current information provided (i) on procedures featured or (ii) by the manufacturer of each product to be administered, to verify the recommended dose or formula, the method and duration of administration, and contraindications. It is the responsibility of the practitioner, relying on their own experience and knowledge of the patient, to make diagnoses, to determine dosages and the best treatment for each individual patient, and to take all appropriate safety precautions. To the fullest extent of the law, neither the Publisher nor the Editors assumes any liability for any injury and/or damage to persons or property arising out or related to any use of the material contained in this book.

The Publisher

Library of Congress Cataloging in Publication Data

Equine breeding management and artificial insemination / [edited by] Juan C. Samper. — 2nd ed.
    p. cm.
Includes bibliographical references and index.
ISBN 978-1-4160-5234-0 (pbk. : alk. paper)
1. Horses—Breeding. 2. Horses—Artificial insemination. I. Samper, Juan. C.
SF291.E68 2009
636.1'082--dc22

2008047525

Vice President and Publisher: Linda Duncan
Publisher: Penny Rudolph
Managing Editor: Jolynn Gower
Senior Developmental Editor: Shelly Stringer
Publishing Services Manager: Patricia Tannian
Senior Project Manager: John Casey
Designer: Kim Denando

Printed in United States of America

Last digit is the print number: 8   7   6   5   4   3   2   1

Contributors

Marco A. Alvarenga, DVM, MSc, PhD
Professor
Department of Animal Reproduction and
    Veterinary Radiology
University of São Paulo State
Botucatu, São Paulo, Brazil

Doug. F. Antczak, VMD, PhD
Professor
Director, Baker Institute
Cornell University
Ithaca, New York

Don R. Bergfelt, MS, PhD
Honorary Fellow
School of Veterinary Medicine
Department of Animal Health
    and Biomedical Sciences
University of Wisconsin
Madison, Wisconsin;
Scientist and Biologist
Office of Science Coordination and Policy
Environmental Protection Agency
Washington, DC

Claire Card, DVM, PhD, DACT
Associate Professor and Director
Department of Large Animal Clinical Sciences
Western College of Veterinary Medicine
University of Saskatchewan
Saskatoon, Saskatchewan, Canada

Elaine M. Carnevale, DVM, MS, PhD
Assistant Professor
Department of Biomedical Sciences
Colorado State University
Fort Collins, Colorado

Tracey S. Chenier, DVM, DVSc, DACT
Assistant Professor
Large Animal Theriogenology
Department of Population Medicine
Ontario Veterinary College
University of Guelph
Guelph, Ontario, Canada

Isabel Gomez, DVM
Resident Veterinarian
P.S. Pferdehaltung
Lewitz, Germany

John P. Hurtgen, DVM, MS, PhD, DACT
Owner
Nandi Veterinary Associates LLC
New Freedom, Pennsylvania

Fernanda da Cruz Landim-Alvarenga, DVM, MSc, PhD
Professor
Department of Animal Reproduction and Veterinary Radiology
University of São Paulo State
Botucatu, São Paulo, Brazil

Charles C. Love, DVM, PhD, DACT
Associate Professor
Department of Large Animal Medicine
Texas A&M University
College Station, Texas

Sarah K. Lyle, DVM, MS, DACT
Clinical Instructor
Department of Veterinary Clinical Sciences
School of Veterinary Medicine
Louisiana State University
Baton Rouge, Louisiana

Phil Matthews, DVM
Director
Equine Reproduction Center
Peterson and Smith Equine Hospital
Ocala, Florida

Sue M. McDonnell, MS, PhD
Equine Behavior Laboratory
Section of Medicine and Reproduction
School of Veterinary Medicine
New Bolton Center
University of Pennsylvania
Kennett Square, Pennsylvania

Stuart Meyers, DVM, MS, PhD, DACT
Professor
Department of Anatomy and Physiology and Cell Biology
School of Veterinary Medicine
University of California
Davis, California

Dale Paccamonti, DVM, MS, DACT
Professor or Theriogenology
Department of Veterinary Clinical Sciences
Louisiana State University
Baton Rouge, Louisiana

Deborah A. Parsons, DVM, DACVIM
Parsons Equine Internal Medicine Services
Langley, British Columbia, Canada

Nelson Pinto, DVM
College of Veterinary Medicine
Large Animal Teaching Hospital
Auburn University
Auburn, Alabama

Jonathan F. Pycock, BVetMed, PhD, DESM, MRCVS
Director
Equine Reproductive Services
Messenger Farm
Malton, North Yorkshire, United Kingdom

Fernando L. Riera, DVM
Director
Centro de Reproduccion Equina
Doña Pilar
Lincoln, Argentina

Jacobo Sebastian Rodriguez, MV
Theriogenology Resident
Veterinary Clinical Sciences
Washington University
Pullman, Washington

Roberto Sanchez, DVM
Resident Veterinarian
P.S. Pferdehaltung
Lewitz, Germany

Harald Sieme, DVM, Dr Med Vet
Director and Professor
Equine Reproductive Services
University Veterinary Foundation of Hanover
Hanover, Germany

Kim A. Sprayberry, DVM, DACVIM
Internist
Department of Internal Medicine
Hagyard Equine Medical Institute
Lexington, Kentucky

†John V. Steiner, DVM, DACT
Department of Theriogenology
Hagyard Equine Medical Institute
Lexington, Kentucky

Tom A. E. Stout, MA, Vet MB, PhD, MRCVS, DECAR
Professor of Equine Medicine and Reproduction
Department of Equine Sciences
Utrecht University
Utrecht, The Netherlands

Ahmed Tibary, DMV, MS, PhD, DSc, DACT
Professor
Veterinary Clinical Sciences
Washington State University
Pullman, Washington

Norman W. Umphenour, DVM
Resident Veterinarian, Ashford Stud
Versailles, Kentucky

†Deceased

This book is dedicated to the broodmare.
With the help of equine theriogenologists, her offspring are the foundation of
equine practice and provide work for all equine practitioners.

PREFACE

Theriogenology. It is difficult word to pronounce let alone to understand. There is no denying that it is a strange word. However, when one learns that an animal gynecologist, obstetrician, andrologist, and blood stock or genetic advisor can be summarized into the word *theriogenologist,* then the term becomes not so difficult to understand. Most veterinarians soon after graduation will practice this discipline to some extent, and a good proportion of them will choose to dedicate their entire career to it. Our discipline continues to grow, since it is the basis for reproduction, production, and productivity of all species, yet the number of faculty positions in theriogenology has been diminishing despite its importance and the increasing interest in this field among students and veterinarians around the world. Is it possible that veterinary schools will relinquish the teaching of this important discipline to field veterinarians, with these institutions losing on the advancement of science within our discipline and depriving students of the advantages of learning at these centers? Is it possible that veterinarians will surrender the practice of veterinary medicine to professionals in other fields because universities cannot fulfill the market's needs? Is it possible that we as theriogenologists have not done a good enough job of explaining to colleagues and producers what the practice of reproductive medicine represents to the animal industry?

The second edition of *Equine Breeding Management and Artificial Insemination* was assembled with the hope of fulfilling two major objectives. First, to define what a theriogenologist is and what he or she can bring to the practice of veterinary medicine. Second, to try to bridge the gap between the scientist and the field veterinarian or breeder so that the information that is generated in laboratories and that sometimes seems remote to our daily practice can be easily understood and applied. To achieve these objectives, 27 chapters were written by a group of authors that are well regarded for their practical, scientific knowledge and background. A theriogenologist, who is a veterinarian that practices reproductive medicine, should be able to practice and discuss with a great degree of confidence each one of these chapters with breeders, owners, and producers.

A great deal of emphasis has been placed on the management aspect of reproduction. This second edition of *Equine Breeding Management and Artificial Insemination* has been expanded to complete the circle, incorporating the management of the breeding process, the pregnant mare, foaling, post-foaling, and the care of the newborn. We know that success or failure in reproduction is attributable in great part to the management practices that are in place during the breeding process. That is why with improper interference we can render very fertile animals infertile, whereas with proper management, others that have limited reproductive capacity can reproduce with seemingly less effort. Although it seems that breeding subfertile animals using the available reproductive techniques would perpetuate a problem, breeding decisions, particularly in horses, are seldom based on reproductive potential.

Today's equine industry is heterogeneous, and motivations for breeding are equally varied, ranging from sentimental to economic. It is therefore imperative that as theriogenologists we understand the industry in which we work, the motivations of owners to breed, and the economic implications that our work has. Without this clear understanding it will be difficult to connect with owners or breeders, and the decisions that we make and the advice we give might not be in the best interest of their or their animals' needs.

It is my sincere hope that those that read this book realize that the practice of our specialty, although sometimes appearing trivial and mundane, has many exciting facets that are and will continue to be the basis for the production and reproduction of all species. The refinement of assisted reproductive techniques, coupled with the information available from the equine genome, will provide important and exciting avenues that our profession will need to incorporate into the practice of reproductive medicine.

Juan C. Samper

ACKNOWLEDGMENTS

I would like to start by thanking the authors of the individual chapters for the timely delivery and the quality of the work that you have produced. I know that all of you are very busy, and taking the time to review the literature and write your chapters was yet another burden that at times appears unappreciated. However, I am sure that the students, veterinarians, and breeders that read this book appreciate the time and effort that you have devoted to your particular subject.

I would like to thank all of my clients for their friendship and support over the years—my colleagues and friends that are not chapter authors but have contributed immensely to this book through frequent discussions and thoughtful insight. Thanks to my wife and the mother of our four daughters, Cristina, Paula, Ana Maria, and Sofia, for their continuous support, patience, and understanding and for providing a loving family environment to work in.

I would also like to thank the staff from Elsevier: Penny Rudolph, Publisher, John Casey, Senior Project Manager, Shelly Stringer, Senior Developmental Editor, and Brandi Graham, Editorial Assistant. Your help, support, and above all, your patience made this venture easier to accomplish. A very special thank you to Jolynn Gower, Managing Editor, who started the project with me. Your guidance and patience during the initial stages were critical to the start and the completion of this book in a timely fashion.

CONTENTS

Teaching consists of causing or allowing people to get into situations from which they cannot escape except by thinking

Equine Breeding Management and Artificial Insemination

Anatomy and Physical Examination of the Stallion

Tracey S. Chenier

This chapter discusses the normal anatomy of both external and internal genitalia of the stallion, including the scrotum, testes, epididymides, spermatic cords, penis, prepuce, ampullae, vesicular glands, prostate gland, and bulbourethral (BU) glands. A brief overview of the relevant findings of physical examination and ultrasonographic examination is included in each section.

MANAGEMENT OF BREEDING STALLIONS

Equine practitioners involved with the care of breeding stallions should consider the importance of frequent and routine examinations of those stallions. A thorough understanding of the physical anatomy of the stallion places the clinician in a better position to monitor the health and reproductive status of the stallions under his or her care. Familiarity with the appearance and palpation findings of normal structures is imperative for detecting what can be subtle deviations from normal. As part of routine management, all normal breeding stallions should receive a complete breeding soundness examination at least twice yearly. An initial examination should occur in advance of the breeding season to allow time to address any potential problems. Stallions with ongoing problems should be examined monthly to monitor progression of disease conditions. This examination should include a thorough physical examination; palpation and ultrasound of the scrotum, testes, and spermatic cords; careful inspection of the erect penis and sheath; and rectal examination with ultrasound of the accessory glands. Additional tests such as routine blood panels for complete blood count, profile, and hormonal tests might be considered in individual cases. Every ejaculate should be examined for color, semen volume, total number of sperm, motility. and morphology. Total number of sperm and morphology are especially important as indicators of testicular health. Early detection of problems can allow management changes to prolong the fertility of stallions with many conditions.

EXTERNAL GENITALIA

The Scrotum

The scrotum of the stallion is located high in the inguinal region and is slightly pendulous. It forms two distinct pouches that contain, protect, and thermoregulate the testes, epididymides, spermatic cords, and cremaster muscles. The testes are located in the scrotum to maintain testicular temperature at several degrees below core body temperature, a necessity for normal spermatogenesis.[1,2] Thermography of scrotal contents of stallions has demonstrated a scrotal skin temperature of 33°C, with testis contents at 30.5° to 32.5°C.[1]

The wall of the scrotum consists of four layers: (1) skin, (2) tunica dartos, (3) scrotal fascia, and (4) parietal vaginal tunic.[3-6] The scrotal skin is thin, generally hairless, and slightly oily, containing numerous sebaceous and sweat glands, which assist in testis thermoregulation.[3,7] The tunica dartos layer is adherent to the scrotal skin and consists of muscular and fibroelastic tissue. It lines both scrotal pouches and extends into the median septum, seen externally as the median raphae of the scrotum. The degree of contraction or relaxation of this layer allows alterations in the size, shape, and position of the scrotum in relation to the body wall, thereby aiding testis thermoregulation. The scrotal fascia, a loose connective tissue layer between the tunica dartos and parietal vaginal tunic, allows the testes and associated parietal tunic layer to move freely within the scrotum.[5] The innermost layer of the scrotum, the parietal vaginal tunic, is an evagination of the parietal peritoneum through the inguinal rings, which forms during testicular descent. This layer forms a sac that lines the scrotum and is closely apposed to the visceral vaginal tunic, the outer layer of the testis. The vaginal cavity is the space between the parietal and visceral layers of the vaginal tunic. It normally contains a very small amount of viscous fluid to allow some free movement of the testis within. The vaginal cavity is a potential space within which considerable fluid may accumulate as a result of a variety of causes.

The scrotum of the normal stallion should appear slightly pendulous, globular, and generally symmetric (Fig. 1-1). Normal variations may be observed in the positioning of the testes if one is relatively anterior to or ventral to the other. The skin should have no evidence of trauma, scarring, or skin lesions. Palpation of the scrotum of a normal stallion reveals a thin and pliable covering, which slides loosely and easily over the testicles and epididymides within.

The Testes

Testicular Descent

The testicles normally descend into a scrotal position between the last 30 days of gestation and the first 10 days postpartum (Fig. 1-2).[7,8-11] In some colts, the testes may descend into the inguinal region and remain there for some time before fully descending into the scrotum. The hormonal factors involved in testicular descent in the stallion are poorly understood. Research in the rat has demonstrated the involvement of androgens and luteinizing hormone (LH) in the process. The timing of testicular descent coincides with significant rises in endogenous gonadotropins. It appears that an intact hypothalamic-pituitary axis, adequate LH levels, and several physical factors must be present for normal testicular descent to occur. In midgestation,

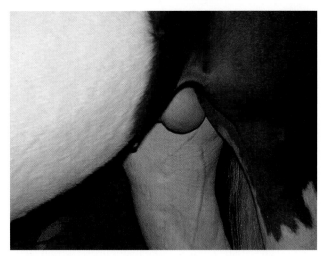

Figure 1-1. The scrotum of the stallion is slightly pendulous, with the testes held in a horizontal position. Frequently one testicle may be held much higher to the body wall than the other, as shown.

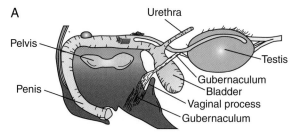

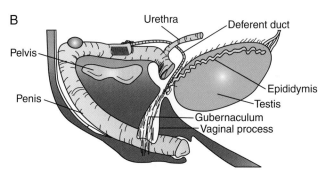

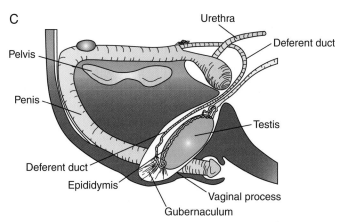

Figure 1-2. Stages of testicular descent into the scrotum of the horse fetus. **A,** Fetus at 75 days of gestation. **B,** Fetus at 175 days of gestation. **C,** Fetus near term (330 days of gestation). (From Varner DD, Schumacher J, Blanchard T, et al: *Diseases and Management of Breeding Stallions.* Goleta, CA: American Veterinary Publications, 1991.)

the abdominal fetal testis hypertrophies significantly, resulting in the developing gonad resting close to the vaginal ring. The developing gubernaculum and abdominal pressure hold the testes in place until late gestation, despite considerable decrease in the size of the gonads later in gestation. The caudal ligament, which attaches the epididymis to the caudal pole of the testis, initially lengthens faster than the rest of the gubernaculum, resulting in the epididymis being drawn into the vaginal ring and inguinal canal. Dilation of the vaginal ring and inguinal canal, combined with abdominal pressure and traction from the gubernaculum, eventually draws the testes into the ring as well.

Failure of the testes to descend into a normal scrotal position is termed *cryptorchidism*. Unilateral cryptorchidism is far more common than bilateral cryptorchidism in horses. Only 14% of cryptorchid stallions had a bilateral condition.[10] At birth, the testes are often located within the inguinal ring. Further contraction of the gubernaculum results in the testes being drawn into the scrotum. In a newborn colt, palpation of the prominent gubernaculum and/or epididymis within the scrotum may be mistaken for a testis. Diagnosis of cryptorchidism is attained by manual palpation of scrotal contents. Rectal palpation and careful inguinal palpation may assist in identification of an abdominally or inguinally retained testis. Ultrasonography has also been recommended as a diagnostic tool for this.[12] In horses with bilaterally retained testicles or apparent geldings with stallion-like behavior, hormonal profiles may be useful in diagnosis of a retained testis.[13,14] Baseline testosterone (T) levels have been suggested as a method to diagnose retained testicular tissue in an apparent gelding.[13,15] However, low wintertime T values in normal stallions, a relatively high percentage of nondiagnostic values, and false-negative values are problems with the test. The use of a single measurement of plasma total estrogens or conjugated estrogens (ES), without human chorionic gonadotropin (hCG) stimulation, also appears to be reliable in the diagnosis of cryptorchidism in colts older than 3 years of age.[13] A stimulation test using hCG reduces the number of nondiagnostic test results obtained with both ES and T measurement. To perform the hCG stimulation test, a baseline blood sample is collected immediately prior to injection of 5000–10,000 IU of hCG intravenously. Follow-up blood samples for T or ES are obtained 60 and 120 minutes later. A fivefold or greater increase in T indicates

that a retained testicle is present. One study demonstrated that the increase in T after hCG stimulation peaked 2–3 days after injection,[14] so it may be advisable to take additional samples at 24 and 48 hours following injection. One study demonstrated that T, but not ES, values increased following the hCG stimulation test. Since the testis of colts younger than 3 years of age produces significantly less ES, false-negative results may occur when ES is measured.[13]

Hormonal therapy to induce testis descent in a cryptorchid stallion is controversial, and no studies exist on its efficacy. LH therapy is commonly used to try to stimulate testis descent in boys with inguinally retained testis. In rats, hCG treatment was able to reverse the blocking effect of estradiol treatment on testicular descent, suggesting a role for LH in the process. One recent study evaluated the ability of the testis of prepubertal colts to respond to hCG hormone injections.[16] Colts of 180–200 days age were given 2500 IU hCG intramuscularly twice weekly for 4 weeks. Treatment resulted in significant increases in testosterone values by 48 hours post-injection. The testis volume in treated colts was greater at the end of therapy (16.4 cm^3 vs. 22.5 cm^3)

whereas untreated colts showed no significant change in testis volume. This study suggests a possible mechanism by which LH therapy for cryptorchidism might be efficacious. However, controlled studies and clinical trials involving hCG or LH therapy for cryptorchidism are lacking. In stallions, twice-weekly treatment for 4 weeks with 2500 IU to 10,000 IU of hCG has been suggested. The author has used this treatment on a low number of cases with unilateral inguinally retained testis, without apparent efficacy. The timing of therapy is generally too late, given the very early closure of the inguinal rings in colts.

Normal Testes

The testes of a normal stallion are palpable as two oval structures of nearly equal size lying horizontally within the scrotal pouches, with the tail of the epididymis directed caudally (Fig. 1-3). Normal orientation of the testis is ascertained by palpation of the tail of the epididymis and the ligament of the tail of the epididymis (or caudal ligament of the epididymis). This structure is a remnant of the gubernaculum, the fetal ligament that is believed to play a role in guiding the testis into the scrotum. The ligament is palpable as a 5- to 19-mm fibrous nodule, attaching the tail of the epididymis to the caudal pole of the testis.[5] It is particularly large in newborn colts and, upon palpation, may be mistaken for a testis within the scrotum. On occasion, examination of a normal stallion may identify rotation of one or both testes, up to 180 degrees. This finding was seen in 3%–4% of "normal" light horse stallions presented for a breeding soundness examination in one study.[17] Rotation may be more common in certain breeds; 9 of 23 Welsh pony stallions (39%) examined in another report exhibited testis rotation.[18] The authors of the latter study commented that the high incidence appeared to be related to specific family lines. Testis rotation is believed to occur in about 15% of Paso Fino stallions (Samper, personal communication, 1997).

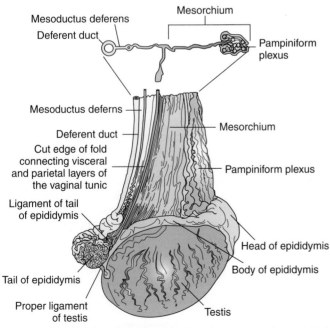

Figure 1-3. Lateral view of the right testis of a stallion. (From Dyce KM, Sack WO, Wensing CJG: *Textbook of Veterinary Anatomy.* Philadelphia: WB Saunders, 1987.)

Opinions differ as to the importance of rotated testicles and whether the condition should be considered a criterion for failing a stallion during a breeding soundness examination. Some clinicians do not place tremendous importance on rotations and would not fail such a stallion if all other parameters of the breeding soundness examination were normal. However, the presence of the condition should be noted clearly on the stallion's record, and it should be communicated clearly to the owner. Testis rotation is often transient, and a subsequent examination may find the testis in normal orientation. Testis rotation must be differentiated from true testicular or spermatic cord torsion, in which stallions demonstrate signs of colic and palpation reveals a painful and swollen testicle.

Within the scrotum, the testis is encapsulated by the tunica albuginea, a layer of tough collagenous tissue and smooth muscle, which is fused externally to the visceral layer of the vaginal tunic. The tunica albuginea sends supportive trabeculae into the testicular parenchyma, dividing the testis into lobules.[5-7] Its muscular content is thought to play a role in intratesticular sperm transport and determination of testicular tone.[2] Unlike the bull and other species, the testis of the stallion does not contain an axially oriented mediastinum or rete testis.[3,5,6] The mediastinum testis is a partial separation within the testis consisting of fibrous tissue continuous with the tunica albuginea. In the stallion, it is located at the cranial pole of the testis, where the excurrent ducts leaving the testis cross the tunica albuginea and enter the head of the epididymis.[6,7] This results in a mediastinum testis that is less prominent grossly on cut section and difficult to identify ultrasonographically. The microanatomy of the testis is described in Chapter 2.

Testicular tone is described as the degree of turgidity of the testicle; the testicle should be firm to turgid but resilient on palpation. Deviation from the normal toward a softer or firmer testis may be associated with degenerative, neoplastic, or traumatic conditions of the testis. Testicular degeneration is an acquired condition in which damage to the germinal epithelium results in eventual atrophy of the epithelium and, grossly, of the testis.[7] In general, early in the course of testicular degeneration, the affected testis is softer than normal and may be enlarged. As the disease progresses, the degenerating testicle becomes small and firm as testicular parenchyma is replaced with fibrous tissue. Wrinkling of the scrotum and tunic may be evident.[7] Testicular conditions may affect only one testis; therefore, comparison of the size and consistency of the two testes of any individual stallion is imperative. Changes in testicular tone or consistency are likely best determined by sequential examinations of the stallion over time, allowing the clinician to monitor the severity and rate of change as the disease progresses. Regular physical examinations of breeding stallions are an important part of routine stallion management and may allow early detection of problems that may significantly impact fertility.

Testicular Size and Volume

Each testis of a postpubertal stallion weighs between 150 and 300 grams[9] and measures approximately 50–80 mm wide, 60–70 mm high, and 80–140 mm long.[6] Testicular size varies among stallions depending on breed, season, age, and reproductive status.[1,19-21] Table 1-1 gives the recommended minimum testicular measurements for light horse stallions. Table 1-2 gives the recommended minimum testicular measurements for miniature stallions. Testis parenchymal weight correlates highly with daily sperm production (DSP)[17,20,22-24] and therefore is a useful predictor of a stallion's breeding potential. However, because parenchymal weight cannot

Table 1-1 | **Mean Testicular Measurements of 43 Light Horse Stallions**

MEASURE MEAN	RECOMMENDED MINIMUM (SD)
Left width (mm)	57.8 (5.2)
Left length (mm)	103.1 (8.2)
Right width (mm)	55.8 (5.8)
Right length (mm)	107.5 (8.0)

Adapted from Thompson DL, Pickett BW. Squires EL, et al. Testicular measurements and reproductive characteristics in stallions. *J Reprod Fertil* 27(Suppl):13-17, 1979.

Table 1-2 | **Testicular Measurements of Miniature Stallions by Stallion Size (n = 216)**

TESTIS MEASUREMENT	RECOMMENDED MINIMUM IN MM (+/- SD) SMALL/MEDIUM (72–96 CM)	RECOMMENDED MINIMUM IN MM (+/- SD) LARGE (97–104 CM)
Left width	39.0 (0.05)	43.13 (0.07)
Left length	63.74 (0.08)	70.30 (0.10)
Right width	38.3 (0.05)	43.00 (0.07)
Right length	62.64 (0.08)	69.20 (0.10)

Adapted from Paccamonti DL, Buiten AV, Parlevliet JM, et al: Reproductive parameters of miniature stallions. *Theriogenology* 51:1343-1349, 1999.

Table 1-3 | **Total Scrotal Width—Recommended Minimum Guideline**

	2-3 YEARS	4-6 YEARS	> 7 YEARS
Minimum	81 mm	85 mm	95 mm
Range	81-111 mm	85-115 mm	95-124 mm

Adapted from Thompson DL, Pickett BW Squires EL, et al. Testicular measurements and reproductive characteristics in stallions. *J Reprod Fertil* 27(Suppl):13-17, 1979.
Determined by 2 SDs below mean value; 95% of study population had TSW measurements at or above this value. Study population consisted of 48 light horse stallions.

Table 1-4 | **Calculated Total Scrotal Width Measurements for Miniature Stallions by Stallion Size (n = 216)***

MINIATURE HORSE SIZE (HEIGHT IN CM)	TOTAL SCROTAL WIDTH MEAN (MM)
Small/Medium (72–96 cm)	72.5
Large (97–104 cm)	79.5

Adapted from Paccamonti DL, Buiten AV, Parlevliet JM, et al: Reproductive parameters of miniature stallions. *Theriogenology* 51:1343-1349, 1999.
*TSW was calculated using the equation TSW = 1.74 + 0.696 (LW + RW).

be measured in the live stallion, estimates must be used. In the bull, scrotal circumference is an extremely important measure used during reproductive evaluation and has been shown to be correlated with daily sperm output (DSO).[25] Measurement of scrotal circumference is difficult in the stallion because the testes are held close to the body wall. However, total scrotal width (TSW) can be measured using calipers. TSW correlates well with testis parenchymal weight ($r^2 = 0.83$) and DSP ($r^2 = 0.75$).[20,24] Caliper measurements should be used judiciously based on their inherent potential sources of error, including caliper sensitivity, operator technique, and testis location within the scrotum.[20,22,24] Taking the average of several measurements helps increase repeatability and accuracy. An additional concern of the value of the TSW measure is the reliability of a single linear measurement, such as width, in estimating the true size of the testicles (three-dimensional structures).[22] Even though TSW is not likely the optimal measurement for use in estimating testis size, it is easily and quickly obtained with minimal, inexpensive equipment. Table 1-3 gives a guideline of the minimum acceptable TSW for light horse stallions by age. Table 1-4 gives the calculated TSW measurements from a study of 216 miniature stallions.

The testes should also be measured individually using calipers for length, width, and height in an effort to estimate their size.[1,7,22,26] Individual testicular measurements correlate well with parenchymal weight, with r^2 values ranging from 0.57 to 0.82.[21,24] Correlation estimates for individual testicular measurements and DSO range from 0.52 to 0.76.[20,24] Testis measurements can be assessed by either caliper (Fig. 1-4) or ultrasonographic (Fig. 1-5) measurement.[22,27] Ultrasonographic measurements may be more accurate in that they are less likely to be affected by sources of error, although proper placement of the probe across the testis to ensure that a cross-sectional image is obtained is critical. Deviation toward an oblique image dramatically affects measurements obtained with this method. Testicular volume,

rather than dimensions, has been suggested to more accurately predict DSO.[22] Because a testis approximates the shape of an ellipsoid, the following formula is used to convert length, width, and height measurements into testicular volume[22]:

$$\text{Testis Volume} = 4/3\pi(\text{length}/2)(\text{width}/2)(\text{height}/2)$$

or,

$$\text{Testis Volume} = 0.5233 \times H \times L \times W \text{ in cm}$$

Love[28] also recommends using this volume to predict the expected DSO of the stallion, using the following formula:

$$\text{Predicted DSO} = [0.024 \times (\text{vol L} + \text{vol R})] - 0.76$$

Predicted DSO can be compared with actual DSO as estimated by semen collection during the routine breeding soundness examination. A stallion whose actual DSO goes below that predicted for his testicular size should be further evaluated for disease conditions of the testes, epididymides, and accessory glands. The expected number of sperm per gram of testicle is 16–20 million/gm. If a stallion has sperm production problems or sperm delivery problems, a clinician can calculate expected DSP and actual total sperm per ejaculate. If expected DSP is the same as sperm collected, 100% spermatogenic efficiency in indicated. On the other hand, if expected DSP is lower than sperm collected (<100% spermatogenic efficiency), excurrent duct blockage, testicular degeneration, or inadequate semen collection/evaluation is possible. If expected DSP is more than sperm collected (>100% spermatogenic efficiency), collection of accumulated sperm or semen counting error could be possible.

Testicular measurements are an important part of the physical examination of any breeding stallion. Because testicular size is likely as heritable in stallions as it is in bulls,[17,22,29] stallions with scrotal width measurements that are less than the aforementioned

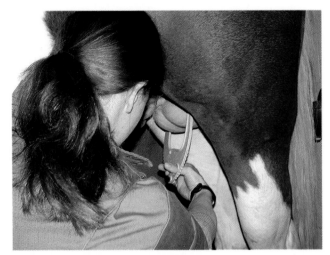

Figure 1-4. Measurement of the total scrotal width (TSW) of a stallion using calipers. The testes are pushed ventrally into the scrotal sac and the TSW measured across the widest point.

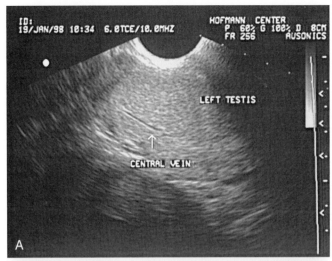

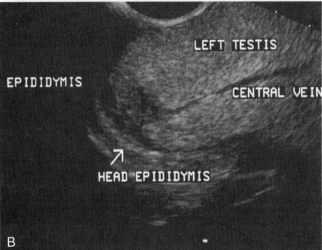

Figure 1-5. A, Ultrasound image of the left testis. Note the homogeneous nature of the testicular parenchyma. **B,** Enlarged view at most cranial aspect of testis. The central vein is seen as it courses into the spermatic cord. The head of the epididymis is also visible. (Courtesy of S. Meyers, University of California, Davis, CA.)

guidelines should not be recommended for breeding purposes. However, for stallions selected for breeding based on performance or conformation characteristics rather than on fertility characteristics, it may be more useful to use testis measurements as a management tool. Veterinarians may caution owners that a stallion with small testicles will have lower sperm production and may not perform well with a large book of mares. However, by creating realistic owner expectations, modifying stallion management such as frequency of breeding, and/or increasing the frequency of examination of the mares so that they are bred only once close to ovulation, the veterinarian or manager can optimize the fertility of such a stallion.

Epididymides and Excurrent Duct System

Each epididymis is a highly convoluted but unbranched duct approximately 70 meters long that has a grossly distinct head, body, and tail.[5-7] The head of the epididymis is a flattened structure that lies dorsomedially along the cranial border of the testis and is closely attached to it (see Fig. 1-3). The body, or corpus, lies along the dorsolateral aspect of each testis and continues as the tail, or cauda—the large, prominent structure attached to the caudal pole of the testis. The tail of the epididymis is anchored by the ligament of the tail of the epididymis. The deferent duct, the excretory duct for sperm, attaches to the tail of the corresponding epididymis, runs along the medial aspect of the testis, and ascends via the spermatic cord through the vaginal ring into the pelvis. Each deferent duct widens into its corresponding ampullary gland and eventually terminates at the colliculus seminalis of the pelvic urethra. The colliculus seminalis is a rounded prominence situated on the ventromedial wall of the urethra about 5 cm caudal to the urethral opening from the bladder.[5] It is the site at which the ducts of the accessory sex glands empty into the urethra. Whereas the deferent ducts are not externally palpable in stallions, all portions of the epididymis are usually palpable through the scrotal wall. The head of the epididymis may be difficult to ascertain because of its flattened nature and because the cremaster muscle lies on top of it.[7,30]

The specific absorptive and secretory functional aspects of each segment of the stallion epididymis remain the subject of considerable debate and investigation. The histologic structure of the epididymis changes as it continues through its different

regions, with epithelial height being greatest proximally and smooth muscle components greatest distally.[2,31,32] As sperm are transported from the excurrent ducts into the head, along the body, and into the tail, they undergo a number of morphologic and physiologic changes that ultimately render them motile and fertile.[2,33-35] Specific maturational changes include (1) the capacity for progressive motility, (2) shedding of the cytoplasmic droplet, (3) plasma and acrosomal membrane alterations, (4) DNA stabilization, and (5) metabolic changes. The tail of the epididymis generally serves to store the matured sperm.

Spermatic Cord and Vascular Supply to the Testis

Each spermatic cord is enveloped in the parietal layer of the vaginal tunic, which extends distally from the internal inguinal ring. Within each cord is the corresponding deferent duct, testicular artery, testicular veins, lymphatic vessels, and nerves. The cremaster muscle is situated in the caudolateral borders of each spermatic cord (see Fig. 1-3).[5,6]

The testicular artery, a branch of the abdominal aorta, descends through the inguinal ring into the cranial border of the spermatic cord in a tortuous manner and divides near the testis into several branches to supply the testis and epididymis. These small branches, embedded in the tunica albuginea, enter the parenchyma via the trabeculae and septa of the testis.[3-5] A corresponding network of veins leaves the testis and surrounds the testicular artery in a tortuous manner, forming the pampiniform plexus. The testicular vein continues from the plexus to join the caudal vena cava.[3-5] This arrangement of artery and veins, as in other species, is responsible for much of the thermoregulation of the testis in the stallion. Blood temperature within the branches of the testicular vein is lowered to less than core body temperature by evaporative heat loss. The arrangement of the cooler venous blood surrounding the testicular arterial blood functions as a countercurrent heat exchanger, resulting in transfer of heat from the testicular arterial blood to the venous side. As a result, blood within the testicular artery is several degrees cooler upon reaching the testicle (Fig. 1-6).[1,7]

Abnormal distention of the veins of the pampiniform plexus is termed *varicocele*. Whereas this is a frequent condition in male humans, it is extremely rare in stallions.[7] Palpation of the spermatic cord of an affected stallion reveals the dilated and often tortuous vessels. Varicoceles are usually not painful and most often involve only one side of the spermatic cord. Although they are thought to result in altered spermatogenesis by effects on thermoregulation,[2] varicoceles have been identified in stallions with normal semen parameters.[7]

Ultrasonography of the Scrotum, Testes, Epididymides, and Spermatic Cords

Ultrasound examination is a useful diagnostic adjunct to physical examination of the scrotum and testes. It enables the clinician to assess palpable changes as well as to identify nonpalpable changes that may be present. Ultrasound is particularly useful for differentiating testicular, epididymal, and scrotal disease in cases of generalized scrotal enlargement where specific structures become difficult to palpate. This section describes the normal ultrasonographic appearance and briefly describes some of the conditions that may be confused with normal structures. For more information, refer to texts that specifically detail disease conditions.[7,27]

Because the testes of a stallion are held horizontally and close to the abdominal wall, ultrasonographic examination is somewhat more difficult than in the ruminant species. A confident and experienced stallion handler providing adequate restraint is essential. Examination is usually easier after semen collection when the stallion is relaxed. A 5.0-, 7.5-, or 10.0-MHz linear array transducer provides good-quality images for evaluation of normal structures. Curvilinear or sector transducers provide better image quality for evaluation of the epididymal structures. Application of a liberal amount of ultrasound coupling gel improves image quality by maximizing probe-to-skin contact. Examination is best attempted with one hand pushing one testis high into the scrotum while the other hand holds the transducer probe across the testis being examined. If the probe is placed in a vertical orientation across the testis axis, a cross-sectional image is attained (see Fig. 1-5). The examination is usually begun at the cranial end of the testis and the probe is slowly moved caudad.

Visualization of the scrotum reveals a thin, echogenic, uniform layer. Minimal, if any, fluid is visible between the scrotal skin and testicular parenchyma in the normal stallion (see Fig. 1-5). In the cranial one third of the scrotum, the head of the epididymis, testicular parenchyma, blood vessels of the spermatic cord, and

central vein are visualized. As the probe is moved caudad, the central vein and spermatic cord vessels disappear, and the head of the epididymis continues into the body of the epididymis. The head and body of the epididymis appear as heterogeneous areas just below the spermatic cord when the probe is positioned as described. As the probe continues farther caudad, the body of the epididymis becomes indistinct. With the exception of the central vein, the testicular parenchyma appears uniformly echogenic and relatively homogeneous. The central vein appears as a small anechoic area within the testicular parenchyma at the cranial one third of the testis and should not be mistaken for a pathologic lesion (see Fig. 1-5). Dilation of the central vein may be seen in cases of varicocele or spermatic cord torsions and is usually accompanied by detectable dilations of the vessels of the spermatic cord.[27] Well-defined and hypoechoic lesions within the parenchyma are suggestive of testicular tumors (Fig. 1-7).

Once the most caudal aspect of the testis is reached, rotating the probe to face cranially, but still remaining in a vertical position, allows examination of the tail of the epididymis. This structure appears as a heterogeneous area, described by some authors as having a "Swiss cheese–like" appearance (Fig. 1-8).[27] Identification of the epididymal tail may be of assistance in diagnosis of testicular torsion. In cases of 360-degree torsions, the tail of the epididymis is still directed caudad. However, when the deferent duct encircles the spermatic cord by 360 degrees, the resulting increased upward tension on the ligament of the tail of the epididymis pulls the tail of the epididymis dorsally.[27]

The spermatic cord is most easily visualized by placing the probe horizontally across the cord, just proximal to the body of the testis (Fig. 1-9). The arrangement of the pampiniform plexus results in the mottled, heterogeneous appearance of the spermatic cord, and the testicular artery and veins are identified in cross-sectional images.

The Penis and Prepuce

The penis of the stallion is composed of a root, a body, and a glans penis and is of the musculocavernous type (Fig. 1-10).[1,3,5,6] The penis is supported at its root by the suspensory ligaments of the penis and the ischiocavernosus muscles. The penile root arises at the ischial arch in the form of two crura, which fuse distally to form the single and dorsal corpus cavernosum penis, and is enclosed by a thick tunica albuginea. The cavernous spaces making up the erectile tissue of the penis are the corpus cavernosum, corpus spongiosum, and corpus spongiosum glandis. Engorgement of these spaces with blood from branches of the internal and external pudendal arteries and obturator arteries is responsible for erection.[3,4] The cavernous spaces within the penis are continuous with the veins responsible for drainage. The corpus spongiosum originates at the pelvis at the bulb of the penis and distally surrounds the penile urethra within a groove on the ventral side of the penis. It continues distally over the free end of the penis to form the glans penis (corpus spongiosum glandis). The corpus spongiosum glandis is responsible for the distinct bell shape of the stallion's penis that is seen following coitus. The urethral process is distinctly visible at the center of the glans penis and is surrounded by an invagination known as the fossa glandis. Accumulations of smegma secretions, known as *"beans,"* are lodged in the dorsal diverticulum of the fossa glandis, the urethral sinus. Careful examination and cleaning of this area are imperative during the reproductive evaluation of a stallion (Figs. 1-11 and 1-12).

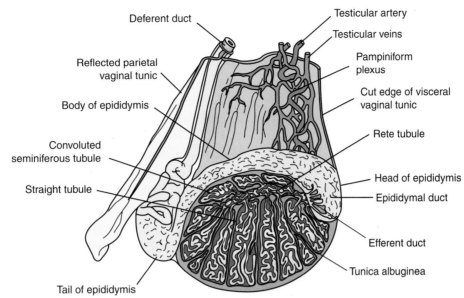

Figure 1-6. Diagrammatic view showing the location of straight tubules and the rete testis in the stallion testis. The straight tubules converge in a group of interconnecting rete tubules that penetrate the tunica albuginea and fuse with the efferent ducts. The efferent ducts merge into the epididymal duct. The testicular artery becomes highly coiled in the pampiniform plexus. After emerging from the pampiniform plexus, the testicular artery passes along the dorsal aspect of the testis to the caudal pole where it starts to branch to vascularize the parenchyma. Venous drainage of the parenchyma is via the central vein and superficial testicular veins. After leaving the testis, the veins form an anastomosing plexus of veins (termed the *pampiniform plexus*) that is in intimate contact with the testicular artery. About 7–10 cm above the testis, the veins converge into the testicular vein. (From Pickett BW, Amann RP, McKinnon AO, et al: *Management of the Stallion for Maximum Reproductive Efficiency: II,* 2nd ed. Animal Reproduction Laboratory General Series Bulletin 05. Fort Collins, CO: Colorado State University, 1989.)

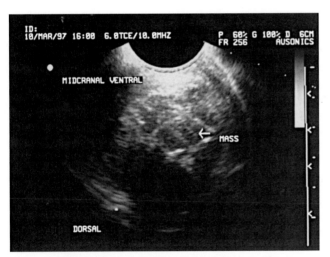

Figure 1-7. Ultrasound image of testicular seminoma.

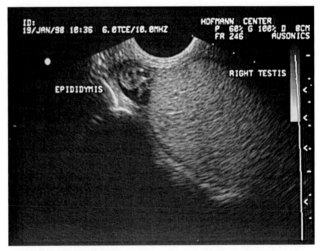

Figure 1-8. Ultrasound image of epididymis. (Courtesy of S. Meyers, University of California, Davis, CA.)

The bulbospongiosus muscle lies ventral to the urethra and along the entire length of the penis (Fig. 1-13). Arising as a direct continuation of the urethralis muscle, its smooth rhythmic contractions assist in moving the penile urethral contents (semen and urine) distally. Rhythmic pulsations of the bulbospongiosus muscle are distinctly felt during ejaculation if a hand is placed on the ventral aspect of the penis during collection. The paired retractor penis muscles also run ventrally along the length of the penis and attach at the glans penis. These smooth muscles function to return the penis to the sheath following detumescence.

The prepuce is formed by a double fold of skin and resembles scrotal skin in that it is essentially hairless and well supplied with sebaceous and sweat glands.[5-7] It functions to contain and protect the non-erect penis. The external part of the prepuce, or sheath, begins at the scrotum and displays a marked raphe that is continuous with the scrotal raphe. This external layer extends some distance cranially before reflecting dorsocaudad to the abdominal wall to form the preputial orifice.[5] The internal layer of the prepuce extends caudad from the orifice to line the internal side of the sheath, then reflects craniad toward the orifice again before reflecting caudad to form the internal preputial fold and preputial ring (see Fig. 1-12). It is this additional internal fold that allows the marked lengthening (approximately by 50%) of the stallion's penis during erection. During erection, the preputial orifice is visible at the base of the penis just in front of the scrotum, and the preputial ring is visible approximately midshaft of

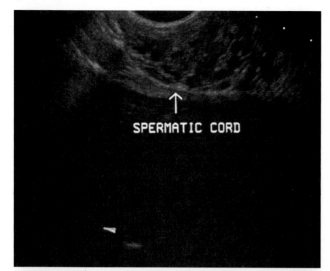

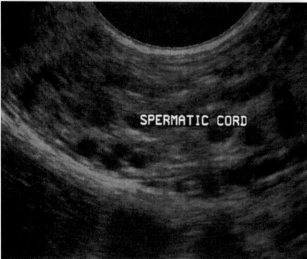

Figure 1-9. Ultrasound images of the normal spermatic cord of the stallion. The hypoechoic areas are the pampiniform plexus. (Courtesy of S. Meyers, University of California, Davis, CA.)

the penis (Fig. 1-14). Located distal to the preputial ring during erection is the internal layer of the internal preputial fold.

The penis and prepuce of a breeding stallion are best examined following teasing with an estrus mare, when the stallion can be observed to drop the penis and attain a full erection. The prepuce and penis should be free of vesicular, proliferative, or inflammatory lesions, such as those found in cases of coital exanthema, squamous cell carcinoma, or cutaneous habronemiasis. Removal of smegma accumulations may be required for a complete examination of the skin surfaces. Ultrasound of the penis of the stallion is not generally used in routine examination; however, this modality may be useful in the diagnosis of suspected penile hematoma or fibrosis following injury.

INTERNAL GENITALIA

Accessory Sex Glands

The prostate gland, seminal vesicles, BU glands, and ampullae are collectively referred to as the accessory sex glands (Fig. 1-15). The fluid portion of semen produced by the accessory glands is referred to as the seminal plasma. Seminal plasma consists of proteins, carbohydrates, lactic acid, glycerylphosphorylcholine

and other substrates that are involved in many aspects of sperm metabolism and function.[2,36,37] Seminal plasma constituents vary between individual stallions as well as by season.[37] The proteins found in seminal plasma originate from the accessory sex glands and the epididymis and have undergone considerable study to try to elucidate their role and association with fertility. Compared with other mammalian species, the seminal plasma protein content in stallion semen is relatively low, at about 10 mg/ml.[38] Membrane-binding seminal plasma proteins are involved in the movement of sperm through the female tract, maintenance of viable sperm at the oviductal reservoir, capacitation, oocyte penetration, and fertilization.[37,38] The heparin-binding proteins SP-1 and SP-2, which account for about 70% of seminal plasma proteins in the stallion, are involved in sperm capacitation. The cysteine-rich secretory, or CRISP, proteins play a role in sperm-oocyte fusion and inhibit tyrosine phosphorylation required for capacitation. To some degree, these proteins are thought to play a role in suppressing capacitation of sperm until they reach the oviductal sperm reservoir. CRISP proteins have also been associated with fertility of individual stallions.[38] One study associated CRISP3 gene polymorphisms with fertility in Hanoverian stallions.[39] Whereas exposure to seminal plasma appears to be important for sperm function, long-term exposure to seminal plasma components in fact may be detrimental to sperm survival for some stallions.[36,38,40-43] Characterization of proteins in seminal plasma of fertile and subfertile stallions suggests that concentrations of certain specific proteins in subfertile stallions are increased.[39,44,45] Other workers have demonstrated that a few of the seminal plasma proteins vary with post-thaw motility of cryopreserved sperm, although the value of these protein levels in predicting a stallion's response to sperm freezing was very low.[36] Seminal plasma also appears to modulate the inflammatory response of the mare's endometrium to sperm following insemination or natural mating.[46] The role of specific seminal plasma constituents, including proteins, is currently the topic of considerable investigation. Increasing our understanding of the physiology of this component of semen may lead to better understanding of the variability of stallions in response to chilled semen and frozen semen technologies.

Examination and Ultrasonography of Accessory Glands

Reproductive examination of all stallions should include rectal palpation and ultrasonography of the accessory sex glands. Most stallions tolerate this procedure well with adequate restraint in stocks, and tranquilization is not usually necessary. Some stallions are more tractable following ejaculation; however, the accessory glands are generally more difficult to evaluate at that time because of reductions in diameter and fluid content. Pozor et al.[47] demonstrated considerable variability in the size, shape, and ultrasound appearance of the accessory sex glands of normal stallions, both among stallions and within individual stallions examined over time. Much of this variability can be attributed to differences in sexual stimulation and frequency of ejaculation among stallions.

Ampullary Glands

The ampullary glands are the enlarged distal portions of the deferent ducts measuring 1–2 cm in diameter and 10–25 cm in length (see Fig. 1-15).[7,30] Palpable along the midline of the pelvic floor over the neck of the bladder, they converge caudad and pass beneath the prostate gland but lie dorsal to the pelvic urethra. At their distal ends, they continue through the wall of

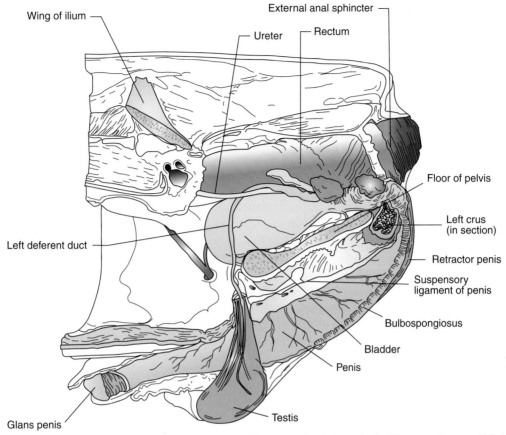

Figure 1-10. The reproductive organs of the stallion in situ. (From Dyce KM, Sack WO, Wensing CJG: *Textbook of Veterinary Anatomy.* Philadelphia: WB Saunders, 1987.)

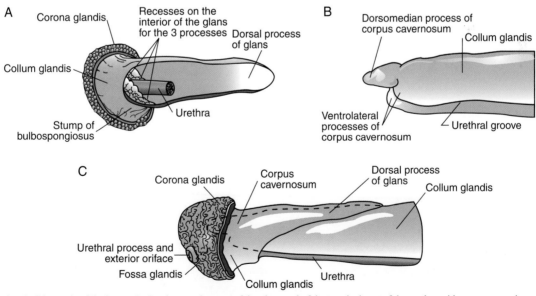

Figure 1-11. Distal end of the penis of the horse. **A,** Caudoventral aspect of the glans and of the terminal part of the urethra with corpus spongiosum; **B,** ventrolateral aspect of corpus cavernosum; **C,** lateral aspect of tip of penis; the skin of the penis has been removed proximal to the corona glandis. (From Nickel R: Male genital organs. In Nickel R, Schummer A, Seiferle E, et al: *The Viscera of Domestic Animals.* New York: Springer-Verlag, 1973.)

the urethra, opening into the colliculus seminalis alongside the excretory ducts of the seminal vesicles. Some authors do not consider the ampullae to be accessory sex glands, rather simply storage depots for sperm.[46] However, the ampullae are not simply a dilation of the lumen of the deferent ducts, and they may be considered glands because of the many branched tubular glands located within the thickened wall.[2,5,31]

Each ampulla is identified ultrasonographically by the hypoechogenic central lumen surrounded by a uniformly echogenic wall and a hyperechogenic outer muscular layer

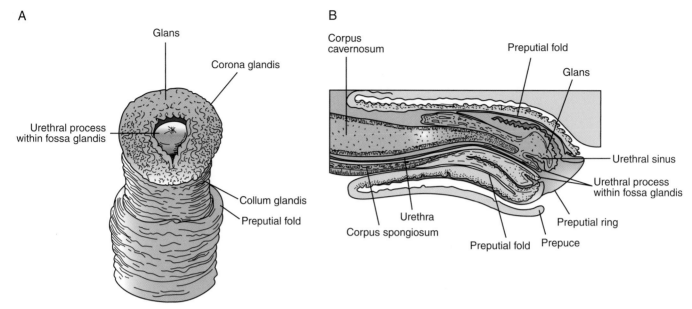

Figure 1-12. Extremity of penis exposed **(A)** and within prepuce in median section **(B)**. (From Dyce KM, Sack WO, Wensing CJG: *Textbook of Veterinary Anatomy.* Philadelphia: WB Saunders, 1987.)

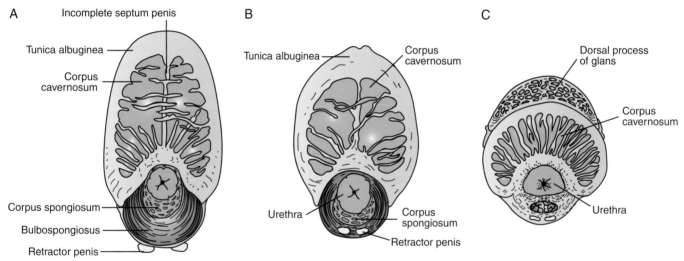

Figure 1-13. Transections of the penis, directly distal to the root **(A)**, midshaft **(B)**, and in its free part **(C)**. (From Dyce KM, Sack WO, Wensing CJG: *Textbook of Veterinary Anatomy.* Philadelphia: WB Saunders, 1987.)

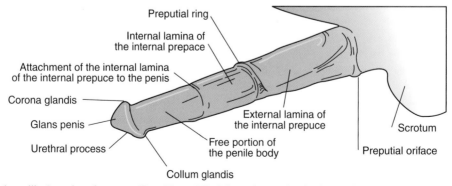

Figure 1-14. Structures of the stallion's penis and prepuce. (From Varner DD, Schumacher J, Blanchard T, et al: *Diseases and Management of Breeding Stallions.* Goleta, CA: American Veterinary Publications, 1991.)

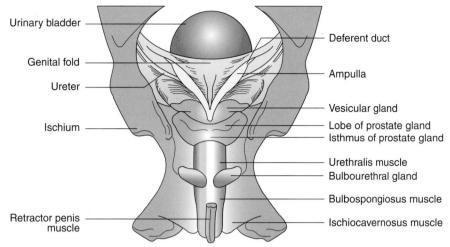

Urinary bladder —
Genital fold —
Ureter —
Ischium —
Retractor penis muscle —

— Deferent duct
— Ampulla
— Vesicular gland
— Lobe of prostate gland
— Isthmus of prostate gland
— Urethralis muscle
— Bulbourethral gland
— Bulbospongiosus muscle
— Ischiocavernosus muscle

Figure 1-15. Drawing showing a dorsal view of the pelvic portion of the reproductive tract. The connective tissue and most of the genital fold, which support the pelvic portion of the tract, were dissected away. (From Pickett BW, Amann RP, McKinnon AO, et al: *Management of the Stallion for Maximum Reproductive Efficiency: II,* 2nd ed. Animal Reproduction Laboratory General Series Bulletin 05. Fort Collins, CO: Colorado State University, 1989.)

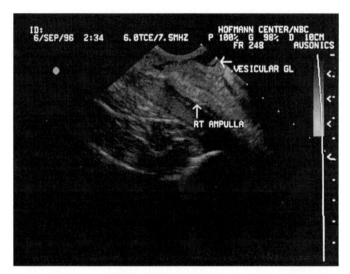

Figure 1-16. Ultrasound image of the right ampullary gland of a stallion. A small hypoechogenic line representing the glandular lumen is visible. The vesicular gland is seen lying dorsally in this image. (Courtesy of S. Meyers, University of California, Davis, CA.)

(Fig. 1-16).[47] Hypoechogenic areas may be seen within the walls and probably represent the glandular areas. In many stallions, the uterus masculinus, a remnant of the müllerian duct system, is visible ultrasonographically as one or two cystic structures located between the ampullae.[47] Because the ampulla is primarily a sperm storage area, stallions that have large testicular size and are not sexually active could have spermiostasis and in extreme cases ampullary blockage that can be unilateral or bilateral. In stallions with ampullary blockage, dilation of the glandular lumen may or may not be seen. These stallions are usually presented with a history of infertility or subfertility, and they often display ejaculatory dysfunction. Clinical examination usually reveals oligozoospermia or azoospermia, morphologic abnormalities (predominantly tailless heads), and palpable enlargement of the distal ampulla.[47] This condition may render a stallion virtually infertile if undiagnosed. Recommendations for treatment include ampullary massage per rectum and repeated semen collection following injection of low doses of oxytocin.[48]

Vesicular Glands

The vesicular glands are paired, pyriform, thin-walled structures lying lateral to the ampullae, predominantly within the genital fold (see Fig. 1-15). They may on occasion extend far cranially to hang over the brim of the pelvis.[47] Sexual stimulation results in dilation and elongation of the vesicular glands, up to 12–20 cm long and 5 cm in diameter.[3,7] The distal ends of the glands converge, passing under the prostate as they parallel the ampullae toward their termination at the urethra. The excurrent ducts of the vesicular glands open lateral to the excurrent ducts of the ampullae at the colliculus seminalis of the urethra. Secretions of the vesicular glands make up the gel fraction of the ejaculate.[7,49] Season influences the output of the vesicular glands, with gel fraction volume being highest during the physiologic breeding season.[1] The vesicular glands are generally difficult to palpate rectally, especially if the examination is performed following semen collection. Palpation of the vesicular glands may be easier when they are enlarged after considerable teasing of the stallion with an estrous mare. The glands are also readily palpable in instances of pathologic enlargement.

Ultrasonographically, the vesicular glands appear in longitudinal section as flattened oval to triangular sacs, depending on the degree of sexual activity (Fig. 1-17).[47] The thin, echogenic wall surrounds a generally uniformly anechoic lumen. In some stallions, echogenic particles are seen within the lumen fluid. Increased echogenicity of vesicular gland fluid is associated with the highly viscous gel fraction produced by some stallions.[47]

Although rare, infection of the seminal vesicles can be unilateral or bilateral. Most often, bacterial infection of the seminal vesicles is not accompanied by clinical signs, although some stallions exhibit ejaculatory dysfunction evidenced as apparent pain on ejaculation with reluctance to breed.[7] The presence of polymorphonuclear cells in the ejaculate warrants further investigation including rectal palpation and ultrasound of the accessory glands and urethroscopy. The vesicular glands may be enlarged, firm, and painful on palpation if the condition is acute. Gland size alone and character of seminal vesicle fluid on ultrasound examination cannot be considered accurate indicators of infection, because the glands are extremely variable in size and appearance, both across and within stallions.[47] Diagnosis of seminal vesiculitis is best made by rectal palpation, observation of large numbers of neutrophils in

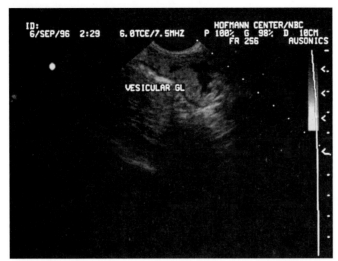

Figure 1-17. Ultrasound image of the vesicular gland. (Courtesy of S. Meyers, California, Davis, CA.)

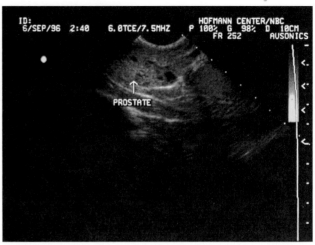

Figure 1-18. Ultrasound image of the prostate gland. Multiple hypoechogenic dilations are seen. Also see Figure 1-20. (Courtesy of S. Meyers, University of California, Davis, CA.)

the semen, bacterial culture of semen, and endoscopy of the urethra and seminal vesicles.[7,50] Collection of semen with an open-ended artificial vagina may aid in localizing the source of bacterial contamination in suspect cases[7]; however, direct culture of the seminal vesicles during endoscopy increases the clinician's confidence in the significance of organisms cultured.[50,51]

Treatment is difficult and prognosis guarded. Reported treatments include systemic treatment with antibiotics, or alternatively, addition of extenders containing appropriate antibiotics to the semen of the affected stallion. Endoscope-aided direct lavage followed by antibiotic instillation into the vesicular gland lumen is likely the preferred treatment for seminal vesiculitis in stallions.[50,51]

Prostate Gland

The prostate gland of the stallion consists of a central isthmus and two lateral lobes that extend along the caudolateral borders of each vesicular gland (see Fig. 1-15). Although not always palpable per rectum, the prostate is lobulated or nodular and firm, distinguishing it from the smooth, thin-walled vesicular glands. Each prostatic lobe measures 5–9 cm long, 2–6 cm wide, and 1–2 cm thick.[6,7] Multiple ductules from the prostate enter the lumen of the urethra lateral to the colliculus seminalis. Prostatic secretions appear to contribute to the sperm-rich fraction of the ejaculate.[7,49] The prostate gland is easily identified ultrasonographically, with its two symmetric and homogeneously echogenic lobes distinctly seen. Hypoechoic dilations within the gland parenchyma of each lobe are usually evident (Fig. 1-18).[47] These hypoechogenic spaces are smaller within the isthmus of the gland, and the size of these spaces is known to vary with the frequency of ejaculation and degree of sexual stimulation.[47]

Bulbourethral Glands

The BU glands attach to the dorsal surface of the pelvic urethra, about 8 cm caudal to the prostate gland (see Fig. 1-15). They are not usually palpable per rectum because they are covered by the urethralis and bulboglandularis muscles,[3,5] but they are easily evaluated ultrasonographically.[47] Similar to the prostate gland, multiple ductules from the BU glands enter the medial aspect of the urethra distal to the prostatic ductules. BU gland

secretions make up the majority of the presperm or first fraction of the ejaculate[49] and likely function to cleanse the urethra before ejaculation.[1] Similar to boars, the BU gland secretions of stallions have been found to have considerable lipase enzyme activity, which can be potentially detrimental to sperm motility over time under cooled storage conditions, at least for some stallions.[52] Ultrasonographically, the BU glands appear as oval structures with multiple small hypoechogenic spaces throughout the parenchyma. A thin hyperechogenic line representing the gland wall is surrounded by a hypoechogenic layer representing the bulboglandularis muscle surrounding the gland (Fig. 1-19).[47] With ultrasound, a sectional image at the level of the prostatic isthmus demonstrates the anatomic relationship of the pelvic urethra, ampullae, and prostate gland (Fig. 1-20).

Endoscopic Evaluation of the Pelvic and Penile Urethra

The pelvic urethra is generally quite narrow, except in the region of the colliculus seminalis just caudal to the prostate, where it widens considerably to allow for the deposition of accessory sex gland fluids during ejaculation. The erectile stratum cavernosum and the striated urethralis muscle surround the pelvic urethra and cause pulsations of the structure when rubbed with the fingers during rectal examination.[5,6] Endoscopic examination of the urethra is indicated in cases of hemospermia or in cases in which obstruction of accessory sex gland ducts is suspected. Hemospermia caused by ulceration of the urethral mucosa and exposure of the underlying cavernous tissue may be visualized endoscopically. These lesions may be most readily identified in the region of the colliculus seminalis.[53] Evaluation of the pelvic urethra, accessory sex gland duct openings, and bladder is recommended. Care should be taken to assess the urethral mucosa as the endoscope is passed forward, because some irritation and erythema of the mucosal lining are often the result of the endoscopic examination. A false diagnosis of urethritis may result if the mucosa is assessed as the endoscope is withdrawn. Refer to appropriate texts for information on equipment and technique.[53-55]

Endoscopically, the colliculus seminalis is identified as a rounded prominent structure, found on the medial aspect of the dorsal wall of the urethra, approximately 5 cm caudal to the

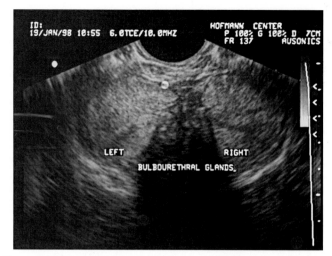

Figure 1-19. Ultrasound image of the bulbourethral glands (enlarged view). Hypoechogenic spaces are extremely small in this stallion but are observed to increase in size following teasing. (Courtesy of S. Meyers, University of California, Davis, CA.)

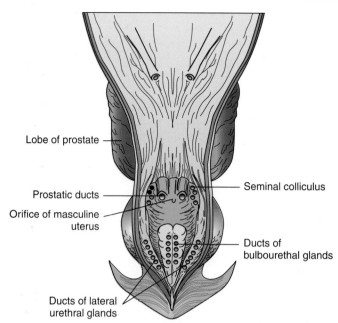

Figure 1-21. Pelvic urethra and caudal part of bladder of horse slit ventrally and laid open. Openings of ductus deferens and duct of seminal vesicle. (From Sisson S: Equine urogenital system. In Getty R, ed: *Sisson and Grossman's Anatomy of the Domestic Animal,* 5th ed. Philadelphia: WB Saunders, 1975.)

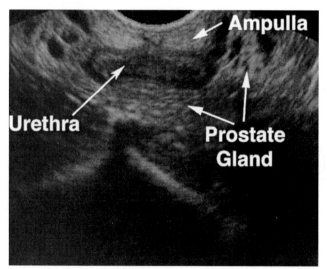

Figure 1-20. Dorsoventral sectional image at the level of the prostatic isthmus, which is seen lying ventral to the urethra. The two lateral lobes of the prostate gland, with their larger hypoechogenic dilations, are visible on each side of the urethra. The ampullary glands are clearly visible dorsal to the urethra in this image. Endoscopically, the colliculus seminalis is identified as a rounded prominent structure, found on the medial aspect of the dorsal wall of the urethra, approximately 5 cm caudal to the internal opening of the urethra from the bladder (Figs. 1-21 and 1-22). If present, a small orifice of the uterus masculinus may be visualized centrally on the colliculus seminalis. On each side of the colliculus is an ejaculatory duct orifice, a small slitlike diverticulum within which the ampullary ducts and ducts of the seminal vesicle open (Fig. 1-23). By passing the endoscope into this orifice, the practitioner can visualize and evaluate the seminal vesicles (Fig. 1-24).[50]

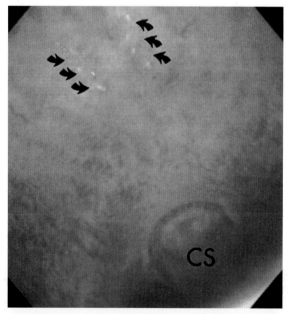

Figure 1-22. Endoscopic view, ampullar portion. The arrows represent the urethral opening of the bulbourethral glands just caudal to the colliculus seminalis (*CS*) (From Traub-Dargatz JL, Brown CM: *Equine Endoscopy,* 2nd ed. St Louis: Mosby, 1997.)

internal opening of the urethra from the bladder (Figs. 1-21 and 1-22). If present, a small orifice of the uterus masculinus may be visualized centrally on the colliculus seminalis. On each side of the colliculus is an ejaculatory duct orifice, a small slitlike diverticulum within which the ampullary ducts and ducts of the seminal vesicle open (Fig. 1-23). By passing the endoscope into this orifice, the practitioner can visualize and evaluate the seminal vesicles (Fig. 1-24).[50] Samples can be taken for culture

with endoscopic culturettes if seminal vesiculitis is suspected. The prostatic ductules are seen as two groups of small openings lateral to the ejaculatory orifices. The BU gland ductules are similarly grouped about 2.5–3 cm distal to the prostatic openings and lie dorsally and closer to the midline (see Figs. 1-21 and 1-22). The openings of the urethral glands are seen laterally on the widened pelvic portion of the urethra at the level of the BU gland openings.[5]

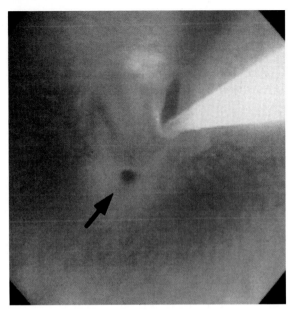

Figure 1-23. Endoscopic view, ejaculatory duct. (From Traub-Dargatz JL, Brown CM: *Equine Endoscopy,* 2nd ed. St Louis: Mosby, 1997.)

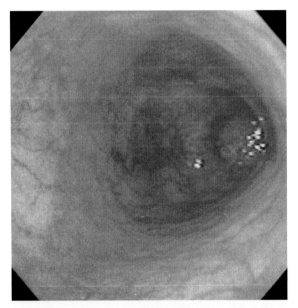

Figure 1-24. Endoscopic view, seminal vesicles. (From Traub-Dargatz JL, Brown CM: *Equine Endoscopy,* 2nd ed. St Louis: Mosby, 1997.)

NEUROENDOCRINE ANATOMY AND FUNCTION

The control of stallion reproductive physiology is complex and includes the hypothalamus, pituitary gland, pineal gland, vomeronasal organ, and testes (Fig. 1-25). Like a well-directed orchestra, all of the individual parts must be functioning and communicating with one another for the overall "performance" to be acceptable. Failure of any one of the parts or links results in reduced reproductive potential for the stallion. The hypothalamus exerts the primary hormonal influence over reproductive function.[20] Located at the base of the brain, the hypothalamus is connected by the infundibulum to the pituitary gland (or hypophysis), which is in turn divided into an anterior and a posterior lobe. Gonadotropin-releasing hormone (GnRH) is released in a pulsatile manner by the hypothalamus in response to both neural and hormonal inputs.[1,56] Tactile, visual, auditory, and olfactory stimuli are important regulators of stallion behavior and reproductive physiology. Exposure of stallions to mares has been shown to increase GnRH and LH concentration at the level of the pituitary.[57] The vomeronasal organ is a duct lying beneath the nasal mucosa, connected by the incisive duct to the ventral nasal meatus.[30] The flehman response or lip curl exhibited by stallions investigating mares is thought to direct air across the openings of the vomeronasal glands, which in turn may convey olfactory information from pheromones to the hypothalamus.[30,58] Although its function is poorly understood, the vomeronasal organ and flehman response are obvious elements of the social interactions of horses with one another.

The importance of the pineal gland, and the resulting influence of season, is less obvious in stallions than in mares, because stallions continue to produce sperm throughout the year, regardless of season. However, stallions do exhibit a circannual rhythm.[59] Testicular size, semen production, libido, and hormone concentrations vary by season in the stallion, with maximal values obtained in the spring and summer months.[59] Normal seasonal variations in reproductive parameters continue despite constant exposure of stallions to 16 hours of darkness for up to 20 months.[59-61] Similar to mares, exposure of stallions to 16 hours of constant light, beginning in December (northern hemisphere) results in earlier attainment of peak reproductive characteristics.[60,61] However, stallions exhibit a photorefractory state. Prolonged exposure to artificially lengthened days does not maintain peak reproductive characteristics, and lighted stallions display an earlier than normal regression of testicular size and accompanying changes in semen characteristics.[60,61] Stallions also appear to require a period of increased darkness before a response to increased light can occur, apparently representing a "resetting" of the circannual rhythm.[59] This is a crucial consideration in the management of stallions breeding in two hemispheres.

GnRH produced by the hypothalamus is transported via the hypothalamic-pituitary portal vessels to the anterior pituitary where it regulates the production and release of the two gonadotropic hormones, LH and follicle-stimulating hormone (FSH). These gonadotropic hormones act on the cells of the testis, regulating spermatogenesis and steroidogenesis. FSH regulates production of a variety of compounds by Sertoli cells that are important for the production of sperm. These include androgen-binding protein, estrogen, growth factors, inhibin, and activin. The latter two protein hormones appear to feed back to the anterior pituitary to regulate FSH release.[1,62] Sertoli cells function to regulate seminiferous tubular fluid, maintain the blood–testis barrier, and support the developing germ cells.[62] LH regulates the Leydig cells of the testis, stimulating the production of the steroid hormones testosterone, dihydrotestosterone, and ES. Testosterone attains high local concentrations within the testis, which are essential for normal spermatogenesis.[56] The steroid hormones also regulate accessory gland function and maintain libido by systemic actions via the bloodstream.[1,7] Testosterone and estrogen feed back on the hypothalamus and anterior pituitary gland to regulate LH release.[1,30, 62] Detailed information on stallion endocrinology and behavior is presented in Chapters 3 and 4.

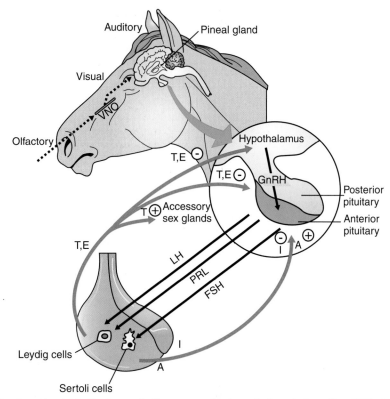

Figure 1-25. Proposed positive *(+)* and negative *(–)* feedback control of hormone production and release in the stallion. *VNO,* Vomeronasal organ; *GnRH,* gonadotropin-releasing hormone; *LH,* luteinizing hormone; *PRL,* prolactin; *FSH,* follicle-stimulating hormone; *T,* testosterone; *E,* estrogens; *I,* inhibin; *A,* activin. Potential external influences on hypothalamic secretion are also depicted. (Adapted from Pickett BW, Amann RP, McKinnon AO, et al: *Management of the Stallion for Maximum Reproductive Efficiency:* II. Animal Reproduction Laboratory General Series Bulletin No. 05. Fort Collins, CO: Colorado State University, 1989, p 1.)

REFERENCES

1. Pickett BW, Amann RP, McKinnon AO, et al. In: Management of the Stallion for Maximum Reproductive Efficiency: II. Animal Reproduction Laboratory General Series Bulletin No. 05. Fort Collins, CO: Colorado State University, 1989.
2. Setchell BP, Maddocks S, Brooks DE: Anatomy; vasculature, innervation and fluids of the male reproductive tract. In Knobil E, Neill ID, eds: *The Physiology of Reproduction*, 2nd ed. New York: Raven Press, 1994, pp 1063-1175.
3. Dyce KM, Sack WO, Wensing CIG: *Textbook of Veterinary Anatomy.* Philadelphia: WB Saunders, 1987.
4. Sack WO: Isolated male reproductive organs. In Sack WO, ed: *Rooney's Guide to the Dissection of the Horse*, 6th ed. Ithaca, NY: Veterinary Textbooks, 1991, pp 75-78.
5. Sisson S: Equine urogenital system. In Getty R, ed: *Sisson and Grossman's Anatomy of the Domestic Animal*, 5th ed. Philadelphia: WB Saunders, 1975.
6. Nickel R: Male genital organs. In Nickel R, Schummer A, Seiferle E, et al: *The Viscera of Domestic Animals*. New York: Springer-Verlag, 1973, pp 340-350.
7. Varner DD, Schumacher I, Blanchard T, et al: *Diseases and Management of Breeding Stallions*. Goleta, CA: American Veterinary Publications, 1991.
8. Bergin WC, Gier HT, Marion GB, Coffman JR: A developmental concept of equine cryptorchidism. *Biol Reprod* 3:82-92, 1970.
9. Arighi M: Testicular descent and cryptorchidism. In Samper JC, Pycock JF, and McKinnon AO: *Current Therapy in Equine Reproduction.* St Louis: Saunders, 2007, pp 185-194
10. Hayes EM: Epidemiological features of 5009 cases of equine cryptorchidism, *Equine Vet J* 18:467, 1986.
11. Levy JB, Husmann DA: The hormonal control of testicular descent, *J Androl* 16(6):459-463, 1995.
12. Jann HW, Rains JR: Diagnostic ultrasonography for evaluation of cryptorchidism in horses. *J Am Vet Med Assoc* 196:297, 1990.
13. Cox JE, Redhead PH, Dawson FE: Comparison of the measurement of plasma testosterone and plasma oestrogens for the diagnosis of cryptorchidism in the horse. *Equine Vet J* 18:179-182, 1986.
14. Silberzahn P, Pouret E, Zwain I: Androgen and oestrogen response to a single injection of hCG in cryptorchid horses. *Equine Vet J* 21(2):126-129, 1989.
15. Cox JE: Experience with a diagnostic test for equine cryptorchidism. *Equine Vet J* 7:179-182, 1975.
16. Brendemuehl J: Effects of repeated human chorionic gonadotropin administration on serum testosterone and testicular volume in prepubertal Thoroughbred colts. *Anim Reprod Sci* 89:199-201, 2005.
17. Pickett BW, et al: Seminal characteristics and total scrotal width (TSW) of normal and abnormal stallions. Proc 34th Annual AAEP Convention, San Diego: 1988, pp 485-518.
18. Colenbrander B, Puyk H, Zandee A, Parlevliet J: Evaluation of the stallion for breeding. *Acta Vet Scand* 88(Suppl):29-37, 1992.
19. Kenney RM, Hurtgen J, Pierson R, et al: Theriogenology and the equine. II. The stallion, *Soc Theriogenol* 1983, pp 88-90.
20. Thompson DL, Pickett BW, Squires EL, et al: Testicular measurements and reproductive characteristics in stallions. *J Reprod Fertil* 27(Suppl):13, 1979.
21. Bums PJ, Jawad MJ, Weld JM, et al. Effects of season, age and increased photoperiod on reproductive hormone concentrations and testicular diameters in Thoroughbred stallions. *Equine Vet Sci* 4(5):202-208, 1984.
22. Love CC, Garcia MC, Riera FR, et al: Use of testicular volume to predict daily sperm output in the stallion. Proc 36th Annual AAEP Convention, Lexington, KY: 1990, p 15.
23. Gebauer MR, Pickett BW, Faulkner LC, et al: Reproductive physiology of the stallion. VII. Chemical characteristics of seminal plasma and spermatozoa. *J Anim Sci* 43:626-632, 1976.
24. Gebauer MR, Pickett BW, Voss JL, Swierstra EE: Reproductive physiology of the stallion: Daily sperm output and testicular measurements. *J Am Vet Med Assoc* 165(8):711-714, 1974.
25. Willet EL, Ohms JI: Measurement of testicular size and its relation to production of spermatozoa by bulls. *J Dairy Sci* 40:1559, 1957.

26. Pickett BW: Reproductive evaluation of the stallion. In McKinnon AO, Voss JL, eds: *Equine Reproduction*. Malvern, PA: Lea & Febiger, 1993.

27. Love CC: Ultrasonographic evaluation of the testis, epididymis, and spermatic cord of the stallion. *Vet Clin North Am Equine Pract* 5:167-182, 1992.

28. Love CC, Garcia MC, Riera FR, Kenney RM: Evaluation of measures taken by ultrasonography and caliper to estimate testicular volume and predict daily sperm output in the stallion. *J Reprod Fertil Suppl* 44:99-105, 1991.

29. Coulter GH, Rounsaville TR, Foote RH: Heritability of testicular size and consistency in Holstein bulls. *J Anim Sci* 43:9-12, 1976.

30. Little TY, Holyoak GR: Reproductive anatomy and physiology of the stallion. *Vet Clin North Am Equine Pract*, 1992, pp 1-30.

31. Banks WJ: *Applied Veterinary Histology*, 2nd ed. Baltimore: Williams & Wilkins, 1986.

32. Johnson L, Amann RP, Pickett BW: Scanning electron microscopy of the epithelium and the spermatozoa in the equine excurrent duct system. *Am J Vet Res* 39:1428, 1978.

33. Johnson L, Amann RP, Pickett BW: Maturation of equine epididymal spermatozoa. *Am J Vet Res* 41:1190-1196, 1980.

34. Amann RP: Maturation of spermatozoa. Proc ICAR Meeting, Dublin, Ireland: 1988, pp 321-328.

35. Amann RP: Function of the epididymis in bulls and rams. *J Reprod Fertil* 34:115-131, 1987.

36. Lindholmer CH: The importance of seminal plasma for human sperm motility. *Biol Reprod* 10:533-542, 1974.

37. Killian GJ: Fertility factors in seminal plasma. Proc 14th Technical Conference on Artificial Insemination and Reproduction, National Association of Animal Breeders. Milwaukee, WI: April 24-25, 1992.

38. Nishikawa Y: Studies on the preservation of raw and frozen horse spermatozoa. *J Reprod Fertil* 23(Suppl):99-104, 1975.

39. Pickett BW, Sullivan JJ, Pace MM, Rememenga EE: Effect of centrifugation and seminal plasma on motility and fertility of stallion and bull spermatozoa. *Fertil Steril* 26:167-174, 1975.

40. Palmer E: L'insemination artificielle des juments: bilan de 5 annees de recherches et d'utilisation pratizue. Le cheval, reproduction, selection, alimentation exploitation. Paris: INRA, 1984, pp 133-147.

41. Topfer-Petersen E, Ekhlasi-Hundrieser M, Kirchhoff C, et al: The role of stallion seminal proteins in fertilization. *Anim Reprod Sci* 89:159-170, 2005.

42. Amann RP, Cristanelli MI, Squires EL: Proteins in stallion seminal plasma, *J Reprod Fertil* 35(Suppl):113-120, 1987.

43. Hamann H, Jude R, Sieme H, et al: A polymorphism within the equine CRISP3 gene is associated with stallion fertility in Hanoverian Warmblood horses. *Anim Genet* 38:259-264, 2007.

44. Brandon CI, Heusner GL, Caudle AB, Fayrer-Hosken RA: Two-dimensional polyacrylamide gel electrophoresis of equine seminal plasma proteins and their correlation with stallion fertility. Proc Society for Theriogenology, Montreal, Quebec: 1997.

45. Troedsson MH: Uterine response to semen deposition in the mare. Proc Society for Theriogenology, Montreal, Quebec: 1995, pp 130–135.

46. Gebauer MR, Pickett BW, Faulkner LC, et al: Chemical characteristics of seminal plasma and spermatozoa of stallions. *J Anim Sci* 43(3):626-630, 1976.

47. Pozor AM, McDonnell SM: Ultrasound evaluation of stallion accessory sex glands. Proc Society Theriogenology, Kansas City, MO: 1996, pp 294-297.

48. Carver DA, Ball BA: Lipase activity in stallion seminal plasma and the effect of lipase on stallion spermatozoa during storage at 5 degrees C. *Theriogenology* 58(8):1587-1595, 2002.

49. Love CC, Riera FL, Oristaglio RM, Kenney RM: Sperm occluded (plugged) ampullae in the stallion. Proc Society for Theriogenology, San Antonio, TX: 1992, pp 117–123.

50. Mann T, Leone E, Polge C: The composition of stallion semen. *J Endocrinol* 13:279, 1956.

51. Schott HC, Yarner DD: Endoscopic examination of the urinary tract. In Traub-Dargatz IL, Brown CM, eds: *Equine Endoscopy*, 2nd ed. St Louis: Mosby, 1997, pp 187-203.

52. MacPherson ML: Male Genital Endoscopy Short Course: Advanced Current Topics in Stallion Veterinary Practice. Philadelphia: University of Pennsylvania, New Bolton Center, October, 1997.

53. Sullins KE, Traub-Dargatz JL: Endoscopy of the equine urinary tract. *Compend Contin Educ Pract Vet* 6:663, 1984.

54. Traub-Dargatz IL, Brown CM: *Equine Endoscopy*, 2nd ed. St Louis: Mosby, 1997.

55. Traub-Dargatz IL, McKinnon AO: Adjunctive methods of examination of the urogenital tract. *Vet Clin North Am Equine Pract* 4:339-358, 1988.

56. Sharpe RM: Regulation of spermatogenesis. In Knobil E, Neill ID, eds: *The Physiology of Reproduction*, 2nd ed. New York: Raven Press, 1994.

57. Irvine CHG, Alexander SL: The effect of sexual arousal on gonadotropin releasing hormone, FSH, and LH secretion in the stallion. *J Reprod Fertil Suppl* 44:85-92, 1991.

58. Lindsay FE, Burton FL: Observational study of "urine testing" in the horse and donkey stallion. *Equine Vet J* 15:330, 1983.

59. Clay CM, Clay IN: Endocrine and testicular changes associated with season, artificial photoperiod, and the peri-pubertal period in stallions. *Vet Clin North Am Equine Pract* 8:31-56, 1992.

60. Clay CM, Squires EL, Amann RP, Pickett BW: Influences of season and artificial photoperiod on stallions: Testicular size, seminal characteristics and sexual behavior. *J Anim Sci* 64:517-525, 1987.

61. Clay CM, Squires EL, Amann RP, Nett TM: Influences of season and artificial photoperiod on stallions: Luteinizing hormone, follicle-stimulating hormone and testosterone. *J Anim Sci* 66:1246-1255, 1988.

62. Bardin CW, et al: The Sertoli cell. In Knobil E, Neill ID, eds: *The Physiology of Reproduction*, 2nd ed. New York: Raven Press, 1994, pp 1291-1333.

REPRODUCTIVE ENDOCRINOLOGY OF THE STALLION

JANET F. ROSER

It is well established in many mammalian species, including the stallion, that normal spermatogenesis depends on a functional hypothalamic-pituitary-testicular (HPT) axis, which involves secretion of pituitary hormones into the peripheral circulation that act at the level of the testis. Subsequently, testicular hormones are secreted back into the blood and act as classic feedback regulators on hypothalamic and pituitary hormones.[1,2] Historically, the major hormones involved have been gonadotropin-releasing hormone (GnRH) produced and secreted from the hypothalamus; luteinizing hormone (LH) and follicle-stimulating hormone (FSH), produced and secreted from the anterior pituitary; androgens and estrogens produced and secreted from the testicular Leydig cells; and estrogens and inhibin produced and secreted from the testicular Sertoli cells. However, recent evidence suggests that a paracrine–autocrine system at the level of the testes is also involved in normal reproductive function.[3-8] The specific nature and relative contribution of the various factors involved in the endocrine–paracrine–autocrine control of reproductive function in normal stallions are not well defined, nor have they been elucidated in the idiopathic subfertile or infertile stallion.[9] My laboratory has been engaged in characterizing the HPT in fertile, subfertile (idiopathic oligospermia), and infertile (idiopathic azoospermia) stallions.[10-24] Our studies have not only identified endocrine factors and mechanisms important for normal reproductive function, but also demonstrated specific hormonal alterations in pituitary and testicular function among fertile, subfertile, and infertile stallions. Although these observations suggest both a pituitary and testicular dysfunction of an endocrine nature, until recently it has not been apparent which reproductive organ has the primary defect or whether paracrine–autocrine factors play a role in reproductive function. Studies in my laboratory suggest that the primary defect is at the level of the testes but that the nature of the dysfunction is not related to a change in LH receptor–binding kinetics.[20,21,23] Associated with receptor activity and signal transduction is the paracrine–autocrine modulation of these endocrine events. Paracrine–autocrine systems in the testes have been well characterized in other species and appear to be an important component of normal testicular function, including regulation of steroidogenesis and spermatogenesis.[3-8] This chapter summarizes current information regarding the nature of the multiple endocrine–paracrine–autocrine systems that may be necessary for normal reproductive function in the stallion and their impact on stallion fertility.

THE PINEAL GLAND AND THE HYPOTHALAMIC–PITUITARY–TESTICULAR AXIS

Sharp and Cleaver[25] have written an excellent review chapter on the pineal gland and melatonin, a hormone that regulates GnRH production and secretion in the stallion. In addition, an outstanding review of the physiology and endocrinology of the stallion by Amann[2] describes the involvement and interaction of the classic hormones that make up the HPT axis to control spermatogenesis in this species. Findings in recent studies have added to our knowledge of the dynamics of the pineal gland–HPT axis, including additional hormones that may be involved in controlling testicular function in the stallion.[26] The interactions of the pineal gland, brain opioids, thyroid gland, and the HPT axis of the stallion is presented in Fig. 2-1.

Pineal Gland and Melatonin

The classic reproductive endocrine system in a seasonal breeder, such as the stallion, starts at the level of the pineal gland and the secretion of melatonin.[25] Melatonin is controlled by light signals received by the retina and transmitted via the optic nerve to the pineal gland.[25] The final action of this indoleamine at the level of the central nervous system is a modulation of GnRH secretion, but it does not act directly on GnRH neurons; rather, its action involves a complex neural circuit of interneurons that includes at least dopaminergic, serotoninergic, and aminoacidergic neurons.[27] In addition, this network appears to undergo morphological changes between seasons.[27] With decreasing light, the pineal gland produces more melatonin, which inhibits the release of GnRH, resulting in a decrease in the gonadotropins, steroids, and testicular activity.[25] The endocrine events leading to maximum reproductive capacity in the stallion are initiated when day lengths are still short, albeit increasing.[28] Increasing the period of light suppresses melatonin synthesis by modulating the activity of its biosynthetic enzymes[29]; in turn, GnRH, LH, and FSH are released and testicular activity resumes.[30] Cleaver and co-authors[31] reported that exposure of mares to constant light resulted in a marked decrease in circulating melatonin concentrations and an increase in hypothalamic GnRH content. It has been demonstrated that exogenous melatonin decreases plasma testosterone concentrations in stallions.[32] Elevated melatonin levels have been found in men with primary hypogonadism or infertility with oligospermia or azoospermia.[33,34] Acute suppression of LH levels has been reported in healthy men as

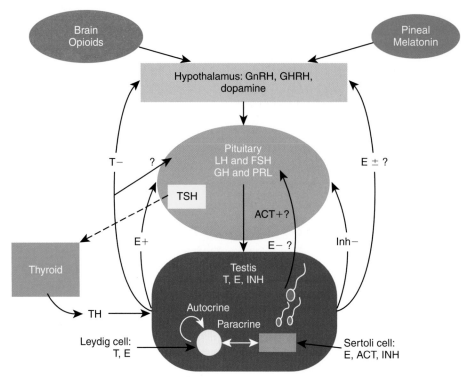

Figure 2-1. Hypothalamic-pituitary-testicular (HPT) axis of the stallion. Melatonin from the pineal gland and opioids from the brain regulate gonadotropin-releasing hormone *(GnRH)* in a negative fashion. GnRH regulates the release of luteinizing hormone *(LH)* and follicle stimulating hormone *(FSH)* from the anterior pituitary. The major regulator of Leydig cells is LH. The major endocrine products of the Leydig cells are testosterone *(T)* and estrogens *(E)* in the adult stallion. The major regulator of the Sertoli cells is FSH. Estrogen, inhibin *(INH)*, and probably activin *(ACT)* in the stallion are the major endocrine products of the Sertoli cells. Growth hormone–releasing hormone *(GHRH)* regulates production and secretion of growth hormone *(GH)* from the anterior pituitary. Dopamine negatively regulates the release of prolactin *(PRL)* from the pituitary. Thyroid-stimulating hormone *(TSH)* is produced in the anterior pituitary and regulates the release of thyroid hormones from the thyroid gland *(TH)*. The role of growth hormone, prolactin, and thyroid hormone on testicular function in the stallion is unclear. Testosterone inhibits GnRH but has no action on LH release at the level of the pituitary. Its role in regulating FSH at the level of the pituitary is unclear. Estrogen modulates GnRH-induced LH release, but its action on FSH release at the pituitary and GnRH at the hypothalamus is unclear. Inhibin feeds back on the pituitary to inhibit the release of FSH. Activin has been shown to positively modulate the release of FSH at the level of the pituitary in other species, but its action in the stallion is unknown.

well.[35] Inhibition of sperm motility in normal semen has also been observed following melatonin administration in vitro and in vivo.[36,37]

HPT Axis

As observed in other species, under appropriate stimuli, the hypothalamus of the stallion releases GnRH in a pulsatile fashion, which, in turn, stimulates the production and pulsatile release of the gonadotropins.[38,39] LH stimulates the production and release of both testosterone (T) and estrogens from the Leydig cells in the adult stallion.[19] In contrast and as demonstrated in the stallion and other species, FSH binds to the Sertoli cell to release estrogen, inhibin, activin, androgen-binding protein (ABP), transferrin, insulin-like growth factor-1 (IGF-1) and other factors needed for spermatogenesis.[2,40-43] Although it has been reported that prolactin plays a role in testicular function in the boar,[44] ram,[45] rodent,[46,47] and human,[47] it is unclear whether it has any function in the stallion testes.[19]

Testicular proteins and steroid hormones feed back to the hypothalamus and pituitary via the peripheral circulation to modulate the discharge of GnRH, LH, and FSH.[1,2] A study by Muyan and co-authors[15] clearly demonstrated that estrogens, particularly estradiol-17β (E₂), and not the androgens, modulate LH release from stallion pituitary cells. The results demonstrated that estradiol significantly enhanced the GnRH-induced LH release

from equine pituitary cells incubated in culture, whereas testosterone and dihydrotestosterone had no effect. Most likely, the major role of testosterone in the stallion is a negative feedback effect on the release of GnRH at the level of the hypothalamus, as has been demonstrated in other male species.[48] In terms of estrogen, its function at the hypothalamus in the stallion is still unclear. Although it has been shown to have both negative and positive feedback effects in other species,[48,49] its mechanism of action at the hypothalamus in the stallion is yet to be revealed. Thompson and co-authors[50] demonstrated that treatment with estradiol decreased circulating FSH levels, increased circulating LH levels, and decreased GnRH-induced FSH secretion in long-term geldings. Thompson and Honey[51] further demonstrated a role of estradiol on FSH secretion when they reported that immunization of colts against estradiol increased circulating FSH levels without changing LH levels. These studies do not identify the site of action of estradiol, however. Estradiol could be acting at the hypothalamus to change the amplitude and frequency of GnRH and thus the ratio of LH and FSH secreted from the pituitary as observed in the rat and primate,[52,53] or estradiol could be acting at the level of the pituitary to modulate GnRH-induced LH and FSH release as observed in other species, including the horse.[15,49,54] Because inhibin inhibits FSH secretion at the level of the pituitary in several mammalian species,[55] inhibin may act in conjunction with estrogen or testosterone in the stallion to control FSH secretion. In the stallion, both FSH and inhibin exhibit similar seasonal changes; peripheral FSH and inhibin increase in the spring and decrease in the fall.[16,56] Inhibin and activins are members of the transforming growth factor super family of growth and differentiation factors.[57] They consist of glycosylated polypeptide dimers involving subunits linked by a disulfide bond. In the case of inhibin, the subunits consist of an alpha (α) subunit linked to a beta (β) subunit, either β_A or β_B. Activin consists of two β subunits linked by a disulfide bond, either $\beta_A\beta_A$, $\beta_B\beta_B$, or $\beta_A\beta_B$. The subunits have been localized in both the Leydig and Sertoli cells by immunocytochemistry.[55-57] Not much is known about the role of activin in the stallion. In other species, activin appears to be stimulated by FSH from Sertoli cells and to act at the level of the pituitary to release FSH.[55] Inhibin/activin β_A subunit mRNA activity has been demonstrated to be expressed in the endometrial glands of the mare during pregnancy.[58] One could surmise that activin is also localized in the testicular somatic cells of the stallion given the fact that activins like inhibins consist of β subunits that have been localized in equine Leydig and Sertoli cells.[56] Studies investigating activin activity at the level of the hypothalamus, pituitary gland, and testes in the stallion have not been done.

Prolactin, Thyroid Hormone, and Growth Hormone

Prolactin, thyroid hormone, and growth hormone (GH) have been reported to affect testicular function in other species. Prolactin appears to play a role in inducing transcription of the estrogen receptor.[59] It has been shown to affect androgen-sensitive tissues and, together with LH and GH, control synthesis of LH receptors in the testes, activate androgen synthesis, and affect spermatogenesis.[44-46] Thyroid hormone is crucial to the onset of adult Leydig cell and Sertoli cell differentiation.[60,61] Hypothyroidism during testicular development leads to proliferation of the testicular somatic cells and larger testes.[60,61] One critical molecular target of thyroid hormone in the Leydig cell may be the steroidogenic acute regulatory (StAR) protein, which is responsible for cholesterol transport across the outer mitochondrial membrane in Leydig cells.[61] Lack of thyroid hormone leads to a decrease in StAR mRNA and protein, causing a decrease in testosterone production.[61] In Sertoli cells, thyroid hormone stimulates lactate secretion as well as mRNA expression of Müllerian-inhibiting substance, aromatase, estradiol receptor, and androgen-binding protein.[62] Thyroid hormone receptors have been identified in sperm, in developing germ cells, and in Sertoli, Leydig, and peritubular myoid cells.[62] GH appears to affect testicular function by modulating gonadal steroid synthesis and gametogenesis.[63] It has been demonstrated that GH mediates the release of pituitary LH as well as the synthesis and release of testicular IGF-1.[64] GH deficiency is associated with abnormally small testes,[65] and in humans can result in reduced or absent sperm motility. GH treatment can increase plasma IGF-1 concentrations and restore sperm motility.[66] GH resistance is associated with reduced fertility in men.[67] GH may alter gametogenesis by affecting testosterone synthesis, since testosterone is necessary for sperm production and mRNA-encoding GH receptors are present in rat Leydig cells.[68] GH increases basal or hCG-stimulated testosterone production in GH-deficient men.[69]

Although prolactin and thyroid hormone fluctuate with the season in the stallion and mare, respectively,[70,71] the role of these hormones on reproductive function in the stallion is yet to be determined. Prolactin did not appear to stimulate testosterone production in equine Leydig cells in culture,[19] and the seasonal changes and effects of thyroid hormone have not been investigated in the stallion. In the mare, thyroid function was not associated with infertility.[72] GH does not appear to fluctuate with season in the stallion.[73] However, treatment with a somatostatin analogue (GH inhibitor) caused a transient decrease in semen motility and hCG-induced testosterone release, suggesting a role for GH in the regulation of testicular function in stallions.[73] A direct effect of GH on Leydig cell steroidogenesis in culture was not observed.[74]

Opioids

In the stallion as well as other species, it appears that seasonal changes in GnRH/LH release are partly regulated by opioids.[75] Opioids are secreted from the brain, travel to the hypothalamus, and cause a decrease in GnRH release during the winter months.[75] Aurich and co-authors[76] showed that treatment with an opioid antagonist naloxone caused an acute LH release in stallions outside of, but not during, the breeding season. The opioidergic regulation of LH release appears to require the presence of the gonads.[77]

ENDOCRINE AND TESTICULAR CHANGES ASSOCIATED WITH SEASON

Historically, the stallion has been classified as a "long-day breeder" because maximum reproductive capacity is attained during periods of increasing day length. During the spring and summer, there is an increase in testicular size and weight, sperm production and output, libido, and plasma concentrations of LH, FSH, testosterone, E_2, inhibin, and prolactin.[16,56,71,78-81] The endocrine events involved in initiating testicular recrudescence in the stallion have not been adequately characterized but appear to start with a photoinducible decrease in melatonin from the pineal gland, which, in turn, allows for an increase in hypothalamic GnRH and a subsequent increase in pituitary LH and FSH release into the peripheral circulation, although reports on seasonal or photoinducible changes in FSH release are conflicting.[25,81-85] Increasing plasma concentrations of gonadotropins, and perhaps prolactin and thyroid hormone, act on the testicular Leydig and Sertoli cells to increase production of T, E_2, and inhibin and spermatogenesis in the stallion. Although the hypothalamic-pituitary-gonadal (HPG) axis of the stallion is stimulated by photoperiod in a similar fashion as the HPG of the mare,[86] it is unclear why ~75% of mares shut down completely while stallions have the capacity to continue to breed throughout the non-breeding season, albeit with lower sperm numbers per ejaculate.[87] In the stallion, opioidergic neuromodulators affect GnRH and dopaminergic neuromodulators affect prolactin release.[88] Major interactions between dopaminergic and opioidergic systems in the regulation of LH and prolactin release do not seem to exist in the male horse.[88] The signaling pathway of these neuromodulators could be different between the mare and stallion. In addition, follicular development, oocyte maturation, and ovulation require an intricate network of shifting hormones and local factors whereas the dynamics involved in the process of spermatogenesis require a more subtle input. Perhaps from an evolutionary standpoint, the stallion's HPT axis is less sensitive to changes in day length in order to ensure maximum breeding efficiency throughout the year.

A comprehensive 2-year study by Clay and Clay[85] on the effects of season and photoperiod on endocrine and testicular function in stallions has revealed that the stallion, like other mammalian species, has an endogenous circannual cycle in testicular function that is entrained by an external environmental rhythm or zeitgeber (time-giver), or photoperiod.[82] In this study, stallions exposed to 8 hours of light and 16 hours of dark (8:16) for 20 months starting in July continued to display a significant seasonal cycle in testicular size, sperm output, and peripheral hormone levels similar to the control group exposed to naturally occurring changes in day length. Thus, stallions maintained on continuous short days have the capacity to recrudesce despite the lack of exposure to a stimulatory photoperiod. On the other hand, testicular recrudescence was accelerated earlier in the season compared with control subjects when stallions were exposed to an 8:16 photoperiod for 20 weeks beginning in July and then 16:8 for 15 months thereafter, indicating that seasonal sexual recrudescence can be photoinducible. In addition, the study demonstrated that continued exposure to a stimulatory photoperiod does not maintain a heightened reproductive capacity indefinitely and testicular regression does ensue. Cox and co-authors[89] found that increasing day length using artificial lights at the end of the breeding season in the northern hemisphere significantly decreased testosterone concentrations, suggesting a negative impact on the fertility of stallions being transported to the southern hemisphere. Therefore, shorter day length in autumn may provide a critical trigger in resensitizing the stallion to the photoinducible events of long days. This concept may be important to keep in mind when shipping stallions, especially those with marginal fertility, from the northern hemisphere to the southern hemisphere for breeding purposes. To maintain peak reproductive performance in these stallions throughout the year, it may be important to put them on an intermittent lighting regimen by alternating intervals of short and long days. Further research in this area is warranted.

SPERMATOGENESIS, STEROIDOGENESIS, AND TESTICULAR FUNCTION: ENDOCRINE-PARACRINE-AUTOCRINE FACTORS

Endocrine Factor

The process of spermatogenesis, steroidogenesis, and testicular function is regulated by a complex interplay of endocrine, paracrine, and autocrine signals.[3-8,90-99] The master control is GnRH that signals the pituitary to produce LH and FSH. LH binds to receptors on testicular Leydig cells to produce testosterone, a steroid hormone that diffuses into the seminiferous tubules. Within the seminiferous tubules only Sertoli cells possess receptors for testosterone and FSH and thus these cells are the major targets of the ultimate hormonal signals that regulate Sertoli cell factors that support spermatogenesis. Reports clearly indicate that testosterone is essential for maintenance and restoration of spermatogenesis in the adult testes.[99] Although there is general agreement that FSH is of critical importance in the initiation and expansion of spermatogenesis in mammals during puberty,[100] the role of FSH in the regulation of spermatogenesis in the adult mammal is still controversial.[101] Spermatogenesis has been shown to be maintained or restored quantitatively by testosterone alone in adult rats actively immunized against GnRH, suggesting that FSH is not required for those events in the adult rat.[102] However, there is strong evidence to suggest that, in the human and non-human primate, under certain conditions, FSH synergizes with testosterone to maintain quantitatively normal spermatogenesis in the adult.[1,103] The controversy

has led to a very basic physiological question: Why have two hormones to regulate spermatogenesis, rather than just one? One reason may be that each hormone has differential effects on sperm production. According to Zirkin and co-authors,[101] in nearly all mammals, testosterone alone acting as a local factor is capable of maintaining qualitatively complete spermatogenesis, whereas the role of FSH may be to influence the quantity of spermatozoa produced at the premeiotic and postmeiotic levels, depending on the species. In addition, the increasing volume of data with regard to the involvement of local paracrine-autocrine modulation of spermatogenesis not only suggests a more complicated story, but also supports the conceptual argument that one hormone or local testicular factor alone cannot do the job as efficiently as several. Other hormones such as insulin, vasopressin, and oxytocin have been implicated as endocrine factors that regulate testicular function.[90] Estrogen, a product of testosterone, has recently been determined to have significant importance in regulating steroidogenesis and spermatogenesis.[93,94]

The role of FSH and testosterone in the development and maintenance of spermatogenesis in the stallion is not entirely clear. Endocrine profiles of colts prior to and during puberty suggest a differential role of FSH and testosterone on spermatogenesis.[2] Prior to puberty, serum FSH concentrations in the colt peaked at about 40 weeks of age, remained relatively high, and then increased again at the time of puberty (~83 weeks). Interestingly, serum concentrations of LH also peaked at around 40 weeks of age, declined to baseline, and then rose again at the time of puberty. Testosterone levels prior to puberty remained low and did not increase at 40 weeks in conjunction with the LH or FSH rise but then rapidly peaked at the time of puberty. These findings suggest that FSH in the colt may be the hormone critical for Sertoli cell development and proliferation prior to puberty, whereas testosterone triggers Sertoli cell differentiation and maturation necessary for gene expression of various paracrine factors important for germ cell development. In adult stallions FSH may have more of a minor role on maintenance of spermatogenesis since it has been reported that FSH receptor numbers in rats decline in the adult Sertoli cell,[104] and seasonal changes of FSH are not always apparent in the stallion.[81,84,85] In the adult stallion, estrogen and not testosterone may play a major role in Sertoli and germ cell function. When stallions were given a GnRH antagonist, testosterone levels were not affected and only the decline in LH, FSH, and estradiol concentrations could be correlated with morphological evidence of testicular degeneration.[105] The concept that testosterone may not be the critical hormone in supporting spermatogenesis in the stallion is also substantiated by a study carried out investigating the plasma hormone concentrations of fertile, subfertile, and infertile stallions. Plasma inhibin, E_2, and estrogen conjugates (ECs) were significantly lower and gonadotropins significantly higher in idiopathic infertile stallions, whereas plasma T levels did not change.[22]

Paracrine-Autocrine Factors

In addition to the endocrine control of LH and FSH on testicular function and sperm production, local testicular steroids, proteins, and peptides called *paracrine-autocrine factors* coordinate the various functions of the different testicular cell types and/or modulate the testicular actions of pituitary gonadotropins according to local conditions and requirements (Fig. 2-2). Paracrine factors are produced by one cell and act on a different cell

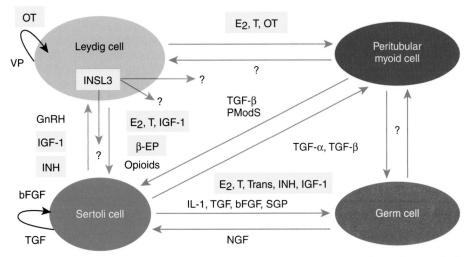

Figure 2-2. Paracrine-autocrine regulation of testicular function. Many of the local interactions in the equine testis are unknown. The figure presents a hypothetical paracrine-autocrine system based on what has been observed in other species: Gonadotropin-releasing hormone *(GnRH)*, insulin-like growth factor-1 *(IGF-1)*, insulin-like peptide 3 *(INSL3)*, inhibin *(INH)*, activin *(ACT)*, beta endorphin *(β-EP)*, transferrin *(Trans)*, basic fibroblast growth factor *(bFGF)*, transforming growth factor *(TGF)*, transforming growth factor beta *(TGF-β)*, transforming growth factor alpha *(TGF-α)*, interleukin-1 *(IL-1)*, sulphated glycoprotein *(SGP)*, nerve growth factor *(NGF)*, peritubular modifying substance *(PModS)*, oxytocin *(OT)*, vasopressin *(VP)*, testosterone *(T)*, estradiol *(E₂)*. Those factors highlighted in yellow have been identified in the stallion testis.

type, whereas autocrine factors are produced by one cell and act on the same cell type. Potential paracrine-autocrine regulators of testicular function and spermatogenesis of proven physiological significance include such factors as estrogen, testosterone, inhibin, activin, GnRH-like peptides, growth factors like IGF-1 and transforming growth factor alpha and beta (TGF-α and β), oxytocin, vasopressin, pro-enkephalins, enkephalins, proopiomelanocortin (POMC), and POMC-derived peptides such as β-endorphins (β-EPs), cytokines, transferrin, sulfated glycoprotein-l (sGP-l) and sGP-2, insulin-like peptide 3 (INSL3) and PmodS, a paracrine factor secreted from peritubular myoid cells that modulates Sertoli cell function.[3-8,90-99] It is beyond the scope of this chapter to discuss the roles of each of these local factors, so only those that have been investigated in the stallion will be reviewed: IGF-1, transferrin, inhibin, activin, estrogen, testosterone, INSL3, POMC, and β-EPsand oxytocin.

Insulin-Like Growth Factor-1(IGF-1)

A publication by Gnessi and co-authors[7] provides an overview of the expression, localization, production, and testicular function of IGF-1 in mammalian species. IGF-1, a single-chain polypeptide, is present in peritubular myoid cells, Sertoli cells, and Leydig cells. Receptors for IGF-1 have been found on the cell membrane of germ cells, Leydig and Sertoli cells, and myoid cells. IGF-1 receptors can be up-regulated by LH, FSH, and GH, with LH being the most important factor. The actions of IGF-1 can be modified by its binding protein (IGFBP), which may enhance or inhibit the effects of IGF-1. IGF-1 stimulates the proliferation of prepubertal Sertoli cells and has a small mitogenic effect on immature Leydig cells. IGF-1 stimulates testosterone production and potentiates hCG-induced testosterone formation. Furthermore, IGF-1 is believed to be involved in spermatogenesis. IGF-1 stimulates spermatogonial DNA synthesis and has a maintaining effect on premeiotic DNA synthesis in the rat under *in vitro* conditions, and IGF-1 induces the differentiation of mouse type A spermatogonia. More recently, IGF-1 has been shown to have anti-apoptotic effects on Leydig cells and germ cells.[106,107]

IGF-1 has been identified in testicular tissue and in seminal fluid in the stallion.[24,108] Hess and Roser[24] reported that in colts less than 2 years of age, IGF-1 concentrations in plasma and testicular extracts were higher than in the other age groups and were higher in the breeding season than in the non-breeding season. Seasonal changes in IGF-1 were not observed in stallions older than 2 years of age. No significant differences in plasma or testicular extract concentrations of IGF-1 were found among fertility groups. The results of this study demonstrate that plasma and testicular IGF-1 levels are high in stallions younger than 2 years of age and then decline and plateau in stallions older than 5 years of age, suggesting that IGF-1 may be involved in testicular development. Circulating and intra-testicular levels of IGF-1 do not appear to correlate with declining fertility in stallions tested, suggesting that IGF-1 may not be a reliable biomarker for the diagnosis of subfertility and infertility using those biological samples.[24] However, there is some evidence to suggest that measurement of IGF-1 in seminal plasma may be a good indicator of fertility.[108] A positive but variable relationship between IGF-1 and sperm morphology and motility was noted. Stallions with high levels of IGF-1 in seminal plasma achieved higher pregnancy rates in mares, suggesting that IGF-1 may play a role in sperm function. Using equine testicular cell culture techniques, Roser[43] observed that the highest IGF-1 production rates in Leydig cells appears to be during puberty, whereas highest production rates in Sertoli cells occur prior to puberty. Although LH and GH do not appear to regulate IGF-1 in Leydig cells, FSH does appear to stimulate IGF-1 from Sertoli cells but only prior to puberty.[43] IGF-1 does not appear to stimulate a steroidogenic response from equine Leydig cells in culture.[74] Preliminary studies in our laboratory indicate that IGF-1 may have anti-apoptotic effects on equine Leydig and Sertoli cells.

Transferrin

An excellent review by Sylvester and Griswold[109] discusses the physiology of transferrin in the mammalian testes. Transferrin is an iron-binding protein that delivers iron as a nutritional component to germ cells. Sertoli cells synthesize transferrin and, when bound to iron, secrete the complex into the adluminal space. The adluminal testicular iron-bound transferrin is then available to receptors on spermatocytes. Histological examination of testes from mutant mice lacking normal transferrin revealed a decreased number of germ cells and a greatly reduced level of spermiation. Transferrin has been identified in human seminal plasma, and evidence indicates that the measurement of seminal fluid transferrin may be an indicator of the function of Sertoli cells in intact human males. In bulls there was a strong positive correlation between sperm output and transferrin concentrations in seminal fluid, suggesting that transferrin production should be a good indicator of Sertoli function and spermatogenic potential in bulls.[110]

In the stallion, transferrin is produced by Sertoli cells with the highest production rate occurring at the time of puberty.[42] Ongoing studies in our laboratory in collaboration with Dr. Joyce Parlevliet (Utrecht University, The Netherlands) are investigating seminal plasma transferrin concentrations in stallions with various degrees of fertility.

Androgens and Estrogens

In other species it has been demonstrated that androgens and estrogens regulate the function of Sertoli cells, Leydig cells peritubular myoid cells, and germ cells by binding to their respective receptors and eliciting a cellular response.[8,94,111-114] By acting through its receptors in Sertoli cells, testosterone appears to be responsible for maintaining an adequate blood-testis barrier function[115] and inducing meiosis and postmeiotic development of germ cells.[8,113] Testosterone has been shown to inhibit germ cell apoptosis.[116] There also appears to be an androgen action on Sertoli cells that modulates their gene expression, proliferation, and differentiation.[8,113] Studies using a tissue-specific knock-out mouse with the androgen receptor gene deleted demonstrated an alteration in the expression of several key steroidogenic enzymes in Leydig cells, suggesting that testosterone is an autocrine factor regulating its own production.[117] The androgen receptor knock-out mouse also demonstrated an arrest of spermatogenesis, predominantly at the round spermatid stage.[117]

Increasing evidence over the last decade has clearly established the importance of estrogen as a paracrine-autocrine factor in regulating testicular function.[93,94,118] The production of estrogen comes from the enzymatic conversion of androgens to estrogens by the aromatase enzyme. According to the literature reviewed by O'Donnell and co-authors[94] and Hess and Carnes,[118] the production of estrogen from the different testicular cell types changes with age and species. For example, during the early stages of testicular development in the rat, basal aromatase activity is found in both the immature Leydig and Sertoli cells with the Sertoli cells being more active in producing estrogen than the Leydig cells. However, aromatase appears to have an age-dependent pattern of expression in the rat. As the animal matures, the Leydig cell basal aromatase activity increases 3- to 4-fold, although the Sertoli cells do continue to express aromatase during their maturation. In other species, it appears that the amount of aromatase activity is equally present in both the adult Sertoli and Leydig cells. Of interest is that germ cells express aromatase activity during different stages of development and into maturity, which suggests that sperm themselves could control the levels of estrogen present in the luminal fluid and epididymis. The localization of estrogen receptors in testicular cells varies depending on the species, developmental stage of the cell, and type of receptor.[93,94,118] Although two different receptors have been identified, estrogen receptor alpha (ERα) and estrogen receptor beta (ERβ), the differences in their mechanisms of action are still not clear except that certain cell types are regulated by one receptor or the other. In general, according to O'Donnell and co-authors,[94] it appears that both ERα and ERβ are localized in Leydig cells, whereas ERβ is mostly confined to Sertoli cells and developing germ cells.

Changes in intra-testicular testosterone and estrogen concentrations during testicular development and stages of fertility have been investigated in the stallion.[22] Intra-testicular concentrations of estradiol and ECs increased with testicular maturation, whereas there was no age effect on testosterone concentrations. There was no difference detected in intra-testicular concentrations of estradiol, ECs, and testosterone among the fertile, subfertile, and infertile groups of stallions, although plasma concentrations of the estrogens but not testosterone were significantly lower in the infertile group. By using in vitro equine testicular cell culture techniques, studies have demonstrated that increasing doses of equine LH stimulate the production of testosterone and estrogens from Leydig cells and increasing doses of FSH influence the production of estrogen from Sertoli cells.[19,41] By using immunocytochemistry techniques, it appears that aromatase expression changes with age in the stallion such that both Leydig cells and Sertoli cells stain positive for aromatase prior to and during puberty, but in the adult stallion, positive staining remains in Leydig cells but to a lesser extent in the Sertoli cells.[119,120]

In the stallion testis, estrogen and androgen receptors have been localized in equine Leydig, Sertoli, or germ cells.[112,121] The stallion makes more estrogens than androgens in the testis as demonstrated in studies investigating basal levels of the steroids using blood samples obtained by catheterization of the testicular vein.[122] Taken together, the studies just mentioned demonstrate an important regulatory role of estrogens in testicular cell function and spermatogenesis.

Inhibin and Activin

de Kretser and co-authors[123] have written a recent overview of inhibin and activin. Inhibin and activin are glycoproteins of the transforming growth factor superfamily produced mainly by the Sertoli cells, but subunits have been localized in Leydig and germ cells depending on the stage of testicular development and mammalian species. Both proteins have endocrine, paracrine, and autocrine functions. As discussed previously, inhibin and activin are released into the peripheral circulation and regulate pituitary FSH. Whereas in the testis, inhibin and activin receptors, co-receptors, and intracellular signaling molecules have been identified in the various somatic cell types and the germ cells,[97] evidence indicates that inhibin and activin act as paracrine factors influencing Leydig cell steroidogenesis,[124-126] as well as spermatogenesis.[127,128] The paracrine role of activin appears to be an inhibitory one on steroidogenesis in Leydig cells.[126] Activin also appears to have an autocrine role in stimulating follistatin and inhibin from Sertoli cells.[123] In rat testes activin has age-dependent effects on Sertoli cell division and affects the development of germ cells in the male.[129,130] In human males, measurement of inhibin B levels in the peripheral circulation appears to be useful as an indicator of functional spermatogenesis and as a marker for male fertility.[131]

In the stallion, inhibin has been demonstrated in testicular tissue and its subunits predominantly located in both the Leydig and Sertoli cells.[16,56] Intra-testicular inhibin concentrations were significantly lower in colts less than 1 year of age compared with pubertal and adult stallions.[22] Changes in hormone levels based on fertility status were different between plasma concentrations and intra-testicular concentrations in stallions. In plasma, inhibin, estradiol, and ECs were significantly lower and testosterone higher in idiopathic infertile stallions but no change was observed in idiopathic subfertile stallions compared with fertile stallions. In contrast, intra-testicular steroid concentrations did not change among fertility groups. However, intra-testicular levels of inhibin tended to be lower in subfertile stallions and were significantly lower in infertile stallions, suggesting that intra-testicular inhibin may be an early marker for declining fertility in stallions. This phenomenon is similar to what has been observed in the peripheral circulation of human males. Plasma concentrations of inhibin B were significantly lower in men with fertility problems, suggesting that inhibin may be a good biomarker for declining fertility.[131]

Insulin-like Peptide 3 (INSL3)

The insulin-like peptide hormone INSL3 (previously known as insulin-like factor [RLF]) is a major new circulating hormone in the male.[132,133] It is produced almost exclusively by the Leydig cells of the testis, with anorchid men having undetectable circulating levels of the hormone.[134] INSL3 is made by both fetal and adult-type populations of Leydig cells, but only when these have attained their mature phenotype.[135] Various studies have indicated that the INSL3 gene and protein are expressed constitutively once Leydig cells are mature, thus making INSL3 an excellent marker of Leydig cell differentiation status.[135,136] It has been used in this context to study changes in testicular function in seasonally breeding animals[137,138] and during aging,[139] as well as to identify unequivocally Leydig cells within testis sections[140] and in primary culture.[141] Although INSL3 appears to be constitutively expressed in adult species, a recent finding using male patients with hypogonadotropic hypogonadism clearly showed that INSL3 production and secretion was dependent on LH.[134]

Currently, little is known about the function of INSL3 in the testis. INSL3 produced by prenatal Leydig cells is essential for the trans-abdominal part of testis descent via stimulation of outgrowth and differentiation of the gubernaculum, as shown in rodents.[142,143] Disruption of the INSL3 gene causes bilateral cryptorchidism.[142,143] The receptor for INSL3 has been recently identified as the novel G-protein coupled receptor (GPCR) LGR8, also known as Great.[144,145] Studies have demonstrated that the observed expression of LGR8 transcripts in the gubernaculum and the INSL3 stimulation of cAMP production by these cells were consistent with the common cryptorchid phenotypes of this ligand-receptor pair in earlier transgenic mouse studies.[144,145] Recently it has been demonstrated that LGR8 is expressed in meiotic and particularly postmeiotic germ cells and in Leydig cells, although not in Sertoli or peritubular cells.[133] The recent finding of LGR8 expression in germ cells and the suppression of apoptosis through binding of INSL3 to LGR8 suggest a paracrine role of INSL3 in germ cell survival.[146] Human male patients with testicular disorders oftentimes have reduced or absent circulating levels of INSL3.[134]

Recent studies by Klonisch and co-authors[147] have identified INSL3 and its receptor LGR8 in the testis of the horse. Equine INSL3 (eINSL3) was identified as a marker of Leydig cells in prepubertal and postpubertal equine testis. The localization of eINSL3 transcripts in Leydig cells was independent of the location of the testis in the animal, whether it is found in the abdomen or scrotum. By contrast, eINSL3 gene activity in testicular Leydig cells appeared to be reduced in cryptorchid testes, despite the presence of multiple Leydig cells. No INSL3 or LGR8 mutations have so far been identified in cryptorchid stallions. Interestingly, however, it was demonstrated that in unilateral cryptorchid stallions, INSL3 expression is down-regulated and LGR8 expression up-regulated in the cryptorchid versus the descended testis.[147] A debate still exists regarding whether unilateral cryptorchidism significantly affects stallion fertility. However, in artificial insemination (AI) stallions, the 50% reduction in sperm production may become relevant if the stallion is used frequently or is a marginal breeder. In the equine testis, Klonisch and co-authors[147] also detected eINSL3 expression despite marked differences in the functional state of the seminiferous epithelial cell cycle. However, the quantitative differences they observed in postpubertal normal as compared with cryptorchid and prepubertal testes suggest regulatory mechanisms that affect INSL3 production in testicular Leydig cells. Klonisch and co-authors[147] also demonstrated the expression of eLGR8 transcripts in the equine testis, indicating that the testes were a target tissue for the actions of eINSL3. Preliminary studies in our laboratory demonstrate an increase in basal production of INSL3 in equine Leydig cells cultured for 24 hours and after treatment with eLH (Fig. 2-3). Further studies are ongoing.

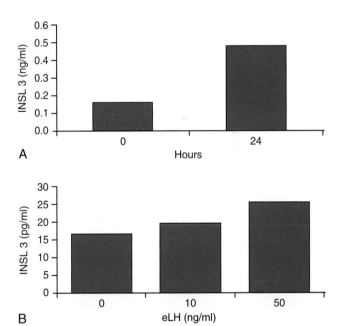

Figure 2-3. **A,** Average concentrations of INSL3 in equine Leydig cell culture media at time 0 and 24 hours (n = 2). Testes from two colts, ages 1 and 2 years old, were processed for Leydig cell cultures as described by Hess and Roser.[74] Equine Leydig cells (1 × 10⁶/ml) were cultured for 0 and 24 hours and media were analyzed for INSL3 concentrations using a human INSL3 EIA kit (Phoenix Pharmaceutical, Inc, Burlingame, CA). Preliminary results suggest that equine Leydig cells produce INSL3. **B,** Concentrations of INSL3 in equine Leydig cell culture media after incubation with increasing amounts of purified equine LH. Testis from a 1-year-old colt was processed for a Leydig cell culture as described by Hess and Roser.[74] Equine Leydig cells (1 × 10⁶/ml) were incubated with increasing doses of purified equine LH (Papkoff 262B, UC Davis) for 24 hours. Culture media were analyzed for INSL3 using a human INSL3 RIA kit (Phoenix Pharmaceutical, Inc, Burlingame, CA). Preliminary data suggest that INSL3 in Leydig cells is regulated by LH in the young colt.

Proopiomelanocortin (POMC) and β-Endorphin

POMC is a precursor protein that contains the sequence for several bioactive peptides, including adrenocorticotropin (ACTH), β-EP, and melanocyte-stimulating hormone (MSH). A review by Bardin and co-authors[148] indicates that the Leydig cell appears to be the only testicular cell that produces POMC-derived peptides and that there is evidence that LH may be involved in the production of these peptides. Studies indicate that POMC-derived peptides have differential effects on the function of the Sertoli cells. ACTH- and MSH-like peptides are stimulatory whereas β-EP is inhibitory.

Recently, Soverchia and co-authors[149] investigated the presence of POMC and β-EP in equine testicular and epididymal tissue. POMC gene expression was not found in either testicular or epididymal tissue. However, using immunocytochemistry techniques, Soverchia and co-authors[149] demonstrated the presence of β-EP in both the testis and epididymis in the stallion.

Oxytocin (OT)

OT is recognized as having endocrine and paracrine roles in male reproduction. OT and its receptor have been localized in the testes of several mammalian species.[150] Evidence supports the role of OT as a paracrine factor inducing contractility of the seminiferous tubules most likely involving the peritubular myoid cells.[150] OT may have a role in modulating Leydig cell steroidogenesis.[150]

The role of OT in the stallion has been investigated by Watson and co-authors.[151] By using radioimmunoassays, Watson and co-authors detected OT in seminal fractions, in washed lysed sperm, and in extracts from the testis and epididymis. With the use of immunocytochemistry, immunostaining for OT was present in occasional interstitial cells in the testis and in the epididymal epithelium and smooth muscle, but the authors concluded that the staining was due to binding of OT to its receptor in these tissues, suggesting that in the stallion OT is not locally produced in the testis or epididymis.

IDIOPATHIC SUBFERTILITY AND INFERTILITY IN STALLIONS—THE NATURE OF A HORMONAL IMBALANCE: CAUSE OR RESULT?

Subfertility or infertility in breeding stallions contributes to low pregnancy rates per cycle (<20%–30%/cycle; normal: >50%/cycle) and low pregnancy rates per season (<60%/season; normal: >80%/season), resulting in substantial financial loss in the equine industry.[9,152] There are a number of conditions associated with subfertility or infertility in stallions such as mismanagement, anabolic steroid treatment, infection, fever, tumors, injury, disease, behavior, and hormonal imbalance.[9,152-159] A number of these problems can be diagnosed and treated appropriately. In addition, a stallion with subnormal semen parameters could be managed more closely (e.g., bred closer to the time of ovulation, bred to mares selected for fertility, and bred to a limited number of mares) such that the stallion would have normal fertility rates. However, the stallion with a hormonal imbalance that is associated with testicular degeneration is difficult to manage, particularly if the cause of the problem is unknown. These stallions come under the category of idiopathic subfertility/infertility. The exact nature of the condition and the hormone imbalance that ensues may be a function of pathophysiological

events in the testes associated with the paracrine-autocrine system.[90,160] Typically, these stallions with idiopathic testicular dysfunction display low motility (≤20%–30% progressive motility) and marginal morphology (<60% normal morphology) along with a slight change in testicular consistency. These stallions may not show a hormonal imbalance at first, but in time, they demonstrate an increase in circulating FSH, a decrease in circulating estrogens, and a decrease in circulating inhibin (personal observations). Testicular volume starts to decline. Peripheral concentrations of LH and testosterone remain normal until sperm concentrations significantly decline. By the time the stallion is infertile, gonadotropins are high, steroids and inhibin are low, and the testes have significantly decreased in size and changed in consistency.[9,26] Therapy with hormones such as GnRH, equine chorionic gonadotropin (eCG), human chorionic gonadotropin (hCG), or FSH has been clinically implemented, but with limited success.[9,26,156,161,162] Controlled studies have demonstrated that treatment with GnRH does not dramatically improve seminal characteristics or conception rates, regardless of the therapeutic regimens used.[17,162,163] Giving anabolic steroids is contraindicated.[158] Although studies have not shown definitively that nutritional supplementation beyond that which is required enhances reproductive efficiency in the stallion,[164] a recent study indicates that feeding a DHA-enriched nutraceutical increased sperm motility parameters in cooled stored semen and frozen-thawed semen.[165] Until the pathophysiology of the problem is clearly understood, most therapies have a higher risk than benefit. Currently, careful management may be the only answer to getting the most out of a subfertile stallion.

A comprehensive understanding of the endocrine-paracrine-autocrine regulation of testicular function in the stallion would enable the clinician to identify, evaluate, and manage the idiopathic subfertile and infertile stallion. Such an understanding includes a clear perception of the normal cell-to-cell interactions in the testes and the abnormal mechanisms that may arise. A significant percentage of subfertile and infertile stallions has been diagnosed with testicular degeneration marked by progressive reduction and softening of the testes along with poor seminal parameters.[152] These stallions make up a heterogeneous population of poor breeding performers with unknown pathophysiology. Evidence suggests that the primary cause of reproductive failure in idiopathic subfertile and infertile stallions starts at the level of the Sertoli cell.[26,43] Abnormalities then spread to the germ cells and Leydig cells and eventually move up to the hypothalamus and pituitary. In these cases, the first clinical sign of a hormonal imbalance is an increase in circulating FSH levels, although an analysis of testicular tissue retrieved by a testicular biopsy procedure[166] may show an initial decline in intra-testicular inhibin.[22] By the time high plasma concentrations of FSH are observed, there is little hope of reversing the process. The hormonal imbalance may be the result of other pathophysiological events.

ENDOCRINE FUNCTION IN STALLIONS WITH POOR FERTILITY

Historically, clinicians relied on baseline concentrations of reproductive hormones in the stallion to help diagnose breeding unsoundness. For example, low levels of testosterone were observed in azoospermic stallions.[167] Burns and Douglas[157] made the first association between elevated plasma concentrations of FSH and subfertility in stallions. Two studies indicated that circulating plasma levels of FSH and estrogens, and not LH and T, could be good markers to predict future changes in fertility,[9,13] whereas another group of investigators suggested that measurement of serum levels of estrogens and testosterone may help in the diagnosis of infertile stallions when other methods are not available.[168] Whitcomb and co-authors[12] presented data on the presence of what appears to be a circulating bio-inactive LH isoform in stallions with poor breeding performance.

In addition to measuring basal levels of reproductive hormones in stallions with poor fertility, GnRH challenge testing involves giving a bolus or intermittent doses of synthetic GnRH to diagnostically assess pituitary and testicular responsiveness.[13,14] In humans, the GnRH challenge test appears to be of some value in revealing intrinsic differences in acute gonadotroph and Leydig cell stimulation between normal men and men with reproductive disorders.[169-175] When stallions were challenged with repetitive pulses of exogenous GnRH, different pituitary and testicular responses were observed between fertile and subfertile stallions, which appeared to be dependent on season and gonadal status.[10,13] The pituitary and testes of fertile stallions appeared to be more responsive to pulsatile administration of GnRH in the non-breeding season than the breeding season.[10] In contrast, the pituitary responsiveness to repetitive pulses of GnRH in subfertile stallions was significantly reduced during the non-breeding season and was not affected by seasonal changes.[13]

When stallions were subjected to a single dose of GnRH in a subsequent study in the non-breeding season, responsiveness was observed to be normal.[14] In this study, the capacity of the Leydig cells to respond to a discrete dose of GnRH (via endogenous LH) was monitored and shown to be significantly reduced. The results of the studies just mentioned suggest that the low testicular response in subfertile stallions may be due to (1) a dysfunctional hypothalamic-pituitary axis producing bio-inactive LH, or (2) a primary testicular disorder.

HYPOTHALAMIC-PITUITARY DISORDER OR PRIMARY TESTICULAR DISORDER?

As discussed, previous studies have demonstrated that idiopathic subfertility and infertility may be associated with normal to high plasma gonadotropin levels (particularly FSH), a circulating form of a biologically inactive LH isoform, decreased pituitary and testicular responsiveness to GnRH, and low plasma estrogen levels in the presence of normal concentrations of plasma testosterone.[12-14] Although these observations suggest both a pituitary and a testicular dysfunction, it is not apparent which reproductive organ has a primary defect or how one organ might affect the demise of the other. Two studies, however, point to a primary testicular problem. In one study, a group of subfertile stallions had a significantly lower testosterone response to a challenge of hCG (10,000 IU) than did the fertile group.[20] In another study, no significant differences were observed in pituitary function of fertile, subfertile, and infertile stallions 1 year after castration with or without steroid therapy or after GnRH treatment.[23] Taken together, these studies suggest that the original malfunction leading to a decline in fertility may not be at the level of the hypothalamus or pituitary but at the level of the testes.

To further explore testicular function in idiopathic subfertile and infertile stallions, two studies were carried out whereby testicular tissue from fertile, subfertile, and infertile stallions was assessed for LH receptor–binding activity and inhibin concentrations. The first study demonstrated that the number of LH receptors and receptor affinity did not change with fertility status, suggesting that a testicular disorder is most likely present at the post-receptor level.[21] The second study indicated that, in stallions with poor fertility, intra-testicular inhibin concentrations declined early on, before changes in intra-testicular steroid hormones were observed, suggesting that an early paracrine-autocrine dysfunction may occur at the level of the Sertoli cell.[22] If inhibin acts as a paracrine factor influencing Leydig cell steroidogenesis and germ cell function, as suggested in the literature in rat and hamster models,[124,125,127,128] then an increase or decrease in testicular inhibin may directly affect steroid production and eventually spermatogenesis. Other paracrine-autocrine factors have been identified in equine testes such as testosterone, estrogen, transferrin, IGF-1, INSL3, and β-EP, as described previously. Based on studies described herein in mammalian species including the stallion, these factors may be important in modulation of normal steroidogenesis and spermatogenesis as well as potential fertility biomarkers in the male horse.

In conclusion, idiopathic subfertility and infertility in the stallion may involve an initial decline in important testicular factors that are necessary for local interactions among Leydig cells, Sertoli cells, and germ cells (Fig. 2-4).

DIAGNOSTIC INVESTIGATION OF ENDOCRINE-PARACRINE-AUTOCRINE PARAMETERS IN IDIOPATHIC SUBFERTILE AND INFERTILE STALLIONS

If idiopathic subfertility and infertility are most likely associated with a primary testicular disorder, then identifying, isolating, and characterizing the disorder at the testicular level seems the most logical diagnostic approach. Recent evidence demonstrates that a testicular biopsy procedure can be a relatively safe diagnostic tool to identify testicular factors and function.[166,176] Several parameters of the specimens collected by the biopsy procedure can be evaluated (Figs. 2-5 and 2-6). This diagnostic tool and others can be useful in providing veterinarians information on the state and stage of fertility in a breeding stallion. Following

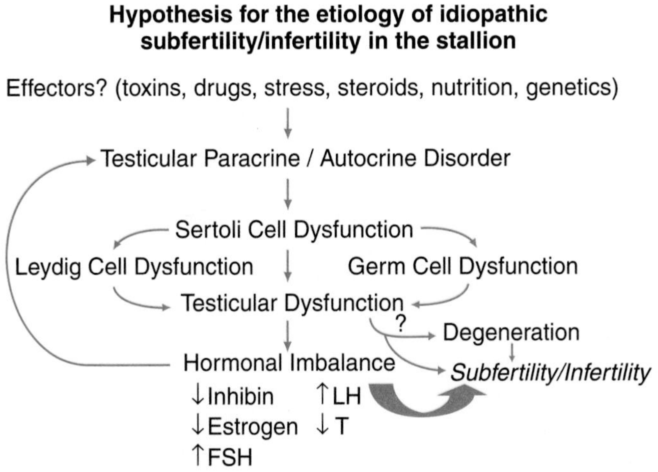

Hypothesis for the etiology of idiopathic subfertility/infertility in the stallion

Effectors? (toxins, drugs, stress, steroids, nutrition, genetics)

Testicular Paracrine / Autocrine Disorder

Sertoli Cell Dysfunction

Leydig Cell Dysfunction   Germ Cell Dysfunction

Testicular Dysfunction

Degeneration

Hormonal Imbalance   Subfertility/Infertility

↓Inhibin   ↑LH
↓Estrogen   ↓T
↑FSH

Figure 2-4. Hypothesis of events that may occur following an initial decline in paracrine-autocrine testicular factors owing to effectors such as toxins, drugs, stress, steroids, and nutritional or genetic abnormalities. *FSH,* Follicle-stimulating hormone; *LH,* luteinizing hormone; *T,* testosterone.

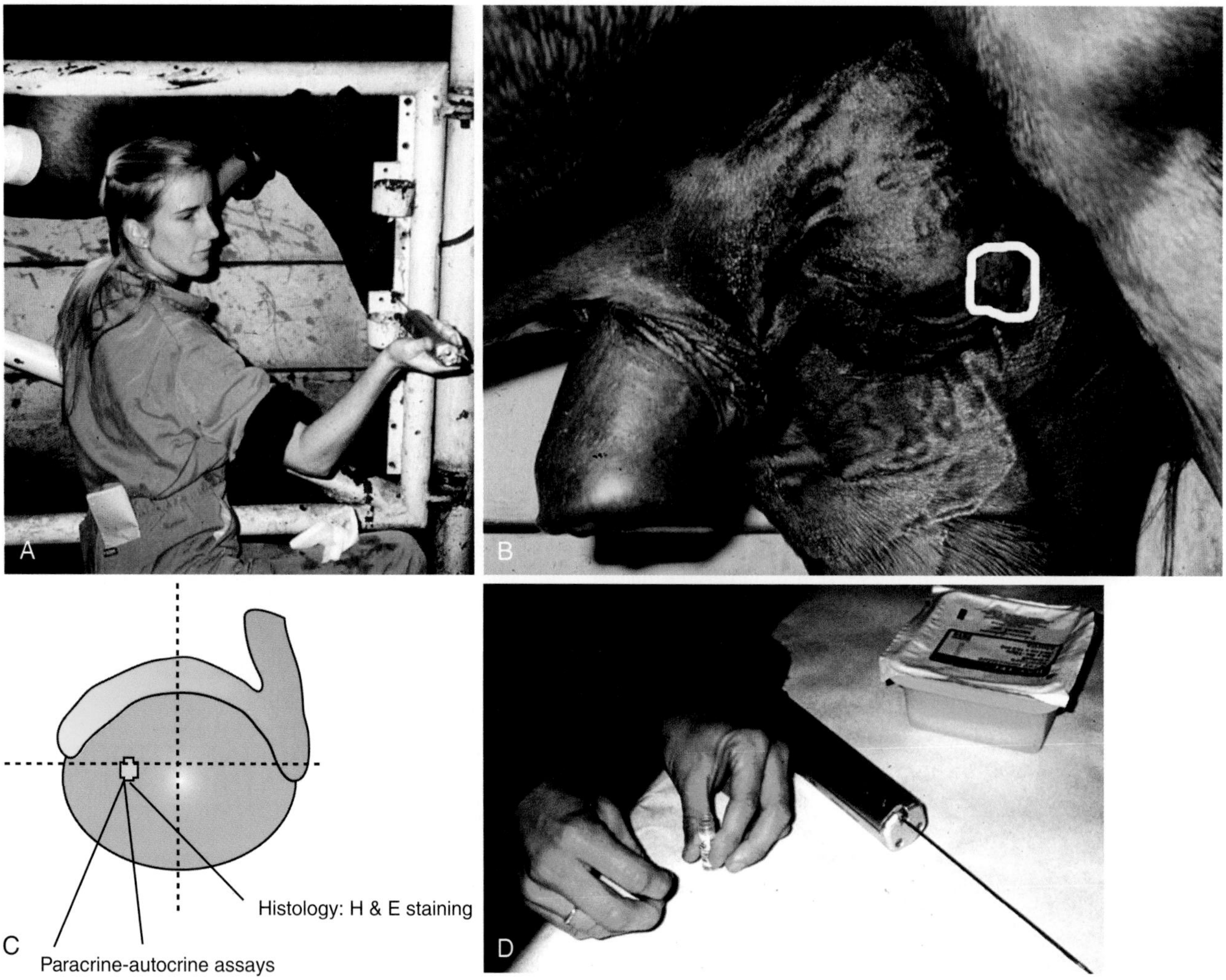

Figure 2-5. A and **B,** Biopsy procedure. Biopsy procedure was performed as a standing procedure in the stocks. Stallions were sedated with detomidine HCl 20–40 μg/kg and butorphanol tartrate at 0.1 mg/kg of body weight. The scrotum was aseptically prepared with iodine scrub. A local subcutaneous anesthesia was applied with 2% lidocaine. A small incision was made in the center of the cranio-lateral quarter of the left testis. Holding the testis down in the scrotum, the practitioner placed a sterile 14-gauge split needle coupled to a spring-loaded Biopty instrument through the incision against the tunica vaginalis. The instrument was fired, and the needle was projected into the testicular parenchyma and then subsequently removed. Two other samples were collected through the same incision but at slightly different angles. **C,** Biopsy sampling and assay procedures. A small incision was made in the center of the cranio-lateral quarter of the left testis. One sample was fixed in Bouin's solution and processed for H&E staining. The other two samples were placed in vials with 1 ml of phosphate buffered saline and frozen at −70°C for future paracrine-autocrine measurements. **D,** Biopsy sample stored in cryostat vial for future paracrine-autocrine assays.

are diagnostic protocols to evaluate endocrine-paracrine and autocrine disorders in the colt or stallion:

1. **Semen evaluation.** This procedure requires two collections obtained 1 hour apart from sexually active stallions. In sexually rested stallions, specimens are collected daily for 7 days and the semen parameters are averaged in the last two ejaculates. Low motility and abnormal morphology are usually observed in subfertile stallions (those with <60% pregnancy rates per season) in the first and second collections. In addition to these abnormalities, infertile stallions (those with 0% pregnancy rates) commonly have a low number of sperm in the ejaculate. Semen can be spun down at 2500 rpm and seminal fluid evaluated for such steroids and proteins as androgens, estrogens, IGF-1, and transferrin.

2. **Testicular biopsy (Fig. 2-5**, *A-F*)**.** This procedure provides a direct measurement of endocrine-paracrine-autocrine factors in testicular tissue.[166,176] Three biopsy punches are obtained using a spring-loaded Biopty instrument attached to a 14-gauge split needle (Biopty Instrument, Bard Inc, Covington, GA) under mild sedation, using a stanchion to secure the stallion. After the scrotum is aseptically prepared with an iodine scrub and blocked using a 2% lidocaine-HCL solution, a small incision is made in the scrotum in the center of the craniolateral quarter of the most affected testis. The Biopty instrument is placed through the incision against the tunica vaginalis, subsequently fired with the needle projecting into the testicular parenchyma, and then removed. Two subsequent samples are collected through the same incision but at slightly different angles. Two punches are each placed in 1.2 mL of phosphate-buffered saline and snap-frozen in dry ice and alcohol or liquid nitrogen and stored frozen until processed for measurement of testicular factors. The third sample is placed in Bouin's solution for 6 hours, transferred to 50% alcohol, and submitted for histological examination.

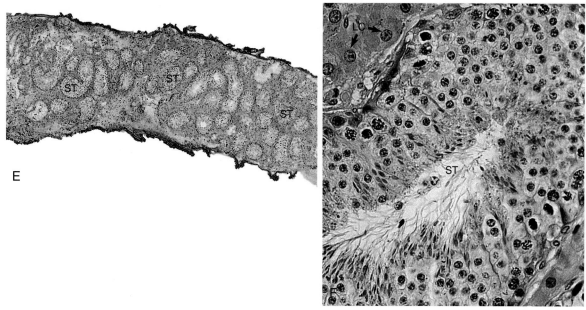

Figure 2-5, cont'd. E and **F,** Histology of biopsy specimens using H&E staining. **E,** At low power, notice staining of many seminiferous tubules *(ST)*. **F,** At high power, single seminiferous tubule *(ST)* with Sertoli and germ cells can be seen. Leydig cells *(LC)* can be seen at the periphery of the tubule.

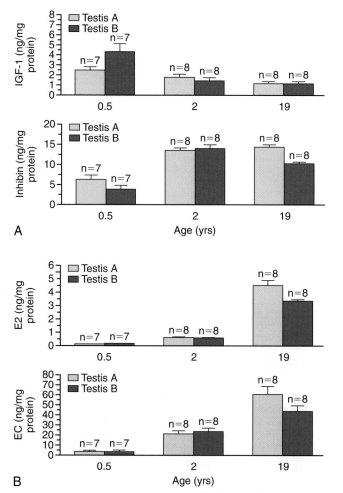

Figure 2-6. Intra-testicular concentrations of insulin-like growth factor-1 *(IGF-1)*, inhibin, estradiol *(E2)*, and estrogen conjugates *(EC)* measured from tissue taken by biopsy punches from the testes of a 6-month-old, a 2-year-old, and a 19-year-old horse. *n,* number of biopsy punches.

3. **Serum or plasma concentrations of FSH, LH, estradiol, inhibin, and testosterone.** Secretion of hormones can be episodic throughout the day, so it is important to get an average baseline. Six venous blood samples are recommended, once every hour on the same day between 10:00 am and 3:00 pm. Alternatively, if only a rough estimate of baseline values is needed, a simpler approach is to take three blood samples, one each day for 3 days taken between 9:00 and 10:00 AM. Usually a 10-ml blood sample is adequate. Either serum or plasma samples can be used. Variations in values can be caused by age, season, laboratory protocols, and fertility status. A stallion with declining fertility usually shows changes in hormone levels in the following order: (1) increasing levels of FSH, (2) decreasing levels of estradiol and inhibin, (3) decreasing levels of LH, and (4) decreasing levels of testosterone. These changes may take a few months or a few years depending on the testicular disorder.

4. **Three-pulse GnRH challenge test.** To assess pituitary responsiveness, a series of small challenges of GnRH are needed. A single challenge is not sufficient to assess pituitary responsiveness in stallions with primary testicular disorder. Three small doses of GnRH, 5 μg/dose, should be given intravenously (IV), 1 hour apart in the non-breeding season starting at 9:00 AM. Blood samples should be obtained every 10 minutes starting at 30 minutes before the first injection, 0–60 minutes after the first injection, 0–60 minutes after the second injection, and 0–60 minutes after the third injection. The entire process should take 210 minutes. Blood samples should be analyzed for LH. Compared with fertile stallions, subfertile stallions have a significantly lower response to the second and third injection of GnRH in the non-breeding season only.[13]

5. **Single-pulse GnRH challenge test.** To assess pituitary and testicular responsiveness, a single dose of 25 μg of GnRH should be given IV at 9:00 AM in the non-breeding season. An abnormal response to a single challenge may help in the diagnosis of a pituitary disorder in stallions with tumors or hypogonadotropic hypogonadism or a testicular disorder in

stallions with testicular dysfunction. Blood samples should be collected 30 minutes before the injection, immediately before the injection, and every 30 minutes after the injection up to 120 minutes. Blood samples should be analyzed for LH and testosterone. Compared with fertile stallions, subfertile stallions have a similar LH response but the testosterone response is lower in the non-breeding season.[14]

6. **hCG challenge.** To assess only testicular responsiveness, a single dose of hCG (10,000 IU) should be given IV at 9:00 AM. This procedure can be performed in either the breeding or non-breeding season. Blood samples should be collected 30 minutes before, immediately before, and every 30 minutes after the injection up to 3 hours after treatment. Blood samples should be analyzed for testosterone. A study on fertile, subfertile, and infertile stallions indicated that only the infertile stallions had a poor testosterone and estradiol response to hCG.[20]

REFERENCES

1. Matsumoto A: Hormonal control of spermatogenesis. In Burger H, de Kretser D, eds: *The Testis.* 2nd ed., New York: Raven Press, 1989, pp 181-196.
2. Amann RP: Physiology and endocrinology. In McKinnon AO, Voss JL, eds: *Equine Reproduction.* Philadelphia: Lea & Febiger, 1993, pp 658-685.
3. Heindel JJ, Treinen KA: Physiology of the male reproductive system: endocrine, paracrine and autocrine regulation. *Toxicol Pathol* 17:411, 1989.
4. Jegou B, Sharpe RM: Paracrine mechanisms in testicular control. In de Kretser D, ed: *Molecular Biology of the Male Reproductive System.* New York: Academic Press, 1993, pp 271-310.
5. Skinner MK: Secretion of growth factors and other regulatory factors. In Russell LD, Griswold MD, eds: *The Sertoli Cell.* Clearwater, FL: Cache River Press, 1993, pp 237-247.
6. Jegou B, Pineau C: Current aspects of autocrine and paracrine regulation of spermatogenesis. In Mukhopadhyay AK, Raizada MK, eds: *Tissue Renin-Angiotensin Systems.* New York: Plenum Press, 1995, pp 67-86.
7. Gnessi L, Fabbri A, Spera G: Gonadal peptides as mediators of development and functional control of the testis: an integrated system with hormones and local environment. *Endocr Rev* 18:541, 1997.
8. Holdcraft RW, Braun RE: Hormonal regulation of spermatogenesis. *Int J Androl* 27:335, 2004.
9. Douglas RH, Umphenour N: Endocrine abnormalities and hormonal therapy. *Vet Clin North Am Equine Pract* 8:237, 1992.
10. Roser JF, Hughes JP: Prolonged pulsatile administration of gonadotropin-releasing hormone (GnRH) to fertile stallions. *J Reprod Fertil Suppl* 44:155, 1991.
11. Seamans MC, Roser JF, Linford RL et al: Gonadotropin and steroid concentrations in jugular and testicular venous plasma in stallions before and after GnRH injection. *J Reprod Fertil Suppl* 44:57, 1991.
12. Whitcomb RW, Schneyer AL, Roser JF, Hughes JP: Circulating antagonist of luteinizing hormone associated with infertility in stallions. *Endocrinology* 128:2497, 1991.
13. Roser JF, Hughes JP: Seasonal effects on seminal quality, plasma hormone concentrations and GnRH-induced LH response in fertile and subfertile stallions. *J Androl* 13:214, 1992.
14. Roser JF, Hughes JP: Dose-response effects of GnRH on gonadotropins and testicular steroids in fertile and subfertile stallions. *J Androl* 13:543, 1992.
15. Muyan M, Roser JF, Dybdal N, Baldwin DM: Modulation of gonadotropin-releasing hormone-stimulated luteinizing hormone release in cultured male equine anterior pituitary cells by gonadal steroids. *Biol Reprod* 49:340, 1993.
16. Roser JF, McCue P, Hoye E: Inhibin activity in the mare and stallion. *Domest Anim Endocrinol* 11:87, 1994.
17. Roser JF, Hughes JP: Use of GnRH in stallions with poor fertility: A review. Proc 40th Annual AAEP Convention. *Vancouver, BC::*23, 1994.
18. Eisenhauer KM, McCue PM, Nayden DK et al: Localization of aromatase in equine Leydig cells. *Domest Anim Endocrinol* 11:291, 1994.
19. Eisenhauer KM, Roser JF: Effects of lipoproteins, eLH, eFSH and ePRL on equine testicular steroidogenesis in vitro. *J Androl* 16:18, 1995.
20. Roser JF: Endocrine profiles in fertile, subfertile and infertile stallions: Testicular response to hCG in infertile stallions. *Biol Reprod Monogr* 1:661, 1995.
21. Motton DD, Roser JF: HCG binding to the testicular LH receptor is similar in fertile, subfertile and infertile stallions. *J Androl* 18:411, 1997.
22. Stewart BL, Roser JF: Effects of age, season and fertility status on plasma and intratesticular immunoreactive (Ir) inhibin concentrations in stallions. *Domest Anim Endocrinol* 15:129, 1998.
23. Roser JF, Tarleton M, Belanger JM: Pituitary response to steroid replacement therapy in fertile, subfertile and infertile stallions after castration. *J Reprod Fertil Suppl* 56:61, 2000.
24. Hess ME, Roser JF: The effects of age, season and fertility status on plasma and intratesticular insulin-like growth factor I concentration in stallions. *Theriogenology* 56:723, 2001.
25. Sharp DC, Cleaver BD: Melatonin. In Mckinnon AO, Voss JL, eds: *Equine Reproduction.* Philadelphia: Lea & Febiger, 1993, pp 100-108.
26. Roser JF: Endocrine diagnostics and therapeutics for the stallion with declining fertility. In Samper JC, Pycock JF, McKinnon AO, eds: *Current Therapy in Equine Reproduction.* St Louis: Saunders Elsevier, 2007, pp 244-251.
27. Malpaux B, Migaud M, Tricoire H, Chemineau P: Biology of mammalian photoperiodism and the critical role of the pineal gland and melatonin. *J Biol Rhythms* 16:336, 2001.
28. Clay CM, Squires EL, Amann RP, Nett TM: Influence of season and artificial photoperiod on stallions: luteinizing hormone, follicle stimulating hormone and testosterone. *J Anim Sci* 66:1246, 1988.
29. Minneman KP, Wurtman RJ: Effects of pineal compounds on mammals. *Life Sci* 17:1189, 1975.
30. Fraschini F, Collu R, Martini L: Mechanisms of inhibitory action of pineal principles on gonadotropin secretion. In Walstenholm GEW, Knight J, eds: *The Pineal Gland.* London: Churchill Livingstone, 1971, pp 259-273.
31. Cleaver BD, Grubaugh WR, Davis SD et al: Effect of constant light exposure on circulating gonadotrophin levels and hypothalamic gonadotrophin-releasing hormone (GnRH) content in the ovariectomized pony mare. *J Reprod Fert Suppl* 44:259, 1991.
32. Argo CM, Cox JE, Gray JL: Effect of oral melatonin treatment on the seasonal physiology of pony stallions. *J Reprod Fert Suppl* 44:115, 1991.
33. Karasek M, Pawlikowski M, Nowakowska-Jankiewicz B et al: Circadian variations in plasma melatonin, FSH, LH, and prolactin and testosterone levels in infertile men. *J Pineal Res* 9:149, 1990.
34. Luboshitzky R, Shen-Orr Z, Ishai A, Lavie P: Melatonin hypersecretion in male patients with adult-onset idiopathic hypogonadotropic hypogonadism. *Exp Clin Endocrinol Diabetes* 108:142, 2000.
35. Luboshitzky R, Shen-Orr Z, Shochat T et al: Melatonin administered in the afternoon decreases next-day luteinizing hormone levels in men: lack of antagonism by flumazenil. *J Mol Neurosci* 12:75, 1999.
36. Irez TO, Senol H, Alagoz M et al: Effects of indoleamines on sperm motility in vitro. *Hum Reprod* 7:987, 1992.
37. Luboshitzky R, Shen-Orr Z, Nave R et al: Melatonin administration alters semen quality in healthy men. *J Androl* 23:572, 2002.
38. Irvine CHG: Gonadotropin-releasing hormone. *J Equine Vet Sci* 3:168, 1983.
39. Irvine CHG, Alexander SL: A novel technique for measuring hypothalamic and pituitary hormone secretion rates from collection of pituitary venous effluent in the normal horse. *J Endocrinol* 113:183, 1987.
40. Griswold MD: Protein secretion by Sertoli cells: general considerations. In Russell LD, Griswold MD, eds: *The Sertoli Cell.* Clearwater, FL: Cache River Press, 1993, pp 195-200.
41. Dean KJ, Roser JF: Inhibin and estradiol production by cultured equine Sertoli cells. *Proc 16th Equine Nutr Physiol Symp*:190-191. Raleigh, NC, 1999, pp 190-191.
42. Bidstrup LA, Dean DJ, Pommer AC, Roser JF: Transferrin production in cultured Sertoli cells during testicular maturation in the stallion. *Biol Reprod Suppl* 66:493, 2002.
43. Roser JF: Endocrine and paracrine control of sperm production in stallions. *Anim Reprod Sci* 68:139, 2001.
44. Jedlinska M, Rozewiecka I, Ziecik AJ: Effect of hypoprolactinaemia and hyperprolactinaemia on LH secretion, endocrine function of testes and structure of seminiferous tubules in boars. *J Reprod Fertil* 103:265, 1995.
45. Regisford EGC, Katz LS: Effects of bromocriptine-induced hyperprolactinaemia on gonadotrophin secretion and testicular function in rams *(Ovis aries)* during two seasons. *J Reprod Fertil* 99:529, 1993.
46. Hondo E, Kuromaru M, Sakai S et al: Prolactin receptor expression in rat spermatogenic cells. *Biol Reprod* 52:284, 1995.

47. Bartke A: Hyperprolactinemia and male reproduction. In Paulson J, Negro-Vilar A, Lucena E, Martini L, eds: *Andrology. Male Fertility and Sterility*. New York: Academic Press, 1986, pp 101-123.

48. Tilbrook AJ, Clarke IJ: Negative feedback regulation of the secretion and actions of gonadotropin-releasing hormone in males. *Biol Reprod* 64:735, 2001.

49. Fink G: The G.W. Harris Lecture. Steroid control of brain and pituitary function. *Q J Exp Physiol* 73:257, 1987.

50. Thompson DL Jr., Pickett BW, Squires EL, Nett TM: Effect of testosterone and estradiol-17β alone and in combination on LH and FSH concentrations in blood serum and pituitary of geldings and in serum after administration of GnRH. *Biol Reprod* 21:1231, 1979.

51. Thompson DL Jr., Honey PG: Active immunization of prepubertal colt against estrogens: hormonal and testicular responses after puberty. *J Anim Sci* 59:189, 1984.

52. Barraclough CA, Wise PM, Turgeon J, et al: Recent studies on the regulation of pituitary LH and FSH secretion. *Biol Reprod* 20:86, 1979.

53. Knobil E: The neuroendocrine control of the menstrual cycle. *Prog Hormone Res* 36:53, 1980.

54. Baldwin DM, Roser JF, Muyan M, et al: Direct effects of free and conjugated steroids on GnRH-stimulated LH release in cultured equine pituitary cells. *J Reprod Fertil Suppl* 44:327, 1991.

55. Vale W, Bilezikjian LM, Rivier C: Reproductive and other roles of inhibins and activins. In Knobil E, Neill JD, eds: *The Physiology of Reproduction*. 2nd ed., New York: Raven Press, 1994, pp 1861-1871.

56. Nagata S, Tsunoda N, Nagamine N, et al: Testicular inhibin in the stallion: cellular source and seasonal changes in its secretion. *Biol Reprod* 59:62, 1998.

57. Loveland KL, Dias V, Meachem S, et al: The transforming growth factor-beta super family in early spermatogenesis: potential relevance to testicular dysgenesis. *Int J Androl* 30:377, 2007.

58. Yamanouchi K, Sugawara Y, Tojo H, Takahashi M: Expression of inhibin/activin subunit genes in reproductive organs of pregnant mare and equine fetus. In Kawashima S, Kikuyama S, eds: *Advances in Comparative Endocrinology I*. Bologna, Italy: Monduzzi Editore, 1997, p 487.

59. Frasor J, Gibori G: Prolactin regulation of estrogen receptor expression. *Trends Endocrinol Metab* 14:118, 2003.

60. Mendis-Handagama C, Ariyaratne S: Prolonged and transient neonatal hypothyroidism on Leydig cell differentiation in the postnatal rat testis. *Arch Androl* 50:347, 2004.

61. Cooke PS, Holsberger DR, Witorsch RJ et al: Thyroid hormone, glucocorticoids, and prolactin at the nexus of physiology, reproduction, and toxicology. *Toxicol Appl Pharmacol* 194:309, 2004.

62. Maran RRM: Thyroid hormones: their role in testicular steroidogenesis. *Arc Androl* 49:375, 2003.

63. Zachman M: Interrelations between growth hormone and sex hormones—physiology and therapeutics consequences. *Horm Res* 38:1-8, 1992.

64. Chandrashekar V, Bartke A: The role of growth hormone in pituitary and testicular function in adult mice. *Biol Reprod Suppl* 58:98, 1998.

65. Spiteri-Grech J, Nieschlag E: The role of growth hormone and insulin-like growth factor I in the regulation of male reproductive function. *Horm Res Suppl* 1:22, 1992.

66. Breier BH, Vickers MH, Gravance CG, Casey PJ: Therapy with growth hormone: major prospects for the treatment of male subfertility?. *Endocrinol J Suppl* 45:53, 1998.

67. Laron Z, Klinger B: Effect of insulin-like growth factor-I treatment on serum androgens and testicular penile size in males with Laron syndrome (primary growth hormone resistance). *Eur J Endocrinol* 138:176, 1998.

68. Kanzaki M, Morris PL: Growth hormone regulates steroidogenic acute regulatory protein expression and steroidogenesis in Leydig cell progenitors. *Endocrinology* 140:1681, 1999.

69. Shoham Z, Conway GS, Ostergaard H et al: Cotreatment with growth hormone for induction of spermatogenesis in patients with hypogonadotropic hypogonadism. *Fertil Steril* 57:1044, 1992.

70. Thompson DL Jr., Johnson L, Wiest JJ: Effects of month and age on prolactin concentrations in stallion serum. *J Reprod Fert Suppl* 35:67, 1987.

71. Johnson AL: Serum concentrations of prolactin, thyroxine and triiodothyronine relative to season and the estrous cycle in the nonpregnant mare. *J Anim Sci* 62:1012, 1986.

72. Meredith TB, Dobrinski I: Thyroid function and pregnancy status in broodmares. *J Am Vet Med Assoc* 224:892, 2004.

73. Aurich JE, Kranski S, Parvizi N: Somatostatin treatment affects testicular function in stallions. *Theriogenology* 60:263, 2003.

74. Hess MF, Roser JF: A comparison of the effects of equine luteinizing hormone (eLH), equine growth hormone (eGH) and human recombinant insulin-like growth factor (hrIGF-I) on steroid production in cultured equine Leydig cells during sexual maturation. *Anim Reprod Sci* 89:7, 2005.

75. Gerlach T, Aurich JE: Regulation of seasonal reproductive activity in the stallion, ram and hamster. *Anim Reprod Sci* 58:197, 2000.

76. Aurich C, Schlote S, Hoppen H-O: Effects of the opioid antagonist naloxone on release of luteinizing hormone in mares during the anovulatory season. *J Endocrinol* 142:139, 1994.

77. Aurich C, Sieme H, Hoppen H: Involvement of endogenous opioids in the regulation of LH and testosterone release in the male horse. *J Reprod Fertil* 102:327, 1994.

78. Pickett BW, Amann RP, McKinnon AO et al: *Management of the Stallion for Maximum Reproductive Efficiency: II. Animal Reproduction Laboratory General Series Bulletin No. 05*. Fort Collins, CO: Colorado State University, 1989.

79. Harris JM, Irvine CHG, Evans MJ: Seasonal changes in serum levels of FSH, LH, testosterone and semen parameters in stallions. *Theriogenology* 19:311, 1983.

80. Thompson DL Jr., Pickett BW, Nett TM: Effect of season and artificial photoperiod on levels of estradiol-17β and estrone in blood serum of stallions. *J Anim Sci* 47:184, 1978.

81. Thompson DL Jr., Johnson L, St George RL, Garza F Jr.: Concentrations of prolactin, luteinizing hormone and follicle stimulating hormone in pituitary and serum of horses: effects of sex, season and reproductive state. *J Anim Sci* 63:854, 1986.

82. Sharp DC, Cleaver BD, Davis SD: Photoperiod. In McKinnon AO, Voss JL, eds: *Equine Reproduction*. Philadelphia: Lea & Febiger, 1993, pp 179-185.

83. Burns PJ, Jawad MJ, Edmundson A et al: Effect of increased photoperiod on hormone concentrations in thoroughbred stallions. *J Reprod Fertil Suppl* 32:103, 1982.

84. Johnson L, Thompson DL Jr.: Age-related and seasonal variation in the Sertoli cell population, daily sperm production and serum concentrations of follicle-stimulating hormone, luteinizing hormone and testosterone in stallions. *Biol Reprod* 29:777, 1983.

85. Clay CM, Clay JN: Endocrine and testicular changes associated with season, artificial photoperiod, and the peri-pubertal period in stallions. *Vet Clin North Am Equine Pract* 8:31, 1992.

86. Sharp DC: Environmental influences on reproduction in horses. *Vet Clin North Am Equine Pract* 2:207, 1980.

87. Pickett BW: Factors affecting sperm production and output. In McKinnon AO, Voss JL, eds: *Equine Reproduction*. Philadelphia: Lea & Febiger, 1993, pp 689-704.

88. Aurich C, Gerlach T, Aurich JE, et al: Dopaminergic and opioidergic regulation of gonadotropin and prolactin release in stallions. *Reprod Domest Anim* 37:335, 2002.

89. Cox JE, Redhead PH, Jawad NMA: The effect of artificial photoperiod at the end of the breeding season on plasma testosterone concentrations in stallions. *Austr Vet J* 65:239, 1988.

90. Spiteri-Grech J, Nieschlag E: Paracrine factors relevant to the regulation of spermatogenesis-a review. *J Reprod Fertil* 98:1, 1993.

91. Le Roy C, Lejeune HA, Chuzel F et al: Autocrine regulation of Leydig cell differentiated functions by insulin-like growth factor I and transforming growth factor beta. *J Steroid Bioch Mol Biol* 69:379, 1999.

92. Hull KL, Harvey S: Growth hormone: a reproductive endocrine-paracrine regulator? *Rev Reprod* 5:175, 2000.

93. Abney TO: The potential role of estrogens in regulating Leydig cell development and function: a review. *Steroids* 64:610, 1999.

94. O'Donnell L, Robertson KM, Jones ME, Simpson ER: Estrogen and spermatogenesis. *Endo Rev* 22:289, 2001.

95. Huhtaniemi I, Toppari J: Endocrine, paracrine and autocrine regulation of testicular steroidogenesis. In Mukhopadhyay AK, Raizada MK, eds: *Tissue Renin-Angiotensin Systems*. New York: Plenum Press, 1995, pp 33-54.

96. Petersen C, Soder O: The Sertoli cell – A hormonal target and 'super' nurse for germ cells that determines testicular size. *Horm Res* 66:153, 2006.

97. Weldt C, Sidis Y, Keutmann H, Schneyer A: Activins, inhibins and follistatins: from endocrinology to signaling. A paradigm for the new millennium. *Exp Biol Med* 227:724, 2002.

98. Huleihel M, Lunenfeld E: Regulation of spermatogenesis by paracrine/autocrine testicular factors. *Asian J Androl* 6:259, 2004.

99. Weinbauer GF, Nieschlag E: Hormonal control of spermatogenesis. In de Kretser D, ed: *Molecular Biology of Male Reproductive System*. New York: Academic Press, 1993, pp 99-142.

100. Russell LD, Alger LE, Nequin LE: Hormonal control of pubertal sper-matogenesis. *Endocrinology* 120:1615, 1987.
101. Zirkin BR, Aawoniyi C, Griswold MD et al: Is FSH required for adult spermatogenesis?. *J Androl* 15:273, 1994.
102. Roberts KP, Zirkin BR: Androgen regulation of spermatogenesis in the rat. *Ann N Y Acad Sci* 637:90, 1991.
103. Sharpe RM: Regulation of spermatogenesis. In Knobil E, Neil JD, eds: *The Physiology of Reproduction.* New York: Raven Press, 1994, pp 1363-1434.
104. Bortolussi M, Zanchetta R, Belvedere P, Colombo L: Sertoli and Leydig cell numbers and gonadotropin receptors in rat testis. *Cell Tiss Res* 260:185, 1990.
105. Hinojosa AM, Bloeser JR, Thomson SR, Watson ED: The effect of a GnRH antagonist on endocrine and seminal parameters in stallions. *Theriogenology* 56:903, 2001.
106. Colon E, Zaman F, Axelson M et al: Insulin-like growth factor-I is an important antiapoptotic factor for rat Leydig cells during postnatal development. *Endocrinology* 148:128, 2007.
107. Ozkurkcugil C, Yardimoglu M, Dalcik H et al: Effect of insulin-like growth factor-1 on apoptosis or rat testicular germ cells induced by testicular torsion. *BJU Int* 93:1094, 2004.
108. Macpherson ML, Simmen RC, Simmen FA et al: Insulin-like growth factor I and insulin-like growth factor binding protein-2 and -5 in equine seminal plasma: association with sperm characteristics and fertility. *Biol Reprod* 67:648, 2002.
109. Sylvester SR, Griswold MD: The testicular iron shuttle: a "nurse" func-tion. *J Androl* 15:381, 1994.
110. Gilmont RR, Senger PL, Sylvester SR, Griswold MD: Seminal transfer-rin and spermatogenic capability in the bull. *Biol Reprod* 43:151, 1990.
111. Sierens JE, Sneddon SF, Collins F et al: Estrogens in testis biology. *Ann N Y Acad Sci* 1061:65-76, 2005.
112. Bilinska B, Wiszniewska B, Kosiniak-Kamysz K et al: Hormonal status of male reproductive system: androgens and estrogens in the testis and epi-didymis. In vivo and in vitro approaches. *Reprod Biol Suppl* 1:43, 2006.
113. Dohle GR, Smit M, Weber RF: Androgens and male fertility. *World J Urol* 21:341, 2003.
114. Kotula M, Tuz R, Frczek B, et al: Immunolocalization of androgen receptors in testicular cells of prepubertal and pubertal pigs. *Folia Histochem Cytobiol* 38:157, 2000.
115. Meng J, Holdcraft RW, Shima JE, et al: Androgens regulate the permeabil-ity of the blood-testis barrier. *Proc Natl Acad Sci USA* 102:16696, 2005.
116. Singh J, O'Neill C, Handelsman DJ: Induction of spermatogenesis by androgens in gonadotropin-deficient (hpg) mice. *Endocrinology* 136:5311, 1995.
117. Xu Q, Lin HY, Yeh SD, et al: Infertility with defective spermatogenesis and steroidogenesis in male mice lacking androgen receptor in Leydig cells. *Endocrine* 32:96, 2007.
118. Hess RA, Carnes K: The role of estrogen in testis and the male repro-ductive tract: a review and species comparison. Anim Reprod 1:5, 2004.
119. Sipahutar H, Sourdaine P, Moslemi S et al: Immunolocalization of aro-matase in stallion Leydig cells and seminiferous tubules. *J Histochem Cytochem* 51:311, 2003.
120. Hess MF, Roser JF: Immunocytochemical localization of cytochrome P450 aromatase in the testis of prepubertal, pubertal and postpubertal horses. *Theriogenology* 61:293, 2004.
121. Clement H, Conley A, Mapes S, Roser J: Immunolocalization of estrogen receptor α, estrogen receptor β, and androgen receptors in the equine testis. *Biol Reprod Proc*:114, 2002.
122. Seamans MC, Roser JF, Linford RL et al: Gonadotrophin and steroid concentrations in jugular and testicular venous plasma in stallions before and after GnRH injection. *J Reprod Fertil Suppl* 44:57, 1991.
123. de Kretser DM, Buzzard JJ, Okuma Y et al: The role of activin, follistatin and inhibin in testicular physiology. *Mol Cell Endocrinol* 225:57, 2004.
124. Hsueh AJ, Dahl KD, Vaughan J, et al: Heterodimers and monodimers of inhibin subunits have different paracrine actions in the modulation of luteinizing hormone-stimulated androgen biosynthesis. *Proc Natl Acad Sci U S A* 84:5082, 1987.
125. Lin T, Calkins JK, Morris PL, et al: Regulation of Leydig cell function in primary culture by inhibin and activin. Endocrinology 125:2134, 1989.
126. Lejeune H, Chuzel F, Sanchez P, et al: Stimulating effect of both human recombinant inhibin A and activin A on immature porcine Leydig cell functions in vitro. Endocrinology 138:4783, 1997.
127. van Dissel-Emiliani FM, Grootenhuis AJ, de Jong FH, de Rooij DG: Inhibin reduces spermatogonial numbers in testes of adult mice and Chinese hamsters. *Endocrinology* 125:1899, 1899.

128. Hakovirta H, Kaipia A, Soder O, Parvinen M: Effects of activin-A, inhibin-A and transforming growth factor-beta 1 on stage specific deoxyribonucleic acid synthesis during rat seminiferous epithelial cycle. *Endocrinology* 133:1664, 1993.
129. Boitani C, Stefanini M, Fragale A, Morena AR: Activin stimulates Sertoli cell proliferation in a defined period of rat testis development. *Endocrinology* 136:5438, 1995.
130. Meehan T, Schlatt S, O'Bryan MK, et al: Regulation of germ cell and Sertoli cell development by activin, follistatin, and FSH. *Dev Biol* 220:225, 2000.
131. Kumanov P, Nandipati K, Tomova A, Agarwal A: Inhibin B is a better marker of spermatogenesis than other hormones in the evaluation of male factor infertility. *Fertil Steril* 86:332, 2006.
132. Ivell R, Bathgate R: The reproductive biology of the relaxin-like factor (RLF/INSL3). *Biol Reprod* 67:699, 2002.
133. Ivell R, Hartung S, Anaud-Ivell R: Insulin-like factor 3: where are we now? *Ann N Y Acad Sci* 1041:486, 2005.
134. Bay K, Hartung S, Ivell R, et al: Insulin-like factor 3 serum levels in 135 normal men and 85 men with testicular disorders: relationship to the luteinizing hormone-testosterone axis. *J Clin Endocrinol Metab* 90:3410, 2005.
135. Balvers M, Spiess AN, Domagalski R, et al: Relaxin-like factor expression as a marker of differentiation in the mouse testis and ovary. *Endocrinology* 139:2960, 1998.
136. Sadeghian H, Anand-Ivell R, Balvers M, et al: Constitutive regulation of the Insl3 gene in rat Leydig cells. *Mol Cell Endocrinol* 124:10, 2005.
137. Ivell R, Balvers M, Anand RJK, et al: Differentiation-dependent expression of 17beta-HSD type 10 in the rodent testis: effect of aging in Leydig cells. *Endocrinology* 144:3130, 2003.
138. Hombach-Klonisch S, Schon J, Kehlen A, et al: Seasonal expression of INSL3 and Lgr8/Insl3 receptor transcripts indicates variable differentia-tion of Leydig cells in the roe deer testis. *Biol Reprod* 71:1079, 2004.
139. Paust HJ, Wessels J, Ivell R, Mukhopadhyay AK: The expression of the RLF/INSL3 gene is reduced in Leydig cells of the aging rat testis. *Exp Gerontol* 37:1461, 2002.
140. Caprio M, Fabbrini E, Ricci G, et al: Ontogenesis of leptin receptor in rat Leydig cells. *Biol Reprod* 68:1199, 2003.
141. Anand RJ, Paust HJ, Altenpohl K, Mukhopadhyay AK: Regulation of vascular endothelial growth factor production by Leydig cells in vitro: the role of protein kinase A and mitogen activated protein kinase cascade. *Biol Reprod* 68:1663, 2003.
142. Nef S, Parada LF: Cryptorchidism in mice mutant for Insl3. *Nat Genet* 22:295, 1999.
143. Zimmermann S, Steding G, Emmen JM, et al: Targeted disruption of the Insl3 gene causes bilateral cryptorchidism. *Mol Endocrinol* 13:681, 1999.
144. Overbeek PA, Gorlov IP, Sutherland RW, et al: A transgenic insertion causing cryptorchidism in mice. *Genesis* 30:26, 2001.
145. Kumagai J, Hsu SY, Matsumi H, et al: INSL3/Leydig Insulin-like peptide activates the LGR8 receptor important in testis descent. *J Biol Chem* 277:31283, 2002.
146. Kawamura K, Kumagai J, Sudo S, et al: Paracrine regulation of mam-malian oocyte maturation and male germ cell survival. *Proc Natl Acad Sci USA* 101:7323, 2004.
147. Klonisch T, Steger K, Kehlen A, et al: INSL3 ligand-receptor system in the equine testis. *Biol Reprod* 68:1975, 2003.
148. Bardin CW, Shaha C, Mather J, et al: Identification and possible func-tion of pro-opiomelanocortin-derived peptides in the testis. *Ann N Y Acad Sci* 438:346, 1984.
149. Soverchia L, Mosconi G, Ruggeri B, et al: Proopiomelanocortin gene expression and β-endorphin localization in the pituitary, testis and epididymis of stallion. *Mol Reprod Dev* 73:1, 2006.
150. Thackare H, Nicholson HD, Whittington K: Oxytocin—its role in male reproduction and new potential therapeutic uses. *Hum Reprod Update* 12:437, 2006.
151. Watson ED, Nikolakopoulos E, Gilbert C, Goode J: Oxytocin in the semen and gonads of the stallion. *Theriogenology* 51:855, 1999.
152. Blanchard TL, Varner DD: Testicular degeneration. In McKinnon AO, Voss JL, eds: *Equine Reproduction.* Philadelphia: Lea & Febiger, 1993, pp 855-860.
153. De Vries PJ: Diseases of the testes, penis, and related structures. In McKinnon AO, Voss JL, eds: *Equine Reproduction.* Philadelphia: Lea & Febiger, 1993, pp 878-884.
154. Pickett BW: Reproductive evaluation of the stallion. In McKinnon AO, Voss JL, eds: *Equine Reproduction.* Philadelphia: Lea & Febiger, 1993, pp 755-768.

155. Pickett BW: Sexual behavior. In McKinnon AO, Voss JL, eds: *Equine Reproduction*. Philadelphia: Lea & Febiger, 1993, pp 809-820.

156. Amann RP: Effects of drugs or toxin on spermatogenesis. In McKinnon AO, Voss JL, eds: *Equine Reproduction*. Philadelphia: Lea & Febiger, 1993, pp 831-839.

157. Burns PJ, Douglas RH: Reproductive hormone concentrations in stallions with breeding problems: case studies. *J Equine Vet Sci* 5:40, 1985.

158. Wallach SJ, Pickett BW, Nett TM: Sexual behavior and serum concentrations of reproductive hormones in impotent stallions. *Theriogenology* 19:833, 1983.

159. Schumacher J, Varner DD: Neoplasia of the stallion's reproductive tract. In McKinnon AO, Voss JL, eds: *Equine Reproduction*. Philadelphia: Lea & Febiger, 1993, pp 871-877.

160. Fabbri A, Ulisse S, Moretti C, et al: Testicular paracrine mechanisms and unexplained infertility. In Spera G, Gnessi L, eds: *Unexplained Infertility: Basic and Clinical Aspects*. New York: Raven Press, 1989, pp 111-120.

161. Dowsett KF: Seminal abnormalities. In Robinson NE, ed: *Current Therapy in Equine Medicine*, 2nd ed. Philadelphia: WB Saunders, 1987, pp 564-566.

162. Brinsko SP: GnRH therapy for subfertile stallions. *Vet Clin North Am Equine Pract* 12:149, 1996.

163. Blue BJ, Pickett BW, Squires EL, et al: Effect of pulsatile or continuous administration of GnRH on reproductive function of stallions. *J Reprod Fertil Suppl* 44:145, 1991.

164. Hintz HF: Feeding the stallion. In McKinnon AO, Voss JL, eds: *Equine Reproduction*. Philadelphia: Lea & Febiger, 1993, pp 840-842.

165. Brinsko SP, Varner DD, Love CC et al: Effect of feeding a DHA-enriched nutraceutical on the quality of fresh, cooled and frozen stallion semen. *Theriogenology* 63:1519, 2005.

166. Faber NF, Roser JF: Testicular biopsy in stallions; diagnostic potential and effects on prospective fertility. *J Reprod Fertil Suppl* 56:31, 2000.

167. Sato K, Miyake M, Tunoda N, et al: Relationship between the semen characteristics and serum testosterone and estrogen levels in three-year-old colts. *Jpn J Zootech Sci* 52:447, 1981.

168. Inoue J, Cerbito WA, Oguri N, et al: Serum levels of testosterone and oestrogens in normal and infertile stallions. *Int J Androl* 16:155, 1993.

169. Marshall JC, Harsoulis P, Anderson DC, et al: Isolated pituitary gonadotrophin deficiency: gonadotrophin secretion after synthetic luteinizing hormone and follicle stimulating hormone-releasing hormone. *BMJ* 4:643, 1972.

170. Bell J, Spitz I, Slonim A, et al: Heterogeneity of gonadotropin response to LHRH in hypogonadotropic hypogonadism. *J Clin Endocrinol Metab* 36:791, 1973.

171. Mortimer CH, Besser GM, McNeilly AS, et al: Luteinizing hormone and follicle stimulating hormone-releasing hormone test in patients with hypothalamic-pituitary-gonadal dysfunction. *BMJ* 4:73, 1973.

172. Mecklenburg RS, Sherins RJ: Gonadotropin response to luteinizing hormone-releasing hormone in men with germinal aplasia. *J Clin Endocrinol Metab* 38:1005, 1974.

173. Turner D, Turner EA, Schwarzstein L, Aparicio NJ: Response of luteinizing hormone and follicle-stimulating hormone to different doses of synthetic luteinizing hormone-releasing hormone by intramuscular administration in normal and oligospermic men: Preliminary report. *Fertil Steril* 26:337, 1975.

174. Bain J, Moskowitz JP, Clapp JJ: LH and FSH response to gonadotropin releasing hormone (GnRH) in normospermic, oligospermic and azoospermic men. *Arch Androl* 1:147, 1978.

175. Dony JMJ, Smals AGH, Rolland R, et al: Differential effect of luteinizing hormone-releasing hormone infusion on testicular steroids in normal men and patients with idiopathic oligospermia. *Fertil Steril* 42:274, 1984.

176. Roser JF, Faber NF: Testicular biopsy. In Samper JC, Pycock JF, McKinnon AO, eds: *Current Therapy in Equine Reproduction*. St Louis: Saunders, 2007, pp 205-211.

SEMEN COLLECTION IN STALLIONS

JOHN P. HURTGEN

Many factors influence libido, mating ability, and semen collection in stallions. These factors may be hereditary, environmental, or learned patterns and are highly influenced by management of the stallion. The efficient collection of high-quality semen is very important in an artificial insemination or semen preservation program. Semen collection is also part of the breeding soundness evaluation of stallions before or after purchase. An integral part of the diagnostic work-up on a stallion with known or suspected infertility is the collection of semen. The collection process itself may in fact be the cause of poor fertility or inferior semen quality.

THE SEMEN COLLECTION AREA

The area used for semen collection should be spacious, dust free, clean, and free of distracting noises, animals, and people. The size of the breeding shed should be designed with safety in mind for both people and animals in case a mount is uncooperative or a stallion is unruly. Stallions with low libido or reluctance to mount are frequently encouraged to mount an estrous mare if the mare can be walked slowly forward or led in a large circle. The well-trained, experienced stallion can be safely handled in a 20-square-foot breeding area, but the novice or unpredictable stallion or mount mare should have an area of at least 30 square feet. In addition, the flooring surface should afford the stallion good traction even when the flooring is wet. Many stallions paw, strike, or kick out while teasing a mare, while being washed, or after dismounting. Loose dirt, stone dust, and shavings should be avoided because some stallions paw debris and dust onto the washed, damp penis just before mounting. If the collection area is dusty, the area should be wetted on a regular basis. The distance from the semen collection area to the laboratory should be minimized.

Collection of semen in an outdoor area is acceptable in most cases but on occasion may be compromised because other animals, people, and vehicles cause distraction. Ambient temperature may also have a marked effect on the rate at which the temperature of the artificial vagina (AV) declines during cold weather periods, or it may have an adverse effect on semen quality during hot weather. Semen collection may need to be halted during storms or rain. Semen collection in an outdoor, grassy area affords the stallion, mare, and handlers the best footing, is usually free of dust, and allows for plenty of space for safety.

METHODS OF SEMEN COLLECTION

Semen can be collected from stallions in four ways: (1) use of a condom, (2) pharmacologically induced ejaculation, (3) use of an AV, or (4) manual manipulation of the penis. Under certain circumstances, it may be necessary to use any one of these methods. However, for routine collection of semen for commercial use, the collection of semen using an AV is the method of choice.

The Condom

Semen collected using the condom method is heavily contaminated by bacteria and debris. This method also requires that a mount mare be in estrus and increases the risk of contamination of the stallion's penis by vaginal entry or urination or defecation during natural breeding. Many stallions do not tolerate breeding while wearing a condom. Condom and semen loss are also common. However, an occasional stallion accustomed to natural service may be intolerant of semen collection with an AV until adequately trained.

Pharmacologically Induced Ejaculation

Numerous schemes have been published for the ex copula ejaculation of stallions using xylazine, imipramine, xylazine and imipramine, and prostaglandin.[1-3] Semen collected in this fashion is of low volume and very high concentration. The resulting ejaculate can be used for cryopreservation or artificial insemination of mares in a cooled semen shipment program. However, the inability to obtain ejaculates on a predictable schedule limits the commercial usefulness of these methods. In experimental ponies, semen was collected in 10 of 24 attempts using imipramine and xylazine.[3]

Under very selected cases of debility in the stallion, it may be possible to obtain semen specimens with the aid of pharmacologic agents.[4] Under farm conditions, semen is obtained in about 25% to 30% of the attempts. It is important that the stallion be kept quiet and undisturbed. Intravenous treatment should be done in a quiet manner. One such successful scheme is to administer 2.0 mg/kg imipramine hydrochloride intravenously. An occasional stallion may appear to hallucinate after the IV use of imipramine. If erection and ejaculation are not induced within 10–15 minutes, xylazine is administered intravenously at the rate of 0.2–0.3 mg/kg. With the use of imipramine and xylazine, ejaculation occurs in association with erection and masturbation.[3] If xylazine is used alone to induce ejaculation, masturbation and erection do not occur in association with ejaculation. Ejaculation usually occurs as the stallion enters or recovers from the period of sedation or sleep.[5] This method of semen collection was used in a cooled, shipped semen program for a stallion with severe tenosynovitis of a rear leg. Although successful about 25% of the time, the procedure was time-consuming and unpredictable for mare owners. Anecdotal evidence suggests that the use of 0.5-ml detomidine hydrochloride (Pfizer Animal Health, NY, NY) IM can induce ex copula ejaculation.

The Artificial Vagina

Semen collection using an AV is the most widely used method of semen collection from stallions. Many models of equine AVs are available. These are fitted with a water jacket that allows for the passive control of the internal temperature of the liner, usually 44° to 48°C. In most cases, the internal diameter of the AV can be modified by the addition of water or air to the water jacket. A lubricant is manually added to the innermost liner of the AV to alter the degree of friction during breeding. Lubricants containing bacteriostatic or spermicidal compounds should not be used to lubricate the AV because these compounds are detrimental to sperm motility.[6] Petroleum jelly (Vaseline) or methylcellulose (H-R Lubricating Jelly, Carter Products, Division of Carter-Wallace, Inc, New York, NY) can be safely used. A recent clinical trial compared the effect of four different "nonspermicidal" lubricants on the longevity of sperm motility.[7] Three of the four lubricants tested were detrimental to sperm motility. The lubricant Pre-Seed (Ing-fertility, Valleyford, WA) did not suppress motility compared with controls. Possible reasons for the detrimental effect of lubricants include hyperosmolarity and unphysiologic pH. Careful selection of lubricant as well as the amount used are important factors in the semen collection process. Most commercially available AVs can be modified to allow the incorporation of a filter into the semen collection system, if desired, so that dirt, debris, and gel can be removed from the semen sample. Otherwise, the entire ejaculate can be filtered after collection, or the gel can be aspirated from the sample using a syringe. Sperm losses during the collection process have been determined with one model of AV.[8,9] Most of the sperm lost during collection is accounted for in the filter and in the gel fraction of semen. Between 25% and 30% of sperm in an ejaculate can be lost in the gel and filter. Polyester filters tend to absorb seminal fluid and therefore reduce sperm recovered in the gel-free ejaculate. Nylon filters do not absorb fluid but allow considerable trapping of sperm in the gel fraction.[10]

Ideally, the AV is constructed to maintain the desired AV temperature for a significant period, to allow the direct ejaculation into the semen receptacle, and to allow for ease of handling and manipulation by the operator. If the AV is large and heavy, the operator may have difficulty positioning the AV for tall stallions, for stallions not trained to the AV, or when the mount mare moves during collection. It is best if the AV can be held in one hand, at the appropriate position, while the other hand is used to deflect the base of the penis to the side of the phantom or mount mare. This is particularly helpful in stallions that thrust with significant force. Deflecting or stabilizing the base of the penis is stimulatory to most stallions and may help prevent preputial hematomas during the collection process.

Semen collection failures are frequently associated with inappropriate AV positioning for the particular stallion, an AV that has dropped in temperature below a "critical" point for the stallion, the phantom mount set too low, and the use of excess pressure in the AV. The AV should be held parallel to the ventral abdomen of the stallion and in direct alignment with the base of the stallion's penis. In this manner, ventral or lateral bending of the penile shaft is avoided.

In certain circumstances, it may seem necessary to elevate the internal temperature of the AV to 50°C for stallions with difficulty ejaculating into the AV. However, an effort should be made to have the horse ejaculate directly into the semen receptacle or coned portion of the AV liner to avoid heat shock to the sperm.

Sperm cells exposed to excess heat from the AV liner exhibit a circling-type motility, have reduced sperm longevity in raw and extended semen, and may be rendered infertile. Exposure of semen to elevated temperatures for as little as 10–20 seconds is sufficient to cause heat shock damage.

Manual Manipulation of the Penis

Ejaculates collected by manual manipulation of the penis are similar to ejaculates collected in an AV.[11,12] This method of collection has not received widespread acceptance because of the training and dexterity required by the person collecting the ejaculate, and many stallions fail to ejaculate unless well trained for this method of collection. A major advantage of this method of collection is that only one or two individuals are necessary for semen collection. The stallion is usually not in direct contact with a tease mare. Specialized equipment or facilities are not necessary for semen collection by the manual stimulation method.

With manual stimulation of the glans penis for semen collection, the stallion remains standing on the ground or is trained to mount a phantom. The horse is teased until erection occurs. The stallion's penis is washed with warm water because this process is also stimulatory to the stallion. The stallion may be trained for collection in his stall, an open barn aisle, or a corner of the breeding shed. An estrous mare is usually nearby, but mare stimulation for the stallion is altered based on stallion response. Once full erection is achieved, a plastic sleeve or bag is placed over the penis. One hand of the operator cups and stimulates the glans penis to achieve favorable thrusting and glans engorgement by the stallion. The opposite hand is used to stimulate the base of the penis and urethra. A very warm towel is sometimes placed at the base of the penis to increase stimulation. Training a stallion for this method of collection may require considerable patience, whereas other stallions readily accept the procedure. Stallions trained for this method of semen collection become habituated to the routine of sights, sounds, and activities surrounding semen collection. These stallions may require very little stimulation by a mare.

SELECTION OF AN ARTIFICIAL VAGINA

All AVs used for semen collection from stallions are basically similar in that they have a water jacket that allows variation in the internal temperature and pressure of the AV liner. The specific characteristics of individual AV types vary in the overall length of the AV, its diameter, ease of filling the water jacket, ease of handling, weight of the AV, and location of ejaculation within the AV by the stallion.[13] Commonly used AV models include the Missouri, Colorado, Hanover, Nishikawa, HarVet, and Polish models.

The Missouri model AV (Nasco, Fort Atkinson, WI, or Veterinary Concepts, Spring Valley, WI) is commonly used in the United States (Fig. 3-1). Many breeding farms with multiple stallions have one of these AVs for each stallion. This model of AV can be readily cleaned. This AV does not need to be assembled for each use because the water jacket is formed by two molded layers of rubber. A single rubber cone leads from the water jacket for attachment of a semen receptacle. The AV is held by a leather case with leather handle. Addition of water or air to the water jacket allows for adjustment in AV temperature and pressure. In most instances, the glans penis of the stallion is

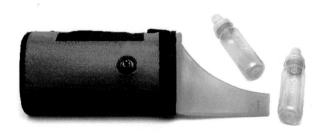

Figure 3-1. Missouri model artificial vagina. (Courtesy of Nasco, Fort Atkinson, WI.)

beyond the warm water jacket at the time of ejaculation, so heat shock damage to sperm is avoided. A plastic bag or baby bottle can be attached to the AV for use as a semen receptacle. A filter can also be incorporated into the semen receptacle.

The Colorado model AV (Animal Reproduction Systems, Chino, CA, or Lane Manufacturing Co, Denver, CO) is substantially longer, larger in diameter, and heavier than other AVs when ready for use (Fig. 3-2). The AV consists of a solid outer plastic casing and is assembled by adding two layers of rubber liners to the casing to form the water jacket. This AV maintains the working temperature for stallions for a significantly longer period. Because of the weight and size of this AV, some operators have difficulty holding it in the most appropriate position for some stallions. A significant shortcoming of the Colorado model AV is that most stallions ejaculate midway along the length of the warm water liner, exposing sperm cells to high temperatures. The operator needs to be extremely cautious when using this AV to avoid heat shock to sperm. Disposable filters and liners are available for the Colorado model AV to remove gel and reduce bacterial contamination from the rubber liners. A disposable but multiple-use variation of the Colorado model AV is shown in Figure 3-3. Shorter versions of the original Colorado AV are also available.

The Hanover model AV (Minitube of America, Verona, WI) is commonly used in Europe (Fig. 3-4). It is shorter and smaller in diameter than the Colorado AV and is made of a hard rubber casing and inner rubber liner. This AV should work well for most stallions. Ejaculation occurs at or near the end of the water jacket.

The Nishikawa (Japanese) model AV is no longer available in the United States, although replacement liners (replacement liners for AV, Lane Manufacturing Co, Denver, CO) are still available. This AV is lightweight and easy to handle, and most stallions ejaculate directly into the semen receptacle. The AV consists of an aluminum casing with a single latex liner. Therefore, a small puncture to the AV liner readily allows water into the semen collection bag. The AV also has a pop-off valve that allows the escape of water under pressure during ejaculation. When using this AV, the pop-off valve opening should be sealed (Fig. 3-5).

The HarVet model AV (Veterinary Concepts, Spring Valley, WI) closely resembles the Nishikawa AV in that it is lightweight and is of similar size with a plastic casing (Fig. 3-6). This AV is designed to be used with disposable AV liners that form a semen receptacle at its distal end, therefore avoiding the water leakage problem of the Nishikawa AV.

The Polish model or open-ended model AV is substantially different from the other models (Fig. 3-7). Using the open-ended AV, the process of ejaculation can be visualized, and individual jets of presperm, sperm-rich, or gel fraction of semen can be collected.[14,15] This AV has been invaluable in the diagnosis of hemospermia, urospermia, internal genital tract infection, and ejaculatory failure. In addition, this AV has been useful in obtaining semen for commercial use from stallions with hemospermia and urospermia, because most affected stallions ejaculate the blood or urine after the initial jets of sperm-rich semen. The open-ended AV has also been useful in a cryopreservation program to obtain sperm-rich and essentially bacteria-free ejaculates from stallions.[14-16] This method of collection can be used to obtain "clean" ejaculates from stallions that are untrained and intolerant of penile cleansing. The Polish AV also allows the use of high internal AV temperatures without risking sperm cell damage because the ejaculate is usually emitted directly into a funnel with an attached receptacle held by a second person.

A commercial source for the open-ended AV is not currently available in the United States. Most open-ended AVs are homemade from plastic or polyvinyl chloride tubing. An open-ended AV can also be made by removing the coned portion of the Missouri model AV and using only the innermost rubber liner to form a water jacket. An open-ended AV can also be made from the Lane or Colorado model AV by shortening its overall length from 60 cm to 40 cm. The internal coned liner is not used when using the shortened Lane or Colorado model AV as an open-ended model.

Sterile, plastic disposable liners have become commercially available for most types of AVs. The purpose of these disposable liners is to reduce the risk of chemical residue exposure of the semen from the AV liner cleaning process. In addition, the disposable liner allows the use of the same AV by multiple stallions. However, many stallions object to these liners, and the number of mounts per ejaculation increases. A 1-mil thickness plastic liner is one to which the stallions will not object. Breakage of the plastic liner may occur during thrusting, and complete eversion of the liner may occur during dismount. If stallions ejaculate on first entry into an AV fitted with a disposable liner, the bacterial contamination of semen is sharply reduced. However, as the number of entries into the AV or the number of thrusts in the AV increases, the bacterial contamination of semen also increases.[16] Additionally increased thrusting and entries into the AV will result in increased bulbourethral gland secretion being collected with the sperm. This presperm fluid is detrimental to the sperm. The AV should be cleaned immediately after use. The AV should be rinsed with volumes of hot water, and dirt, debris, and smegma should be wiped from it. If disposable liners are not used, the rubber liners should be immersed in 70% alcohol for at least 1 hour, rinsed with volumes of hot water, and hung in a dust-free, dry environment. Soaps and disinfectants should not be used on the rubber equipment to avoid accumulation of chemical residue by the rubber. Without the use of disposable AV liners or thorough cleansing of the AV and its liners, the AV may become contaminated by *Pseudomonas, Klebsiella, Escherichia coli, Taylorella equigenitalis,* or other harmful bacteria and in turn may contaminate subsequent semen samples and inoculate the penile surface of the stallion. For these reasons, many farms maintain an individual AV for each stallion at the breeding farm.

SELECTION OF A MOUNT

Semen can be collected from the stallion while he is mounted on a behaviorally estrous mare, phantom mare, or breeding mount or while he is standing on the ground.

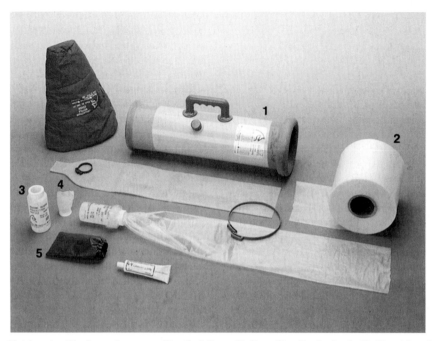

Figure 3-2. Colorado model artificial vagina. The figure shows case *(1)*, roll of disposable liner *(2)*, collection bottle *(3)*, filter *(4)*, and protective cover for bottle *(5)*. (Courtesy of Animal Reproduction Systems, Chino, CA.)

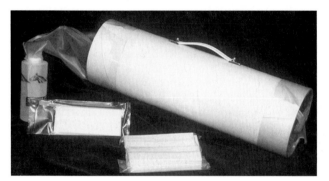

Figure 3-3. Lane disposable model artificial vagina.

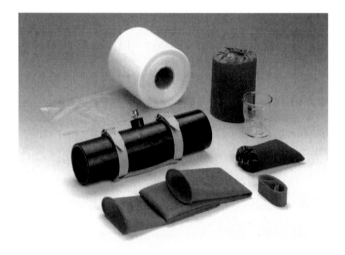

Figure 3-4. Hanover model artificial vagina displaying inner disposable liner and collection glass. (Courtesy of Minitube of America, Verona, WI.)

Estrous Mare

Selection of a suitable mount mare is frequently dependent on the experience and breeding mannerisms of the stallion. For example, the novice, inexperienced stallion may need to be taught to mount the mare from the rear quarters. This requires a disciplined, cooperative mount and one that will tolerate being mounted from the side. Some stallions vocalize loudly in the breeding shed and may frighten maiden or timid mares. The mount mare needs to tolerate a certain amount of nipping and biting of the neck, shoulders, flank region, and hocks to be suitable for some stallions. Mares with foals at their sides are frequently protective of their foals and less cooperative than barren mares. The mount mare should also be an appropriate size match for the stallion.

For routine breeding farm activities, the reliance on an estrous mare as a mount has significant shortcomings. In addition, in a cooled, shipped semen program, the breeding farm may not have access to non-pregnant mares, particularly at the end of the breeding season. Therefore, some breeding farms maintain one or more ovariectomized mares as mount mares. These mares

should be selected as candidates based on their size, tolerant attitude toward handling, and strong estrous behavior signs as intact mares. A mare with gonadal dysgenesis (XO) may be a good mount mare candidate without having to be ovariectomized. Most ovariectomized mares perform well as mount mares while being restrained with a twitch or lip chain placed on the upper gum. In some cases, a low dose of estrogen (2–5 mg estradiol cypionate) may need to be administered at intervals of 3 days to 3 weeks to maintain receptivity by the mare.

During the semen collection process, the mount mare is usually restrained using a twitch. Hobbles applied to the rear pasterns or hocks may also be used, but the novice, untrained stallion may become entangled in the hobbles if the collection procedure does not go as planned. The long hairs at the base of the mount mare's tail should be wrapped to prevent the tail from interfering with deflection and entry of the penis into the AV.

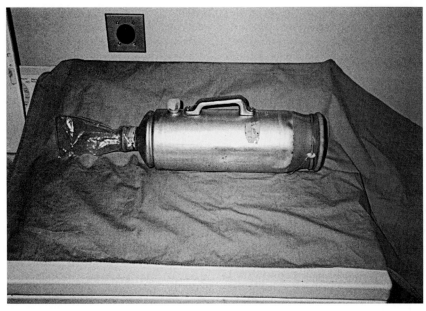

Figure 3-5. Aluminum case or Nishikawa model artificial vagina.

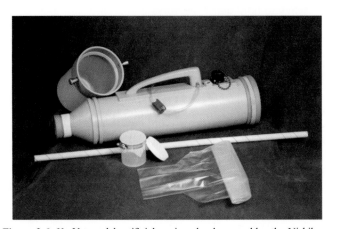

Figure 3-6. HarVet model artificial vagina closely resembles the Nishikawa artificial vagina.

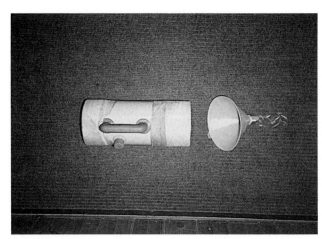

Figure 3-7. Open-ended or Polish model artificial vagina with collection funnel and attached collection bag. This artificial vagina was made by shortening a full-size Colorado artificial vagina.

Phantom Mare

Because of the lack of readily available mount animals, the increased expertise required of an additional horse handler, and the increased safety risks encountered while using a mount mare, many farms prefer to train the breeding stallions to mount a phantom or dummy mare for semen collection (Fig. 3-8). Most stallions, including novice stallions, readily accept the phantom as a mount during semen collection. The working area around the phantom should be dust free and allow good footing by the stallion. Adequate space should surround the phantom for the safety of the handlers and to allow a "tease" mare to be positioned alongside or in front of the phantom. Many stallions are trained to mount the phantom even when the tease mare is not near the phantom.[17]

When collecting semen from a stallion using the phantom, the stallion should approach the mount in a controlled fashion, mount the rear of the phantom, and use his forelegs to stabilize himself by grasping the padded barrel of the mount. The penis should be quickly deflected to the side of the phantom. With the operator on the stallion's left side, the operator's right hand is used to deflect and stabilize the base of the stallion's penis. This practice minimizes potential injury to the penis and prepuce during thrusting by the stallion. Some phantom mounts are fitted with the Lane or Colorado model AV inserted into the posterior diameter of the phantom (Breeding Mount, Equine Breeders Services, Inc, Penrose, CO). Stallions regularly used for live cover breedings are the most difficult to train to accept the phantom as a suitable mount. For this reason, it is necessary in certain circumstances to have access to an estrous mare.

The breeding phantom is usually made of a hollow cylinder with closed ends. The barrel is covered with 1–2 inches of firm padding. The padded cylinder is then covered by a tough, nonabrasive cover that is free of wrinkles. Stallions that repeatedly mount and dismount a phantom abrade the medial aspects of the forelegs and knees. The stallion should be taught to dismount the phantom in a controlled manner by backing off the mount rather than making a side dismount. The diameter of the body of the phantom should be 20–24 inches total. The legs of the

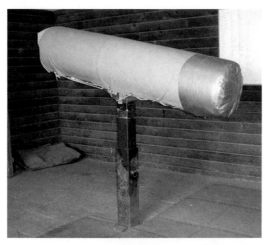

Figure 3-8. Phantom mare or mount used for semen collection from stallions. The mount was handmade and is adjustable for the height and angle of the body. The body of the phantom is set at a slight incline. A rubber mat can be placed on the floor behind and alongside the phantom for cleanliness and cushioning for sore-footed stallions.

phantom should be kept away from the mounting end of the phantom to avoid injury to the stallion's hind legs during breeding and dismount. The mount should be adjustable for height, and the angle of the phantom should be adjustable to accommodate older stallions, stallions with hock problems, and stallions of varying stature.

Ground Collection from the Standing Stallion

The usefulness of semen collection from the standing stallion has become apparent in the past few years, even though this method of collection has been used in selected stallions for nearly 35 years.[17] This technique may be particularly beneficial in stallions with tarsal arthritis, rear fetlock or tendon injury, laminitis, or hind limb weakness associated with the nervous system form of rhinopneumonitis or equine protozoal myelitis. The technique is useful in the normal stallion in that the need for an estrous mare is usually eliminated, risk of injury to the horse by the mare is prevented, and one less handler is needed. This method of semen collection has been most useful on small farms that stand a stallion at stud using a fresh, cooled semen breeding program and that have only two or three mares, which are usually pregnant. At these sport horse and show horse farms, it is difficult to have adequate experienced help for handling mares and stallions for breeding and semen collection.

The stallion is brought to the breeding shed or barn aisle that is free of equipment, or he is left in his stall. The stallion is exposed to an estrous or non-estrous mare or to a gelding sufficient to cause the stallion to achieve an erection. The "tease" animal may be free in a stall or 5–10 m away, being held on a lead shank. The stallion's penis is washed with clear, very warm water. With the stallion positioned against a smooth wall to prevent lateral movement, or with him in front of a solid wall to prevent his forward movement, the warm, lubricated AV is placed on the horse's erect penis. The stallion is encouraged to

search and thrust into the AV. Once the stallion has engaged in the AV, the collection person's right hand is used to stimulate additional urethral pulsations while the AV is held against the stallion's abdomen with the left hand. The stallion handler may help support the stallion by pushing against the stallion's shoulder with the right hand.

Stallions may stand on their hind legs while ejaculating, walk slowly forward while ejaculating, or continue to stand with all four feet on the ground. The handler should not discourage the horse from walking forward or standing up. Once horses are trained in the procedure, they usually stand flat footed with arched back and a head-down posture. At first application of the AV to the standing stallion, a few stallions may kick out or want to nip or bite at the handler. The veterinarian should inform the stallion and mare handlers of how the process works and of the likely responses by the stallion before the initiation of this method of semen collection. After a successful collection, the procedure should be repeated in 1–2 days, preferably in the same location with the same handler and collection person.

At some farms, this method of collection has become the main method for semen collection. The AVs most suited for this method of collection are the Nishikawa, Hanover, HarVet, and Missouri models. The Lane or Colorado models are too large and heavy to hold under the horse during thrusting. For safety, the person collecting semen from the standing stallion should maintain shoulder contact with the stallion.

SEMEN COLLECTION PROCEDURE

Preparation and planning are the keys to the efficient collection of semen from stallions and to ensure proper handling of the semen immediately after collection. The laboratory should be prepared so that the equipment and any extenders used in semen handling after collection are clean and at the desired temperature (35°–37°C). The AV is then assembled and prefilled with warm water (usually at 48°–52°C) because AV equipment quickly decreases the temperature during equilibration.

A suitable area for semen collection is selected. If an estrous mare is to be used as a mount mare, she has been prepared. The mare's tail is wrapped and her perineal area washed to prevent undue contamination of the stallion's penis during mounting. The mare is adequately restrained. At this point, the stallion is brought to the collection area. Once the stallion has achieved full erection, the penis is cleansed with clear, warm water. The urethral diverticula are wiped clean to further reduce bacterial contamination of the semen. The penis is wiped dry, if necessary, using clean, soft toweling.

The final temperature of the AV is adjusted, if necessary, to 45°–48°C for most stallions. The inner liner is lightly lubricated using a non-spermicidal lubricating gel, and the AV pressure is adjusted.

The stallion is presented to the mare's side and is encouraged to mount after achieving a full erection and after the mare has demonstrated her receptivity. For safety reasons, the mare and stallion handlers should be on the same side of the mount mare as the person collecting the stallion. After the stallion has mounted, the erect penis is directed into the AV using the hand placed on the ventral surface of the stallion's penis. This hand continues to stabilize and deflect the base of the stallion's penis during thrusting and ejaculation. The AV should be held to accommodate the stallion. This usually involves holding the AV parallel to the stallion's ventral abdominal wall. Just before the stallion ejaculates, strong urethral pulsations can be felt with the right hand. Once ejaculation begins, the AV should be tilted downward to allow rapid entry of semen into the collection vessel to avoid heat shock to the sperm.

Semen collection from the stallion mounted on a phantom is conducted in the same manner as previously discussed. As soon as the stallion dismounts, the semen is taken to the laboratory for processing and evaluation.[13,18]

Selection of an appropriate estrous mare or a phantom, preparation and restraint of the mount mare, adequate sexual stimulation of the stallion, and selection of an AV to supply proper temperature and pressure desires of the stallion are all required for the efficient collection of high-quality semen. Safety of the animals and handlers is of great importance when working with breeding stallions. Many modifications to the traditional method of semen collection using an AV have been developed and are well suited to a variety of circumstances. For example, the ground collection method of semen collection has become quite commonplace and safe. At some clinics, the open-ended AV is used exclusively to obtain ejaculates free of gel and bacterial contamination.

REFERENCES

1. McDonnell SM: Ejaculation: physiology and dysfunction. *Vet Clin North Am Equine Pract* 8:57-70, 1992.
2. McDonnell SM, Garcia MC, Kenney RM, et al: Imipramine-induced erection, masturbation and ejaculation in male horses. *Pharmacol Biochem Behav* 27:187-191, 1987.
3. McDonnell SM, Odion MJ: Imipramine and xylazine-induced ex copula ejaculation in stallions. *Theriogenology* 41:1005-1010, 1994.
4. Turner RMO, McDonnell SM, Hawkins IF: Use of pharmacologically induced ejaculation to obtain semen from a stallion with a fractured radius. *J Am Vet Med Assoc* 206:1906-1908, 1995.
5. McDonnell SM, Love CC: Xylazine-induced ex copula ejaculation in stallions. *Theriogenology* 36:73-76, 1991.
6. Froman DP, Amann RP: Inhibition of motility of bovine, canine and equine spermatozoa by artificial vagina lubricants. *Theriogenology* 20:357-361, 1983.
7. Samper JC, Garcia A, Burnett K: The effect of different lubricants on longevity of motility and velocity of stallion spermatozoa. *Theriogenology* 68:4196, 2007.
8. Gebauer MR, Pickett BW, Voss J, et al: Reproductive physiology of the stallion. Daily sperm output and testicular measurements. *J Am Vet Med Assoc* 165:711, 1974.
9. Pickett BW, Gebauer MR, Seidel GE, et al: Reproductive physiology of the stallion: spermatozoal losses in the collection equipment and gel. *J Am Vet Med Assoc* 165:708, 1974.
10. Amann RP, Loomis PR, Pickett BW: Improved filter system for an equine artificial vagina. *J Equine Vet Sci* 3:120-125, 1983.
11. Crump J, Crump J: Stallion ejaculation by manual stimulation of the penis. *Theriogenology* 31:341-346, 1988.
12. McDonnell SM, Love CC: Manual stimulation collection of semen from stallions: training time, sexual behavior and semen. *Theriogenology* 33:1201-1210, 1990.
13. Love CC: Semen collection techniques. *Vet Clin North Am Equine Pract* 8:111-128, 1992.
14. Tischner M, Kosiniak K: Techniques for collection and storage of stallion semen with minimal secondary contamination. *Acta Vet Scand Suppl* 88:83-90, 1992.
15. Tischner M, Kosiniak K, Bielanski W: Analysis of the pattern of ejaculation in stallions. *J Reprod Fertil* 41:329-335, 1974.
16. Clement F, Vidament M, Guerin B: Microbial contamination of stallion semen. *Biol Reprod Monogr* 1:779-786, 1995.
17. Kenney RM, Cooper WL: Therapeutic use of a phantom for semen collection from a stallion. *J Am Vet Med Assoc* 165:706-707, 1974.
18. Hurtgen JP: Evaluation of the stallion for breeding soundness. *Vet Clin North Am Equine Pract* 8:149-165, 1992.

STALLION SEXUAL BEHAVIOR

SUE M. MCDONNELL

This chapter reviews normal and abnormal breeding behavior of domestic stallions. Included are practical considerations for routine management of stallions as well as for the retraining of behaviorally challenging stallions.

NORMAL BEHAVIOR OF DOMESTIC STALLIONS

Descriptions of reproductive behavior of equids under free-running conditions are available in a number of resources.[1,2] These can be very instructive toward understanding the basic nature of stallions and how behavior varies under domestic breeding conditions.

Most domestic stallions are handled under halter for live breeding or collection of semen. Compared with the full complement of harem formation and maintenance behaviors typical of a harem stallion under free-running conditions, the behavior of a domestic stallion bred under halter is typically limited to the immediate precopulatory interactions. Key elements of normal stallion behavior are listed in Box 4-1. To the extent allowed, these may include vocalization to the female, limited olfactory and tactile investigation, and flehmen response. Most stallions interact with an estrous mare as soon as allowed, achieve erection within 2 minutes of contact, and are ready to mount a receptive mare or dummy mount within 5–10 seconds after erection is achieved. Copulatory behavior of stallions includes mounting, insertion, thrusting, ejaculation, and dismount. Once mounting occurs, copulatory behavior of halter-bred stallions proceeds similarly to that of free-running stallions of any of the equid species. Most stallions ejaculate after six to eight organized pelvic thrusts. For most stallions on well-managed breeding farms, the entire breeding process, including washing of the penis, is usually accomplished in 1–2 minutes. With consistent good handling and a good stimulus mare, most stallions are remarkably consistent over time in their breeding behavior. Monitoring of the details of a stallion's typical breeding behavior can be useful in early detection of problems. The most useful aspects to monitor include erection latency, number of mounts, thrusts, and palpable ejaculatory pulses. On many farms, live cover breedings or semen collections are videotaped, which provides a valuable record in case behavior problems arise.

Most stallions quickly learn the breeding routine to which they are exposed. They respond to conditioned stimuli associated with the breeding process, and they may breed efficiently with little or no teasing or contact with a mare. Others, still quite normal, may require considerable opportunity to interact with mares to become aroused. Some stallions that are bred under rigid protocols can appear to become "ritual-bound." Any change in breeding routine may appear to disturb their response, usually temporarily. With patience and good handling, most ritual-bound stallions can usually adapt to procedural changes, even after years of a fixed regimen. Once these horses accept a new routine, occasional minor changes in routine can be useful in teaching the horse to be more flexible. In contrast to the ritual-bound stallion, some stallions tend to get "bored" with fixed breeding routines and clearly benefit from reasonable variety in breeding-stimulus mares, breeding location, handlers, and order of procedures. In extreme cases, stallions seem to need something new every few days to sustain their interest.

Starting a Stallion in the Breeding Shed

The handling of stallions for breeding is an art. Box 4-2 summarizes the important characteristics of good stallion handling, as well as common errors. It is also helpful to have a designated breeding area that is out of the way of farm traffic and that has plenty of room for both the animals and the personnel. In many cases of stallion-handling difficulties, human fear of the stallion, in general or specifically during breeding, is the primary challenge to overcome. Schooling for handling tough horses is probably the best way to become an excellent stallion handler, so such a situation is a good opportunity for development.

Almost all stallions are capable of learning the few basics of handling and manipulation required for organized, safe in-hand breeding or semen collection. These include maintaining attention to the handler, taking necessary direction from the handler during teasing, being tolerant of genital manipulation and washing of the penis, waiting for direction from the handler to mount, and maintaining orderly mount and dismount. Behaviors that are unacceptable and unsafe and that can be easily eliminated include biting or kicking of the mare or handler and rushing or charging to mount the mare. All of these goals can be achieved in any stallion with thoughtful arrangement of the breeding situation, positive reinforcement for desirable responses, and judicious direction and correction. Harsh beating, explosive disciplinary sessions, overcorrecting at the head, and jerking and shanking to hold the horse's attention are all unnecessary, usually

Box 4-1	**Normal Behavior of Domestic Stallions**
Immediate interest and interaction with a mare in estrus
Erection within 2 minutes
Mount readiness within 5 to 10 seconds after erection
Ejaculation on first mount
Total breeding time of 2 to 5 minutes

Box 4-2 | **Important Aspects of Good Stallion Handling**

Willingness to work with the stallion in a nonsexual situation to establish mutual respect and to establish working commands to stop, stand, and back

Firm, respectful direction of the sexually aroused stallion; calmly using simple, clear physical or verbal cues

Recognition that vocalization, prancing, arched neck are pre-copulatory behavior to be allowed and celebrated

Use of positive reinforcement with sparse and judicious aversive conditioning; appreciation that punishment is a dangerous teaching tool

Appreciation that stallions vary in the degree of restraint and control required

Provision of ample room to remove a stallion from a situation if things get out of hand

Recognition that much of what is asked of the stallion is natural and much is not

Common errors

Ditzing with the stallion to "hold his attention"
Allowing the stallion to circle
Not allowing the stallion to touch the mare during teasing
Allowing the stallion to charge or leap at the mare for mounting
Overcorrecting rearing
Punishing mounting without erection
Rushing the stallion to dismount after ejaculation
Using delayed or explosive discipline that only delays learning

Box 4-3 | **Specific Procedures for Introducing a Stallion To Washing of the Penis**

The handler of the stallion positions the stallion to stand under control, for example, parallel to a padded wall. The stallion handler stands on the near side almost in front of the stallion, but out of the way of a strike.

The washing technician approaches at the shoulder of the stallion, running the back of the left hand along the neck, shoulder and abdomen of the horse until standing with the left shoulder of the technician touching the side of the stallion. The erect penis is firmly grasped with the left hand midway along the shaft. It is gently directed toward the handler.

If the stallion moves away, the technician should attempt to move with the horse, without flinching or otherwise reacting. The stallion needs to learn two things: (a) The procedure is not going to hurt him (it actually quickly appears pleasant to most stallions), and (b) nothing the stallion does will avoid the procedure. In other words, his movement does not stop the washing of the penis.

If the stallion kicks, explosive punishment should be avoided. Gentle discouragement and continuation of the job so that the stallion gets to know that it can be pleasant and that it leads to the opportunity to breed is usually the best strategy for all but the most dangerously resistant stallions.

If the stallion should thrust forward or the glans penis should flower from the stimulation, no discipline is necessary. Gently deflecting the penis downward toward the back legs naturally reduces the tumescence. Cooler wash water is less likely to stimulate thrusting or flowering. It is useful for most handlers to appreciate that the horse is not misbehaving, just responding positively to this unnatural procedure.

All that is necessary to adequately cleanse the penis is gentle massage along the shaft to loosen flaky debris, with warm water splashed from a cup or towel onto the penis. Up and down stroking motion abrades the surface and is unnecessary.

Some horses resent having hot water splashed on their hind legs or abdomen and scrotum. With experience most technicians can effectively deliver a vigorous splash of water to the penis without hitting the belly or legs.

The glans penis is deflected with the thumb to rinse out the fossa and any smegma "bean."

The base of the penis is an area with heavy smegma accumulation that cannot be effectively cleansed. It is often best left undisturbed.

Care should be exercised to allow water run-off to flow toward the base rather than the glans penis, which was just cleaned.

The penis is dried by wrapping and blotting with a clean cloth or paper towel from glans to base direction. This keeps the glans cleanest. Rubbing abrades the delicate tissues and is unnecessary.

Nondisposable fabrics are generally too abrasive. Air-drying for a minute or two is also adequate.

Common mistakes

Ditzing with the head of the horse during washing of the penis
Startling the stallion by simply grasping the penis without warning
Too light or too rough handling of the penis
Abrading the penis by vigorous rubbing of the shaft
Splashing water on the belly, scrotum, or hind legs
Overreacting each time the horse flinches or lifts a leg, teaching him that he can control human behavior

delaying the learning process. For some stallions, such handling can create serious behavior and libido problems.

Box 4-3 outlines the steps used at our clinic to introduce stallions to washing of the penis. Even for stallions that initially appear most resentful of manipulation, training to tolerate washing can be done safely within a short period (usually two to three 5-minute sessions) using simple positive reinforcement for increasing tolerance. The horse needs to learn as quickly as possible that this procedure does not hurt, that it may even be pleasant, and that avoidance will not interrupt procedure. Safe positioning of the handler and technician so that the work can proceed quickly and so that the technician can stay with the horse through episodes of mild resistance can greatly facilitate the process. Beyond the breeding hygiene reasons, the lessons of waiting for a procedure before breeding as well as tolerating genital manipulation and examination are valuable basic training for a stallion.

Starting a Stallion on a Dummy Mount

Some stallions mount a dummy when initially presented, sometimes even without a mare in the vicinity. So it is worth trying a stallion without a mare just in case he is one of the few who take to the dummy immediately. Other stallions require more stimulation and some training. Except for stallions with seriously inadequate libido or physical disability, almost all stallions can learn to mount a dummy of appropriate design. Some may take several training sessions lasting 10–20 minutes each. Box 4-4 summarizes the key features of dummy mount design, with particular attention to factors affecting behavior.

There is no one correct way to introduce or train a stallion to a dummy mount. The mare and stallion handlers are critical to the success of this training. The best results can be expected

Box 4-4	Key Features of a Breeding Dummy Mount

Single pedestal (safest in event of fall)
Smooth, snug, "cool" cover (to avoid abrasions)
Sturdy, quiet when mounted
Ample head room, front and side clearance (some horses hesitant to mount if too crowded)
Especially secure footing, without a pit worn at the rear
Grasping grooves or "mane"
Angled or level makes little difference for most stallions
Other accoutrements unnecessary
Note: Self-service or adjustable dummies typically do not meet many of these key features. Penis injuries are common with self-service dummies.

Box 4-5	Steps for Training a Stallion to a Dummy Mount

Stimulate the stallion to readiness to mount using a stimulus mare at a distance from the dummy; gently walk the stallion from directly behind the dummy.

Place the mare alongside the dummy and tease across the rear of the dummy.

Allow the stallion to mount the mare for semen collection a few times near the dummy to get the stallion comfortable with breeding in that location, then remove the mare.

Lead the mare with the stallion following/teasing from behind, diverting the mare at the last moment to the side and bumping the stallion's chest into the rear of the dummy.

If the stallion seems ready to mount, but hesitates, stimulate the penis by placing the artificial vagina or warm compresses on the glans while the stallion is teasing.

with positive encouragement and with athletic positioning and movement of the stallion and mare, without frustrating or abusing the stallion. Our usual procedure is to progress through the steps outlined in Box 4-5. Each is tried several times before going to the next. Once the stallion has successfully mounted and ejaculated on the dummy a few times, the mare or other special procedures used during training may be gradually eliminated.

Pasture Breeding

Most domestic stallions also can easily adapt to pasture breeding. Stallions that are turned out to pasture with mares, even after years of in-hand breeding or semen collection, usually immediately perform all of the harem formation and maintenance behaviors typical of wild equids. Also, stallions that have been pasture-bred for years usually readily adapt to breeding under halter or to semen collection. There are some special concerns for pasture breeding. It is best to have ample space and safe facilities, including good footing, to accommodate some expected commotion, especially when the animals are first introduced. If a group of mares are to be bred at pasture, it is best if all are co-mingled as a band before or at the time the stallion is first introduced. Sometimes the stallion and more often the mares of an established band tend to reject mares that are later added. Care must be taken to control the stallion when removing a mare, since most stallions will attempt to keep the mare. If mares are removed temporarily, they may be rejected when returned. Breeding injuries may not be any more frequent than for hand breeding and tend to go unnoticed, and mares may suffer complications at pasture.

FACTORS AFFECTING STALLION BEHAVIOR

Season and Hormones

Reproductive hormones of the stallion show a seasonal pattern consistent with reduced reproductive function during fall and winter. Whereas most stallions show sexual interest and respond adequately during fall and winter, most breeding stallions display a measurable decrease in sexual behavior vigor and endurance during fall and winter compared with the spring and summer natural breeding season months.

Stimulus Mare

Most stallions respond adequately to any mare in estrus. Others show clear preferences for a particular mare or type of mare. Clinical observations suggest that mare characteristics such as color, size, breed, age, lactation status, and days from ovulation may affect sexual interest and response of certain stallions. An important mare factor that is often overlooked in artificial insemination programs is that almost all stallions respond more vigorously to stimulus mares in natural estrus than to ovariectomized stimulus mares or to a dummy mount. It is also interesting and not widely appreciated that almost all stallions respond more vigorously when provided with more than one stimulus mare. Occasionally, a stallion does not respond adequately unless provided two or more estrous mares from which to "choose."

Sociosexual Environment

Evidence is accumulating that reproductive physiology of stallions includes mechanisms for modulation by social conditions.[2] In semi-feral herds, bachelor or harem social status influences a stallion's reproductive hormones. Bachelor stallions have low levels of plasma testosterone; their aggressive behavior is of a playful, sparring nature; and they form close affiliative relationships among males. Harem stallions have higher levels of testosterone, their intermale aggressive behavior is of the serious type, and they generally repel any mature male intruders. When a stallion becomes a harem stallion, testosterone levels rise and remain higher than when a bachelor. If a stallion loses his harem, his testosterone decreases to bachelor levels. These effects of transition can occur at any time of the year.

Evidence is also accumulating that effects of sociosexual environment seem to be similarly operational in domestically managed stallions.[3] In brief, housing conditions, whether with other stallions or as the only stallion with other mares, appear to simulate the bachelor and harem social conditions. Access to teasing and breeding also seems to be a positive influence on testosterone levels of stallions.

General Management and Handling

Management and handling of stallions vary considerably throughout the horse-breeding industry. In general, stallions are flexible in adjusting to a variety of management and breeding practices. As with general health and semen production, for most stallions there is a tangible benefit to ample exercise, adequate exposure to natural light, and firm but judicious and consistent handling. For all stallions, breeding vigor is affected by frequency of breeding and teasing frequency. However, there is wide variation among stallions in breeding frequency, which maintains optimal libido and copulatory efficiency. Some stallions can maintain adequate libido at the rate of one to three ejaculations per day, 7 days a week. In some, problems develop if they are bred more than three to five times weekly.

STALLION BEHAVIOR PROBLEMS

The most common problems related to stallion behavior can be categorized as breeding behavior problems, behavior issues and problems of performance stallions, and residual stallion-like behavior in geldings.

The Breeding Stallion

Inadequate Sexual Interest and Arousal (Libido)

Specific stallion libido problems include slow starting novices, slow or sour-experienced stallions, and specific aversions or preferences.[1] Most of these problems are man-made. Stallions that have been disciplined for showing sexual interest in mares during their performance career are discouraged from showing spontaneous erection and masturbation, or those that are mishandled during breeding under halter, often experience a difficult transition to a breeding career. When exposed to a mare for teasing, such a stallion may simply stand quietly, appear anxious and confused, or even savage the mare. Most stallions with such experience-related libido problems respond well to behavior therapy alone or in combination with anxiolytic medication. These stallions typically respond best to continued exposure to mares, initially with minimal human presence, and then with gradual introduction of quiet, respectful, patient, positive reinforcement–based handling. These stallions appear to respond favorably to reassurance for even small increments of improvement. Tolerance of minor misbehavior, rather than punishment, is often a rewarding strategy. The anxiolytic drug diazepam (0.05 mg/kg slow intravenous [IV] 5–7 minutes before breeding) is useful in about half of such cases as an adjunct to behavior modification.

Some libido problems are hormone related and can improve with management aimed at increasing exposure to mares and reduced exposure to other stallions. This typically increases androgen levels and general confidence, as well as sexual interest and arousal.[3,4]

Specific Erection Dysfunction

Libido-independent erection dysfunction is rare in stallions. The majority of erection dysfunction that does occur is related to traumatic damage of the corpora cavernosa. Common causes include stallion ring injuries, drug-related paralyzed penis and paraphimosis, kick injuries, and other breeding accidents. A considerable number of such accidents involve "self-serve" dummy mounts and thermometers left in the lumens of artificial vaginas.

An interesting and often confusing type of erection dysfunction involves the folding back of the penis within the prepuce. The behavioral hallmark of this situation is a stallion that appears aroused and ready to mount, without a visible erection. The stallion may also appear uncomfortable or intermittently distracted, pinning the ears, kicking toward the abdomen, or stepping gingerly on the hind legs. Close visualization reveals a rounded, full-appearing prepuce, with the skin stretched taut. Resolution usually requires removing the stallion from the mare until the penis detumesces. Once the penis is fully withdrawn, application of a lubricating cream to the prepuce facilitates subsequent normal protrusion. This situation tends to repeat occasionally with particular stallions. We have observed this condition repeating in stallions with particularly profuse smegma production, as well as in stallions in which the penis and sheath is fully cleansed one or more times daily for breeding. The tendency for the penis to fold back on itself within the prepuce may be related to having too much or too little smegma lubrication.

Mounting and Thrusting Problems

Many breeding behavior problems, particularly ejaculatory dysfunction, appear to involve neurological or musculoskeletal problems that affect the stallion's ability to mount and thrust. Many such stallions can continue breeding with therapy aimed at reducing discomfort and accommodating disabilities during breeding, including adjustments to the breeding schedule aimed at reducing the total amount of work. We have found that long-term treatment with oral phenylbutazone (2–4 mg/kg orally twice daily) often works well to keep such stallions comfortable for breeding.

Specific Ejaculation Dysfunction

Whereas any libido, erection, or mounting and thrusting problem can result in failure to ejaculate, there are also stallions in which the dysfunction seems to be specific to ejaculation. Specific ejaculation problems can include apparent failure of the neural ejaculatory apparatus, physical or psychological pain associated with ejaculation, and genital tract pathology.[5,6] A variety of management changes and pharmacological aids that can enhance ejaculatory function in such instances are outlined in Box 4-6.

Rowdy Breeding Stallions

Rowdy, misbehaved breeding stallions in most cases represent a human–animal interaction problem. Most can be overcome with judicious, skillful, respectful training.[7] As with dogs, the rare exception of even the most misbehaved, mishandled stallion can become retrained in 1 or 2 hours total training time. As with the training of pets, the handler typically needs more actual training time than the animal. Successful modification of unruly behavior of a breeding stallion holds the special challenge of eliminating undesirable behaviors without suppressing normal sexual behavior. A common misunderstanding of handlers is that vocalization, prancing gait, and normal sexual enthusiasm should be discouraged. Simple handler education (e.g., that vocalization is not particularly associated with dangerous or undesirable behavior) can be productive. Some handlers benefit from systematic desensitization to the shrill sexual call of stallions. This can be done using audiotapes or videotapes of breeding or teasing of a vocal stallion that is being handled by an expert stallion handler.

Even the most strong, vigorous, and misbehaved breeding stallion can be retrained using simple positive and negative reinforcement, with very little or no punishment. It can be done in a safe and systematic manner without abuse or commotion, usually within a few brief sessions. Some of the most challenging stallions may benefit from initially being allowed several

Box 4-6 | Management and Pharmacologic Aids to Facilitate Ejaculation

Management Aids

To Enhance Sexual Arousal

Prolonged teasing under conditions that yield the highest safe level of arousal

Breeding schedule for maximum arousal

Natural estrus stimulus and mount mares

Stable (no side-to-side movement) mount mare, or dummy necessary

Minimal distractions in the breeding area

Established breeding routine rich with conditioned stimuli for maximum arousal

Encouragement and positive reinforcement

To Reduce Back and Hind Limb Pain and Accommodate Musculoskeletal Deficiencies

Mount mare or dummy of appropriate height and conformation

Mare or dummy down-grade from stallion to reduce weight on hind limbs

Semen collection on the ground (artificial vagina or manual stimulation)

Weight loss to reduce work of hind limbs, particularly during breeding

Pain treatment

Lateral support at the hips during mount

Good footing (grass or dry athletic surface)

To Increase Positive Stimulation of the Penis

Pressure and temperature of artificial vagina that yields best response

Hot compresses applied to the base of the penis

Pharmacologic Aids

To Enhance Sexual Arousal

GnRH: 50µ Cystorelin SC 1 and 2 hours before breeding

Diazepam: 0.05 mg/kg slow IV

To Lower Ejaculatory Threshold

Imipramine: 500–1000 mg orally in grain

To Induce Ejaculation

Xylazine: 0.66 mg/kg IV

Imipramine: 2.2 mg/kg IV

Prostaglandin F 2α, 0.01 mg/kg IM

GnRH, Gonadotropin-releasing hormone; *SC*, subcutaneously; *IV*, intravenously; *IM*, intramuscularly.

breedings in rapid succession. With reduced urgency to breed, it may be easier to maintain the stallion's attention for teaching the breeding shed procedures and manners. Our clinical approach to systematic behavior modification of unruly stallions and example case reports from our clinic have been detailed elsewhere.[7]

Frenzied Stallions

Distinct from simple rowdiness, some stallions, like some mares or geldings, are hyperactive or even "frenzied." Reproductive hormones may or may not be a factor. Important factors are genetics, experience, sociosexual environment, housing, diet, and exercise. Most of these stallions can benefit from more roughage and less grain in the diet, organized and pasture exercise, and

consistent housing in a quiet area. L-tryptophan supplementation (1–2 gm twice daily in feed) can have a calming effect on such stallions.

THE PERFORMING STALLION

Stud-Like Behavior During Training or Performance

Despite the strong male sex drive of most stallions, their sexual and aggressive behavior is remarkably amenable to control during performance situations with simple behavior modification. Consistent, firm, judicious, and skillful training is typically all that is necessary even for the most energetic and strong-willed stallions. The principles for stallion training are similar to those of any animal training; however, the size and strength of the stallion necessitate a higher skill level of the trainer. Even though physical size and strength in the trainer may be helpful, they are not necessary for handling and training stallions. Unlike with the rowdy breeding stallion, behavior problems of performance stallions are usually addressed to trainers rather than to veterinarians. The veterinarian may become involved when asked to provide pharmacological aids to managing rowdy performance stallions or to provide advice on effectiveness of castration. Progesterone is also used to help quiet sexual drive in stallions. Certainly tranquilizers, both long- and short-acting, are used widely in the show and racing industries. However, medication without good handling and training is rarely satisfactory in controlling stallion behavior.

Most rowdy performing stallions can also benefit from the opportunity to breed. Providing clear signals distinguishing breeding time and performing time can help most stallions learn and abide the difference.

Combining Breeding and Performing

With the wide acceptance of cooled-shipped semen and the growth of the hunter-jumper segment of the horse industry, more people are considering breeding a stallion while he is still performing. Opinions vary among owners and trainers concerning whether stallions should combine breeding and performance careers. A commonly expressed concern is that a stallion will lose interest in performance or become more difficult to handle once he has had breeding experience. Another commonly expressed concern is that the physical demands of mounting and breeding can adversely affect high-level dressage or jumping performance. Also, some breeding farm managers believe that performance demands will limit a stallion's fertility. On the other hand, some trainers believe that stallions become more poised and manageable, both for breeding and for performance, when the two careers are combined. None of these beliefs have been scientifically tested. Examples of all of these outcomes can be found. Important factors include individual stallion variation, the level and demands of each career, and, most importantly, the attitudes and expectations of owners, trainers, and breeding managers. With a positive attitude, a good understanding of a few behavior and reproductive management principles, and reasonable organization, the outcome is typically excellent.

Residual Stallion-Like Behavior in Geldings

Castration, regardless of the age or previous sexual experience, does not always eliminate stallion-like behavior in horses. If given the opportunity, as many as half of geldings will show stallion-like behavior to mares; many will herd mares and even mount and appear to breed. Similarly, even though castration does tend to "mellow" most horses, it does not eliminate general misbehavior. Traditional behavior modification is usually much more effective in controlling sexual and aggressive behavior in a gelding under saddle or in-hand than it is with an intact stallion.

Also, treatment aimed at quieting sexual and aggressive behavior, such as progesterone treatment, is typically more effective in geldings than in intact stallions.

REFERENCES

1. McDonnell SM: Normal and abnormal sexual behavior. *Vet Clin North Am Equine Pract* 8:71-89, 1992.
2. McDonnell SM: The Equid Ethogram: a practical field guide to horse behavior. Lexington KY: Eclipse Press, 2003. The Equid Ethogram video companion DVD available at www.HorseBehaviorDVD.com.
3. McDonnell SM, Murray SC: Bachelor and harem stallion behavior and endocrinology. *Biol Reprod Monogr* 1:577, 1995.
4. McDonnell SM: Stallion behavior and endocrinology. What do we really know? Proc 41st Annual AAEP Convention, Lexington, KY: 1995.
5. McDonnell SM: Ejaculation: physiology and dysfunction. *Vet Clin North Am Equine Pract* 8:57-70, 1992.
6. Martin BB, McDonnell SM, Love CC: Effects of musculoskeletal and neurologic diseases on breeding performance in stallions. *Compend Contin Educ Pract Vet* 20:1159, 1998.
7. McDonnell SM, Diehl NK, Oristaglio Turner RM: Modification of unruly breeding behavior in stallions. *Compend Contin Educ* 17(3):411, 1994.

Sperm Physiology

Chapter 5

Stuart A. Meyers

SPERMATOGENESIS

Spermatogenesis is the process of sperm production by the seminiferous epithelium during which spermatogonial stem cells generate spermatocytes, which differentiate, multiply, and generate spermatozoa. This occurs within the seminiferous tubules, which are the major constituent of the testicular parenchyma in the stallion's testis. Seminiferous tubules comprise a myoid cell layer surrounding the basal lamina, which surrounds a complex of somatic and germ cells. The Sertoli cell is a somatic cell that serves a structurally and physiologically supportive role to each successive generation of germ cells. Each sperm cell and its precursors are physically embedded between or in contact with the Sertoli cells such that each Sertoli cell contacts a large number of germ cells at various stages of development. Sertoli cells are spaced along the tubule, and specialized tight junctional complexes between neighboring Sertoli cells form the epithelial portion of the blood-testis barrier. This provides isolation of the diploid spermatogonia and preleptotene spermatocytes from subsequent haploid postmeiotic spermatocyte cell types, spermatids, and the released spermatozoa.[1] The final product of spermatogenesis, the spermatozoon, is the last of numerous successive cellular generations that result from a repeatable sequence of developmental events within the tubule. The culmination of the process is the release from Sertoli cells of spermatids into the lumen of the convoluted portion of the seminiferous tubules and subsequent passage of the spermatozoa into the straight portion of the tubules, tubuli efferentes, and caput epididymis.

Spermatogenesis consists of three developmental phases: (1) spermatocytogenesis (mitotic divisions of spermatogonia), (2) meiosis, and (3) spermiogenesis (maturation and differentiation of spermatids). Amann[9] indicated that the three phases correspond to durations of approximately 19.4, 19.4, and 18.6 days, respectively, leading to a total duration of spermatogenesis in stallions of approximately 57–58 days.

Beginning with spermatocytogenesis, the A_1-type spermatogonia divide mitotically to (1) produce daughter cells that are committed to completion of spermatogenesis and (2) repopulate the uncommitted stem cell population (A_o) to maintain a progenitor population capable of continuing the spermatogenic cell lineage. The latter is localized to the seminiferous epithelium nearest the basement membrane (Fig. 5-1). The A_1 spermatogonia mitotically divide at regular intervals to enter spermatogenic cell development (approximately every 12.2 days), differentiating into at least five subtypes (A_{1-3}, B_1, B_2) prior to the appearance of preleptotene primary spermatocytes,[3] which undergo the first meiotic division. The spherical secondary spermatocytes resulting from completion of meiosis then undergo morphologic differentiation. The resulting spermatids have a characteristic elongated cellular shape, condensed nucleus, and axoneme for motility. Each generation of spermatogonia and spermatocytes is intimately linked by intercytoplasmic bridges and undergoes synchronous cellular division and differentiation. Consequently, the cells advance toward the seminiferous epithelial lumen and away from the basement membrane with each successive cell division. This culminates in the synchronous release of each generation of spermatids into the tubular lumen in the process known as spermiation, which occurs at approximately 12.2-day intervals, coinciding with the entry of A_1 spermatogonia into the cellular differentiation process.[3]

Cross-sections of equine seminiferous tubules have revealed eight consistent cellular associations, or stages, of spermatogenesis, which account for essentially all of the developmental stages during spermatogenesis. Thus, in a given section of seminiferous tubule, each time all eight stages are completed in sequence, spermatozoa have been released into the seminiferous tubular lumen. This is known as the cycle of the seminiferous epithelium and has been described in detail for the stallion.[3-5]

Seasonal variations in numbers of spermatogonia, spermatocytes, and daily production of sperm have been described.[4,5] Moreover, seasonal and age-related changes in Sertoli cells and Leydig cells may also contribute to variations in sperm production. Testicular parenchymal volume has been associated with sperm production such that, in most species studied, spermatogenic efficiency may be measured. For mature stallions, approximately $18–20 \times 10^6$ sperm per gram of testicular parenchyma has been estimated to be the daily production of sperm.[6]

SPERM TRANSPORT IN THE STALLION

As sperm are produced by the seminiferous tubules and released into the tubular lumen following spermiation, they are passively transported into the rete testis. This area is an extensively branched, centrally located storage reservoir for sperm and rete testis fluid. Both ends of each seminiferous tubule empty into the rete. The rete testis fuses with the 10–20 efferent tubules (vasa efferentia), which, in turn, fuse with the epididymal duct at the origin of the caput epididymis. The efferent tubules become progressively more convoluted as they reach the caput epididymis and merge into a single epididymal duct in which the sperm are received.[7]

The Epididymis

For purposes of description, the epididymis has been divided arbitrarily into three major anatomic regions with indiscreet borders: (1) caput (head), (2) corpus (body), and (3) cauda (tail); however,

47

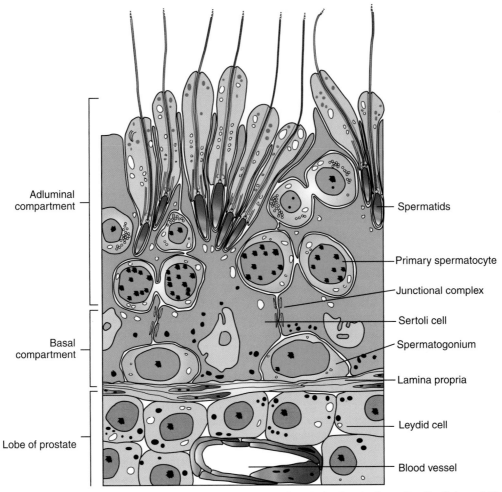

Adluminal compartment

Basal compartment

Lobe of prostate

Spermatids

Primary spermatocyte

Junctional complex

Sertoli cell

Spermatogonium

Lamina propria

Leydid cell

Blood vessel

Figure 5-1. Drawing of a section of a stallion seminiferous tubule showing the relationship of germinal cells and adjacent Sertoli cells in seminiferous epithelium. Spermatogonia, primary spermatocytes, secondary spermatocytes, and spheric spermatids all develop in the space between two or more Sertoli cells and are in contact with them. Primary spermatocytes are moved by the Sertoli cells from the basal compartment through the junctional complexes and into the adluminal compartment. During elongation of spermatids, they are repositioned by the Sertoli cells to become embedded within long pockets in cytoplasm of individual Sertoli cells. Note the intercellular bridges between adjacent germinal cells in the same cohort or generation. (From Pickett BV, Amann RP, McKinnon AO, et al: Management of the Stallion for Maximum Reproductive Efficiency. II. Animal Reproduction Laboratory Bulletin No. 05. Fort Collins: Colorado State University, 1989.)

several additional functionally distinct regions, or zones, have been described.[2,8] Additional sperm maturation occurs during epididymal transit, evidenced by the knowledge that caput epididymal sperm are incapable of fertilization and demonstrate little or no motility, whereas those residing in and leaving the cauda epididymis are fully fertile for most species studied. The latter also display a percentage of progressively motile sperm that is similar to that of ejaculated sperm.[2,8]

In the caput, the secretions of the epididymal epithelium essentially replace the rete testis fluid that accompanies the entering sperm and that is absorbed by the epididymal epithelium. Additional changes in epididymal fluid character occur as the sperm progress caudally through the epididymis. Changes in membrane phospholipids, proteins, and carbohydrates have been described in various regions of the epididymis.[9] Sperm movement through the epididymis is thought to be independent of sperm motility factors and is more reliant on epididymal epithelial factors such as luminal ciliary activity and smooth muscular activity from the epididymal duct wall.[10] This wall has a well-developed smooth muscle component

that becomes progressively more prominent caudally along the length of the duct. The cauda epididymis is richly innervated by sympathetic neurons associated with smooth muscle cells.[10] By contrast, the caput has sympathetic neurons but the nerve terminals are fewer and more likely to be associated with the microvasculature. It has been suggested that sperm passage from the caput to corpus epididymis takes approximately 4.1 days; however, transit time through the cauda is not known with certainty for the stallion because frequency of ejaculation modifies such transit.[11] Total sperm transit time through the epididymis has been estimated at approximately 10 days for stallions. Frequent ejaculation may decrease transit time of sperm through the cauda by several days, resulting in decreased average storage time of individual sperm compared with that of sexually rested stallions.[2]

From the cauda epididymis, where the majority of sperm are stored, sperm enter the ductus deferens and remain there until smooth muscular contractions at ejaculation propel them to the pelvic and penile urethral regions. It has been estimated that the majority of extragonadal sperm are stored within the cauda

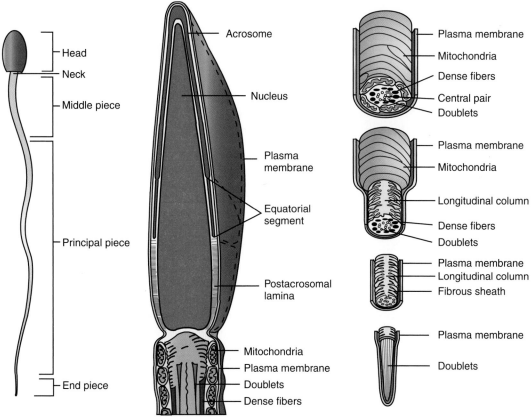

Figure 5-2. Diagrams of a stallion spermatozoon. The entire spermatozoon is overlaid by the plasma membrane, which usually is in apposition with the underlying structures and is anchored to the caudal margin of the head, at the annulus, and along the longitudinal columns of the principal piece. The head includes the nucleus (containing the genetic information in highly condensed DNA), the bag-like acrosome (containing enzymes necessary for fertilization), a specialized portion of the acrosome termed the *equatorial segment,* and the post-acrosomal lamina. The neck is the point of attachment of the tail to the head, by a ball-and-socket arrangement. The central pair and nine doublets of microtubules, which constitute the axoneme, are surrounded by nine dense fibers. All extend from the neck region, through the middle piece and principal piece, into the end piece where they terminate at slightly different sites. Because these dense fibers are tapered, the tail becomes progressively thinner. The doublets are the contractile elements, which contract differentially to induce a sliding motion and flex the tail in a helical pattern. This propels the spermatozoon. Mitochondria are membranous structures where most of the energy necessary for spermatozoal motion is produced. The longitudinal columns and fibrous sheath of the principal piece and the dense fibers provide the rigidity necessary for normal motion of the tail. Dimensions of stallion spermatozoa are approximately as follows: head length, 7 µm; middle piece length, 10 µm; middle piece diameter, 0.9 µm; principal piece length, 40 µm; principal piece diameter, 0.6 <0.5 µm; and end piece length, 4 µm. (Modified from Amann RP, Pickett BW: Principles of cryopreservation and a review of cryopreservation of stallion spermatozoa. *J Equine Vet Sci* 7:145-173, 1987.)

epididymis and ductus deferens. Of the total sperm stored, approximately 61% is located within the cauda epididymis.[12]

THE EQUINE SPERM CELL

The equine sperm cell, like other mammalian sperm, is a highly specialized cell, consisting of a head, middle piece, principal piece, and end piece (Fig. 5-2). The posterior border of the sperm head and the middle piece are joined at the neck region, which is itself a highly specialized structure. Equine sperm heads are flattened, paddle-shaped cells with dimensions of approximately 60–65 µm in overall length; head length, 6–7 µm; middle piece length, 10 µm; principal piece length, 40 µm; end piece length, 4–5 µm. The sperm head width is approximately 3.5–4.0 µm at the equatorial segment of the acrosome, the widest dimension of the cell.[9]

Normal sperm function is essential during gamete transport in the male and female and relies critically on the coordinated function of several cellular organelles. This discussion focuses on several of the critical sperm cell organelles: the plasma membrane, the acrosome, the nucleus, and the flagellum.

The Plasma Membrane

The entire sperm cell is covered by the plasma membrane, which is a typical phospholipid bilayer incorporating cholesterol, complex carbohydrates, and proteins. Cholesterol likely serves as a membrane-stabilizing substance.[13] Some of the proteins are embedded within the lipid layers to varying extents, but others are localized to the outer lipid leaflet and are associated with the glycocalyx. Certain transmembrane proteins have been reported to span the lipid bilayer as ion channels, pores, receptors, and signal transduction components. Proteins that function as receptors for various hormones and extracellular matrix components are localized on the outer lipid layer and glycocalyx, although transmembrane receptor proteins are likely to exist.[13] Proteins make up about 50% of total membrane molecular weight.[13] The plasma membrane appears to be anchored to underlying structures in the region of the sperm acrosome, post-acrosomal lamina, and neck region.

The plasma membrane overlying the sperm head has been subdivided into specialized surface domains, notably the acrosomal and postacrosomal regions.[14] In the acrosomal region, the anterior portion has been described as the marginal segment and includes the peripheral rim of the cell and lies anterior to the principal segment, which is the major acrosomal area. The posterior part of the acrosome is called the *equatorial segment* and is the area in which sperm-zona pellucida binding is initiated during the early stages of fertilization. The marginal, principal, and equatorial segment domains comprise what is often called the *acrosomal cap*. The postacrosomal region of the plasma membrane is the region between the posterior margin of the equatorial segment of the acrosome and the neck of the sperm cell. At the junction of the neck and middle piece is the posterior ring, which probably forms a tight seal between cytoplasmic compartments of the head and tail of the sperm (Fig. 5-3).[14]

An interesting feature of the sperm cell is that of differential surface composition of membrane-associated constituents. It has been reported that the plasma membrane overlying the head differs in lipid and protein content from that of the sperm tail. In addition, the net negative charge of the sperm has been more closely associated with the tail than the head.[14] Furthermore, the use of fluoresceinated lectin-binding sites and colloidal iron has demonstrated that surface-associated carbohydrates differ with respect to cellular location.[15,16] In stallion sperm, similar findings have been reported with respect to surface carbohydrate variations.[15]

The Acrosome

The acrosome lies between the plasma membrane in the anterior head region and the nuclear envelope and has its own set of membranes: the inner acrosomal membrane bordering the nuclear envelope and the outer acrosomal membrane, which is overlaid by the plasma membrane and fuses with that structure during acrosomal exocytosis, or the acrosome reaction. The acrosome is derived from the Golgi complex of the spermatid. The acrosome consists of a protein matrix core and contains numerous hydrolytic and glycolytic enzymes, which are important for fertilization. Although not described for stallion sperm specifically, the most well-known acrosomal enzymes in other species are proacrosin-acrosin, hyaluronidase, β-galactosidase, various proteinases, neuraminidases, esterases, arylsulfatase, and phospholipases A and C, as well as numerous phosphatases and regulatory enzymes and proteins. It is likely that stallion sperm have many of these enzyme systems.

The Nucleus

The nucleus of the sperm cell consists of chromatin-containing genomic DNA, which is densely packed and closely associated with the major nuclear proteins known as *protamines*. The latter are low-molecular-weight proteins (27–65 amino acids) that are highly basic and rich in arginine and cysteine residues. Numerous disulfide bonds serve to stabilize the DNA-protamine complexes. Chromatin from normal sperm are somewhat resistant to acid-denaturation, which forms the basis of the sperm chromatin structure assay.[17,18] Using this flow cytometric assay, it has been shown in numerous species, including horses, that males with subnormal fertility or infertility demonstrate characteristic fluorescence patterns of their sperm cell populations.[17,18] This is based on the failure of large numbers of sperm within ejaculates from subfertile or infertile males to resist acid denaturation (see Chapter 6). The test is usually confirmatory for large numbers of abnormal sperm in ejaculates and has been shown to have a significant inverse relationship with percentage of morphologically normal sperm.[17]

The Flagellum

The sperm tail, or flagellum, comprises four regions, which are tapered caudad: the neck (connecting piece), middle piece, principal piece, and end piece. The flagellum furnishes the motile force that is essential to propel the sperm through the female genital tract to arrive at the site of fertilization in the ampulla of the mare's oviduct.

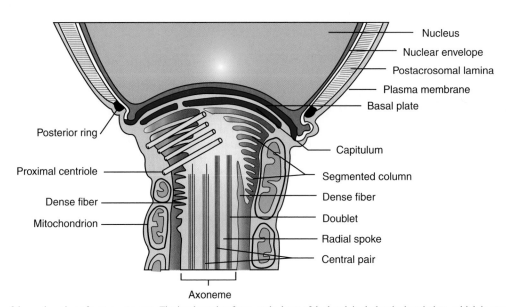

Figure 5-3. Diagram of the neck region of a spermatozoon. The implantation fossa, at the base of the head, includes the basal plate, which is attached to the capitulum, the most proximal structure of the principal piece. The capitulum consists of the cranial segments of the segmented columns, which are coupled to the dense fibers. When the tail is detached from the head, usually it is because of separation of the basal plate and capitulum. (From McKinnon AO, Voss JL: Equine Reproduction. Malvern, PA: Lea & Febiger, 1993.)

The neck, or connecting piece of the flagellum, contains several specialized structures, specifically, the segmented columns and the capitulum (see Fig. 5-3). The capitulum forms the cranial border of the flagellum at the implantation fossa and is composed of proteins that are rich in disulfide bonds. In stallion sperm, the implantation fossa may be off-center, which results in the well-known abaxial tail attachment for a significant percentage of sperm within an ejaculate. This is not considered to be abnormal for this species; most stallions have significant numbers of sperm with abaxial tails in their ejaculates. An implication of abaxial tail placement is that sperm with such tail implantation tend to swim in broad circular motions, which many observers would define as abnormal or, at least, non-progressive motion in a non-equid species. However, in stallions, some degree of circular or semi-circular movement is acceptable because of abaxial attachment of the tail. In these sperm, an observer would note that the sperm motion tracks often reverse or straighten as the sperm cell flips over such that the abaxial attachment is reversed.

The segmented columns serve as the origin of the nine longitudinal outer dense fibers that provide rigidity and resiliency to the flagellum and extend to the end of the principal piece in most species, including the horse. The dense fibers surround the central axoneme, which is composed of nine pairs of doublet microtubules (A and B) surrounding a central pair of microtubules, resulting in a 9 + 9 + 2 arrangement (Fig. 5-4). The central axoneme is derived from the distal centriole of the cell. In the region of the middle piece, the outer dense fibers are surrounded by the mitochondrial sheath, whereas in the principal piece, the dense fibers are surrounded by the fibrous sheath. In the end piece, the 9 + 2 microtubular arrangement continues about half the distance and then is lost gradually in the remaining end piece.[9,14]

The overall significance of the arrangement of the flagellar microtubular system is that the sequential and coordinated contraction of neighboring doublets in conjunction with anchorage of the doublets and dense fibers allows bending of the flagellum. This coordinated contraction along with the sequential sliding of the doublet along the axoneme results in the typical whip-like movement of the flagellum.[9] Specific pairings of doublets occur (e.g., 1 and 4, 6 and 9), in which each pair contracts in a sequential circular wave around the nine pairs of doublets such that coordination of flagellar motion results in sperm cell motility.

The mitochondrial sheath consists of a double helical arrangement of mitochondria in end-to-end formation. Stallion sperm commonly have about 50 helical turns of mitochondria.[9] Mitochondria produce and store energy in the form of adenosine triphosphate, which is used by the axoneme for development of coordinated flagellar motion originating from the neck region.

SPERM CAPACITATION AND THE ACROSOME REACTION

Capacitation of Sperm

It has been shown for numerous species that sperm must undergo the poorly understood process of capacitation as a prerequisite for most events of fertilization, including cumulus penetration, zona pellucida binding, penetration, the acrosome reaction, and fusion with the oocyte.[16] Although the mechanisms associated with capacitation have not been elucidated for stallion sperm, it seems likely that some of the properties that have been described for other mammalian sperm may hold for stallion sperm. There is evidence that sperm transport and capacitation in vivo are interrelated,[16] and this linkage may be critical for controlling the migration to the oviduct of sperm cells that are competent to fertilize.

Prior to fertilization, the sperm undergoes the largely undefined process of "'capacitation,'" as independently observed by Austin[19] and Chang[20] in 1951, which is essential for sperm to acquire fertilizing ability. In nature, this occurs in the female genital tract after ejaculation, but capacitation can occur in vitro.

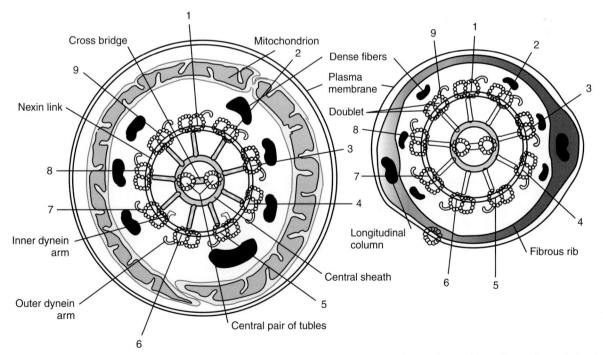

Figure 5-4. Diagram of the middle piece (left) and the principal piece (right) showing the plasma membrane, mitochondria or fibrous ribs, and nine dense fibers arranged around the axoneme, consisting of nine doublets and the central pair. Dense fibers and doublets are numbered as designated. Passing distally through the principal piece, the dense fibers become thinner and terminate; dense fibers 1, 5, and 6 are the longest. (From McKinnon AO, Voss JL: *Equine Reproduction*. Malvern, PA: Lea & Febiger, 1993.)

The initial event in sperm capacitation is a rise in intracellular calcium, bicarbonate, and hydrogen peroxide, which collectively activate adenylyl cyclase to produce cyclic AMP (cAMP). The stimulation of cAMP then activates protein kinase A, which begins to phosphorylate a number of proteins.[21,22] Visconti and co-authors[22-25] have correlated mouse, human, and bovine sperm capacitation with an increase in protein tyrosine phosphorylation of a variety of protein substrates of Mr 40,000–120,000. It has been suggested that protein tyrosine phosphorylation mediates a variety of cellular functions such as growth regulation, cell cycle control, cytoskeleton assembly, ionic current regulation, and receptor regulation[23-25] and is an essential downstream component of capacitation.

In addition to phosphorylation of membrane and cytosolic proteins, the best documented changes in sperm physiology during capacitation are those that involve the sperm membranes. There is considerable evidence to suggest that, during capacitation, there is alteration or removal of coating substances from the sperm surface.[16] These coating substances, known as decapacitating factors, are components from seminal plasma that inhibit the fertilizing ability of capacitated sperm. Sperm washing procedures may initiate the removal of sperm surface coats in vitro, and, during sperm transport through female genital tract secretions, these substances may be physically sheared from the sperm plasma membrane.[26] Cholesterol regulates the orientation, fluidity, and thickness of membrane lipids, and the role of cholesterol in sperm capacitation has received considerable attention.[27,28] It has been demonstrated that albumin and high-density lipoproteins in culture medium or in the female tract remove cholesterol from the sperm membrane. This loss of cholesterol from the sperm plasma membrane is thought to increase the fluidity of the membrane, thus making the membrane more fusogenic with the outer acrosomal membrane during the acrosome reaction. There is evidence that d-mannose–binding lectins are involved in the binding of human sperm to the zona pellucida[29] and that the expression of these lectins on the sperm surface depends on loss of sperm membrane cholesterol during capacitation.[30]

Several studies have indicated that in vitro sperm interaction with oviductal epithelium results in modulation of sperm viability, motility, and intracellular calcium regulation.[31,32] This oviductal epithelial binding in oviductal storage sites may prevent premature capacitation and acrosomal exocytosis in vivo. Changes associated with in vitro capacitation have been observed to cause release of the epithelium-bound sperm, suggesting that capacitated sperm may be less capable of binding to oviductal storage sites in vivo.[33] This suggests that it is likely that an oviductal storage site for sperm provides a specialized metabolic rate for sperm once they arrive at the oviductal site of fertilization. This would allow the sperm cells to remain viable while awaiting the descent of the oocyte following ovulation. This is consistent with the prolonged period of estrus in mares and with reports of single breedings as early as 6 days before ovulation that have resulted in mare pregnancies.[34]

The Acrosome Reaction

It is generally believed that the acrosome reaction of the fertilizing sperm must take place at or near the zona pellucida and that the natural stimulus for this event may involve molecules associated with the oocyte or its investments. Because acrosome reactions at other times or locations may render sperm infertile, prolonged acrosomal stability of sperm in vivo may ensure that sperm reaching the oocyte are competent to fertilize, regardless of their period of residence in the female tract.

The acrosome reaction can occur only following completion of capacitation and can be induced in vitro by a variety of chemical and biological agents, including zona pellucida proteins, calcium ionophores, glycosaminoglycans, and progesterone[16,35-37] As a result of binding to ZP-3, the sperm receptors aggregate.[38] A signal transduction cascade follows receptor aggregation and may involve a guanosyl nucleotide regulating (G) protein and phospholipase C (PLC).[39] In the initial stages (within 1 minute of sperm stimulation), calcium ion influx into the cell occurs, and the acrosomal matrix swells as a prelude to fusion and vesiculation of the plasma membrane and outer acrosomal membrane. As membrane vesicles form, the acrosomal matrix is thought to leak from the matrix area as pores essentially form between areas of vesicle formation. Consequently, acrosomal enzymes and structural elements are released into the immediate vicinity of the anterior sperm head and acrosome.

In this mouse-derived model of the acrosome reaction,[16,35-37] PLC acts on membrane phosphatidyl inositol diphosphate (PIP_2) to produce inositol triphosphate (IP_3), which releases intracellular Ca^{2+}, and diacylglycerol (DAG). The DAG is known to promote protein phosphorylations. Phosphorylation of IP_3 produces IP_4, which may open voltage-dependent membrane Ca^{2+} channels.[40] Increased intracellular Ca^{2+} is thought to facilitate membrane fusion by promotion of phase transition and separation of membrane phospholipid. The activated G protein may act on membrane phospholipid to produce fusogenic lipids such as lysophosphatidyl choline, arachidonic acid, and phosphatidic acid. Calcium may also act through the adenylate cyclase pathway to elevate cyclic adenosine monophosphate, which is required for protein phosphorylation and the Na^+/H^+ flux that elevates intraacrosomal pH.[41] Other models suggest that receptor-ligand interactions open sperm membrane ion channels for Ca^{2+},[42] or they suggest that progesterone binds and aggregates membrane steroid receptors to allow Ca^{2+} influx.[43] The mechanism of progesterone and zona pellucida induction of acrosome reactions in stallion sperm is unknown; however, in porcine and human sperm, the progesterone effect has been attributed to a sperm chloride ion channel/gamma-aminobutyric acid (GABA) receptor,[44] whereas the zona effect has been attributed in stallion sperm to a sperm galactosyltransferase protein.[45]

Investigations into Capacitation and Acrosome Reactions in Stallion Sperm

Various incubation media and sperm preparation methods have been used in studies of stallion sperm capacitation. Most studies have assessed capacitation by the ability of stallion sperm to penetrate a relatively small number of zona-free hamster oocytes[46] or bind to zona-intact horse oocytes.[47] Only a few studies have assessed the mechanisms involved in the equine zona-induced acrosome reaction.[46,48]

Although a few studies have evaluated the acrosomal status of stallion sperm as a measure of capacitation, most of these assessments did not include a supravital stain and thus could not distinguish between viable acrosome-reacted sperm and sperm that had lost their acrosomes in the process of degeneration. Varner and colleagues,[49] using Toyoda's medium and heparin sulfate for capacitation followed by treatment with calcium ionophore, reported percentages of acrosome reactions in viable sperm that were comparable with those reported for other species (20%–30% live acrosome-reacted cells). Meyers and co-authors[50,51] demonstrated that stallion sperm could be induced *in vitro* to capacitate using an egg yolk–containing modified Tyrode's medium and could then undergo the acrosome reaction when stimulated by progesterone, equine zona pellucida, or porcine zona pellucida.[52] Progesterone treatment following *in vitro* capacitation resulted in increased acrosome reactions in live sperm from the fertile stallions compared with control-treated sperm. Although variation in magnitude of response to progesterone was evident among stallions, the results suggested that there are functional differences in the ability of sperm from fertile and subfertile males to capacitate and acrosome-react. Similar differences have been reported for sperm of fertile and subfertile human males and have been attributed to the lack of progesterone receptor on sperm or to a nonfunctional receptor.[53] Meizel and co-authors have studied the progesterone-induced acrosome reaction in human sperm[37,54] and in porcine sperm,[55] and they have demonstrated that progesterone acts by elevating intracellular levels of calcium but not through G-protein pathways. A nongenomic progesterone receptor located on or near the sperm plasma membrane may mediate these events in human spermatozoa.[54] Wistrom and Meizel[44] have reported that the progesterone-binding mechanism of human sperm is associated with a chloride ion–channel resembling a GABA receptor. Cheng and co-authors[56] demonstrated the presence of a membrane-associated progesterone receptor in stallion sperm. This receptor is exposed as capacitation proceeds such that more progesterone receptor is available for binding progesterone and stimulating induction of the acrosome reaction. Further, it has been shown that the action of the progesterone receptor is linked with phosphorylation of tyrosine residues during *in vitro* capacitation.[57]

Sperm binding to the zona *in vitro* and induction of acrosome reactions as a consequence of sperm-zona binding have been reported for stallions,[48,51] rams,[58] boars,[59] and bulls.[60,61] Fazeli and colleagues[61] and Pantke and associates[62] suggested that fertility of bulls and stallions may be reflected in the capacity of sperm to bind to the zona; however, acrosome reactions of zona-bound sperm were not evaluated in those studies. Meyers and colleagues[51] demonstrated that sperm from certain subfertile stallions bound homologous zona pellucida to a lesser extent than did sperm from fertile stallions, in agreement with Pantke and associates,[62] but they also reported that acrosome reactions of zona-bound sperm from subfertile males were significantly decreased relative to those of fertile stallions in the study group. Thomas and co-authors[33] and Dobrinski and colleagues[63,64] have demonstrated that equine sperm display prolonged viability and maintenance of basal intracellular Ca^{2+} when attached to equine oviductal epithelial cells (OECs) *in vitro*. These authors have suggested that this oviduct epithelial binding in oviductal storage sites may prevent premature capacitation and acrosomal exocytosis *in vivo*. Changes associated with *in vitro* capacitation have been observed to cause release of the epithelium-bound sperm, suggesting that capacitated sperm may be less capable of binding to oviductal storage sites *in vivo*.[33] When intracellular Ca^{2+} levels increased in OEC-bound equine sperm, the OEC binding decreased accordingly.[64]

Stallion subfertility has been associated with a decreased ability to capacitate *in vitro* and respond to progesterone- and zona pellucida–stimulated acrosome reactions.[50,51] In those studies, progesterone was evaluated for its ability to stimulate acrosome reactions because the equine preovulatory follicle has been reported to secrete progesterone before ovulation and

luteinization[65] and is present in oviductal fluids and within the cumulus of ovulated oocytes of mares *in vivo*. Similarly, bovine and human male fertility has been correlated to acrosome reaction inducibility by progesterone, chondroitin sulfates, and dilauroylphosphatidylcholine liposomes.[53,66]

Additional reports[67-70] have been published in which several stallions were identified with histories of subfertility that failed to acrosome-react following treatment with the calcium ionophore A23187. Other spermatozoal motility and morphological parameters were unable to explain the subfertility in these horses. In these studies, the acrosome reaction was stimulated over a 2- to 3-hour period in seven subfertile stallions. The calcium ionophore A23187 stimulated 60%–80% of acrosome-reacted sperm over this period in control stallions with history of normal fertility whereas the subfertile stallions failed to demonstrate any significant percentages of cells with acrosome reactions.[68,70] Although this method is considered by some to be non-physiological because the A23187 causes an extensive influx of calcium through altered membranes, this Acrosome Responsiveness Assay (ASA) has use as a diagnostic test that may distinguish between stallions with normal and abnormal acrosomal function. A companion study, using the same stallions, recently demonstrated that the molar ratio of cholesterol to phospholipids was notably higher in the sperm and seminal plasma of these subfertile stallions, suggesting a cellular mechanism for poor acrosomal function in this subset of subfertile stallions.[69]

APPLICATION OF SPERM CELL BIOLOGY TO EQUINE BREEDING MANAGEMENT

The development of improved techniques for equine artificial insemination and semen preservation will require an improved understanding of sperm cell biology and biochemistry. Furthermore, an understanding of low-temperature sperm physiology and cryobiology will improve equine fertility because equine breeding programs increasingly include transported and cryopreserved semen. In all domestic species, including horses, pregnancy rates using cooled or cryopreserved semen have been uniformly lower than with artificial insemination of fresh semen. The essential requirements for maintaining stallion sperm *in vitro* while providing metabolic support for spermatozoa are largely unknown. In the horse, the events involved in sperm capacitation and the ability to undergo acrosomal exocytosis (the acrosome reaction) have not been elucidated. Thus, the requirements for protecting sperm for storage *in vitro* while optimizing fertilization capacity have not been determined. In addition, the effects of chilling and freezing on membrane fluidity and, therefore, on some of the functional aspects of the plasma membrane have not been determined for the horse. The consequences of changes in membrane fluidity from low temperatures are likely to be manifest as detrimental changes in Ca^{2+} metabolism, capacitation, signal transduction, acrosomal exocytosis, and fertilization. Understanding of some of these processes, much of which is presently derived from other species, will most likely rely upon specific determination of some of the basic cell functions for the horse.

REFERENCES

1. Bardin W, Cheng C, Mustow N, et al: The Sertoli cell. In Knobil E, Neill J, eds: *The Physiology of Reproduction*, 2nd ed. New York: Raven Press, 1994, pp 1291-1333.
2. Amann R: Physiology and endocrinology. In McKinnon A, Voss JL, eds: *Equine Reproduction*. Philadelphia: Lea & Febiger, 1993, pp 658-685.

3. Johnson L: Spermatogenesis. In Cupps P, ed: *Reproduction in Domestic Animals*, 4th ed. San Diego: Academic Press, 1991, pp 173-219.

4. Johnson L: Seasonal differences in equine spermatocytogenesis. *Biol Reprod* 44:284-291, 1991.

5. Johnson L, Tatum ME: Temporal appearance of seasonal changes in numbers of Sertoli cells, Leydig cells, and germ cells in stallions. *Biol Reprod* 40:994-999, 1989.

6. Johnson L, Thompson DL Jr: Age-related and seasonal variation in the Sertoli cell population, daily sperm production and serum concentrations of follicle-stimulating hormone, luteinizing hormone and testosterone in stallions. *Biol Reprod* 29:777-789, 1983.

7. Setchell B, Maddocks S, Brooks D: Anatomy, vasculature, innervation, and fluids of the male reproductive tract. In Knobil E, Neill JD, eds: *The Physiology of Reproduction*, 2nd ed. New York: Raven Press, 1994, pp 1063-1175.

8. Amann R: Function of the epididymis in bulls and rams. *J Reprod Fertil* 34(Suppl):115-131, 1987.

9. Amann R, Graham J: Spermatozoal function. In McKinnon A, Voss JL, eds: *Equine Reproduction*. Philadelphia: Lea & Febiger, 1993, pp 715-745.

10. Harper M: Gamete and zygote transport. In Knobil E, Neill JD, eds: *The Physiology of Reproduction*, 2nd ed. New York: Raven 'Press, 1994, pp 123-187.

11. Swierstra E, Pickett B, Gebauer M: Spermatogenesis and duration of transit of spermatozoa through the excurrent ducts of stallions. J Reprod Fertil 23(Suppl):53-57, 1975.

12. Amann R, Thompson D, Squires E, et al: Effects of age and frequency of ejaculation on sperm production and extragonadal sperm reserves in stallions. *J Reprod Fertil* 27(Suppl):1-6, 1979.

13. Langlais I, Roberts K: A molecular membrane model of sperm capacitation and the acrosome reaction of mammalian spermatozoa. *Gamete Res* 12:183-224, 1985.

14. Eddy E, O'Brien D: The spermatozoon. In Knobil E, Neill ID, eds: *The Physiology of Reproduction*, 2nd ed. New York: Raven Press, 1994, pp 29-78.

15. Lopez M, deSouza W, Bustos-Obregon E: Cytochemical analysis of the anionic sites on the membrane of the stallion spermatozoa during epididymal transit. *Gamete Res* 18:319-332, 1987.

16. Yanagimachi R: Mammalian fertilization. In Knobil E, Neill ID, eds: *The Physiology of Reproduction*, 2nd ed. New York: Raven Press, 1994, pp 189-317.

17. Kenney R, Evenson D, Garcia M, et al: Relationships between sperm chromatin structure, motility, and morphology of ejaculated sperm and seasonal pregnancy rate. *Biol Reprod Monogr* 1:647-653, 1995.

18. Evenson D, Sailer B, Lost L. Relationship between stallion sperm deoxyribonucleic acid (DNA) susceptibility to denaturation in situ and presence of DNA strand breaks: Implications for fertility and embryo viability. *Biol Reprod Monogr* 1:655-659, 1995.

19. Austin CR: Observations on the penetration of the sperm into the mammalian egg. Austr J Sci Res Biol Sci 4(4):581, 1951.

20. Chang MC: Fertilizing capacity of spermatozoa deposited in Fallopian tubes. *Nature* 168:997-998, 1951.

21. Breitbart H, Naor Z: Protein kinases in mammalian sperm capacitation and the acrosome reaction. *Rev Reprod* 4,151-159, 1999.

22. Visconti PE, Ning X, Fornes MW, et al: Cholesterol efflux-mediated signal transduction in mammalian sperm: cholesterol release signals an increase in protein tyrosine phosphorylation during mouse sperm capacitation. *Dev Biol* 214:429-443, 1999.

23. Visconti PE, Moore GD, Bailey JL, et al: Capacitation of mouse spermatozoa. II. Protein tyrosine phosphorylation and capacitation are regulated by a cAMP-dependent pathway. *Development* 121:1139-1150, 1995.

24. Visconti PE, Galantino-Homer H, Moore GD, et al: The molecular basis of sperm capacitation. *J Androl* 19:242-248, 1998.

25. Visconti PE, Kopf GS: Regulation of protein phosphorylation during sperm capacitation. *Biol Reprod* 59:1-6, 1998.

26. Overstreet I, Katz D, Yudin A: Cervical mucus and sperm transport in reproduction. *Semin Perinatol* 15:149, 1991.

27. Langlais I, Kan F, Granger L, et al: Identification of sterol acceptors that stimulate cholesterol efflux from human spermatozoa during in vitro capacitation. *Gamete Res* 20:185-201, 1988.

28. Parks I, Ehrenwalt E: Cholesterol efflux from mammalian sperm and its potential role in capacitation. In Bavister B, Cummins I, Raldan E, eds: Fertilization in Mammals. Norwell, MA: Serono Symposia USA, 1990, p 155.

29. Benoff S, Cooper GW, Hurley I, et al: Human sperm fertilizing potential in vitro is correlated with differential expression of a head specific mannose-ligand receptor. *Fertil Steril* 59:854-862, 1993.

30. Benoff S, Hurley I, Cooper GW, et al: Fertilization potential in vitro is correlated with head-specific mannose ligand receptor expression, acrosome status, and membrane cholesterol content. *Hum Reprod* 12:2155-2166, 1993.

31. Thomas PG, Ball BA, Miller PG, et al: A subpopulation of morphologically normal, motile spermatozoa attach to equine oviductal epithelial cell monolayers. *Biol Reprod Monogr* 51:303-309, 1994.

32. Dobrinski I, Smith T, Suarez S, et al: Membrane contact with oviductal epithelium modulates the intracellular calcium concentration of equine spermatozoa in vitro. *Biol Reprod Monogr* 56:861, 1997.

33. Thomas P, Ball BA, Brinsko S: Changes associated with induced capacitation influence the interaction between equine spermatozoa and oviduct epithelial cell monolayers. *Biol Reprod Monogr* 1:697-705, 1995.

34. Woods I, Bergfelt D, Ginther OO: Effects of time of insemination relative to ovulation of pregnancy rate and embryonic loss rate in mares. *Equine Vet J* 22:410-415, 1990.

35. Kopf G, Gerton G: The mammalian sperm acrosome and the acrosome reaction. In Wassarman EP, ed: *Elements of Mammalian Fertilization*. Boca Raton, FL: CRC Press, 1991, pp 154-203.

36. Drobnis E: Capacitation and acrosome reaction. In Zinaman M, Scialli AR, eds: *Clinical Reproductive Toxicology and Infertility*. New York: McGraw-Hill, 1992.

37. Osman R, Andria ML, Iones AD, et al: Steroid induced exocytosis: the human sperm acrosome reaction. *Biochem Biophys Res Com* 160:828-833, 1989.

38. Leyton L, Saling P: Evidence that aggregation of mouse sperm receptors by ZP3 triggers the acrosome reaction. *J Cell Biol* 108:2163, 1989.

39. Saling P: How the egg regulates sperm function during gamete interaction: facts and fantasies. *Biol Reprod* 44:246-251, 1991.

40. Florman H, Corron ME, Kim TDH, et al: Activation of voltage-dependent calcium channels of mammalian sperm is required for zona pellucida-induced acrosomal exocytosis. *Dev Biol* 152:304-314, 1992.

41. Working P, Meizel S: Correlation of increased intraacrosomal pH with the hamster sperm acrosome reaction. J Exp Zool 227:97-107, 1983.

42. Harrison R, Roldan E: Phosphoinositides and their products in the mammalian sperm acrosome reaction. *J Reprod Fertil Suppl* 42:51-67, 1990.

43. Thomas P, Meizel S: An influx of extracellular calcium is required for initiation of the human sperm acrosome reaction induced by follicular fluid. *Gamete Res* 20:397-411, 1988.

44. Wistrom C, Meizel S: Evidence suggesting involvement of a unique human sperm steroid receptor/CI-channel complex in the progesterone-initiated acrosome reaction. *Dev Biol* 159:679-690, 1993.

45. Miller C, Fayrer-Hosken R, Timmons T, et al: Characterization of equine zona pellucida glycoproteins by polyacrylamide gel electrophoresis and immunological techniques. *J Reprod Fertil* 96(2):815-825, 1992.

46. Brackett B, Cofone MA, Boice ML, et al: Use of zona-free hamster ova to assess sperm fertilizing ability of bull and stallion. *Gamete Res* 5:217-227, 1982.

47. Blue B, McKinnon AO, Squires EL, et al: Capacitation of stallion spermatozoa and fertilization of equine oocytes in vitro. *Equine Vet J* 8(suppl):111-116, 1989.

48. Ellington J, Ball BA, Yang X: Binding of stallion spermatozoa to the equine zona pellucida after coculture with oviductal epithelial cells. *J Reprod Fertil* 98:203-208, 1993.

49. Varner D, Bowen J, Johnson L: Capacitation and acrosome reaction of equine spermatozoa by heparin. *Mol Androl* 4:81-100, 1992.

50. Meyers S, Overstreet JW, Liu IKM, et al: Capacitation in-vitro of stallion spermatozoa: comparison of progesterone-induced acrosome reactions in fertile and subfertile males. *J Androl* 16:47, 1995.

51. Meyers S, Liu IKM, Overstreet JW, et al: Sperm-zona pellucida binding and zona-induced acrosome reactions in the horse: Comparisons between fertile and subfertile males. *Theriogenology* 46:1277-1288, 1996.

52. Meyers S, Liu IKM, Overstreet JW, et al: Induction of acrosome reactions in stallion sperm by equine zona pellucida, porcine zona pellucida, and progesterone. *Biol Reprod Monogr* 1:739-744, 1995.

53. Tesarik J, Mendoza C: Defective function of a nongenomic progesterone receptor as a sole sperm anomaly in infertile patients. *Fertil Steril* 58:793-797, 1992.

54. Meizel S, Turner K: Progesterone acts at the plasma membrane of human sperm. *Mol Cell Endocrinol* 11:R1-R5, 1991.

55. Melendrez C, Meizel S, Berger T: Comparison of the ability of progesterone and heat solubilized porcine zona pellucida to initiate the porcine sperm acrosome reaction in vitro. *Mol Reprod Dev* 39:433-438, 1994.
56. Cheng FP, Gadella BM, Voorhout WF, et al: Progesterone-induced acrosome reaction in stallion spermatozoa is mediated by a plasma membrane progesterone receptor. *Biol Reprod* 59(4):733-742, 1998.
57. Rathi R, Colenbrander B, Stout TAE, et al: Progesterone induces acrosome reaction in stallion spermatozoa via a protein tyrosine kinase dependent pathway. *Molec Reprod Devel* 64(1):120-128, 2003.
58. Crozet N, Dumont M: The site of the acrosome reaction during in vivo penetration of the sheep oocyte. *Gamete Res* 10:97-105, 1984.
59. Berger T, Turner KO, Meizel S, et al: Zona pellucida-induced acrosome reaction in boar sperm. *Biol Reprod* 40:525-530, 1989.
60. Florman H, First N: The regulation of acrosomal exocytosis I. Sperm capacitation is required for the induction of acrosome reactions by bovine zona pellucida in vitro. *Dev Biol* 128:453-463, 1988.
61. Fazeli A, Steenweg W, Bevers MM, et al: Development of a sperm zona pellucida binding assay for bull semen. *Vet Rec* 132:14-16, 1993.
62. Pantke P, Hyland JH, Galloway DB, et al: Development of a zona pellucida-sperm binding assay for the assessment of stallion fertility. *Biol Reprod Monogr Equine Reprod* 1:681-688, 1995.
63. Dobrinski I, Thomas P, Ball B: The oviductal sperm reservoir in the horse: functional aspects. Proc Annu Meeting, Society for Theriogenology, Kansas City, MO: 1996.
64. Dobrinski I, Suarez S, Ball B: Intracellular calcium concentration in equine spermatozoa attached to oviductal epithelial cells in vitro. *Biol Reprod* 54:783-788, 1996.
65. Linford R, McCue P, Montavon S, et al: Long-term cannulation of the ovarian vein in mares. *Am J Vet Res* 53:1589-1593, 1992.
66. Ax RL, Dickson K, Lenz RW. Induction of acrosome reactions by chondroitin sulfates in vitro corresponds to nonreturn rates of dairy bulls. *J Dairy Sci* 68:387-390, 1985.
67. Varner DD, Thompson JA, Blanchard TL, et al: Induction of the acrosome reaction in stallion spermatozoa: effects of incubation temperature, incubation time, and ionophore concentration. *Theriogenology* 58:303-306, 2002.
68. Bosard T, Love C, Brinsko S, et al: Evaluation and diagnosis of acrosome function/dysfunction in the stallion. *Anim Reprod Sci* 89(1-4):215-217, 2005.
69. Brinsko SP, Love CC, Bauer JE, et al: Cholesterol to phospholipid ratio in sperm of stallions with unexplained subfertility. *Anim Reprod Sci* 99:65-71, 2007.
70. Love C, Bosard TS, Brinsko SP, et al: Acrosomal dysfunction in stallion spermatozoa: what is known. Havemeyer Workshop, Bandera, TX: Sept 22–25, 2006.

SEMEN EVALUATION

HARALD SIEME

The general aim of semen evaluation is to assess the prospects of fertility of individual stallions or individual semen samples such as ejaculates or doses of fresh, cooled-transported, frozen/thawed semen).[1–10]

The target of semen evaluation is to clarify if quantitative and qualitative spermatological parameters are in compliance with the minimum requirements fixed for biological composition of stallion semen. Minimum standards are empirically determined averages with consideration of the standard deviation of spermatological parameters in a fertile stallion population. To define standards, variation, and minimal criteria of stallion semen, Klug[11] and Parlevliet et al.[12] in the Warmblood, Dowsett and Pattie[13] and Pickett et al.[14] in Quarter Horses and Thoroughbreds, and Paccamonti et al.[15] in Miniature stallions reported semen parameters such as volume with and without gel, sperm concentration per cc, total number of spermatozoa per ejaculate, percentage of motile spermatozoa, percentage of morphological normal spermatozoa, and seminal pH. Recommendations regarding semen standards used in artificial insemination are published as "Minimum standard requirements for stallion semen for AI" by the World Breeding Federation for Sport Horses (WBFSH) (Fig. 6-1).

The predictive value of semen analysis in the evaluation of stallion fertility has been reported by numerous investigators.[16–24] The failure to find strong correlations between fertility and quantitative assessments using either standard spermatological parameters or the more sophisticated tests has been reported in several domestic species[25,26] and in the horse.[27–29] The fact that the relationship between sperm quality determined by different assays and stallion fertility is often questionable and might be explained by the use of the limited numbers of examined males and females and the use of inconsistent fertility scores in the studies.[30,31]

Specific indications for semen evaluation exist in AI practice, such as breeding soundness evaluation of stallions, preseasonal and seasonal monitoring of stallion semen quality in AI centers in case of liability claims due to sperm quality, and evaluation of extenders and/or material toxicity tests, or research.[32–35]

Parameters usually included in a conventional evaluation of raw semen quality are either quantitative (e.g., volume gel, gel-free, and total semen volume; sperm concentration per ml; total number of spermatozoa in the ejaculate) or qualitative (e.g., percentages of motile spermatozoa, sperm morphology,[16,18,36–39] longevity of sperm motility after cooled storage,[40] and bacteriological status). Composition of seminal plasma, although not routine, can be performed in cases where stallions have unexplained low motility or longevity.[41–43]

Although these evaluations provide abundant information, it is well accepted that these parameters give only crude information on the fertility of stallions. Prediction of male fertility could be improved if additional parameters based on functional characteristics of spermatozoa are considered.[34] Therefore, several functional tests have been developed and are summarized in this chapter together with established routine tests for analysis of stallion spermatozoa. In commercial AI settings, however, a quick assessment of appearance, volume, concentration, and motility remains the most common evaluation.

ROUTINE MACROSCOPIC EVALUATION (GROSS APPEARANCE) OF STALLION SEMEN

Volume of the ejaculate is dependent on species, breed, age, and environment. Environmental factors affecting seminal volume may include feeding, housing, teasing, soundness, method and frequency of semen collection (collection of total ejaculates or seminal fractions[44]), and time of the year (e.g., small volume during the non-breeding season).[45] In general, species with intrauterine ejaculation (e.g., stallion, boar) release larger ejaculates than species with vaginal ejaculation (e.g., cattle, sheep). Seminal volume is largely influenced by the amount of secretions resp. seminal plasma of the accessory sex glands. The seminal volume should be determined in terms of gel-free volume representing main parts of the sperm-rich fraction of a stallion ejaculate; thus, sperm-free pre-ejaculatory fluid secreted from urethral and bulbourethral glands as well as the stallion-specific gel fraction released by the seminal vesicle glands in the second sperm-poor fraction should be recorded separately. The volume of the semen sample should be measured in a pre-warmed, sterile measuring cylinder. The total volume of the ejaculate should be 60–120 ml and the gel-free volume 30–100 ml. These figures are highly variable between stallions[36] and with season[45] and collection frequency.[16,18,44] Reduced seminal volume can be a result of failure of emission of semen (e.g., ejaculatory failure syndrome, obstruction of deferent ducts).[34,46] Correct measurement of seminal volume in combination with sperm concentration is a prerequisite for calculation of total sperm count of the ejaculate, with the latter being the most important measure determining the amount of producible AI doses.

Macroscopic appearance of the ejaculate depends on its density that is determined by sperm concentration, composition of seminal plasma, and physiological (epithelial cells) or pathological (urine, blood) constituents. Seminal characteristics include fluidity, consistency, and color. The color of the semen sample should be milky white, evenly turbid, without clots, and with no unusual smell. Consistency varies with decreasing sperm number from creamy, milky, whey-like, to watery, and is regarded as an indication of reduced sperm number (oligozoospermia) or absolute

MINIMUM STANDARD REQUIREMENTS FOR STALLION SEMEN FOR AI

Fresh Semen

Minimum of 300 million progressively motile sperm cells

Chilled Semen

Diluted/Fresh

Sperm dose: Minimum of 300 million progressively motile spermatazoa at time of portioning

Insemination within 12 hours of collection

Storage conditions maintained

Progressively motile spermatazoa at time of insemination no less than 35%

Diluted/Transported

Sperm dose: minimum of 600 million progressively motile spermatozoa at time of portioning

Maximum volume 40 cc (dilution1:2)

Insemination 24-36 hours after collection

Storage conditions maintained

Progressively motile spermatozoa at time of insemination no less than 35%

All semen leaving the insemination center has to be treated as diluted/transport semen

Frozen Semen

Volume dose: dependent on manufacturing process

Sperm dose: minimum of 35% progressively motile spermatozoa post-thawing

Minimum of 250 million progressively motile spermatozoa per AI dose post-thawing

A breeding dose for insemination of one mare has to contain a minimum of 3 straws.

Free to sell a single insemination dose

Figure 6-1. Recommendations for commercial stallion semen standards used in AI practice published as "Minimum standard requirements for stallion semen for AI" by the World Breeding Federation for Sport Horses (WBFSH). Available at http://www.wbfsh.org/?GB/Activities/Semen%20standards.aspx.

absence of spermatozoa (azoospermia). The color of stallion semen occurs physiologically as whitish or whitish-gray. Any pink or red coloring may suggest hemospermia (blood in the sperm), which could be detrimental to fertility. Ejaculates showing red (indication of fresh blood), brown (indication of old blood, dirt or contamination), or yellow (urospermia) should be rejected from AI. Color and consistency give important indications of the appropriateness of an ejaculate for use in AI. Odor is examined also as routine laboratory practice, and stallion ejaculates are normally odor neutral ("non olet"); urine odor, putrid odor, and ejaculates with species-specific fecal odor should be discarded.

MICROSCOPIC AND FLOW CYTOMETRIC EVALUATION OF STALLION SEMEN

Sperm Concentration

Sperm concentration, or density, represents the number of spermatozoa per volume unit. It is repeated usually in millions per mm^3 or ml; in stud farm practice the information in millions per ml is customary. Sperm concentration may be measured using a counting chamber with a microscope (hemacytometer) or a spectrophotometer, where the estimate is based on the density of the solution. Concentrations of 100–350 × 10^6/ml are common, depending on the seasonal influences and ejaculation frequency, and usually fall in the range of 50–150 × 10^6/ml when regular (once daily or every second day) semen collections are carried out.

Traditionally sperm concentration is determined by means of cell-counting chambers (hemacytometer method), upon recommendations of the World Health Organization. The Neubauer chamber or hemacytometer is regarded as the golden standard for evaluation of sperm concentration.[47,48] Defined aliquots of the sperm sample are dissolved and immobilized in 10% formol/NaCl solution. After gentle stirring of the sample, the hemacytometer chambers are loaded. According to sedimentation, sperm are counted microscopically in a total of 10 squares out of two chamberfields. Contingent upon sperm sample volume, fixed variables for height, and volume of the hemacytometer chamber, the resulting sperm concentration can be calculated. The accuracy of the procedure depends significantly on precision of pipetting, careful stirring, and absolute number of counted sperm (at least 100).[49] Considering these rules, the hemacytometer method is regarded as a comparably precise method to measure concentration of spermatozoa. However, the amount of time required is disadvantageous.[50] Therefore, this method is often not applied in routine laboratory practice.

In AI centers, more feasible techniques to determine sperm concentration are in use (e.g., photometer or electronic particle counters). The disadvantage of these methods is the missing differentiation between sperm and other cells in the semen sample. A regular species-particular alignment is presupposed when investigations are carried out by photometer or Coulter Counter; these automates represent the method of choice for AI centers where semen of several stallions is collected daily (e.g., SpermaCue, MiniTube, Tieffenbach, Germany; 591B Equine Densimeter, Animal Reproduction Systems, Chino, CA; Accucell, IMV; LÁigle, France).

Additional possibilities arise out of integration of computer-assisted sperm analysis (CASA) (sperm motility analysis) into laboratory practice; these machines can determine sperm concentration and sperm motility simultaneously with adequate accuracy. The use of a flow cytometer in combination with fluorescence dye–marked sperm has been reported as a valuable tool to determine sperm concentration with high precision.[51] Because of methodical and device-related reasons, flow cytometry is expensive. Due to the complexity of sperm preparation, as well as the instrument itself and its cost, it finds application in specialized labs.

Recently, easy-to-use counting equipment has been developed; the NucleoCounter SP-100 (ChemoMetec, Alleroed, Denmark) counts mammalian cell nuclei stained with the DNA-specific fluorescent dye, propidium iodide. Propidium iodide is excluded from viable cells. This is used in the NucleoCounter to estimate the concentration of non-viable cells and the concentration of total cells in a suspension.[52]

Accurate determination of sperm concentration of ejaculates in commercially available AI doses is of high importance in the industry. Efficiency and accuracy of the sperm processing depends on accurate methods to determine sperm concentration particularly when a specific number of spermatozoa in the AI dose is guaranteed when commercializing stallion semen.

The total sperm count (TSC) in an ejaculate is the result of the product between seminal volume and sperm concentration per ml.

Sperm Motility Analysis

Light Microscopy

The activity or motility of spermatozoa is an important functional parameter that is comparatively simple to determine. Motility analysis still remains the easiest and is a major component of every evaluation of semen quality. The objective of estimating sperm motility is to determine the percentage of motile and the proportion of progressively moving spermatozoa. Traditionally, the evaluation has depended on subjective estimates of sperm motility characteristics using a microscope, which is inexpensive and simple to do.

The motility of gel-free semen should be estimated immediately after collection on a pre-warmed microscope slide. Prerequisites are a phase-contrast microscope with a warm surface (37°–40°C). The typical procedure to assess sperm motility is done by placing approximately 2-5-μl droplets on a pre-warmed slide covered with a warm cover-slip and using a phase-contrast microscope at a magnification of 150–200×.[4] Motility is expressed, in percentage form, as oscillatory or progressive (i.e., those that are alive but are moving in a circle around their own axis and those that are actively moving forward). Sperm from a normal fertile stallion should have an immediate progressive motility ≥60%. Abaxial attachment of the midpiece to the sperm head is physiological in stallion spermatozoa and responsible for a circular motion of specific aliquot of stallion semen samples. Therefore, estimating only the progressive motility may underestimate good motility from some stallions. Preferably, semen should be extended before it is analyzed because raw stallion semen tends to agglutinate and individual sperm movement could be difficult.[4] Visual estimation is inexpensive, simple, and accurate if analysis is performed by an experienced technician. Nevertheless, the microscopic evaluation is a subjective procedure that requires experience and a regular control and training of the laboratory personnel. Standardization is indicated and recommendations include incubation of the sample at 37°C for 2 minutes in a waterbath, sperm concentration of 25–50 × 10^6 sp/ml, and chamber 10–20 μl; a minimum of two drops from the suspension should be analyzed. Evaluation of at least four or five fields near the center of the coverslip is recommended.[4,46] Motility at the edges declines more rapidly than in the center as a result of drying and exposure to air. If subjective motility is used experimentally, it should be done blindly, preferably by averaging values of two evaluators. Simultaneously with the evaluation of sperm motility, agglutination incidence of spermatozoa, and number of foreign cells should be recorded.[1,2,24,38,39]

Agglutination is defined as clusters of spermatozoa attached to each other or to a foreign particle. Agglutination is often by the head while the tail is free and still motile. Agglutination of spermatozoa may occur as head to head in a pair-wise or star-shape formation. The degree of agglutination (low, moderate, high) is to be recorded in the evaluation sheet.

External cells and other foreign particles should be recorded in connection with sperm motility and agglutination. Sperm heads are elliptical, with a length of ~6.6 μm and width of ~3.6 μm. The midpiece is on average ~9.8 μm long. All cellular components in the semen are differentiated with regard to type and degree. Frequently, epithelial cells are present and their size is approximately 10 times larger compared to the sperm head. Their polygonal shape makes them easy to distinguish from other cellular material in semen. Epithelial cells originate from urethra, penis, or prepuce and are harmless. Erythrocytes are smaller than sperm heads and they appear as circular discs when observed through the microscope. The causes of hemorrhage must be clarified and the ejaculate excluded from further processing. The proof of leukocytes is always dubious in semen. Differential diagnosis between white blood cells (e.g., neutrophils), which are identifiable due to their size and segmentation of the nucleus, is done by doing a thin smear and triple staining it. Ejaculates containing leukocytes are unsuitable for AI, and a clinical and microbiological investigation of the sperm donor is indicated.

Occasionally cylindrical "round" cells are present in semen. They represent early undifferentiated stages of spermatogenesis. These round cells are tail-less and up to eight times larger than the sperm head. Immature spermatogenic cells vary in size and typically possess round, dark-staining nuclei. This is in contrast to the homogeneous size of white blood cells and the distinctive nuclear characteristics of the neutrophil. These immature "round" spermatogenic cells may appear in the ejaculate in increasing numbers when stallions are affected with early stages of testicular degeneration.[38,39]

Computer-Assisted Sperm Analysis (CASA)

Classical microscopic assessment has the disadvantage that sperm motility estimates can vary among examiners. Computer-assisted sperm analysis (CASA) should offer a more reliable and repeatable means of assessing sperm parameters such as motility.[53]

CASA allows for the objective determination of a variety of motility parameters, sperm concentration, and newest models also have a morphology module, although limited to sperm head morphology.[54]

In 1985 the first commercial CASA system developed specifically for evaluation of sperm motion was called the CellSoft system. The second commercial system developed specifically for evaluation of sperm motion was the Hamilton Thorn Motility Analyzer, HTM-2000, introduced in 1986. The impetus for development of this system was quantification of changes in stallion sperm during storage in the Equitainer. This system had technical advances including an integrated optical system, video display, warming tray, and an automated positioning of the sample to pre-determined locations. The near-infrared illumination and dark-field optics of the initial system soon were replaced in the HTM-S by visible-light illumination and phase-contrast optics.[53] Today several other systems are in the market, such as the Sperm Vision from MiniTube. Video images for computerized sperm motion analysis are obtained from viewing fields of motile sperm using a microscope. A set number, usually 20 to 30 successive video frames were analyzed at a constant rate, typically 30–60 frames per second (Fig. 6-2). When all frames for a given field have been recorded, image-processing computer software detects and tabulates algorithms and distinguishes sperm from non-sperm objects and reconstructs sperm tracks.

This technique is objective and evaluates the motility according to the given criteria.[55–57] It allows analysis of more specific characteristics of spermatozoa. Kinematics as shown in Figure 6-3 are percentages of total motility (MOT) and progressive motility (PMOT), as well as mean straight-line velocity (VSL), mean curvilinear velocity (VCL), average path velocity (VAP), straightness (STR = VSL/VAP), linearity (LN = VSL/VCL), lateral head displacement (LHD). Due to the high cost of the instrument, computerized sperm image analysis systems are used primarily

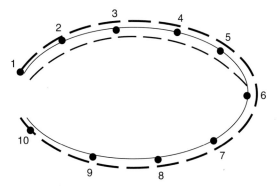

Figure 6-2. Influence of the number of frames analyzed on straightness of a circling spermatozoon. If the track is defined by 6 frames, it can be considered linear; if the track is defined by 10 frames, it can be considered circular. Straight path of spermatozoa is dependent on the number of frames analyzed.

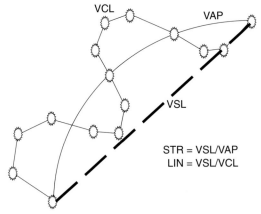

Figure 6-3. Schematic representation of different motility parameters evaluated by computer-assisted sperm analysis (CASA). *VAP,* Path velocity (average velocity of the smoothed cell path [μm/sec]); *VSL,* progressive velocity (average velocity measured in a straight line from the beginning to the end of the track); *VCL,* track speed (average velocity measured over the actual point to point track followed by the cell); *STR,* straightness (average value of the ratio VSL/VAP; STR measures the departure of the cell path from a straight line); *LIN,* linearity (average value of the ratio VSL/VCL; LIN measures the departure of the cell track from a straight line).

in well equipped AI centers, commercial AI organizations, or research facilities. Today, more complex CASA instruments that would overcome the limitations of current instruments, such as being able to simultaneously analyze sperm motion characteristics, sperm viability, and morphology, are in development.[47,52,58] On the other hand, development of any device might be inhibited by perception of an unfavorable cost–benefit ratio.

Each CASA system needs standardization and validation concerning calibration and technical settings (e.g., frame rate, light settings, recognition of spermatozoa by sperm head size and brightness, tail detection, recognition of immotile particles) to provide accurate and repeatable results.[53,57] Potential sources of error should be minimized to allow comparison of data obtained by different systems and groups.[7] However, no international standardization in equipment settings has yet been implemented, which does not allow direct comparison of results between laboratories. Thus, there is an urgent need for users of CASA to agree on standard analysis parameters.[7,53] In addition to having correct settings, repeatability and accuracy of the data within a sample and the relationship between CASA and subjective evaluation of motility by an experienced operator are important factors that must be considered to ensure that the data are accurate. Using an HTM analyzer, Bataille et al.[59] evaluated samples from 62 stallion ejaculates that had been frozen. Their results indicated that the variability within a sample was only 2% in the percentage of rapid sperm (3.5 μm/sec in VAP), and 2 million in sperm concentration when at least 12 measures were realized. The analysis was done on two straws per ejaculate, with two drops per straw and three fields per drop. These authors reported a significant correlation between linearity, mean path velocity, percentage of rapid spermatozoa, and motility analysis determined subjectively with light microscopy. Kirk et al.[28] reported that the mean percentages of motile sperm in cryopreserved stallion semen samples were 26% and 36% when the same samples were evaluated visually and using CASA, respectively. Interestingly, the inter-assay variability was 16% for both tests, and the intra-assay variability was 5% and 10%, respectively, for the two assay methods.

The main factors that affect the CASA results are the type of chamber used for the evaluation and the amount of debris or foreign material in the sample. Most CASA systems use Makler chambers, but semen dries quickly at 37°C; however, newer CASA models are faster and can analyze 400 cells in 2 minutes. Varner et al.[54] demonstrated that field within chamber

accounted for most of the variability in the CASA analysis and recommended that three chambers per ejaculate and three fields per chamber be evaluated, which would result in the analysis of approximately 500 cells per sample. The SpermVision system analyzes motility of semen samples with the help of a standardized ready-to-use Leja Chamber (Leja Products, Nieuw-Vennep, The Netherlands). The ideal sperm concentration is between 25 and 50 ×10^6 sperm/ml. However, time between filling of the chamber and starting the measurements, the duration of the analysis, and selection of and number of measuring positions in the chamber are the most important technical factors to consider.

In addition, the type of extender and ejaculate characteristics are important factors to consider. Sperm agglutination and the presence of non-sperm particles such as egg yolk are factors that can affect the analysis and results. To overcome this problem, many laboratories use (1) clarified egg yolk suspensions obtained by centrifugation,[60] (2) detergents in the extender, such as Equex STM (delta-amino-sodium lauryl sulphate) to solubilize the egg yolk lipids and lipoproteins, (3) non-fat dry milk glucose extender to dilute frozen-thawed semen samples before CASA evaluation, and (4) fluorescence dyes that do not affect motility (e.g., Hoechst 33342) to differentiate sperm cells from egg yolk particles in CASA systems equipped with epifluorescent illumination (e.g., HTM, SpermVision).[47,58]

Motility had a low (0.45) but significant correlation with the first-cycle pregnancy rate of 177 mares inseminated with frozen semen from nine stallions.[61] However, predominant motility of the spermatozoa is poorly correlated with fertility.[18,23,56,62] This seems reasonable because motility is only one attribute of the sperm. Thus, attempts have been made to evaluate several sperm attributes as a means of determining semen quality[58,63–65] or to differentiate between subpopulations of sperm with different motility characteristics.[66] Kirk et al.[28] compared flow-cytometric assays for viability, acrosome status, and mitochondrial membrane potential of frozen-thawed sperm with visual and computer-assisted motility analysis; the results of these assays were correlated with stallion sperm fertility. The ultimate goal of multi-parametric sperm analysis is to be able to distinguish sperm samples that could have good fertilizing potential from those likely to have poor fertility.

Longevity of Spermatozoa

Cooled-stored or frozen-thawed semen samples may be examined on warm microscope slides after different time intervals and under different storage conditions (+5°C, 37°C test of thermoresistancy). Motility estimations under different conditions for frozen-thawed spermatozoa have been proposed: Frozen-thawed sperm have been evaluated at 1°C, for several days until no motile cells are present[67]; at 4°C during 5 days,[68] at 38°C for 3 hours.[69] Longevity of motility is used in 15 centers out of 21 as reported in a survey conducted by Samper and Morris,[70] while four centers incubated sperm at 38°C for 4 hours. Nine centers evaluated semen by incubating at 20°C during 12–48 hours. Acceptable motility thresholds varied among laboratories ranging between 5% and 20%. Today most laboratories would incubate frozen-thawed sperm at 38°C for 2 hours, expecting a minimum of 15% motility after that period. Although visual motility and the straightness of sperm motility conducted 90 minutes after thawing were correlated with seasonal fertility (0.56 and 0.55, respectively), data from no single assay were significantly correlated with first-cycle fertility rates.[28]

Post-Thaw Motility of Stallion Spermatozoa

Samper and Morris[70] reported in their survey of equine AI centers freezing semen that CASA is the basic method for all the centers. Before freezing, 13 of 21 centers required >50% motile sperm, while 8 of 21 required >60% before discarding the semen. After freezing and thawing, the threshold is quite different between centers: 2 centers required a minimum of 25%, 10 centers 30%, 8 centers 35%, and 1 center 40%. Even though motility estimation before freezing is well correlated with motility after freezing and thawing, it cannot be considered as a test to predict poor freezable ejaculates. Vidament[71] summarized 20 years of field results with frozen semen in France and reported that stallions and ejaculates were selected on the basis of CASA measured post-thaw motility; an ejaculate was considered acceptable if motility was ≥35% rapid sperm. In their study a rapid sperm was defined as a motile cell with an average path velocity between 30 and 40 μm/sec.

In a previous study Loomis[72] reported that acceptable ejaculate frozen following the Select Breeders Services freezing protocol was one that yielded post-thaw progressive motility of ≥35% and ≥25% following a 30-minute incubation at 37°C.

In a recent study, Loomis and Graham[73] reported that following incubation, the motility of the extended semen as determined using CASA. A minimum of 400 motile or 1000 total sperm from more than five fields were analyzed for motion characteristics at 60 frames/sec for 40 frames. The stage of the microscope was maintained at 37°C throughout analysis. For this program, a sperm is considered progressively motile if it has a VAP >50 μm/sec and STR value >75%. A sperm with VAP <20 μm/sec is considered non-motile in the calculation of percentage of motile spermatozoa.

Computer-Assisted Sperm Morphometry

Morphometric analysis consists of measuring the length, width, area, and perimeter of the sperm head performed on stained smears by computer-assisted imaging. Morphometric analysis of the sperm head by computer-assisted microscopy is preferably used in specialized laboratories mostly using Feulgen or

hematoxylin stains.[74–77] Software is available by using either the ASMA (automated sperm morphology analysis, Hamilton Thorne Research, Beverly, MA) or SAMBA-TM2005 software (Alcatel TITN, Meylan, France). Several reports have indicated a positive and significant correlation between sperm head size and stallion fertility.[5,78,79]

Sperm Morphology Analysis

A major part of any breeding soundness examination is an evaluation of sperm morphology. It requires specialized equipment (a light microscope equipped with a planapochromatic ×100 oil immersion objective and a condense enabling bright field and differential interference contrast microscopy), expertise and experience of the technician, and often a great deal of time and patience. A minimum of >100 cells per slide should be analyzed and classified.[2,4,8,37–39,80,81]

Many different staining techniques have been devised for examining sperm morphology in stallion.[38,39] Sperm morphology can be evaluated by examining stained smears under bright field microscopy. Stains that are routinely used are: Williams,[82] Karras,[83] Eosin Anilin Blue,[84] nigrosin-eosin,[85] Spermac,[86] and Feulgen[87]). Nigrosin-eosin stain[85] is commonly used because it is effective and simple, spermatozoa are readily visualized, and it is a "live-dead" stain, allowing the practitioner to assess membrane integrity at the same time as morphology. The nigrosin-eosin stain produces a dark background on which the sperm stand out as lightly colored objects. Normal live sperm exclude the eosin stain and appear white, whereas "dead" sperm (i.e., those with loss of membrane integrity) take up eosin and appear pinkish in color. A number of variations of the nigrosin-eosin stain exist.[87] The nigrosin-eosin formulation is prepared by dissolving 5% w/v nigrosin, 0.6% w/v eosin, 3% w/v sodium citrate-dihydrate in water. The pH of the stain is then adjusted to 7.0 and passed through a filter paper.

Furthermore, a technique preferred in many laboratories for evaluating sperm morphology is to visualize sperm under phase-contrast microscopy or preferably under differential interference contrast microscopy. This method allows excellent visualization of sperm defects, but the requirement of 100× objective and excellent microscope optics limits its use to well-equipped laboratories. When one of these methods is used, it is important to allow some time after the preparation of the wet mount for sperm to settle flat on the slide. By running this "wet-mount" technique, the sperm are first fixed (~1:4 ratio) with glutaraldehyde or buffered formol saline[88–90] and can be stored for prolonged periods in that solution. This procedure is particularly useful for assessing acrosomal integrity. In addition, incidence of artifacts is lower compared with stained smears.

It seems obvious that conventional light microscopic evaluation of sperm alone does not fully provide potential indicators of functional impairment in spermatozoal organelles. Thus, Veeramachaneni et al.[38] reported a technique that combined evaluation of sperm under a wet mount and a dry smear stained with toluidine blue for bright field microscopy. Transmission electron microscopy using thin sections stained with uranyl acetate and lead citrate have also been reported. This technique provides information of the ultrastructural morphology of sperm organelles and has proven to be a useful tool to help in the diagnosis of infertility of stallions.[34,91]

Two types of classifications are commonly used. Abnormalities can be classified with regard to the anatomic site of the defect; thus, the head, midpiece, or tail is affected, with some sperm having defects in more than one site.[22,92] The other system classifies defects into primary (failure of spermatogenesis), secondary (failure of maturation), and tertiary (damage occurring during or after ejaculation) categories or abnormalities.[93] Generally, primary defects are the more severe and are thought to originate during spermatogenesis within the seminiferous epithelium of the testis. Disturbances in spermatogenesis are best detected by evaluating sperm morphology; with this in mind, sperm morphology represents one of the most important sperm assays because of its moderate-to-high correlation with fertility in the stallion. Secondary defects are regarded as less serious and thought to arise during epididymal passage and storage. Tertiary defects could be iatrogenic and may occur by mishandling of sperm after ejaculation. Limitations of this classification system are the unknown origin of some sperm defects and the fact that primary defects are not necessarily more deleterious to fertility than secondary defects, a common misinterpretation of this system. Therefore, the utility or physiological basis of this classification scheme is controversial in the literature.

The Society for Theriogenology sperm morphology evaluation form, also called the *differential spermiogram*,[94,95] records the following sperm categories: normal sperm, abnormal acrosomal regions/heads, detached head, proximal droplets, distal droplets, abnormal midpieces, and bent/coiled tails. The presence of teratoid sperm and of other cells (round germ cells, white blood cells, red blood cells, etc.) should also be indicated. Acrosome defects include knobbed, roughed, and detached acrosomes. Head defects include microcephalic (small, underdeveloped, or dwarf), macrocephalic (large or giant), pyriform (narrow at the base), tapered (narrow), nuclear vacuoles (pouches or craters), and multiple heads. Midpiece defects include midpiece reflex (simple bent or folded midpiece), segmental aplasia of the mitochondrial sheath, fractured, swollen (thick, pseudodroplet), roughed (corkscrew), swollen/roughed/broken (Dag-like), disrupted sheet (filamentous), duplicated, and stump tail. Bent or coiled tails refer to those sperm in which both the midpiece and the principal piece are bent or coiled, or the distal part of the principal piece is coiled. The percentage of normal and abnormal detached heads (tailless or separated heads) could be recorded separately.

It has been assumed that certain sperm defects are more important or more deleterious to fertility than others, so only the most deleterious defect is recorded per spermatozoon. However, this assumption has not been justified by scientific data and is therefore not recommended for use in laboratories evaluating sperm.

The classification of sperm defects as major and minor has been accepted by some authors,[96,97] suggesting that major defects cause early embryonic death or prevent fertilization (e.g., acrosomal defects preventing zona binding and subsequent fertilization of the egg, nuclear defects may result in EED or nonfertilization) and minor defects (e.g., abnormalities of the sperm tail) alter sperm motility, so the spermatozoon cannot reach the egg. Some abnormalities are compensable and some are non-compensable.[98] A non-compensable abnormality gives the animal a poor fertility prognosis.

The current method of classification is to record the numbers of specific morphologic defects. However, when more than one abnormality is found on a single spermatozoon, it is an indication of a more severe disturbance of spermatogenesis and possibly a poorer fertility prognosis.[99] This procedure is considered superior to the traditional system because it offers specific information with regard to the semen sample analyzed and avoids erroneous speculations about the origin of these defects. It has been generally accepted that the total number of morphologically normal sperm in ejaculates may provide more information regarding the fertility of a stallion than the percentage or absolute number of morphologically abnormal spermatozoa.

In general, threshold values for the different categories are: >30% sperm head defects, >25% proximal cytoplasmic droplets, >10% premature germ cells, and <30% morphologically normal spermatozoa. The current guidelines from the Society for Theriogenology for stallion breeding soundness evaluation are used to select stallions that could render at least 75% of 40 or more mares pregnant when bred naturally or 120 or more mares when bred artificially. These guidelines have no standard for percentage of normal spermatozoa in the ejaculate, but they state that a satisfactory prospective breeder should produce a minimum of 1 billion morphologically normal, progressively motile sperm in each of two ejaculates collected 1 hour apart.

Fluorophores and Flow Cytometry

Many different fluorescent stainings and combinations of fluorophores have been developed to evaluate different sperm characteristics in several mammalian species (see Morrell,[100] Gadella et al.,[101] and Caiza de la Cueva et al.[102] for review). Fluorescent sperm can be analyzed by fluorescence microscopy or by flow cytometry: proportions of live and dead cells,[103–107] mitochondrial function,[108–110] acrosomal integrity,[111–119] capacitation status,[120–122] intracellular calcium concentration of spermatozoa,[123] and sperm chromatin or DNA content[124–126] have all been evaluated. Although most fluorescent stains can be used in combination with fluorescence microscopy, flow cytometry has become the most used method. Basically, a flow cytometer has a light source, usually a laser or a mercury arc lamp, a sample chamber, flow cell or jet-in-air nozzle, sheath-fluid stream, photodetector or photomultiplier tubes that convert the collected light to electronic signals, a signal-processing system that processes digital signals from analog output, as well as a computer to direct operations, store the collected signals, display data, and drive the sorting process. This in itself provides a method of rapidly analyzing a population of cells into subpopulations and determining any changes relative to the percentage of each.[127] There are several types of lasers available, which differ in the gain medium that is used to amplify light (e.g., argon ion [365, 488, or 514 nm], krypton [567 or 646 nm] and helium-neon [633 nm], mercury arc lamp lasers), specific wavelength emitting solid state laser). Spermatozoa are labeled with a fluorochrome of choice and used in either the viable or fixed state. The choice of fluorochrome is influenced both by the application and the excitation wavelengths available on the flow cytometer.[100,128] Once labeled, spermatozoa are aspirated and made to flow rapidly through the flow cell where they are illuminated by the laser beam; scattered and emitted light is collected by a typical arrangement of lenses, optics, and filters, resulting in the measurement of specific bands of fluorescence. Flow cytometry permits the observation of physical characteristics, such as cell size assessed by the so-called forward scatter, the granularity of cells differentiated by side scatter, and any fluorescence signal emitted by fluorophore-stained spermatozoa that can be collected with photomultiplier tubes. Flow cytometry also has the capacity to detect labeling by multiple fluorochromes associated with individual spermatozoa, meaning that more than one sperm attribute can be assessed simultaneously, which offers the advantage of a more accurate fertility prediction because several sperm attributes can be tested simultaneously. A further advantage of flow cytometric assessment is that large numbers of spermatozoa can be analyzed by high flow rates of 200–800 s^{-1} in a very short period. Routinely a total of 10,000 spermatozoa are analyzed, which is substantially more than the total of 100–200 cells generally observed by microscopic analysis. Thus, flow cytometry is a very rapid and sensitive method for the detection of subtle differences among thousands of spermatozoa that may not be apparent using other techniques. Multiple aspects of sperm function can be assayed simultaneously. The disadvantages of using the flow cytometer for semen analysis are the costs, the need of a skilled operator, and, because of the size and sensitivity of the apparatus, the requirement of a dedicated position in the laboratory.

Sperm Plasma Membrane Integrity and Sperm Viability Assays

The plasma membrane of sperm is composed of three different compartments or regions: the outer acrosomal membrane, the post-acrosomal region of the sperm head, and the middle and principal pieces of the sperm. Thus, to analyze the integrity of these different plasma membrane compartments, classical stains such as eosin-nigrosin[85] and eosin-aniline-blue[84] or fluorophores are used. Fluorescent stains such as propidium iodide, ethidium bromide, diamidino-2-phenylindole [DAPI] or bis-benzimide–Hoechst 33258 bind to and stain the DNA of sperm possessing defects of post-acrosomal plasma membrane of the sperm head. Whereas the integrity of the plasma membrane covering the principal pieces of sperm can be assessed by analysis of sperm motility or the hypo-osmotic swelling test (HOST), the integrity of the plasma membrane covering the acrosome is focused on the integrity of the outer acrosomal membrane using microscopy (DIC), fluorometers, and flow cytometry.[104,129]

Fluorescent staining of spermatozoa to determine viability can be approached in two ways: fluorochromes used to indicate viable (intact plasma membrane) cells and those used to indicate non-viable (damaged plasma membrane) cells. Use of the flow cytometer to determine the proportion of viable spermatozoa can be achieved by the use of fluorochromes (e.g., 6-carboxyfluorescein diacetate [CFDA], calcein AM),[105,117,130,131] which penetrate the plasma membrane and are de-esterified by esterases in viable spermatozoa to non-permeant fluorescent compound that is retained in the cytoplasm, causing them to fluoresce green when exposed to the appropriate wavelength of light. Therefore, only live cells with both active intracellular esterases and intact plasma membranes will fluoresce with these markers. Plasma membrane permeant DNA fluorochromes (e.g., SYBR-14 excitation/emission 488/515 nm wavelength[65,106]) label nuclei of viable cells. SYBR-14 is cell permeable and brightly stains only the nuclei of living cells, emitting green fluorescence in response to excitation. Nucleic acid stains are less variable than enzyme-based stains, and sperm DNA is a preferable target because of its stainability and staining uniformity.

Non-viable cells can be determined using membrane-impermeable nucleic acid stains, which penetrate through a damaged plasma membrane and result in fluorescent signals of nuclei of dead spermatozoa. Fluorochromes staining non-viable cells have been tested for sperm cells each with distinct excitation (ex) and emission (em) properties: phenanthridines (e.g., propidium iodide [PI][102,106,132] ex/em of 488/>620 nm wavelength, ethidium homodimer-1 [EthD-1][115] ex/em of 568/>620 nm wavelength, the cyanine Yo-Pro-1[122] ex/em of 488/515 nm wavelength, and the benzimidazole Hoechst 33258[132] ex/em of 358/488 nm wavelength). PI cannot cross intact cell membranes; it gains access to nuclear DNA only when cell membranes are damaged and non-viable. Bound to nucleic DNA, PI fluoresces red in response to excitation. Wilhelm et al.[62] compared the fertility of cryopreserved stallion spermatozoa with a number of laboratory assessments of semen quality and found that viability, as assessed by flow cytometry using PI, was the single laboratory assay that correlated with stallion fertility. The use of H33258 requires a laser that operates with ultraviolet light excitation, which is not standard on all flow cytometric machines. Alternatively a fluorometer can be used. Another option is the simultaneous analysis of sperm viability using H33258 and sperm motility with modern CASA systems (e.g., HTM-IVOS or SpermVision). As an alternative in the field, if fluorescent microscopy or flow cytometry is not available, simple light microscopic evaluation of background smears stained with eosin-nigrosin can also be used to differentiate between viable and non-viable cells.

Fluorochromes used to assess sperm viability can be used in combination in order to identify live spermatozoa, which are green (stained by CFDA or SYBR-14), and dead, which are red (stained by PI). Harkema and Boyle[105] reported the combination of CFDA/PI, Casey et al.[114] on Hoechst 33258, and Garner and Johnson[106] SYBR-14 for stallion semen analysis. At present, the viability stain(s) most commonly used are combinations of SYBR-14 and PI, sold commercially as LIVE/DEAD Sperm Viability kit (Molecular Probes Inc, The Netherlands) (Fig. 6-4, *top panel*). Live/dead stains typically are of low diagnostic value in cases in which sperm motility is good, since sperm motility is highly correlated with sperm viability in stallions. Thus, despite individual variation between stallions, expectedly 70%–80% of the sperm in a fresh ejaculate from a normal stallion are viable. However, in animals with unexplained high percentages of immotile sperm, combined viability (live/dead) staining may identify an explanation for the pathology. Viability stains can also be used in combination with stains for assessing other components of sperm function by flow cytometry, such as acrosomal integrity (FITC-PNA/SYTO-17/PI)[133] or mitochondrial function (PI/SYBR-14/JC-1).[65]

Functional Integrity of Sperm Plasma Membrane: Hypo-osmotic Swelling Test

Spermatozoa react to hypo-osmolality by developing bent or curled tails. In the classic hypo-osmotic swelling test (HOST) this property is used to characterize membrane integrity by testing osmoregulatory function of the cells. This assay is a relatively simple test to evaluate the functional integrity of the spermatozoal membrane. Jeyendran et al.[134,135] developed this assay for human spermatozoa (Fig. 6-5), and since then the HOST has been used in several species including the stallion.[102,136,137] When spermatozoa are exposed to hypo-osmotic conditions, they will undergo morphological alteration and their size is increased. During HOST, the biochemically active spermatozoa, because of the influx of water, will undergo swelling and increase in volume to establish equilibrium between the fluid compartment within the spermatozoa and the extracellular environment. This volume increase is associated with the spherical expansion of the cell membrane covering the tail, thus forcing the flagellum to coil inside the membrane.

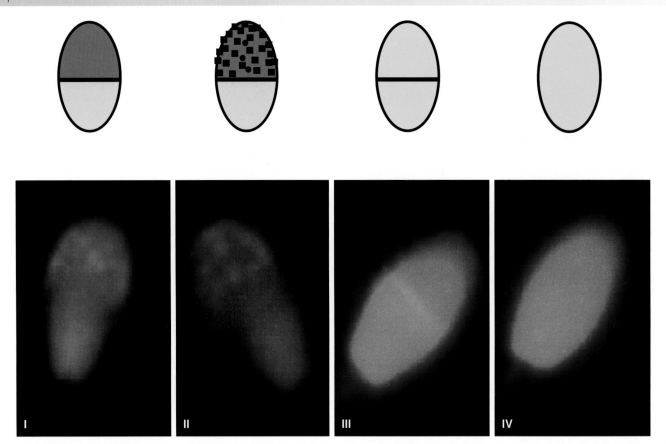

Figure 6-4. Schematic drawing (top panel) and fluorescence microscopy images (bottom panel) of stallion spermatozoa using a standard acrosomal stain. Fluorescein isothiocyanate conjugated to peanut agglutinin FITC-PNA/PI.[116] PNA binds to the outer acrosomal membrane, and has been used successfully to determine the acrosomal status of stallion sperm. Fixed, permeabilized sperm are incubated in the presence of FITC-PNA/PI and then washed. Acrosome-intact sperm will fluoresce evenly across the entire acrosomal cap *(I)*. Sperm in the process of reacting to acrosome show patchy fluorescence over the acrosome *(II)*, whereas those that have acrosome reacted most typically and do not fluoresce over the acrosome *(IV)* or fluoresce only over the equatorial segment *(III)*. Acrosome-intact and reacted sperm can then be counted manually using a fluorescent microscope. Acrosomal responsiveness in sperm of stallions could be determined by running the assay both with and without an inducer of the acrosome reaction and calculating the difference of acrosome reaction rate between both. Alternatively, flow cytometry can be used to count larger numbers of sperm.

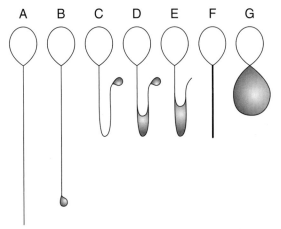

Figure 6-5. Schematic representation of typical morphologic changes of human spermatozoa subjected to hypoosmotic stress. **A,** No change. **B-G,** Various types of tail changes. Tail region showing swelling is indicated by shaded area. (From Jeyendran RS, Van der Ven HH, Perez-Palaez M, Crabo BG, Zaneveld LJD: *J Reprod Fertil* 70: 219, 1984.)

Coiling of the tail begins at the distal end of the tail and proceeds toward the midpiece and head as the osmotic pressure of the suspending media is decreased. The optimal hypo-osmotic medium should exert an osmotic stress large enough to cause an observable increase in volume, but small enough to prevent the lysis of the sperm membrane. Optimal results can be obtained at 50–150 mOsm/L. HOST values are well correlated with progressive motility. French researchers suggested that the HOST performed on fresh semen is the best predictive test of the freezability of stallion semen.[136] Relationship of HOST to fertility in stallions was studied by Neild et al.[138] Katila et al.[139] tested commercially used frozen semen from 31 stallions and compared results with foaling rates of 1085 mares. The HOST was carried out using a 100-mOsm solution and an incubation of 45 minutes at 37°C. A significant correlation was found between foaling rate and HOST performed on sperm immediately after thawing or after an incubation of 3 hours at 37°C.

The traditional HOST considers swollen sperm with curled tails as intact. However, this evaluation is somewhat subjective and is not quantitatively rigorous. Since sperm integrity can be detected only via the possession of curled tails, it is not possible with this test to either determine the percentage of intact sperm under isotonic conditions or distinguish between the intact sperm that have not developed curled tails under hypo-osmotic conditions and defective cells that did swell but then ruptured. However, response to osmotic challenge can be measured quantitatively using an electronic cell counter (Casy1, Schärfe System, Reutlingen)[140]; this system evaluates not only the percentage of swollen cells, but also the swelling level. In this instrument, cell volume is determined by changes in electrical resistance as sperm pass through a capillary pore; the resulting data are expressed on the basis of cell frequency distribution.[140,141]

Capacitation Status and Membrane Fluidity of Spermatozoa

Freshly ejaculated stallion spermatozoa are unable to fertilize unless they undergo a series of biochemical changes referred to as capacitation.[102,142,143] Sperm capacitation involves a series of events including influx of extracellular calcium, increase in cyclic AMP, decrease in intracellular pH, loss of membrane cholesterol, changes in membrane phospholipid content, and exposure of membrane progesterone receptors. These changes are associated with removal of adherent seminal plasma proteins and phospholipid rearrangements within the membrane. The molecular pathways of capacitation appear to vary somewhat among species.[142,144,145] Most importantly, however, capacitation appears to destabilize the sperm's membrane to prepare it for the acrosome reaction, a prerequisite to fertilize an egg.

Frozen-thawed stallion sperm typically possess some of the structural changes of capacitated sperm, thus leading to the hypothesis that the freeze-thaw process leads to premature capacitation of sperm.[146] This has been attributed to be one reason for lower fertility results and shortened longevity of frozen-thawed stallion sperm.

In AI practice, tests to evaluate capacitation status of stallion sperm are carried out either to determine whether sperm are prematurely capacitated (as a result of cooled-storage or cryopreservation) or to determine whether capacitation can occur normally *in vitro* in response to certain fertilization media. Several different tests have been described to evaluate the capacitation status of stallion sperm by assaying functional and structural events during the process of capacitation (including but not limited to hyperactivated motility,[147,148] tyrosine phosphorylation,[149–151] calcium metabolism,[122] and membrane cholesterol/phospholipid changes[152]).

Sperm that have undergone capacitation are said to become hyperactivated and display hyperactivated motility. The proportion of spermatozoa with hyperactive movement can be estimated by subjective microscopic examination or by using CASA systems. Although there are no values that indicate hyperactivation, a significant increase of VCL and amplitude of lateral head displacement (ALH) and a decrease in straightness compared with preincubation values are generally regarded as characteristic signs of hyperactivation.

Tyrosine phosphorylation of proteins within the flagellum occurs during the process of capacitation. Tyrosine phosphorylation has been described in several other mammalian species, including horses, and thus has been established as a diagnostic tool to determine capacitation of spermatozoa. Immunoblotting combined with an antiphosphotyrosine antibody to test for an increase in the number of proteins that are tyrosine phosphorylated has been developed and is currently used in research to study capacitation status in stallion sperm using Western blot techniques[149,153] or flow cytometry.[151]

The chlortetracycline assay (CTC) is used to detect capacitation and acrosome reactions of stallion spermatozoa.[121] In this assay, capacitation status is followed via calcium-mediated changes using the fluorescent antibiotic CTC. CTC traverses the cell membrane of the spermatozoa, enters intracellular compartments containing free calcium, and binds to calcium, resulting in green fluorescence. Differences in binding patterns of CTC allow discrimination between capacitated, non-capacitated, and acrosome intact vs. reacted sperm (Fig. 6-6). The CTC assay requires intense fluorescent microscopic analysis by a skilled person, but on the other hand, simultaneous measurement of both capacitation status and acrosomal status is possible.

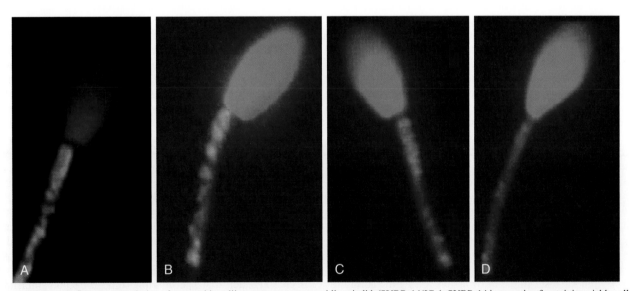

Figure 6-6. Triple-stain fluorescent technique for use with stallion spermatozoa: propidium iodide/SYBR-14/JC-1. SYBR-14 is an option for staining viable cells. This compound is cell permeable and brightly stains only the nuclei of living cells. This compound also fluoresces green in response to excitation. Propidium iodide (PI) is a membrane-impermeable, fluorescent nucleic acid stain. Since PI cannot cross intact cell membranes, it gains access to nuclear DNA only when cell membranes are damaged (i.e., only in non-viable cells). Once bound to DNA, PI fluoresces red in response to excitation. Therefore, non-viable sperm will fluoresce red (**A**). Analyzing mitochondrial function offers a means of assessing the "motility potential" of sperm. This can be performed with stains that attach preferentially to the depolarized membrane of active mitochondria, such as JC-1. Because JC-1 produces a membrane potential-sensitive shift in color pattern, it clearly separates sperm into levels of mitochondrial function. Decreasing mitochondrial potential is depicted in **B** to **D**.

The increase in intracellular free calcium believed to be associated with capacitation can also be detected using fluorophores that penetrate the plasma membrane and change their spectra when bound to calcium (e.g., fluo-3-acetomethoxy ester [fluo-3AM], fura red-AM ester, and indo-1 AM).[123,154]

Membrane changes associated with sperm capacitation, including the loss of membrane cholesterol and phospholipid rearrangements within the membrane, can be assessed using filipin[152] and ideally with the hydrophobic dye Merocyanine-540.[122] M540 is believed to detect a decreased packing order of phospholipids in the outer leaflet of the plasma membrane lipid bilayer, which is believed to occur in capacitated spermatozoa. Harrison and Gadella[155] showed that bicarbonate triggers capacitation of stallion spermatozoa. The merocyanin assay showed that the membrane fluidity changes induced by bicarbonate and detected by M540 precede the calcium influx detected by CTC, making M540 a better method for evaluating the early events of capacitation.[122]

Incorporation techniques using labeled phospholipid analogs and binding proteins (e.g., C6NBD, FITC-conjugated Annexin V) can also be used to investigate the phospholipid changes by binding of Annexin with phosphatidylserine and phosphatidylethanolamine occurring in the plasma membrane of spermatozoa undergoing capacitation.[156]

In practice, data are lacking on normal standard values for percentages of capacitated sperm obtained immediately after semen collection, after cooled storage, or after freeze/thaw, as well as for the percentage of sperm that capacitate in response to certain fertilization media from different stallion populations. Thus, whenever ability of stallion sperm to undergo capacitation is questionable, the results of the test case must be compared with those of a fertile stallion treated under the same conditions.

Acrosomal Integrity and Function of Spermatozoa

The acrosome reaction allows the sperm by exocytotic release of acrosomal enzymes to penetrate the zona pellucida of the egg.[101,111,142] The species-specific zona pellucida protein that serves as a sperm receptor also stimulates a series of events that lead to fusion between the plasma membrane and outer acrosomal membrane.[157,158] Membrane fusion and vesiculation expose the acrosomal contents, leading to leakage of acrosomal enzymes from the sperm's head. As the acrosome reaction progresses and the sperm passes through the zona pellucida, more and more of the plasma membrane and acrosomal contents are lost. By the time the sperm traverses the zona pellucida, the entire anterior surface of its head, down to the inner acrosomal membrane, is denuded. Stallion sperm that lose their acrosomes or have undergone spontaneous acrosome reaction prematurely immediately after semen collection, after cooled storage, or after freezing and thawing are unable to bind to the zona pellucida and thereby are no longer capable of fertilization. Assessment of acrosomal integrity of sperm is one main target of semen analysis. Therefore, assays to analyze acrosomal status were developed in two ways; either by measurement of the initial percentage of acrosome reacted sperm in the test sample or by assays testing the ability to undergo acrosome reaction in response to adequate stimuli.

Most methods available to assess acrosomal integrity are based on the use of dyes or fluorescent markers. These methods are inadequate for evaluating the existence of primary acrosomal defects (e.g., knobbed acrosomes). Intact acrosomes will be labeled with the acrosome-specific dye or fluorophore, whereas sperm with reacted acrosomes will not; this relationship could be determined either by microscopical counting or, in the case of fluorophores, by using a flow cytometer.[112,133]

In general, fluorescent staining of acrosomes can be achieved by two methods: (1) using spermatozoa with alcohol-permeabilized plasma and acrosomal membranes,[116,159] which allow fluorescent-labeled lectins to enter and stain intact acrosomes, or (2) using viable non-permeabilized spermatozoa. The ideal standard acrosomal stain is using fluorescently labeled agglutinins from peas (PSA) or peanut (PNA) plants. The most commonly used method to analyze acrosomal integrity is with a plant lectin labeled by a fluorescent probe (lectins conjugated with fluorescein isothiocyanate [FITC]). PNA (*Arachis hypogea* agglutinin) is a lectin from the peanut plant that binds to β-galactose moieties, which are exclusively associated with the outer acrosomal membrane; thus, FITC-PNA (excitation/emission 488/515 nm wavelength) has been used successfully to determine the acrosomal status of acrosome-intact stallion sperm.[115,116] PSA (*Pisum sativum* agglutinin) is a lectin from the pea plant that binds to α-mannose and α-galactose moieties of the acrosomal matrix. Since PSA cannot penetrate an intact acrosomal membrane, only acrosome-reacted or damaged spermatozoa will stain, which is commonly assessed in combination with fluorescence microscopy.[113,117] Permeabilization of spermatozoal membranes has the disadvantage that acrosomal integrity and viability cannot be assessed simultaneously. However, PNA is believed to display less non-specific binding to other areas of the sperm, thus some laboratories favor this over PSA. FITC-PSA or FITC-PNA labeling of stallion spermatozoa is used in order to determine whether there is an association between the acrosome reaction and the incidence of subfertility in stallions. Acrosome-intact sperm will fluoresce evenly across the entire acrosomal cap. Under a fluorescent microscope, sperm in the process of acrosome reaction show patchy fluorescence over the acrosome, whereas those that have acrosome reacted most typically do not fluoresce or fluoresce only over the equatorial segment (see Fig. 6-6). Acrosome-intact and reacted sperm can be counted manually using a fluorescent microscope, or alternatively, flow cytometry can be used to count larger numbers of sperm.

Monoclonal antibodies specific for an acrosomal antigen can be used to evaluate integrity of acrosomal membranes in combination with indirect immunolabeling techniques. The antigen is localized at the inner surface of the outer acrosomal membrane. Only cells with damaged plasma and acrosomal membranes will bind primary antibody and demonstrate fluorescence after exposure to a secondary antibody (anti-mouse IgG-FITC) when viewed by epifluorescence microscopy.[160]

The acrosome reaction in equine sperm can be induced by exposing capacitated sperm to suitable inducers such as progesterone, calcium ionophore A23187, heparin, and PC12.[62,143,161–164] Induction of the acrosome reaction with calcium ionophore (A23187) is rapid and does not require capacitation of sperm. Ionophores (e.g., A23187) are non-physiological stimuli that induce influx of calcium into the cell. This will result in the acrosome reaction in the major number of intact sperm. It has been suggested that sperm from some infertile/subfertile stallions have a <20% acrosome reaction rate when exposed to ionophore treatment. Others have reported that the drastically reduced ability of spermatozoa to acrosome react when exposed to ionophore A23187 for up to 3 hours was the sole abnormal spermatozoal characteristic in a group of severely subfertile stallions. Acrosome reaction in this group was 6%, compared with

84% in normal stallions.[165] Demonstration of reduced acrosomal responsiveness in sperm of stallions has been a major breakthrough in shedding light on the reason of subfertility in specific candidates. A possible explanation for this condition lies on the fact that the molar ratio of cholesterol-to-phospholipid was 2.5 times greater in the seminal plasma and 1.9 times greater in whole sperm of subfertile stallions compared with fertile stallions.[166] Furthermore, the discovery of an alteration in the cholesterol-to-phospholipid ratio in the sperm of affected stallions may allow further elucidation of the underlying acrosomal problem, and this finding may lead to therapeutic dietetic options in affected stallions.[167] However, prevalence of both phenomena (acrosomal reaction rate, cholesterol-to-phospholipid ratio in the sperm) needs further confirmation on larger numbers of stallions.

Induction of the acrosome reaction with progesterone is the more physiological option.[150,168] There is evidence that the initial percentage of spontaneous acrosome reactions may be higher in subfertile than in fertile stallions. On the other hand, the incidence of a progesterone-induced acrosome reaction was significantly lower in subfertile (6%) compared with fertile (17%) stallions, suggesting that assessment of the induced acrosome reaction may be a useful parameter to assess fertility.[169,170] In addition, the percentage of spermatozoa with exposed progesterone receptors has been reported to correlate highly with fertility of stallions.[171] Therefore, it seems obvious that this approach could serve as an excellent diagnostic assay. On the other hand, this assay is not easy to run and requires that the sperm be capacitated in vitro.

The golden standard to evaluate acrosomal status in the stallion is to perform electron microscopy.[34,91] However, this approach is limited by costs of the microscope, the need for trained personnel, and the limited number of sperm examined per sample. Although this technique has limited use in routine practice, electron microscopical evaluation of acrosomal status can be performed at referral centers.

Regardless of which assay is chosen to evaluate initial acrosomal status or the ability of sperm to acrosome react, normal values have not been validated for large numbers of fertile or subfertile stallion populations. Thus, if any of the tests are to be used in a clinical setting, positive controls from known fertile animals must be run simultaneously.

Oocyte Binding of Spermatozoa

The physiological inducer of the acrosome reaction is the zona pellucida.[158,168] For sperm to bind to the zona pellucida, it must possess an intact acrosome and have capacitated sufficiently to expose their zona binding proteins. Therefore, the ideal test of a sperm's ability to acrosome react is to expose sperm to intact or hemizonae.

Those assays have been developed to test the ability of sperm to bind to homologous[170,172,173] and heterologous[158,174] zona pellucida, and the results had been correlated well with the fertility of some candidate stallions. Unfortunately, this assay is even more difficult, costly, and time consuming than the progesterone-induced acrosome reaction assay. Similar to the progesterone assay, sperm can undergo the zona-induced acrosome reaction only if they have previously been capacitated. In addition, the zona assay requires that a reasonable number of intact or hemizonae be available. Isolation of equine zonae is difficult and costly, and maturation state of the oocytes will have an impact on the results. Furthermore, assays that evaluate the ability of sperm to fertilize oocytes are carried out in vitro[175] under nonphysiological conditions, therefore making these assays of limited practical use.

Mitochondrial Integrity of Spermatozoa

The percentage of normal functional mitochondria is significantly correlated with the percentage of viable and motile sperm.[108,176] In stallions, a relationship between mitochondrial function and motility, as well as some sperm velocity traits (linearity and straightness), has been observed.[65,177] Evidence in other species suggests that glycolysis in the flagellum rather than oxidative phosphorylation by the mitochondria in the midpiece represents an additional source of ATP for axonemal function and sperm motility.[178] Thus, the value of using mitochondrial functional assays as the sole means of testing for flagellar movement potential remains unresolved. Rhodamine 123 (R123) and MitoTracker (MITO) fluorochromes have been used to evaluate mitochondrial function of spermatozoa by labeling a negative potential across the inner mitochondrial membrane.[179] Only actively respiring mitochondria will take up these dyes, causing them to fluoresce green. All functioning mitochondria stain green with R123 and MITO, and consequently no distinction can be made between spermatozoa exhibiting different respiratory rates. R123 is not suitable for use in experiments in which the spermatozoa are treated with aldehyde fixatives, whereas the MITO probes are well retained during the fixation process. The mitochondrial stain 5,5′,6,6′-tetrachloro-1,1′,3,3′-tetraethyl-benzimidazolyl-carbocyanine iodide (JC-1) does permit identification of sperm with varying degrees of mitochondrial function. JC-1 is a lipophilic cationic fluorescent carbocyanine dye that is internalized by all functioning mitochondria, where at low concentrations it is present as a monomer and fluoresces green. In highly functional mitochondria, the concentration of JC-1 inside the mitochondria increases and the stain forms aggregates that fluoresce orange. Thus, JC-1 fluorescence intensity allows division of stallion spermatozoa into subpopulations of sperm with high, moderate, and low mitochondrial membrane potential by fluorescence microscopy (see Fig. 6-4, *bottom panel*). Flow cytometric evaluation can separate highly functioning mitochondria, exhibiting a greater red-to-green ratio, and poorly functioning mitochondria, exhibiting a lower red-to-green ratio.[109,110]

Sperm Chromatin

Sperm chromatin is highly organized and compact and consists of DNA and nucleoproteins that are more condensed than those of somatic or spermatogenic cells. It has been suggested that the high degree of condensation of the sperm chromatin protects the paternal genome during transport through the male and female reproductive tracts, and protects it from environmental stress. A high integrity of sperm chromatin is also necessary for proper fertilization during sperm DNA methylation, decondensation, male pronucleus formation, and subsequent embryo development.[180–186] It has been confirmed in men that reduced sperm chromatin integrity may allow normal fertilization of the egg, but subsequent embryo and fetal development may be impaired.[187] A similar phenomena may exist in the horse, where fertilization rates are very high but pregnancy rates are considerably lower due to a high early pregnancy loss rate.[188,189] This could be due to the fact that sperm with chromatin structure abnormalities are able to fertilize oocytes but fail to sustain proper embryo development and a successful pregnancy. These sperm characteristics as mentioned before are called *uncompensable sperm traits*.[98] The fertility of males with uncompensable sperm traits cannot be changed by increasing the quantity of sperm in the insemination dosage.

Sperm DNA integrity or fragmentation can be evaluated in a variety of ways.[186] The most widely used, statistically robust, and well-established test is called the Sperm Chromatin Structure Assay (SCSA), introduced by Evenson in 1980. Other methods to evaluate chromatin integrity are the Sperm DNA Fragmentation Assay (SDFA), similar to the SCSA; deoxynucleotidyl transferase (Tdt)–mediated dUTP nick end labeling (TUNEL) assay; single cell gel electrophoresis (COMET) assay; and acridine orange staining technique (AOT). Recently, the sperm chromatin dispersion (SCD) test was introduced for evaluating sperm DNA fragmentation. Although these assays have not been used to the same extent as the SCSA in breeding soundness evaluation in the stallion, they are commonly established in human-assisted reproduction technologies.

The SCSA is applied following the procedure described by Evenson and Jost.[125] The ideal sample is native sperm snap-frozen immediately after semen collection and stored in liquid nitrogen until start of the analysis. After thawing, sperm are treated with a low-pH (1.2) detergent solution which will not affect normal DNA but will denature fragmented DNA. Then sperm are stained with purified acridine orange (AO). Cells are analyzed using a flow cytometer after being excited by a laser light source. AO, which is intercalated with double-stranded, native DNA, emits green (515–530 nm) fluorescence, whereas AO associated with single-stranded, denatured DNA emits red ($\geq$630 nm) fluorescence. Thus, sperm chromatin damage can be quantified by detection of the metachromatic shift from green (native, double-stranded DNA) to red (denatured, single-stranded DNA) fluorescence. The ratio of red/red+green yields the percentage of DNA fragmentation, referred to previously as comp alpha-t and recently as Denaturation Fragmentation Index (DFI) (Fig. 6-7, *A*).[125]

Test parameters for sperm DNA integrity are weakly to moderately correlated with conventional examinations of sperm motility, viability, and morphology in men[184,190] and stallions.[126,191,192] Semen samples with normal conventional parameters may have very poor DNA quality that contributes to lowered pregnancy rates. Therefore, testing sperm chromatin integrity offers additional clinical information not provided by conventional semen analysis.

In humans, a threshold of 30% DFI is frequently suggested as a cut-off to distinguish between a potentially fertile vs. infertile semen sample. DFI statistically derived thresholds of 0%–15%, 16%–29%, and >30% correlate with high, moderate, and low *in vivo* fertility potential in men, respectively, indicating that if the DFI is >30%, there is a significantly greater risk for infertility.[184,185,193] A normal sample should have less than 15% of the sperm with DNA damage. These numbers are thresholds, meaning that above 30%, the outcome for most couples resulted in failure to establish a successful pregnancy even though only 30% of the sperm were damaged.[194,195] Negative relationships between percentage of DFI sperm and pregnancy rates could be observed in stallions.[126,191,196] Kenney et al.[191] reported higher rates of sperm chromatin denaturation in semen from subfertile than from fertile stallions (32% vs. 16%) and a negative correlation between denaturation score and seasonal pregnancy rate. In a group of fertile stallions. Love et al.[126] was able to demonstrate variations in SCSA

that correlated moderately with both seasonal and per-cycle fertility rates. They suggested that the SCSA could be used to prospectively rank stallion fertility and to identify changes associated with impending fertility loss. This study reported an average of less than 12% DFI in the group of highly fertile stallions, greater than 15% in the group of stallions with moderate fertility, and greater than 30% in the group of severely subfertile stallions (Fig. 6-7, *B-D*). Interestingly, in groups with a moderate and low fertility score, the stallions exhibit similar percentages of morphologically normal sperm, suggesting that morphological values alone cannot account for the variation in fertility between stallions. Others[196] reported a similar relationship between DFI and pregnancy rate (r = −0.63) in eleven stallions, but in contrast, a significant negative correlation between DFI and percentage of morphological normal sperm was detected.

In summary, the SCSA provides an additional characteristic of sperm quality in stallions that is independent of those parameters routinely evaluated by conventional methods, thereby providing the clinician with an additional test that could explain changes in stallion fertility when other seminal parameters are unchanged. In addition to being a diagnostic aid, the SCSA can also measure alterations in DNA quality caused by environmental changes, such as the effect of seminal plasma, storage time, and extender type.[126,135] SCSA can be used to evaluate the DFI of frozen semen samples; however, cryopreservation of stallion sperm does not seem to result in damage to chromatin integrity of spermatozoa.

In addition to the SCSA test, the SDFA test, used in human laboratories, measures the intensity of the green fluorescence (High DNA Stainability [HDS]) after acridine orange exposure. An abnormal HDS score indicates a high percentage of immature sperm present in semen, which could indicate impaired seminiferous tubule function, Sertoli cell dysfunction, varicocele or illness. Relationship of HDS to fertility is controversial.[190,197,198] Thus, analysis of the clinical significance of an abnormal HDS score has not yet been determined.

DNA fragmentation in spermatozoa can also be assessed using the terminal deoxynucleotidyl TUNEL assay; this assay detects both single- and double-stranded DNA breaks by labeling the free 3′-OH terminus with modified nucleotides in an enzymatic reaction with terminal TdT and can be analyzed microscopically or with flow cytometry.[156]

The COMET assay is a microscopic assay in which sperm are embedded in agarose on a glass slide, lysed, applied to electrophoresis, stained with ethidium bromide, and observed under epifluorescence to score the degree of migration of single and double DNA strand break fragments.[199] Sperm possessing more DNA damage exhibit larger DNA migration areas similar to a comet's tail compared to sperm possessing little DNA damage.

The AOT is a simple microscopic procedure based on the same principle as the SCSA.[187,200] Unfortunately, indistinct colors, rapid fading of fluorescence, and heterogeneous staining of slides makes AOT a test of questionable value in laboratory practice.

A new method, the sperm chromatin dispersion (SCD), was recently introduced for evaluating sperm DNA fragmentation.[201] The SCD test is based on the principle that sperm with fragmented DNA fail to produce the characteristic halo of dispersed DNA loops that is observed in sperm with non-fragmented DNA following acid denaturation and removal of nuclear proteins. The degree of DNA damage in a sperm sample can be quantified using the sperm DNA fragmentation index (sDFI, percentage of fragmented cells) as assessed using the Sperm-Halomax kit

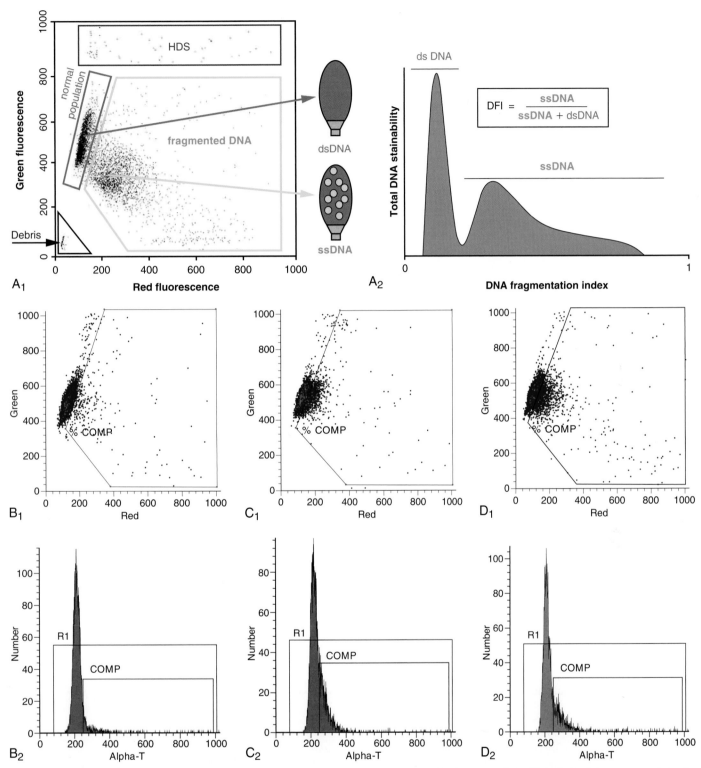

Figure 6-7. Results of sperm chromatin structure analysis (SCSA) according to a procedure described by Evenson and Jost.[125] Analysis of the sperm population is represented in the scattergrams (A_1, B_1, C_1, and D_1), and sperm cell analysis is depicted in the histograms (A_2, B_2, C_2, and D_2). Distribution of sperm cells in the scatterplot (A_1) is from a typical SCSA sample. In the scattergrams, a fertile (B_1), moderately subfertile (C_1), and severely subfertile (D_1) stallion are shown. Percentage of high DFI-sperm (cells outside the main "normal" population [i.e., cells within the face labeled "fragmented DNA" in A1]) indicates those cells that have more red fluorescence (denaturated, fragmented ssDNA) than the main (normal, unfragmented dsDNA) population. Cells labeled "HDS" represent immature cells with high DNA stainability (HDS). Illustrated histograms (A_2, B_2, C_2, and D_2) present distribution of DNA Fragmentation Index (DFI) of the scattergrams. The DFI is a ratio expressed as a percentage of sperm fluorescence, with both unfragmented dsDNA (green fluorescence) and fragmented ssDNA (red fluorescence).

(ChromaCell SL, Madrid, Spain). This assay provides an easy way for estimating DNA fragmentation by direct cell counting under the microscope.

BIOCHEMICAL MARKERS OF STALLION FERTILITY (COMPONENTS OF SEMINAL PLASMA)

Identification of biochemical markers of spermatozoal function may be helpful in fertility diagnostics by characterizing enzymatic and functional composition of specific subcellular domains. Most of these methods have been used in bulls and boars, but constantly increasing numbers of tests have been proposed in the stallion.[202] However, it is necessary to select between enzymes found only in sperm cells, specific domains of sperm cells, seminal plasma, and extenders. These approaches can be distinguished by their specific markers in order to target for specific sperm functions such as caspase for apoptosis,[203,204] protein tyrosine phosphorylation activity,[149,151,153] heparin-binding proteins for capacitation,[43] glutathione peroxidase,[205] bodipy-c_{11},[206–209] reactive oxygen species [ROS] for oxidative stress,[210–212] spermadhesins,[43,213] zonadhesins,[214–216] and cysteine rich proteins 1 and 3 for sperm oocyte interaction.[217–219]

Alkaline phosphatase (AP) represents a classical biochemical marker in seminal plasma of stallions.[46] Detection of high AP activity by standard serum chemistry indicates normal contribution of testicular and epididymal secretions into the ejaculate. Measuring AP can be used as a marker for ejaculation in the stallion and can aid to distinguish azoospermia of testicular origin from azoospermia resulting from ejaculation failure (e.g., plugged ampullae).[220] Fertile stallions have AP activities in seminal plasma over 15000 IU/L. AP activities <100 IU/L indicate that the sample does not contain fluid from the epididymis and testicles.[46,221]

Reactive oxygen species (ROS) such as hydrogen peroxide, superoxide anion and hydroxyl radical in physiological quantities are known to be necessary for cell survival but will result in cell damage at elevated levels.[210] Several redox systems are involved in the physiological control of the sperm cell. However, oxidative stress from excess ROS present from either increased production or reduced antioxidant protection is thought to be a major cause of sperm dysfunction predominantly resulting from lipid peroxidation in the plasma membrane. High levels of unsaturated fatty acids of sperm and inability of a repair mechanism may explain susceptibility of sperm to ROS-mediated injury.[212,222,223] Tests assaying ROS generation are carried out by determination of chemiluminescence, lipid peroxidation, and antioxidant capacity.[224] Morte et al.[225] reported that lipid and protein oxidation may aid in the identification of subfertile stallions during the non-breeding season. In this study levels of ROS production never seemed to result in compromised sperm DNA integrity, indicating that measurements were within physiological levels and/or that there is an efficient antioxidant activity in stallion sperm cells. In contrast, ROS and cryopreservation promoted DNA damage in equine sperm.[226]

GENETIC MARKERS OF STALLION FERTILITY

One promising area for future development is the use of genetic markers to predict fertility.[227–229] The assembly of the horse genome was recently publicly released (http://www.broad.mit.edu/mammals/horse/).[230,231] However, the horse genome was studied on a female and not a male horse; thus the genomic information on the horse Y-chromosome has lagged behind. However there is a significant amount of information that has recently been released.[231a] The availability of mammalian genome sequences represents a valuable source of information that can be mined and explored to devise new hypotheses for reproductive research. Novel tools like the 60K SNP-chip and expression microarray will lay the groundwork for several new research studies.[232] Although reproduction and fertility are complex traits that are influenced by environment to a varying extent, the interpretation of genotypic information needs substantial support by reliable and excellent data describing the phenotype.

The discovery of genetic aberrations that lead to infertility in humans and mice has made great progress. From human genetics and the study of mouse mutants, more than 200 genes are known that affect male fertility. Some of the genetic aberrations discovered in humans or mice are also found in infertile domestic animals. The increasing availability of genome sequences of the horse facilitates the analysis of specific candidate genes found out by human or mouse research in domestic animal species. Information obtained from these new technologies is being applied to male fertility, including that of horses.[228,233]

REFERENCES

1. Colenbrander B, Puyk H, Zandee AR, et al: Evaluation of the stallion for breeding. *Acta Vet Scand Suppl* 88:29, 1992.
2. Jasko DJ: Evaluation of stallion semen. In Blanchard TL, Varner DD, eds: *Vet Clin North Am Eq Pract* 8:129, 1992.
3. Amann RP, Hammerstedt RH: In vitro evaluation of sperm quality: an opinion. *J Androl* 14:397, 1993.
4. Malmgren L: Assessing the quality of raw semen: a review. *Theriogenology* 48:523, 1997.
5. Magistrini M, Guitton E, Le Vern Y, et al: New staining methods for sperm evaluation estimated by microscopy and flow cytometry. *Theriogenology* 48:1229, 1997.
6. Juhasz J, Nagy P, Kulcsar M: Method for semen and endocrinological evaluation of the stallion: a review. *Acta Vet Brno* 69:247, 2000.
7. Katila T: In vitro evaluation of frozen-thawed stallion semen: a review. *Acta Vet Scand* 42:199, 2001.
8. Card C: Cellular associations and the differential spermiogram: making sense of stallion spermatozoal morphology. *Theriogenology* 64:558, 2005.
9. Graham JK, Mocé E: Fertility evaluation of frozen/thawed semen. *Theriogenology* 64:492, 2005.
10. Petrunkina AM, Waberski D, Günzel-Apel AR, et al: Determinants of sperm quality and fertility in domestic species. *Reproduction* 134:3, 2007.
11. Klug E: Untersuchungen zur klinischen Andrologie des Pferdes. Die Bedeutung andrologischer Befunde am Hengst für den Zuchteinsatz, Hannover, *Tierärztl Hochsch,* Habil-Schr, 1982.
12. Parlevliet JM, Kemp B, Colenbrander B: Reproductive characteristics and semen quality in maiden Dutch Warmblood stallion. *J Reprod Fertil* 101:183, 1994.
13. Dowsett KF, Pattie WA: Variation in characteristics of stallion semen caused by breed, age and season of year and service frequency. *J Reprod Fertil* 35:45, 1987.
14. Pickett BW, Voss JL, Bowen RA, et al: Seminal characteristics and total scrotal width (T.S.W.) of normal and abnormal stallions. Proc AAEP: 1988, p 485.
15. Paccamonti DL, Buiten AV, Parlevliet JM, et al: Reproductive parameters of miniature stallions. *Theriogenology* 51:1343, 1999.
16. Bielanski W, Kaczmarski F: Morphology of spermatozoa in semen from stallions of normal fertility. *J Reprod Fertil Suppl* 27:39, 1979.
17. Bielanski W, Dudek E, Bittmar A, et al: Some characteristics of common abnormal forms of spermatozoa in highly fertile stallions. *J Reprod Fertil Suppl* 32:21, 1982.
18. Voss JL, Pickett BW, Squires EL: Stallion spermatozoal morphology and motility and their relationship to fertility. *J Am Vet Med Assoc* 178:287, 1981.
19. Voss JL, Pickett BW, Loomis PR: The relationship between seminal characteristics and fertility in Thoroughbred stallions. *J Reprod Fertil Suppl* 32:635, 1982.

20. Dowsett KF, Pattie WA: Characteristics and fertility of stallion semen. *J Reprod Fertil Suppl* 32:1, 1982.

21. Amann RP: Can the fertility potential of a seminal sample be predicted accurately? *J Andrology* 10:89, 1989.

22. Jasko DJ, Lein DH, Foote RH: Determination of the relationship between sperm morphologic classifications and fertility in stallions: 66 cases (1987–1988). *J Am Vet Med Assoc* 197:389, 1990.

23. Jasko DJ, Little TV, Lein DH, et al: Comparison of spermatozoal movement and semen characteristics with fertility in stallions: 64 cases (1987–1988). *J Am Vet Med Assoc* 200:979, 1992.

24. Graham JK: Analysis of stallion semen and its relation to fertility. *Vet Clin Eq Pract* 12:119, 1996.

25. Rodriguez-Martinez H: Laboratory semen assessment and prediction of fertility: still Utopia? *Reprod Domest Anim* 38:312, 2003.

26. Rodriguez-Martinez H: Can we increase the estimative value of semen assessment? *Reprod Domest Anim Suppl* 41:2, 2006.

27. Colenbrander B, Gadella BM, Stout TAE: The predictive value of semen analysis in the evaluation of stallion fertility. *Reprod Domest Anim* 38:305, 2003.

28. Kirk ES, Squires EL, Graham JK: Comparison of in vitro laboratory analyses with the fertility of cryopreserved stallion spermatozoa. *Theriogenology* 64:1422, 2005.

29. Kuisma P, Andersson M, Koskinen E, et al: Fertility of frozen-thawed stallion semen cannot be predicted by the currently used laboratory methods. *Acta Vet Scand* 48:14, 2006.

30. Magistrini M, Vidament M, Clement F, et al: Fertility prediction in stallions. *Anim Reprod Sci* 42:181, 1996.

31. Amann RP: Weaknesses in reports of "fertility" for horses and other species. *Theriogenology* 63:698, 2005.

32. Pickett BW, Squires EL, McKinnon AO: Procedures for collection, evaluation and utilization of stallion semen for artificial insemination. Anim Reprod Lab Colorado State University. Fort Collins, CO, 1987.

33. Parlevliet JM, Colenbrander BC: Prediction of first season stallion fertility of 3-year-old Dutch Warmbloods with prebreeding assessment of percentage of morphologically normal live sperm. *Eq Vet J* 31:248, 1999.

34. Varner DD, Blanchard TL, Brinsko SP, et al: Techniques for evaluating selected reproductive disorders of stallions. *Anim Reprod Sci* 60-61: 493, 2000.

35. Silva PF, Gadella BM: Detection of damage in mammalian sperm cells. *Theriogenology* 65:958, 2006.

36. Love CC, Varner DD, Thompson JA: Intra- and inter-stallion variation in sperm morphology and their relationship with fertility. *J Reprod Fertil Suppl* 56:93, 2000.

37. Clement F, Ladonnet Y, Magistrini M: Sperm morphology and fertility. *Anim Reprod Sci* 68:362, 2001.

38. Veeramachaneni DN, Moeller CL, Sawyer HR: Sperm morphology in stallions: ultrastructure as a functional and diagnostic tool. *Vet Clin Eq* 22:683, 2006.

39. Brito F: Evaluation of stallion sperm morphology. *Clin Tech Eq Pract* 6:249, 2007.

40. Vidament M, Magistrini M, Palmer E, et al: Equine artificial insemination in French National Studs. *Reprod Dom Anim Suppl* 6:61, 1999.

41. Amann RP, Cristanelli MJ, Squires EL: Proteins in stallion seminal plasma. *J Reprod Fertil Suppl* 35:113, 1987.

42. Calvete JJ, Nessau S, Mann K, et al: Isolation and biochemical characterization of stallion seminal-plasma proteins. *Reprod Dom Anim* 29:411, 1994.

43. Töpfer-Petersen E, Ekhlasi-Hundtrieser M, Kirchhoff C, et al: The role of stallion seminal proteins in fertilisation. *Anim Reprod Sci* 89:159, 2005.

44. Sieme H, Katila T, Klug E: Effect of semen collection practices on sperm characteristics before and after storage and on fertility of stallions. *Theriogenology* 61:769, 2004.

45. Janett F, Thun R, Niederer K, et al: Seasonal changes of semen quality and freezability in the Warmblood stallion. *Theriogenology* 60:453, 2003.

46. Turner RM: Current techniques for evaluation of stallion fertility. *Clin Tech Equine Pract* 4:257, 2005.

47. Tomlinson M, Turner J, Powell G, et al: One-step disposable chambers for sperm cell concentration and motility assessment: how do they compare with the World Health Organization's recommended methods. *Human Reprod* 16:121, 2001.

48. Bailey E, Fenning N, Chamberlain S, et al: Validation of sperm counting methods using limits of agreement. *J Andrology* 28:364, 2007.

49. Christensen P, Stryhn H, Hansen C: Discrepancies in the determination of sperm concentration using Bürker-Türk, Thoma and Makler counting chambers. *Theriogenology* 63:992, 2005.

50. Vanderwall DK: Counting spermatozoa with a hemacytometer. *J Equine Vet Sci* 28:244, 2008.

51. Evenson DP, Parks JP, Kaproth MT, et al: Rapid determination on sperm cell concentration in bovine semen by flow cytometry. *J Dairy Sci* 76:86, 1993.

52. Hansen C, Vermeiden T, Vermeiden JPW, et al: Comparison of FAC-SCount AF system, improved Neubauer hemacytometer, Corning 254 photometer, SpermVision, UltiMate and NucleoCounter SP-100 for determination of sperm concentration of boar semen. *Theriogenology* 66:2188, 2006.

53. Amann RP, Katz DF: Reflections on CASA after 25 years. *J Androl* 25:317, 2004.

54. Varner DD, Vaughan SD, Johnson L: Use of a computerized system for evaluation of equine spermatozoal motility. *Am J Vet Res* 52:224, 1991.

55. Jasko DJ, Lein DH, Foote RH: A comparison of two computer-automated semen analysis instruments for the evaluation of sperm motion characteristics in the stallion. *J Andr* 11:453, 1990.

56. Palmer E, Magistrini M: Automated analysis of stallion semen post-thaw motility. *Acta Vet Scand Suppl* 88:137, 1992.

57. Davis RO, Katz DF: Operational standards for CASA instruments. *J Androl* 14:385, 1993.

58. Wessel MT, Althouse GC: Validation of an objective approach for simultaneous assessment of viability and motility of fresh and cooled equine spermatozoa. *Anim Reprod Sci* 94:21, 2006.

59. Bataille B, Magistrini M, Palmer E: Objective determination of sperm motility in frozen-thawed stallion semen. Correlation with fertility. 16th Journée d'étude du CEREOPA, Paris, France. Anim Breed Abstr, 1990, pp 96-106.

60. Burns PJ, Reasner DS: Computerized analysis of sperm motion: effects of glycerol concentration on the cryopreservation of equine spermatozoa. *J Equine Vet Sci* 15:377, 1995.

61. Samper JC, Hellander JC, Crabo BG: Relationship between the fertility of fresh and frozen stallion semen and semen quality. *J Reprod Fertil Suppl* 44:107, 1991.

62. Wilhelm KM, Graham JK, Squires EL: Comparison of the fertility of cryopreserved stallion spermatozoa with sperm motion analyses, flow cytometric evaluation, and zona-free hamster oocyte penetration. *Theriogenology* 46:559, 1996.

63. Evenson DP, Darzynkiewicz Z, Melamed MR: Simultaneous measurement by flow cytometry of sperm cell viability and mitochondrial membrane potential related to cell motility. *J Histochem Cytochem* 30:279, 1982.

64. Kavak A, Johannisson A, Lundeheim N, et al: Evaluation of cryopreserved stallion semen from Tori and Estonian breeds using CASA and flow cytometry. *Anim Reprod Sci* 76:205, 2003.

65. Love CC, Thompson JA, Brinsko SP, et al: Relationship between stallion sperm motility and viability as detected by two fluorescence staining techniques using flow cytometry. *Theriogenology* 60:1127, 2003.

66. Quintero-Moreno A, Miró J, Teresa Rigau A, et al: Identification of sperm subpopulations with specific motility characteristics in stallion ejaculates. *Theriogenology* 59:2003, 1973.

67. Tischner M: Evaluation of deep-frozen semen in stallions. *J Reprod Fertil Suppl* 27:53, 1979.

68. Müller Z: Practicalities of insemination of mares with deep-frozen semen. *J Reprod Fertil Suppl* 35:121, 1987.

69. Bittmar A, Kosiniak K: The role of selected biochemical components of equine seminal plasma in determining suitability for deep-freezing. *Arch Vet Pol* 32:17, 1992.

70. Samper JC, Morris CA: Current methods for stallion semen cryopreservation: a survey. *Theriogenology* 49:895, 1998.

71. Vidament M: French field results (1985–2005) on factors affecting fertility of frozen stallion semen. *Anim Reprod Sci* 89:115, 2005.

72. Loomis PR: Artificial insemination of horses: where is it going? Proc Ann Conf Soc Theriogenol. Nashville, TN: 1999, pp 325-336.

73. Loomis PR, Graham JK: Commercial semen freezing: Individual male variation in cryosurvival and the response of stallion sperm to customized freezing protocols. *Anim Reprod Sci* 105:119, 2008.

74. Davis RO, Gravance CG: Standardization of specimen preparation, staining, and sampling methods improves automated sperm-head morphometry analysis. *Fertil Steril* 59:412, 1993.

75. Ball BA, Mohammed HO: Morphometry of stallion spermatozoa by computer assisted image analysis. *Theriogenology* 44:367, 1995.

76. Gravance CG, Liu IK, Davis RO, et al: Quantification of normal head morphometry of stallion spermatozoa. *J Reprod Fertil* 108:41, 1996.

77. Card C: Detection of abnormal stallion sperm cells by using the Feulgen stain. Proc AAEP Denver, 44:9, 1998.

78. Casey PI, Gravance CG, Davis RO, et al: Morphometric differences in sperm head dimensions of fertile and subfertile stallions. *Theriogenology* 47:575, 1997.

79. Gravance CG, Champion Z, Liu IK, et al: Sperm head morphometry analysis of ejaculate and dismount stallion semen samples. *Anim Reprod Sci* 47:149, 1997.

80. Dott HM: Morphology of stallion spermatozoa. *J Reprod Fertil Suppl* 23:41, 1975.

81. Veeramachaneni DN, Sawyer HR: Use of semen as biopsy material for assessment of health status of the stallion reproductive tract. *Vet Clin North Am Equine Pract* 12:101, 1996.

82. Williams WW: Technique of collecting semen for laboratory examination with a review of several diseased bulls. *Cornell Vet* 10:87, 1920.

83. Karras W: Spermastudien 1. Mitteilung: Eine Methode zur färeberischen Darstellung der Kopfkappen und des Kolloidüberzuges der Spermien. *Monatshefte Prakt Tierhlkd* 2:162, 1950.

84. Schaaf A: Vitalkleuring van stieren sperma met een oplossing van anilineblauw en eosine. *Tijdschr Diergeneesk* 77:815, 1952.

85. Dott HM, Foster GC: A technique for studying the morphology of mammalian spermatozoa which is eosinophilic in a differential "live-dead" stain. *J Reprod Fertil* 29:443, 1972.

86. Oettle EE: Using a new acrosome stain to evaluate sperm morphology. *Vet Med* 81:263, 1986.

87. Hancock JL, Hovell GJR: The collection of boar semen. *Vet Rec* 71:664, 1959.

88. Lagerlöf N: Morphological studies on the change in sperm structure and in the testes of bulls with decreased or abolished fertility. *Acta Pathol Microbiol Scand Suppl* 19:254, 1934.

89. Casserett GW: One solution stain for spermatozoa. *Stain Technol* 22:125, 1953.

90. Hancock JL: The morphology of boar sperm. *J R Micro Soc* 76:84, 1957.

91. Pesch S, Bostedt H, Failing K, et al: Advanced fertility diagnosis in stallion semen using transmission electron microscopy. *Anim Reprod Sci* 91:285, 2006.

92. Kenney RM, Hurtgen J, Pierson R, et al: Theriogenology and the equine, part II: The Stallion (Society for Theriogenology Manual for Clinical Fertility Evaluation of the Stallion). *J Soc Theriog* 9:1100, 1983.

93. Bielanski W: Characteristics of the semen of stallions. Macro- and microscopic investigations with estimation of fertility. Mém Acad Polon Sci Lettr. *Cl Sci Math Nat* 16:59, 1951.

94. Barth A, Oko A: Evaluation of the spermiogram, abnormal morphology of bull spermatozoa. Ames, IA: Iowa State University Press, 1989, pp 271-279.

95. Varner DD: Introduction of the stallion breeding soundness examination form of the Society for Theriogenology, Proc Soc Theriogenology. San Antonio, TX: 2002, pp 113-116.

96. Blom E: Interpretation of spermatic cytology in bulls. *Fertil Steril* 1:223, 1950.

97. Blom E: The ultrastructure of some characteristic sperm defects and a proposal for a new classification of the bull spermiogram. *Nord Vet Med* 25:383, 1973.

98. Saacke RG, Dalton JC, Nadir S, et al: Relationship of seminal traits and insemination time to fertilization rate and embryo quality. *Anim Reprod Sci* 60–61:663, 2000.

99. Love CC: Stallion semen evaluation and interpretation. Proc Soc Theriogenology. Colorado Springs, CO: 2002, pp 93-102.

100. Morrell JM: Applications of flow cytometry to artificial insemination: a review. *Vet Rec* 129:375, 1991.

101. Gadella BM, Rathi R, Brouwers JF, et al: Capacitation and the acrosome reaction in equine spermatozoa. *Anim Reprod Sci* 68:249, 2001.

102. Caiza de la Cueva FI, Pujol MR, Rigau T, et al: Resistance to osmotic stress of horse spermatozoa: The role of ionic pumps and their relationship to cryopreservation success. *Theriogenology* 48:947, 1997.

103. Garner DL, Pinkel D, Johnson LA, et al: Assessment of spermatozoal function using dual fluorescent staining and flow cytometric analyses. *Biol Reprod* 34:127, 1986.

104. Harrison RAP, Vickers SE: Use of fluorescent probes to assess membrane integrity in mammalian spermatozoa. *J Reprod Fertil* 88:343, 1990.

105. Harkema W, Boyle MS: Use of fluorescent stains to assess membrane integrity of equine spermatozoa. Proc 12th Intern Congr Anim Reprod. The Hague, The Netherlands: 3:1424, 1992.

106. Garner DL, Johnson LA: Viability assessment of mammalian sperm using SYBR-14 and propidium iodide. *Biol Reprod* 53:276, 1995.

107. Merkies K, Chenier T, Plante C, et al: Assessment of stallion permatozoa viability by flow cytometry and light microscope analysis. *Theriogenology* 54:1215, 2000.

108. Garner DL, Thomas CA, Joerg HW, et al: Fluorometric assessments of mitochondrial function and viability in cryopreserved bovine spermatozoa. *Biol Reprod* 57:1401, 1997.

109. Garner DL, Thomas CA: Organelle-specific probe JC-1 identifies membrane potential differences in the mitochondrial function of bovine sperm. *Mol Reprod Dev* 53:222, 1999.

110. Gravance CG, Garner DL, Baumber J, et al: Assessment of equine sperm mitochondrial function using JC-1. *Theriogenology* 53:1691, 2000.

111. Cross NL, Meizel S: Methods for evaluating the acrosomal status of mammalian sperm. *Biol Reprod* 41:635, 1989.

112. Jankovicová J, Simon M, Antalíková J, Horovská L: Acrosomal and viability status of bovine spermatozoa evaluated by two staining methods. *Acta Vet Hung* 56:133, 2008.

113. Farlin ME, Iasko DI, Graham IK, et al: Assessment of *Pisum sativum* agglutinin in identifying acrosomal damage in stallion spermatozoa. *Mol Reprod Dev* 32:23, 1992.

114. Casey PJ, Hillman RB, Robertson KR, et al: Validation of an acrosomal stain for equine sperm that differentiates between living and dead sperm. *J Androl* 14:289, 1993.

115. Cheng FP, Fazeli A, Voorhout WF, et al: Use of PNA (peanut agglutinin) to assess the acrosomal status and the zona pellucida induced acrosome reaction in stallion spermatozoa. *J Andr* 17:674, 1996.

116. Blottner S, Wegner H, Roelants H, et al: Flow cytometric determination of the acrosomal status of bull and stallion spermatozoa after marking with FITC-conjugated PNA (peanut agglutinin), *Tierärztl Umsch* 53:442, 1998.

117. Arruda RP, Souza NL, Marques A, et al: Evaluation of techniques using CFDA/PI, H258/FITC-PSA and Trypan blue/Giemsa for assessment of the viability and acrosomal integrity of cryopreserved equine spermatozoa. *Theriogenology* 57:477, 2002.

118. Bosard TS, Love CC, Brinsko SP, et al: Evaluation and diagnosis of acrosome function/dysfunction in the stallion. *Anim Reprod Sci* 89:215, 2005.

119. Brum AM, Thomas AD, Sabeur K, et al: Evaluation of Coomassie blue staining of the acrosome of equine and canine spermatozoa. *Am J Vet Res* 67:358, 2006.

120. Ward CR, Storey BT: Determination of the time course of capacitation in mouse spermatozoa using a chlortetracycline fluorescence assay. *Dev Biol* 104:287, 1984.

121. Varner DD, Ward CR, Storey BA, et al: Induction and characterization of acrosome reaction in equine spermatozoa. *Am J Vet Res* 48:1383, 1987.

122. Rathi R, Colenbrander B, Bevers MM, et al: Evaluation of in vitro capacitation of stallion spermatozoa. *Biol Reprod* 65:462, 2001.

123. Landim-Alvarenga FC, Graham JK, Alvarenga MA, et al: Calcium influx into equine and bovine spermatozoa during in vitro capacitation. *Anim Reprod* 1:96, 2004.

124. Evenson DP: Flow cytometric analysis of male germ cell quality. *Methods Cell Biol* 33:401, 1990.

125. Evenson D, Jost L: Sperm chromatin structure assay is useful for fertility assessment. *Methods Cell Sci* 22:169, 2000.

126. Love CC: The sperm chromatin structure assay: a review of clinical applications. *Anim Reprod Sci* 89:39, 2005.

127. Cunningham RE: Flow cytometry. In Rapley R, Walker JM, eds: *Molecular Biomethods Handbook*. Totowa, NJ: Humana Press, 1998, pp 653-667.

128. Gillan L, Evans G, Maxwell WMC: Flow cytometric evaluation of sperm parameters in relation to fertility potential. *Theriogenology* 63:445, 2005.

129. Graham JK: Assessment of sperm quality: a flow cytometric approach. *Anim Reprod Sci* 68:239, 2001.

130. Aurich JE, Kühne A, Hoppe H, et al: Seminal plasma affects membrane integrity and motility of equine spermatozoa after cryopreservation. *Theriogenology* 46:791, 1996.

131. Aurich JE, Schönherr U, Hoppe H, et al: Effects of antioxidants on motility and membrane integrity of chilled-stored stallion semen. *Theriogenology* 48:185, 1997.

132. Pintado B, de la Fuente J, Roldan ER: Permeability of boar and bull spermatozoa to the nucleic acid stains propidium iodide or Hoechst 33258, or to eosin: accuracy in the assessment of cell viability. *J Reprod Fertil* 118:145, 2000.

133. Thomas CA, Garner DL, DeJarnette JM, et al: Fluorometric assessments of acrosomal integrity and viability in cryopreserved bovine spermatozoa. *Biol Reprod* 56:991, 1997.

134. Jeyendran RS, Van der Ven HH, Perez-Palaez M, et al: Development of an assay to assess the functional integrity of the human sperm membrane and its relationship to other semen characteristics. *J Reprod Fertil* 70:219, 1984.

135. Jeyendran RS, Van der Ven HH, Zaneveld LID: The hypoosmotic swelling test: an update. *Arch Androl* 29:105, 1992.

136. Vidament M, Cognard E, Yvon J-M, et al: Evaluation of stallion semen before and after freezing. *Reprod Dom Anim* 33:271, 1998.

137. Neild D, Chaves G, Flores M, et al: Hypoosmotic test in equine spermatozoa. *Theriogenology* 51:721, 1999.

138. Neild DC, Chaves MG, Flores M, et al: The HOS test and its relationship to fertility in the stallion. *Andrologia* 32:351, 2000.

139. Katila T, Koskinen E, Andersson M: Evaluation of frozen-thawed semen. Havemeyer Foundation Workshop Advanced Current Topics in Stallion Veterinary Practice Krakow. 2000, pp 54-56.

140. Petrunkina AM, Petzoldt R, Stahlberg S, et al: Sperm-cell volumetric measurements as parameters in bull semen function evaluation: correlation with nonreturn rate. *Andrologia* 33:360, 2001.

141. Petrunkina AM, Harrison RAP, Tsolova M, et al: Signalling pathways involved in the control of spermatozoal cell volume. *Reproduction* 133:61, 2007.

142. Flesch FM, Gadella BM: Dynamics of the mammalian sperm plasma membrane in the process of fertilization. *Biochem Biophys Acta* 1469:197, 2000.

143. Neild DM, Gadella BM, Agüero A, et al: Capacitation, acrosome function and chromatin structure in stallion sperm. *Anim Reprod Sci* 89:47, 2005.

144. Hunter RH, Rodriguez-Martinez H: Capacitation of mammalian spermatozoa in vivo, with a specific focus on events in the fallopian tubes. *Mol Reprod Dev* 67:243, 2004.

145. Brewis IA, Moore HD, Fraser LR, et al: Molecular mechanisms during sperm capacitation. *Human Fertil* 8:253, 2005.

146. Neild DM, Gadella BM, Chaves MG, et al: Membrane changes during different stages of a freeze/thaw protocol for equine semen cryopreservation. *Theriogenology* 59:1693, 2003.

147. Magistrini M, Palmer E: Motility, triple stain and electron microscopic analysis of spermatozoa treated with ionophore A23187 for in vitro fertilization. *J Reprod Fertil Suppl* 44:661, 1991.

148. Mollova M, Atanassov B, Nedkova R, et al: Biochemical and immunochemical characterization of boar sperm flagellar protein with role in hyperactivation/capacitation process. *Reprod Biol* 6:79, 2006.

149. Pommer AC, Rutlant J, Meyers SA: Phosphorylation of protein tyrosine residues in fresh and cryopreserved stallion spermatozoa under capacitating conditions. *Biol Reprod* 68:1208, 2003.

150. Rathi R, Colenbrander B, Stout TAE, et al: Progesterone induces acrosome reaction in stallion spermatozoa via a protein tyrosine kinase dependent pathway. *Mol Reprod Dev* 64:120, 2003.

151. Piehler E, Petrunkina AM, Ekhlasi-Hundrieser M, et al: Dynamic quantification of the tyrosine phosphorylation of the sperm surface proteins during capacitation. *Cytometry* 69:1062, 2006.

152. Flesch FM, Brouwers JF, Nievelstein PF, et al: Bicarbonate stimulated phospholipid scrambling induces cholesterol redistribution and enables cholesterol depletion in the sperm plasma membrane. *J Cell Sci* 114:3543, 2001.

153. Visconti PE, Ning XP, Fornes MW, et al: Cholesterol efflux mediated signal transduction in mammalian sperm: cholesterol release signals an increase in protein tyrosine phosphorylation during mouse sperm capacitation. *Dev Biol* 214:429, 1999.

154. Pena AI, Lugilde LL, Barrio M, et al: Effects of Equex from different sources on post-thaw survival, longevity and intracellular Ca2+ of dog spermatozoa. *Theriogenology* 59:1725, 2003.

155. Harrison RAP, Gadella BM: Bicarbonate-induced membrane processing in sperm capacitation. *Theriogenology* 63:342, 2005.

156. Gadella BM, Miller NGA, Colenbrander B, et al: Flow cytometric detection of transbilayer movement of fluorescent phospholipid analogues across the boar sperm plasma membrane: elimination of labelling artefacts. *Mol Reprod Dev* 53:108, 1999.

157. Cheng FP, Fazeli A, Voorhout WF, et al: Progesterone in mare follicular fluid induces the acrosome reaction in stallion spermatozoa and enhances in vitro binding to the zona pellucida. *Int J Androl* 21:57, 1998.

158. Sinowitz F, Wessa E, Neumüller C, et al: On the species specificity of sperm binding and sperm penetration of the zona pellucida. *Reprod Domest Anim* 38:141, 2003.

159. Blottner S, Warnke C, Tuchscherer A, et al: Morphological and functional changes of stallion spermatozoa after cryopreservation during breeding and non-breeding season. *Anim Reprod Sci* 65:75, 2001.

160. Wöckener A, Schubert HJ: Freezing of maiden stallion semen—motility and morphological findings in sperm cells assessed by various staining methods including a monoclonal antibody with reactivity against an antigen in the acrosome ground substance. *Reprod Dom Anim* 28:265, 1993.

161. Cheng FP, Gadella BM, Voorhout WF, et al: Progesterone-induced acrosome reaction in stallion spermatozoa is mediated by a plasma membrane progesterone receptor. *Biol Reprod* 59:733, 1998.

162. Christensen P, Whitfield CH, Parkinson TJ: In vitro induction of acrosome reactions in stallion spermatozoa by heparin and A23187. *Theriogenology* 45:1201, 1996.

163. Varner DD, Thompson JA, Blanchard T, et al: Induction of the acrosome reaction in stallion spermatozoa—effects of incubation temperature, incubation time, and ionophore concentration. *Theriogenology* 58:303, 2002.

164. Gómez-Cuétera C, Squires EL, Graham JK: In vitro induction of the acrosome reaction in fresh and frozen-thawed equine spermatozoa. *Anim Reprod Sci* 94:165, 2006.

165. Varner DD, Brinsko SP, Blanchard TL, et al: Subfertility in stallions associated with spermatozoal acrosome dysfunction in 2001. Proc AAEP. 2001, pp 227.

166. Brinsko SP, Love CC, Bauer JE, et al: Cholesterol-to-phospholipid ratio in whole sperm and seminal plasma from fertile stallions and stallions with unexplained subfertility. *Anim Reprod Sci* 99:65, 2007.

167. Brinsko SP, Varner DD, Love CC, et al: Effect of feeding a DHA-enriched nutriceutical on the quality of fresh, cooled and frozen stallion semen. *Theriogenology* 63:1519, 2005.

168. Varner DD, Bowen JA, Johnson L: Effect of heparin on capacitation/acrosome reaction of equine sperm. *Arch Andr* 31:199, 1993.

169. Meyers SA, Overstreet JW, Liu IKM, et al: Capacitation in vitro of stallion spermatozoa: comparison of progesterone induced acrosome reactions in fertile and subfertile males. *J Androl* 16:47, 1995.

170. Meyers SA, Liu IKM, Overstreet JW, et al: Sperm-zona pellucida binding and zona-induced acrosome reactions in the horse: comparisons between fertile and subfertile stallions. *Theriogenology* 46:1277, 1996.

171. Rathi R, Nielen M, Cheng FP, et al: Exposure of progesterone receptors on the plasma membranes of stallion spermatozoa as a parameter for prediction of fertility. *J Reprod Fertil Suppl* 56:87, 2000.

172. Fazeli AR, Steenweg W, Bevers MM, et al: Use of sperm binding to homologous hemizona pellucida to predict stallion fertility. *Eq Vet J Suppl* 15:57, 1993.

173. Fazeli AR, Steenweg W, Bevers M, et al: Relation between stallion sperm binding to homologous hemizonae and fertility. *Theriogenology* 44:751, 1995.

174. Yanagimachi R, Yanagimachi H, Rogers BJ: The use of zona-free animal eggs as a test-system for the assessment of the fertilizing capacity of human spermatozoa. *Biol Reprod* 15:471, 1976.

175. Landim-Alvarenga FC, Alvarenga MA, Seidel GE: Penetration of zona-free hamster, bovine and equine oocytes by stallion and bull spermatozoa pretreated with equine follicular fluid, dilauroylphosphatidylcholine or calcium ionophore A23187. *Theriogenology* 56:937, 2001.

176. Thomas CA, Garner DL, DeJarnette JM, et al: Effect of cryopreservation on bovine sperm organelle function and viability as determined by flow cytometry. *Biol Reprod* 58:786, 1998.

177. Papaioannou KZ, Murphy RP, Monks RS, et al: Assessment of viability and mitochondrial function of equine spermatozoa using double staining and flow cytometry. *Theriogenology* 48:299, 1997.

178. Turner RM: Moving to the beat: a review of mammalian sperm motility regulation. *Reprod Fertil Dev* 18:25, 2006.

179. Gravance CG, Garner DL, Miller MG, et al: Fluorescent probes and flow cytometry to assess rat sperm integrity and mitochondrial function. *Reprod Toxicol* 15:5, 2001.

180. Evenson DP, Darzynkiewicz Z, Melamed MR: Relation of mammalian sperm chromatin heterogeneity to fertility. *Science* 210:1131, 1980.

181. Perreault SD, Naish SJ, Zirkin BR: The timing of hamster sperm nuclear decondensation and male pronucleus formation is related to sperm nuclear disulfide bond content. *Biol Reprod* 36:239, 1987.

182. Evenson DP, Jost LK, Varner DD: Relationship between sperm nuclear protamine free-SH status and susceptibility to DNA denaturation. *J Reprod Fertil Suppl* 56:401, 2000.

183. Agarwal A, Said TM: Role of sperm chromatin abnormalities and DNA damage in male infertility. *Hum Reprod* 9:331, 2003.

184. Evenson DP, Jost LK, Marshall D, et al: Utility of the sperm chromatin structure assay as a diagnostic and prognostic tool in the human fertility clinic. *Human Reprod* 14:1039, 1999.
185. Evenson DP, Larson KL, Jost LK: Sperm chromatin structure assay: Its clinical use for detecting sperm DNA fragmentation in male infertility and comparisons with other techniques. *J Androl* 23:25, 2002.
186. Evenson DP, Wixon R: Clinical aspects of sperm DNA fragmentation detection and male fertility. *Theriogenology* 65:979, 2006.
187. Ibrahim ME, Pedersen H: Acridine orange fluorescence as male fertility test. *Arch Androl* 20:125, 1988.
188. Ball BA: Embryonic loss in mares. Incidence, possible causes, and diagnostic considerations. In van Camp SD, ed: *Veterinary Clinics of North America Equine Practice.* vol 263, 1988.
189. Evenson DP, Sailer BL, Jost LK: Relationship between stallion sperm deoxyribonucleic acid (DNA) susceptibility to denaturation in situ and presence of DNA strand breaks: implications for fertility and embryo viability. *Biol Reprod Mono* 1:655, 1995.
190. Evenson DP, Jost LK, Baer RK, et al: Individuality of DNA denaturation patterns in human sperm as measured by the sperm chromatin structure assay. *Reprod Toxicol* 5:115, 1991.
191. Kenney RM, Evenson DP, Garcia MC, et al: Relationship between sperm chromatin structure, motility, and morphology of ejaculated sperm and seasonal pregnancy rate. *Biol Reprod Mono* 1:647, 1995.
192. Love CC, Kenney RM: The relationship of increased susceptibility of sperm DNA to denaturation and fertility in the stallion. *Theriogenology* 50:955, 1998.
193. Larson KL, DeJonge CJ, Barnes AM, et al: Relationship of assisted reproductive technique (ART) outcomes with sperm chromatin integrity and maturity as measured by the sperm chromatin structure assay (SCSA). *Human Reprod* 15:1717, 2000.
194. Larson KL, Brannian J, Hansen K, et al: Relationship between assisted reproductive techniques (ART) outcomes and DNA fragmentation (DFI) as measured by the Sperm Chromatin Structure Assay (SCSA). *Am Soc Reprod Med,* Seattle: Oct 12-17, 2002.
195. Saleh RA, Agarwal A, Nelson DR, et al: Increased sperm nuclear DNA damage in normozoospermic infertile men: a prospective study. *Fertil Steril* 78:313, 2002.
196. Morrell JM, Johannisson A, Dalin AM, et al: Sperm morphology and chromatin integrity in Swedish Warmblood stallions and their relationship to pregnancy rates. *Acta Vet Scand* 50:1, 2008.
197. Payne JF, Raburn DJ, Couchman GM, et al: Redefining the relationship between sperm deoxyribonucleic acid fragmentation as measured by the sperm chromatin structure assay and outcomes of assisted reproductive techniques. *Fertil Steril* 84:356, 2005.
198. Bungum M, Humaidan P, Axmon A, et al: Sperm DNA integrity assessment in prediction of assisted reproduction technology outcome. *Human Reprod* 22:174, 2007.
199. Linfor JJ, Meyers SA: Detection of DNA damage in response to cooling injury in equine spermatozoa using single-cell gel electrophoresis. *J Androl* 23:107, 2002.
200. Tejada RI, Mitchell MS, Norman A, et al: A test for the practical evaluation of male fertility by acridine orange (AO) fluorescence. *Fertil Steril* 42:87, 1984.
201. Garcia-Macias V, de Paz P, Martinez-Pastor F, et al: DNA fragmentation assessment by flow cytometry and Sperm-Bos-Halomax (bright-field microscopy and fluorescence microscopy) in bull sperm. *Int J Androl* 30:88, 2007.
202. Pesch S, Bergmann M, Bostedt H: Determination of some enzymes and macro- and microelements in stallion seminal plasma and their correlations to semen quality. *Theriogenology* 66:307, 2006.
203. Desvousges AL, Dow CA, Hayna JT, et al: Heat shock induces apoptosis in equine spermatozoa. *Anim Reprod Sci* 94:125, 2006.
204. Brum A, Sabeur K, Ball BA: Apoptotic-like changes in equine spermatozoa after separation by density-gradient centrifugation or after cryopreservation. *Anim Reprod Sci* 94:138, 2006.
205. Stradaioli G, Rubei M, Zamparini M, et al: Enzymatic evaluation of phospholipid hydroperoxide glutathione peroxidase (PHGPx) in equine spermatozoa. *Anim Reprod Sci* 94:29, 2006.
206. Neild DM, Gadella BM, Colenbrander B, et al: Lipid peroxidation in stallion spermatozoa. *Theriogenology* 58:295, 2002.
207. Neild DM, Brouwers JFH, Colenbrander B, et al: Lipid peroxide formation in relation to membrane stability of fresh and frozen thawed stallion spermatozoa. *Mol Reprod Dev* 72:230, 2005.
208. Almeida J, Ball BA: Effect of alpha-tocopherol and tocopherol succinate on lipid peroxidation in equine spermatozoa. *Anim Reprod Sci* 87:321, 2005.
209. Guthrie HD, Welch GR: Use of fluorescence-activated flow cytometry to determine membrane lipid peroxidation during hypothermic liquid storage and freeze-thawing of viable boar sperm loaded with 4, 4-difluoro-5-(4-phenyl-1,3-butadienyl)-4-bora-3a, 4a-diaza-s-indacene-3-undecanoic acid. *J Anim Sci* 85:1402, 2007.
210. Aitken RJ: Sperm function tests and fertility. *Int J Androl* 29:69, 2006.
211. Ball BA, Vo AT, Baumber J: Generation of reactive oxygen species by equine spermatozoa. *Am J Vet Res* 62:508, 2001.
212. Guthrie HD, Welch GR: Determination of intracellular reactive oxygen species and high mitochondrial membrane potential in Percoll-treated viable boar sperm using fluorescence-activated flow cytometry. *J Anim Sci* 84:2089, 2006.
213. Rodriguez-Martinez H, Iborra A, Martinez P, et al: Immunoelectron microscopic imaging of spermadhesin AWN epitopes on boar spermatozoa bound in vivo to the zona pellucida. *Reprod Fertil Dev* 10:491, 1998.
214. Gao A, Garbers DL: Species diversity in the structure of zonadhesin, a sperm-specific membrane protein containing multiple cell adhesion molecule-like domains. *J Biol Chem* 273:3415, 1998.
215. Breazeale KR, Brady HA, Bi M, et al: Biochemical properties and localization of zonadhesin in equine spermatozoa. *Theriogenology* 58:359, 2002.
216. Bailey LB, Brady HB, Tardif S, et al: Zonadhesin expression and localization in stallion testes. *Anim Reprod Sci* 94:56, 2006.
217. Schambony A, Hess O, Gentzel M, et al: Expression of CRISP proteins in the male equine genital tract. *J Reprod Fertil Suppl* 53:67, 1998.
218. Reineke A, Hess O, Schambony A, et al: Sperm-associated seminal plasma proteins—a novel approach for the evaluation of sperm fertilizing ability of stallions. *Pferdeheilkunde* 6:531, 1999.
219. Jude R, Giese A, Piumi F, et al: Molecular characterization of the CRISP 1 gene—a candidate gene for stallion fertility. *Theriogenology* 58:417, 2002.
220. Turner RM, Sertich PL: Use of alkaline phosphatase as a diagnostic tool in stallions with azoospermia and oligospermia. *Anim Reprod Sci* 68:315, 2001.
221. Turner RM, McDonnell SM: Alkaline phosphatase in stallion semen characterization and clinical applications. *Theriogenology* 60:1, 2003.
222. Ball BA, Baumber J, Vo A, et al: Effect of oxidative stress on equine spermatozoa. *Anim Reprod Sci* 68:364, 2001.
223. Burnaugh L, Sabeur K, Ball BA: Generation of superoxide anion by equine spermatozoa as detected by dihydroethidium. *Theriogenology* 67:580, 2007.
224. Stradaioli G, Gennevieve A, Magistrini M: Evaluation of lipid peroxidation by thiobarbituric acid test in equine spermatozoa. *Anim Reprod Sci* 68:320, 2001.
225. Morte ME, Rodrigues AM, Soares D, et al: The quantification of lipid and protein oxidation in stallion spermatozoa and seminal plasma: Seasonal distinctions and correlations with DNA strand breaks, classical seminal parameters and stallion fertility. *Anim Reprod Sci* 106:36, 2008.
226. Baumber J, Ball BA, Linfor JJ, et al: Reactive oxygen species and cryopreservation promote deoxyribonucleic acid (DNA) damage in equine sperm. *Theriogenology* 58:301, 2003.
227. Sullivan R: Male fertility markers, myth or reality. *Anim Reprod Sci* 82:341, 2004.
228. Leeb T, Sieme H, Töpfer-Petersen E: Genetic markers for stallion fertility—lessons from humans and mice. *Anim Reprod Sci* 89:21, 2005.
229. Chenoweth PJ: Genetic sperm defects. *Theriogenology* 64:457, 2005.
230. Chowdhary BP, Taudsepp T, Kata SR, et al: The first-generation whole-genome radiation hybrid map in the horse identifies conserved segments in human and mouse genomes. *Genome Res* 13:742, 2003.
231. Tozaki T, Hirota KI, Hasegawa T, et al: Whole-genome linkage disequilibrium screening for complex traits in horses. *Mol Genet Genomics* 277:663, 2007.
231a. Chowdhary BP, Paria N, Raudsepp T: Potential applications of equine genomics in dissecting diseases and fertility. *Anim Reprod Sci* 107:208, 2008.
232. He Z, Chan WYC, Dym M: Microarray technology offers a novel tool for the diagnosis and identification of therapeutic targets for male infertility. *Reproduction* 132:11, 2006.
233. Hamann H, Jude R, Sieme H, et al: A polymorphism within the equine CRISP3 gene is associated with stallion fertility in Hanoverian Warmblood horses. *Anim Genet* 38:259, 2007.
234. Thiessen H: Fluorescence microscopic analysis of the sperm chromatin structure in the stallion. Thesis, Hannover: 2006.

BREEDING MANAGEMENT OF THE THOROUGHBRED STALLION

†JOHN V. STEINER AND NORMAN W. UMPHENOUR

The stallion is perhaps the most important asset of a breeding operation. Therefore, the primary concern of the stallion manager should be to maintain the stallion's health and to maximize the stallion's reproductive capacity. To use the stallion to his maximum capability, the stallion manager must meet the basic needs of the stallion and must understand his behavioral patterns as well as his reproductive limitations. Having one mare who is a poor reproductive performer is unfortunate, but one poorly managed stallion can have a disastrous effect on a breeding program. Because of the impact that the stallions can have on the productivity of a farm, they are judged more critically and culled more extensively than the brood mares.[1]

SELECTION OF STALLIONS

There are basically two criteria for selecting a stallion.[1] The first is that a stallion prospect be a horse that is recognizable. Trying to promote an unknown stallion in the modern Thoroughbred market is difficult. A horse without a pedigree or a good race record is not a stallion prospect.[1] In addition, a stallion prospect must have shown ability on the racetrack because the object is to produce future racehorses. Horses selected as stallions should be able to potentially improve the quality of their offspring in a breeding program. If the stallion passes on desirable traits to a large percentage of his offspring, he is fulfilling an important genetic role. The thoughtful selection of a stallion for a breeding program must take into consideration the goals that the breeding program is intended to achieve.

The selection criteria for a breeding stallion are based mainly on performance, conformation, and pedigree. Although the main purpose of the stallion is to breed and impregnate mares, in general, his reproductive potential is not considered.[2] Therefore, the stallion manager must implement procedures to increase the reproductive efficiency of any stallion regardless of his inherent fertility.[2] The long-term effects on the reproductive performance of the offspring of subfertile stallions are potentially catastrophic.

GENERAL MANAGEMENT OF THE BREEDING STALLION

Feeding Program

A successful breeding program requires a sound feeding program. Feeding is still considered an art, and although a great deal of scientific knowledge has been gained in recent years, the stallion's body condition should be evaluated on a regular

basis and feeding adjustments made as needed. In general, the nutritional needs of a stallion during the breeding season do not appear to be different from his needs during maintenance.[3] A slight increase in energy intake may be necessary or beneficial during the height of the breeding season; however, it is easy to overestimate the nutrients needed by a stallion at this time.[3] Overfed and obese stallions are more common and of greater concern than underfed ones. A maintenance ration consists of enough balanced nutrients to support normal, basic bodily functions.[4] Adequate pasture or good-quality hay can usually meet these requirements, and free access to trace mineralized salt and fresh water is also necessary. Grain as an energy supplement in cold weather or under certain stressful conditions may also be warranted. The stallion's size, condition, activity, and temperament all play a role in his nutritional needs. Therefore, diets should be adjusted for individual stallions.

The healthy stallion consumes 2%–3% of his body weight daily. At least 50% of this should be in the form of roughage. Vitamin A plays an important part in reproduction.[3] A severe deficiency of vitamin A can result in a decrease or cessation of sperm production.[3] Leafy green forages generally supply adequate amounts of vitamin A. Contrary to popular belief, supplementation with vitamin A and E over National Research Council requirements does not improve reproductive performance of stallions. Stallions generally require 10% protein in their feed; younger stallions require 12%–14%. Obesity may adversely affect libido and mating ability. Therefore, the only dietary requirement for efficient sperm production and good breeding performance is a balanced diet that maintains the stallion at his optimum weight. There is no conclusive evidence of any nutrient that is able to increase sperm numbers or quality.

Exercise

Horses naturally are roaming and grazing animals. Therefore, exercise for stallions is an integral part of their management that affects their mental and reproductive well-being. This basic need for exercise is often ignored or underestimated, and nutrition and exercise go hand-in-hand. A stallion needs exercise to remain in good physical condition and to maintain a sharp mental attitude. Exercise can be provided in one of the following ways or in various combinations: (1) turn-out in paddock, (2) riding, (3) lunging, (4) treadmill, (5) swimming, or (6) mechanical walker.

In determining the type of exercise program, the stallion manager must consider the physical condition of the stallion as well as his temperament. Turn-out in a small, 1- to 2-acre paddock should be the least that is done to provide exercise for the stallion.

†Deceased.

If the horse is not very active outside or seems to be gaining weight, a more forced type of exercise may have to be provided, such as riding or lunging, to keep the horse fit and happy. In addition, lack of exercise may lead to vices such as weaving, stall walking, and cribbing.

The amount of exercise time must be tailored to the stallion's personality. Free exercise in a paddock can last as long as 24 hours a day for some horses depending on the weather conditions. Others may do well with just 1–4 hours a day. Riding or driving in a jog cart should be at a slow canter or a jog for 1–2 miles a day. This exercise should be done 6 days a week depending on how easily the horse maintains his condition. The goal is to keep a stallion fit for the breeding shed, not the racetrack, so that he has a good attitude toward his daily duty of covering mares.

The personnel responsible for exercising stallions must be good horsemen or horsewomen so that overwork and injuries can be avoided. If soreness, lameness, or an attitude problem develops, the person responsible should be capable of detecting the problem. The exercise program must be discontinued and the stallion must be completely evaluated before continuing with any exercise.

Regardless of the type of exercise, the horse must have a positive attitude toward the routine. The form of exercise must be safe and minimize the chances of injury to the breeding stallion. Horses that have to go to the breeding shed several times a day must be kept as sound as possible because this may influence their attitude toward covering mares. For the exercise program to be effective, it must complement other aspects of the overall management of the horse (e.g., amount of turn-out, physical condition, and mental attitude).

Housing

An area of recent study is the effect on testosterone levels and seminal parameters by the grouping or housing of stallions. Intermale effects may be involved in behavior-related subfertility seen in some domestic breeding stallions or in the generally lower behavioral vigor and apparent fertility of stabled stallions compared with pasture-bred stallions.[4] Pasture-bred horses generally exhibit high levels of fertility and greater sexual behavior endurance than stabled, hand-bred stallions.[4] In general, stallions that have access to outside and get exercise have increased testosterone levels.

PREVENTIVE MEDICINE

Preventive medicine should cover several areas of care for the overall well-being of the stallion. Foot care, dental care, vaccinations, and deworming should be performed in unison with the other management programs.

Parasite Control

A good parasite control program should incorporate the use of deworming agents and pasture management. Although there are few studies to evaluate the effect of antiparasitic drugs on stallion fertility, most drugs are considered safe unless stated to the contrary by the manufacturer. Regular pasture rotation and harrowing are also part of a parasite control program. Periodic fecal examination for parasite eggs is a good way to monitor the effectiveness of the control measures used. Stallions are generally dewormed every 60 days, with rotation between ivermectin, pyrantel pamoate, and fenbendazole.

Immunization Program

Vaccinations

Most stallions are isolated for 6 months of the year, but during the breeding season, which lasts approximately 5.5 months (150 days), they are exposed to mares from different farms and countries. Stallions used for dual-hemisphere breeding are at greater risk of contracting contagious diseases. Therefore, it is important that an organized vaccination program be considered. At breeding farms, mares come from several farms and different areas, as well as countries, into a central location for breeding. Not only does this put the stallions at risk, but any exposed mare is at risk of spreading disease to many boarding farms.

Breeding stallions should be vaccinated approximately 60 days before the breeding season. In that way, any fever that may occur does not adversely affect semen quality. Generally, most stallions in Kentucky are vaccinated in December against rabies, tetanus, influenza, rhinopneumonitis, botulism, and West Nile virus. Rhinopneumonitis and influenza vaccines are repeated every 2 months. In addition, equine viral arteritis vaccine is required for Thoroughbred stallions in Kentucky with a subsequent 28-day isolation period following vaccination. If appropriate, eastern and western encephalomyelitis vaccine and Potomac horse fever vaccine are generally given in the spring.

Hoof Care

Hoof care should be tailored to the individual stallion. Daily turn-out in a grassy area is conducive to good hoof quality and is another reason to keep stallions out in the paddock as much as possible. Hooves tend to become dryer and more brittle when stallions are kept in a stall, especially when stabled on wood shavings or sawdust.

In general, hooves are trimmed every 6–8 weeks. Some stallions with specific hoof problems may have to be shod. Whenever possible, stallions should not wear shoes because shoes tend to constrict and damage the hoof wall.

Dental Care

Dental examination is conducted routinely once or twice a year or whenever a dental or oral problem is suspected. Routine dental floating is carried out as dictated by the oral examinations. This ensures the proper use of feeds so that body condition is maintained and digestive upsets can be kept to a minimum.

ARTIFICIAL LIGHTING PROGRAM

Horses are considered to be long-day breeders. Reproductive function in the stallion is not arrested during the winter months as it is in most mares. However, certain seminal and hormonal characteristics and many aspects of sexual behavior are affected by day length. Testicular size and weight, daily sperm production, semen volume, hormonal concentrations, and libido are increased during the natural breeding season compared with the non-breeding season.[5]

The breeding season of brood mares is accelerated with an artificial lighting program. Providing stallions with the same artificial lighting program as for mares (16 hours of total light beginning December 1) results in increased testicular size and increased sperm output early in the year (i.e., February).[6] Thoroughbred stallions show distinct seasonal and age-related changes in most of the reproductive parameters studied, and the exposure of such stallions to increased photoperiod produced significant alterations in these changes.[6] In non-lighted stallions in central Kentucky, testicular diameters increased between February and June in young and middle-age stallions. In lighted stallions, testicular diameters were smaller in June than in February or April. Changes in testicular diameter were seen only in young or middle-age stallions, not older stallions, when under light treatment.

Similarly, hormone concentrations are affected by artificial lighting programs. Increased artificial light exposure results in elevated testosterone in February in both young and middle-age stallions, but by March, testosterone decreases and is similar to December levels. This increase is generally short-lived because stallions become refractory to this light stimulation. If the majority of mares are to be bred in February and March (early breeding season), exposing stallions to light may be beneficial. This is not the usual case, however, and a lighting program may not be suitable because the largest number of mares in a stallion's book are generally presented in April and May in the northern hemisphere. Under the stimulation of lights, as the breeding season progresses, testicular size regresses to near that of stallions exposed to only natural day length. Therefore, increased day length by means of an artificial lighting program causes stallions to "peak" earlier than they would have on their own.

BREEDING SOUNDNESS EXAMINATION

The purpose of conducting an examination of a stallion for the evaluation of fertility is to select stallions that can reasonably be expected to be capable of efficiently rendering at least 75% of 40 or more mares pregnant when used in a natural breeding program in one breeding season. In addition, stallions with genetic defects, such as cryptorchidism or umbilical hernia, can be identified. The Society for Theriogenology has published guidelines for the clinical fertility evaluation of the stallion.[7] These guidelines are used to help determine the suitability of a stallion as a breeding prospect. The examination includes a general physical examination, observation of libido and mating ability, and detection of infectious venereal diseases; it also gives insight into semen quality and quantity.

New stallions should have a breeding soundness examination as far in advance of their first breeding season as possible. In addition, experienced stallions should have a breeding soundness examination before the start of each breeding season so that a baseline of semen parameters can be established.

There is no single physical or seminal measurement that is satisfactorily correlated with fertility. The best measure of stallion fertility is the number of pregnancies per cycle. Recently, more and more stallions have been doing "double duty," shuttling between the northern and southern hemispheres and participating in two breeding seasons per year. The full ramifications of this practice are not totally known, but it certainly is increasing the reproductive demands on the stallion. In our experience with "shuttle stallions," there does not appear to be any detrimental effect on semen quality or pregnancy rates. This is only our impression, and as more stallions are moved between the northern and southern hemispheres, change may be noted. In addition, we believe that any effects that are seen (e.g., on libido) are purely the result of an individual's variability.

ESTIMATING A STALLION'S BOOK

There is no simple formula for determining the number of mares to be mated to a given stallion, and a number of factors must be taken into consideration. In 1996, 5200 stallions covered 59,719

mares (Jockey Club Statistics).[8] These coverings resulted in 33,448 foals being born in 1997, a success rate of 56% being reported by the Jockey Club on Live Foal Reports in September of that year (Jockey Club, personal communication, 1997). The number of stallions used to cover the mares decreased by 3.8%, down from 5427 reported in 1995. There was a 0.9% decline from the 60,284 mares reported in 1995. Thoroughbred breeding activity in Kentucky outpaced breeding in all other regions, with 16,895 mares being bred in 1996, producing 11,288 live foals. In 1995, 16,006 mares were bred, producing 10,652 foals. Florida reported 5895 mares bred and 3455 live foals, and California reported 4919 mares bred and 2985 live foals. The percent of live foals increases significantly as book size increases. Only 11% of all Thoroughbred stallions breed 25 or more mares per breeding season, and 1% breed more than 60 mares.[8]

In estimating a stallion's book size, the first consideration lies with the stallion himself. Because the stallion is usually chosen based on pedigree, performance, and conformation, with little or no emphasis placed on reproductive potential, a significant number of stallions enter the breeding pool with poor or marginal fertility. A complete breeding soundness examination and a complete review of past reproduction performance play an integral part in the management process. If a stallion has stood at stud in previous breeding seasons, past reproductive performance records are invaluable. For example, information concerning the number of mares bred, number of covers made, pregnancy rate per cycle, and covers per pregnancy is helpful in evaluating reproductive efficiency.

Libido of the stallion can play a large role in determining the number of mares a stallion can service during a breeding season. This is a genetically acquired trait[4] that can be modified by environment. As discussed previously, testosterone levels can be altered by interaction between stallions and mares and with exercise.[4] Many times, poor libido is a limiting factor in the number of mares a stallion can cover. The number of covers a stallion can make in a day varies with the individual stallion. Factors such as age, physical abnormalities, and testosterone levels play a role. Some stallions can breed two to three times a day, 7 days a week, and some can cover only one mare per day.

The length of the breeding season also plays a role in the number of mares that can be mated. The Thoroughbred season is generally from February 15 to July 15. Therefore, the number of mares that can be presented during this time is somewhat limited in a natural breeding program.

The age and physical condition of the stallion must also be considered. Stallions typically retire to stud at 3–5 years of age. Reproductive capacity is influenced by age. Stallions reach puberty at 12–24 months of age but continue to mature and increase reproductive performance until 5–6 years of age and older. During the breeding season there is seasonal fluctuation of sperm production. In addition, physical problems, especially of the hind legs, may limit the number of mares that the stallion can physically mount and service. Injuries to the penis must also be considered. Penile injuries can occur as a result of trauma (e.g., a kick from a mare). In addition, the use of certain medications such as acepromazine can result in paraphimosis. These conditions must be addressed quickly and aggressively so that a great deal of time is not lost during the breeding season.

Medications that the stallion received in the past during his racing career or drugs that he currently receives may affect his reproductive performance. The effect of most drugs on reproductive performance has not been determined in the stallion, and no drug has been shown to improve sperm quality or sperm production. In our experience, the use of gonadotropin-releasing hormone (GnRH) has not helped remedy conditions such as low sperm numbers or poor motility or morphology of sperm, and no scientific evidence justifies the expense of implementing this therapy for the stallion. However, almost all medications have the potential to adversely affect sperm production. Administration of testosterone or anabolic steroids has been shown to decrease testicular size, reduce sperm production, and depress sperm motility.[5] The negative effect of anabolic steroids on testicular function probably results from interference with endogenous gonadotropin production and release. These effects on reproduction are considered temporary in adult stallions, but the long-term effects on prepubertal testes are unknown. We find that the larger the doses of anabolics and the longer the time administered, the more permanent the effects on the stallion.

One medication that has helped with libido is aqueous testosterone. The aqueous form of testosterone is a suspension and, when used appropriately, will not downregulate the stallion since the testosterone levels will not rise above 4 ng. The protocol for stallions that have little or no libido is to administer 80 mg/1000 lb body weight intramuscularly or subcutaneously every other day. Usually by day 5–12 the stallion "turns on" and has adequate libido. Once the stallion is breeding normally, the injections are discontinued. Many times, this one course of treatment is all that is needed, but there have been several stallions that require this therapy at the beginning of each breeding season.

Semen quality plays an integral role in estimating a stallion's book size. Ideally, daily sperm output (DSO) is determined by daily collections of semen for 8–10 consecutive days to deplete extragonadal sperm reserves. Alternatively, estimation of DSO using testicular volume (TV) can be calculated.[5] TV is based on measurement of each testis:

$$TV = \frac{4}{3}\pi\frac{abc}{2}$$

$$TV = 0.5233 \times (width \times length \times height\ in\ cm)$$

where a is testicular height/2, b is testicular width/2, and c is testicular length/2. When the total volume of the testes is calculated, $DSO = 0.024x - 0.76$, where $x = TV$. Low DSO may require more intense management of the stallion or mares.[5]

Longevity of sperm from a given stallion may play a role in the number of mares that a particular stallion can service. Longevity can be determined by accurate records of insemination, ovulation, and pregnancy rates. Another method, although perhaps more subjective, is to evaluate semen longevity during the breeding soundness examination. This may be evaluated by estimating motility of spermatozoa in a raw semen sample hourly until less than 10% motility is observed or by mixing a semen sample with an appropriate semen extender. Semen is either stored at room temperature or gradually cooled to 5°C.

Sperm motility is evaluated daily. There is no good scientific evidence that correlates sperm longevity in the laboratory with longevity in the mare. In general, the longer the sperm is viable in the mare, the fewer the matings that are needed. For example, with good sperm longevity, a mare can be mated and conceive even if she ovulates 3–5 days or more after mating. Conversely, if a stallion's sperm is viable for only 24 hours in a mare, the mare must be bred within 24 hours before ovulation.

The fertility of the mares presented to a stallion can also affect the season conception rate. Live foal percentage decreases significantly as mare age increases, whereas the live foal percentage does not change with stallion age.[8]

The more evenly mares are presented throughout the breeding season (e.g., equal numbers daily and weekly), the more mares can be presented to the stallion. The even spacing of mare presentation is linked to the distribution of mare status (i.e., percentage of maiden, barren, and foaling mares). Most mares foal between March and May, so if an unusually large proportion of foaling mares are presented to the stallion, it means that a large number of mares are presented in a relatively short time span. In addition, maiden and barren mares are generally bred earlier in the season. However, an unusually large percentage of barren or older mares booked to a stallion may contribute to overuse of the stallion early in the year. In our experience, conception rates for foal heat breedings are generally lower than for subsequent estrous cycles. Therefore, to prevent overuse of the stallion and increase the conception rate, careful selection of mares for foal heat breedings is important. Suggested criteria for breeding mares on foal heat are that the mare (1) must have experienced an easy, trauma-free delivery, (2) must be free of fluid in the uterus as determined by ultrasound examination, (3) must be free of bruising of the cervix and vagina, and (4) must be estimated to ovulate on day 10 or later after foaling. If these criteria are satisfied, a foal heat breeding can reduce the number of mares bred at foal heat.

Management of the mares presented to a stallion must also be considered. Ideally, mares bred to any given stallion are kept at the same farm as the stallion so that their management can be controlled.[9] However, this generally is not the case. Lighting programs for barren, maiden, and early foaling mares may help to more evenly distribute the presentation of the mares to the stallion. In addition, palpation of mares to estimate optimal time of breeding and the use of ovulatory inducing agents, such as human chorionic gonadotropin and GnRH analogs, help keep the number of covers to a minimum, which, in turn, allows a larger number of mares to be bred more efficiently.

For the subfertile stallion, all mares that are booked to him should be examined frequently by one veterinarian at the same farm where the stallion stands. This guarantees a more efficient use of the stallion. Mares may have to be palpated two or more times per day.

In general, the average Thoroughbred stallion can breed twice daily, 7 days per week, during the breeding season. (As discussed, libido and semen parameters can modify this average.) The size of a stallion's book is greatly driven by economic factors. The extremely high purchase prices for some stallions necessitate that large numbers of mares be booked to them or that they receive high stud fees. Once the stallion has offspring, the laws of supply and demand become important, as does the demand for the resultant offspring. A stallion's demand is influenced by the performance of his offspring. A stallion that produces a high percentage of winners from starters, a high percentage of stakes winners, a high percentage of 2-year-old winners, or a major winner is in greater demand than a stallion that does not achieve such a good record. There is a strong demand for the offspring of proven sires. These stallions will breed books of 75–100 mares, but this does not adversely affect the market for offspring of these types of stallions.[10] These stallions generally have proven themselves as producers of superior racehorses, and even though there are larger numbers of offspring, these types of horses are still desirable.

A relatively new phenomenon that has arisen since the mid-1990s is the shuttling of Thoroughbred stallions from the Northern Hemisphere to the Southern Hemisphere. These stallions do "double duty" in any given year, by breeding mares in the Northern Hemisphere breeding season of February 15 to July

15 and then breeding mares in the Southern Hemisphere from September to December. Stallions that shuttle back and forth have come from the United States, Japan, France, Ireland, United Kingdom, and Canada at various times. In 1997, 64 confirmed stallions traveled from the Northern Hemisphere to the Southern Hemisphere. This number varies from year to year since some stallions go out of favor and do not live up to their expectations. In addition, some stallions seem to handle the stress of traveling differently than others and therefore may not be included in the program in subsequent years.

In order to try and evaluate the effects on stallions that become involved in this dual hemisphere breeding, a research project was undertaken in 1997. The project was coordinated by Dr. W.R. Allen from New Market, England and this author (JVS) participated in this project. Stallions included in this project were those that spent at least two consecutive years shuttling between the Northern and Southern Hemispheres. Stallions from the United Kingdom and the United States were included. Three ejaculates of semen were collected by artificial vagina from each stallion near the beginning, middle, and end of the breeding season in both the Northern Hemisphere and Southern Hemisphere. In addition, a blood sample was collected from each stallion every 2 weeks throughout the year to measure hormone levels. A total of seven stallions were included in the United Kingdom and four in the United States. Thirteen stallions served as controls.

Semen sample evaluation failed to reveal any specific differences among individuals in the group. The tendency was for sperm output to increase in the single hemisphere stallions (controls) as the breeding season advanced, especially those in the Northern Hemisphere. This is probably due to the longer day length and the reduction in the number of matings as the breeding season winds down. However, no significant differences were seen in semen parameters based on the small sampling intervals during the breeding season.

Blood analysis did reveal a few interesting features. The dual hemisphere horses showed two apparent peaks in testosterone levels, with the first peak from November to January in the Southern Hemisphere (coinciding with the summer solstice there) and the second peak from May to July in the Northern Hemisphere (summer solstice there). Therefore, there were two peaks for the year instead of the normal one. These stallions were able to respond to the lengthening days in both hemispheres.

The single hemispheres control stallions (North), as expected, only had one peak of testosterone levels (April to June). The Southern Hemisphere controls peaked in the November to January period. When testosterone levels were compared with sperm output, there was no obvious relationship between the two.

This simple but useful study, while interesting, was generally inconclusive and not published. Two interesting points could be made:
1. Semen parameters told us nothing concerning these horses.
2. Testosterone levels peaked twice in shuttle stallions as compared with once in single-hemisphere stallions.

BREEDING PROGRAMS FOR THOROUGHBRED STALLIONS

Introducing a New Stallion to Breeding

New stallion prospects arriving from a racing career to a breeding farm are going into a new phase of their life and in so doing must be acclimated and trained for their new duties. Life at the farm is far different from their life and routine at the racetrack, and a period of adjustment must take place.

Ideally, a stallion prospect should arrive at the breeding farm at least 3 months before the start of the breeding season. At this time, the stallion must become accustomed to his new surroundings and handler. One person should be assigned to handle the stallion at all times so that the handler and horse can get to know each other and so the handler can become aware of the particular stallion's habits and personality. The horse's shoes should be pulled if possible.

A small paddock should be provided for turn-out. On the first few occasions for turn-out, farm personnel should be positioned in the corners of the paddock to help ensure that the stallion does not injure himself. In addition, it may be helpful to sedate the stallion lightly before the first turn-out. A combination of 100 mg of xylazine coupled with 10 mg of butorphanol tartrate intravenously is adequate for this purpose. This is usually administered 5 minutes before turn-out. An alternative regimen is the administration of 15–20 mg of acetylpromazine intravenously 15 minutes before[2] or intramuscularly 45 minutes before turn-out. In valuable stallions, the risk of priapism or paraphimosis should be considered when promazine sedation is used.

When first working with the stallion, it is imperative that the handler be able to control him. A chain shank over the bridge of the horse's nose is usually sufficient, but occasionally it must be placed in the mouth. The stallion must first be taught to stand and back up. Once the stallion can back up on command and the handler feels comfortable with him, the stallion can be introduced to a mare. In addition, the stallion should be walked around the breeding shed area and allowed to become familiar with the sights and smells.

The jump mare must be in estrus or must be an ovariectomized mare that has been administered 5 mg of estradiol cypionate intramuscularly. The mare must have a quiet, tolerant temperament. When first introduced, the stallion should be allowed to tease the mare over a teasing bar so that the stallion's reactions can be observed. The whole experience of introduction should be pleasurable to the stallion, so the minimal restraint and punishment necessary is used.

When introducing the stallion to live cover, the mare is placed in a breeding shed or other sufficiently sized area (e.g., 36 × 40 ft or greater). Again, the mount mare should be in strong behavioral estrus and of quiet temperament. The stallion should enter the breeding area and take notice of the mare. It is not recommended to wash the stallion's penis during this first experience because doing so may distract and startle the horse. The mare is twitched and the left foreleg flexed at the carpus and held flexed with a leather leg strap. Hobbles are used at some farms, but we do not recommend them because of their potential for injury. The stallion is allowed to approach the mare from the left side of the mare's flank and allowed some contact to tease the mare. The stallion is then allowed to move toward the rear quarters and perineum. If the stallion wants to mount at this time, he should be allowed to do so. Preferably, this mounting takes place with the stallion's penis in erection, but if the stallion does not have an erection, he should still be allowed to mount the mare. If the stallion mounts with an erection, he may require some assistance for penile intromission.

Once the stallion has bred a mare, the washing process can be introduced. This is accomplished again by bringing the stallion into the breeding area, letting him achieve an erection, and then backing him into the wash area. The wash area should be a corner of the breeding shed that has been set up for this purpose with proper wall padding. Plain warm water and cotton are used to gently wash the penis. Slow, deliberate steps should be taken in this process. Initially, the stallion may violently object to this process, but, with patience, the stallion will tolerate this well.

Experienced Stallions

The older, experienced stallion that is new to a farm should be introduced to the new farm's breeding environment and procedures. This is necessary for the stallion and for the farm personnel so that they can get to know any idiosyncrasies or problems that the stallion may have. Previous records and history pertaining to the stallion are invaluable in this case.

Breeding Shed Management

The actual management of the daily breeding activities of a stud farm varies depending on the size of the farm, the number of stallions standing at stud, and the number of mares. A farm with large numbers of stallions requires an efficient staff whose sole responsibility is to book mares for the stallions and to make the daily bookings for the stallion.

Most large breeding farms have set times for breeding mares on a daily basis. Generally, there are two or three sessions for breeding per day that are fairly evenly spaced (e.g., 9:00 AM, 2:00 PM, and 7:00 PM).

Mares brought to the breeding farm are first identified and then placed in an area where they can be teased to verify their stage of receptivity. Mares that do not show overt signs of behavioral estrus to the teaser are generally identified and jumped by a shielded teaser before being covered by the stallion to which they are booked.

The mare is taken to the mare washing area, where her tail is wrapped with gauze and the vulva and perineal area washed with mild, non-detergent soap (e.g., Ivory). The mare's perineal area is then thoroughly rinsed and dried. At this time, if the vulva has been sutured so that the opening is too small for normal breeding, the vulva is opened. In addition, if the Caslick's sutures are in place, they are removed to avoid lacerating the stallion's penis. Breeding stitches should also be removed to avoid injury to the stallion.

The mare is next taken to the breeding shed area, where she is twitched and her left carpus is flexed and held with a leather strap. A leather breeding shield is placed over the withers to protect the mare from being bitten by the stallion (Fig. 7-1). The stallion may grasp this shield to help maintain balance.

The stallion is then brought up to breed the mare after having his erect penis washed. Once the stallion has mounted the mare, the leg strap is released so that the mare has the use of all four legs to steady herself. The erect penis may have to be guided into the vagina, and the mare's tail may have to be moved (Fig. 7-2). If there is concern that the stallion's penis is too long for the mare's vagina or for certain maiden mares, a breeding roll may have to be inserted between the mare's perineum and the dorsal surface of the stallion's penis (Fig. 7-3). After ejaculation, the stallion should be allowed to lie on top of the mare. When he indicates he is ready to dismount, it is preferable to walk the mare forward and turn her away from the stallion while the stallion slowly glides off the mare. The stallion should not be forcibly yanked off the mare if possible.

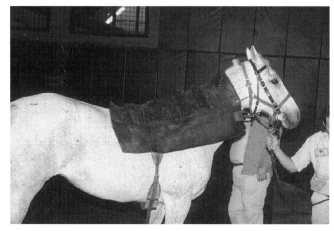

Figure 7-1. A leather breeding shield is placed over the withers to protect the mare from being bitten by the stallion.

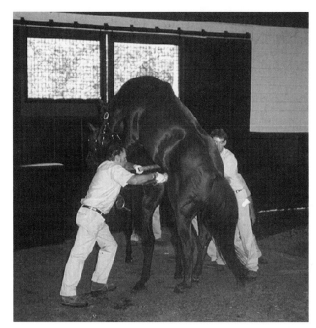

Figure 7-2. The tail may have to be moved so that the erect penis may be guided into the vagina.

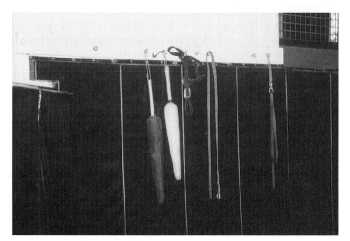

Figure 7-3. Examples of breeding rolls.

After the stallion dismounts, a sample of semen dripping from the penis is collected in a clean, dry container, and this "dismount" sample is viewed on a slide under a microscope to confirm the presence of spermatozoa. If no spermatozoa are seen, the mare is usually covered again.

After the stallion dismounts and the presence of spermatozoa is confirmed, the stallion is backed into the wash area, where his penis is rinsed with water and he is returned to his stall or paddock. Many stud farms also take routine cultures from stallions during the breeding season when large numbers of mares are mated. The penis, urethra, and fossa glandis, as well as the post-ejaculatory urethra, are cultured. This may occur after every 10–15 covers or as deemed necessary.

In addition, various stud farms have prebreeding requirements for mares breeding to their stallions. Generally, uterine cultures are required before first service from barren mares and any mares returning to be bred for a third estrous period. Breeding farms may require a certificate signed by a veterinarian stating that the mare to be bred is suitable for this mating. This may be determined by whatever means the veterinarian decided necessary, such as ultrasound examination of the uterus, uterine cytology and culture, uterine biopsy, or any combination of these techniques.

On many larger farms and on farms with extremely valuable stallions, each cover is recorded to verify that it actually took place and that the correct stallion was bred to the correct mare.

This is another means, along with proper identification of the mare at the time of presentation, to avoid misunderstandings and possible problems.

REFERENCES

1. Taylor I: *Complete Guide to Breeding and Raising Racehorses*. Neenah, WI: The Russell Meerdink Co, 1993, p 257.
2. Varner D, Blanchard T: Stallion management. *Vet Clin North Am Equine Pract* 8:219-235, 1992.
3. Morrow D: *Current Therapy in Theriogenology*. Philadelphia: WB Saunders, 1980.
4. McDonnell SM, Murray SC: Bachelor and harem stallion behavior and endocrinology. *Biol Reprod Monogr* 1:577-590, 1995.
5. Varner DD, Schumacher J, Blanchard TL, Johnson L: *Disease and Management of Breeding Stallions*. Coleta, CA: American Veterinary Publications, 1991, pp 97-115, 211-212.
6. Burns PJ, Douglas R: Effects of season, age and increased photoperiod on reproductive hormone concentrations and testicular diameters in Thoroughbred stallions. *Equine Vet Sci* 4:202, 1984.
7. Kenny RM: *Manual for Clinical Fertility Evaluation of the Stallion*. Hastings, NE: Society for Theriogenology, 1983, pp 3-100.
8. Baker B, McDowell KJ: *Normal Reproduction Performance in Thoroughbred Horses*. Lexington, KY: Maxwell Cluck Equine Research Center, 1988.
9. McKinnon AO, Voss J: *Equine Reproduction*. Philadelphia: Lea & Febiger, 1993, pp 798-808.
10. Conboy S: Large animal reproduction—stallion management. Sixth Annual Hudson Walker Theriogenology Conference. Auburn University: March 4-5, 1995, pp 79-88.

BREEDING MANAGEMENT OF THE WARMBLOOD STALLION

JOHN P. HURTGEN

The Warmblood or show horse breeding stallion is somewhat unique compared with racehorse stallions and stallions shown at halter. The Warmblood stallion frequently competes at an increasingly competitive level from age 3 through 15 years or more. The breeding demands of Warmblood stallions frequently peak at the same time as the horse's show career. It is not unusual for the Warmblood breeding stallion to be in a regular, daily training program, compete in numerous 3- to 7-day-long shows during the year, and be transported hundreds of miles during the course of the breeding and non-breeding seasons. Frequently, the Warmblood stallion is located at a training stable or small farm that is less well-suited for natural mating or on-farm artificial insemination. The use of fresh, cooled semen has become commonplace for the breeding of Warmbloods. The use of frozen semen has also been accepted by most Warmblood breed registries.

Ideal management of the Warmblood breeding stallion needs to be tailored to the individual horse with respect to his training schedule, show date commitments, transportation, adequacy of the farm and its personnel for breeding activities, and the stallion's innate fertility.

NUTRITION

The Warmblood breeding stallion should remain athletic and fit even if he has been retired from active competition. High-quality hay and pasture will meet the stallion's energy and protein requirements in most cases. First or second cutting grass or first cutting grass-alfalfa mixed hay should be available to the horse throughout the day. This will maintain healthy intestinal function, minimize boredom, and reduce the incidence of undesirable stall behaviors. The addition of grain or a vitamin-and-mineral supplement may be necessary to balance the nutrients supplied by hay and pasture.

Vitamin and mineral supplementation of the breeding stallion beyond National Research Council requirements is not necessary and will not improve semen quality.[1]

The feeding program for stallions will need to be evaluated for each horse. If the horse is actively training and competing, he may need to be on a higher plane of nutrition to accommodate his level of exercise. Stallions that are stalled for long periods each day may be more relaxed and content if fed small portions of the ration throughout the course of the day. Fresh water should be available 24 hours per day for all stallions.

A common problem in breeding stallions is excessive weight. Horse owners commonly increase feed intake, particularly grain, during the fall and winter to offset the nutritional demands of cold weather. Feed intake, again, may be increased at the onset of the breeding season. However, many of these stallions are kept indoors during the winter and may even be blanketed. These nutritional changes are usually unwarranted and predispose the horse to laminitis. It is recommended that stallions be weighed each month. An ideal weight for the horse should be determined and maintained with minimal fluctuation. The feeding program should be closely associated with an exercise program. Recent evidence would suggest that feeding docosahexaenoic acid (DHA)–enriched nutraceuticals would have a significant effect on the quality of fresh, cooled, and frozen stallion semen [2]

EXERCISE

Stallions should receive daily exercise. Horses retired from competition should be turned out in a safe paddock or small pasture every day for as long as possible. Most stallions will then remain more athletic and will be more content and satisfied when returned to their stalls. The turn-out protocol, however, will need to be designed for each horse based on paddock behavior, stall behavior, personality, farm breeding schedule, and physical needs or limitations of each horse. If individual stallions do not run and play when turned out, they may need to be exercised on a walking machine, lunged in-hand or free for 30 minutes per day, or ridden under tack or driven in a jog cart three or more times per week for 20–30 minutes per session. The goal of the exercise program is to keep the horse alert, athletic, and content.

When a new stallion is brought to a farm, the farm personnel should be informed about the horse's habits concerning feeding and exercise during the previous month. Management should also be made aware of any physical limitations or conditions affecting the horse, such as prior history of laminitis, tarsitis, navicular syndrome, colic, and objectionable habits. If the new farm management is aware of a stallion's propensity for behavior such as nipping, stall kicking, running the paddock fenceline, stall walking, or weaving, procedures for correcting some of these behaviors may be successful now that the horse's environment has changed. However, some of these behaviors may also begin with the environmental changes. It may take a stallion 1–2 weeks to acclimate to a new farm, personnel, feeding schedule, and other horses.

Many stallion owners are reluctant to turn out stallions during inclement weather (e.g., rain, snow, wind, insect season, heat, or muddy conditions). The breeding farm will still need to allow these horses to exercise. During the heat of the summer, horses can be turned out overnight or after sundown to avoid insect feeding times. Most horses are not adversely affected by rain or snow, unless excessive. An alternative may be to exercise stallions in an indoor arena during severe weather. Blanketing the horse when turned out during bad weather may preserve coat condition. Inclement conditions may persist for many days, so farm managers need to weigh the risks of stall confinement with any risks of turn out. Some farms that stand stallions retired from competition may find that 24-hour-per-day turn out is best for the health of the stallion, provided the horse has access to a run-in shed.

PREVENTIVE HEALTH CARE

The routine health care of the Warmblood breeding stallion is quite similar to that of the other horses on the farm.

Parasite Control

The stallion should be dewormed at regular intervals based on farm needs. No adverse effects from anthelmintics, such as pyrantel pamoate,* fenbendazole,† ivermectin,‡ or moxidectin,§ have been noted in stallions. A frequently used interval for deworming horses is 8 weeks, with the dosage based on the horse's weight. Continuous, daily feeding of pyrantel pamoate¶ has also been safely used in breeding stallions. Periodic examination of fecal specimens should be performed to monitor the efficacy of specific deworming compounds and intervals between treatments.

Dental Examinations

Dental examinations should be conducted on all stallions once per year, or as needed, for each horse. Floating and other dental procedures should be performed as needed to maintain normal mastication and dental arcade alignment. If tranquilization is needed to safely conduct dental examinations and procedures, promazine tranquilizers should not be used due to risk of penile paralysis.[3,4]

Foot Care

The stallion's feet should be evaluated by a competent farrier at regular intervals of 6–8 weeks. Special needs of some horses may require more frequent hoof care. Stallions that receive adequate paddock turn-out usually require minimal hoof trimming. Some stallions need shoes on the front feet only, and some need them on all four feet. For safety reasons, many farms prefer to have stallions barefoot in the front feet during the breeding season unless shoes are necessary for the health of the horse's feet. Hind shoes may be indicated for stallions that are used for live cover or that become sore-footed during the breeding season. Horses that have laminitis, hoof wall cracks, or flat soles may require regular shoeing to remain comfortable.

Vaccinations

The vaccination program for Warmblood stallions should be similar to the immunization program established for the other horses on the breeding farm. Horse population density, age of the horse, degree of non-resident horse exposure, and incidence of specific diseases on a farm are important considerations in development of an immunization program for the stallion. In general, the stallion should be vaccinated against tetanus, eastern and western encephalitis, rabies, and West Nile virus. On many farms, the stallion should also be vaccinated one or more times during the year against the most recent serovars of influenza and rhinopneumonitis viruses. Other vaccines that should be considered on a given farm include botulism, Potomac horse fever (Ehrlichia risticii), and strangles. The efficacy of these vaccines should be judged in relation to the disease risk on a given farm. Encephalitis and Potomac horse fever usually occur in relation to insect- and tick-biting activity. Therefore, these vaccines should be given in late spring in most parts of the United States. However, immunization against the upper respiratory viruses and bacteria should be carried out prior to the onset of the breeding and show season when exposure to other horses will be highest.

Equine arteritis virus can be spread from stallions to mares via respiratory secretions and the semen.[5,6] Approximately 30% of horses previously exposed to equine viral arteritis (EVA) continue to shed EVA virus in their semen. Some of these stallions continue to shed the virus in semen for life. EVA virus infection can cause upper respiratory infections and abortion. The virus from shedding stallions can be passed to seronegative mares during live cover or artificial insemination with fresh, cooled, or frozen semen. Therefore, it is recommended that all stallions to be used for live cover breeding or in an artificial insemination program be serologically tested for exposure to EVA virus before the onset of each breeding season. Stallions that are serologically positive to EVA virus should have an aliquot of semen submitted to an approved diagnostic laboratory to determine the presence or absence of EVA virus in the semen. If the stallion has EVA virus in his semen, he should not be used to breed seronegative mares. Seronegative mares, however, can be safely bred to a virus-shedding stallion following EVA vaccination of the mare. The seropositive stallion that does not shed EVA virus in his semen can be safely used to breed seropositive or seronegative mares without risk of inducing viral infection in the mare.

Seronegative stallions can and, in most cases, should be vaccinated against EVA (e.g., Arvac, Equine Arteritis Vaccine, Fort Dodge Animal Health, Ames, Iowa) before the onset of the breeding season and given boosters annually.[5] This will prevent the stallion from becoming infected with EVA and eliminate the risk of the stallion becoming a shedder of the virus in his semen. Stallions that shed EVA virus in their semen are usually excluded from export to other countries. In addition, fresh or frozen semen from virus-shedding stallions cannot be exported.

The vaccines listed above are considered safe for use in breeding stallions despite the fact that many of these vaccines have not been specifically tested in stallions. A cautionary note concerning EVA vaccination of stallions is that the vaccinated stallion should not be used for breeding during the subsequent 30-day period, since some stallions will shed the vaccine virus in their semen for a short period. EVA vaccination of stallions shedding virus in their semen does not alter their shedding state.

Coggins Testing

Equine infectious anemia is a viral disease of horses. All breeding stallions should be tested annually for EIA.

---

*Strongid Paste, pyrantel pamoate, Pfizer Animal Health.
†Panacur, fenbendazole, Hoechst-Roussel Pharmaceuticals.
‡Eqvalan, ivermectin, Merck AgVet Division.
§Quest, moxidectin, Fort Dodge Animal Health.
¶Strongid C, pyrantel tartrate, Pfizer Animal Health.

BREEDING SOUNDNESS EVALUATION

A thorough breeding soundness evaluation should be performed on the Warmblood stallion prior to purchase. If the stallion is purchased as a competition horse, but some of the value of the horse is residual value as a breeding stallion, the horse should undergo a complete breeding soundness examination. If the stallion is being purchased for breeding, or for both breeding and competition, an evaluation of his breeding soundness should be conducted. Prior to purchase of the Warmblood sport horse, a pre-purchase examination is frequently requested by the purchaser. In the case of the prospective breeding stallion, it may be necessary for the horse to be evaluated by two different clinicians.

A breeding soundness examination should also be performed prior to use of the stallion for breeding in his first year at stud. Specifically, the stallion owner needs to determine the suitability of the stallion for use in a fresh, cooled semen shipment breeding program before this service is advertised or offered to the public. In general, this determination will be based on the stallion's ability to produce adequate numbers of morphologically normal sperm that have the ability to remain progressively motile for 24–72 hours when diluted in an acceptable semen extender and stored at approximately 5°C.[7] The stallion's semen should be free of equine arteritis virus, *Taylorella equigenitalis* (CEM), and other pathogenic bacteria such as *Pseudomonas, Klebsiella,* or *Streptococcus zooepidemicus.*[8] The presence and type of bacteria present in the raw semen samples will assist in appropriate selection of a semen extender containing antibiotics.[9] The extended semen should be cultured to determine the efficacy of the extender-antibiotic combination in eliminating potential reproductive pathogens and minimizing other bacterial organisms. The effect of the extender-antibiotic diluent on sperm viability should also be determined. The most commonly used diluent for equine semen is made of nonfat dry skim milk powder, glucose, and sterile water. Antibiotics frequently added to the extender include ticarcillin, Timentin, penicillin, and amikacin. Antibiotics such as gentamicin and polymyxin B have also been used in equine semen extenders but tend to have a suppressive effect on sperm longevity.[7]

During the breeding soundness evaluation, the stallion's libido, mating behavior, and ejaculatory pattern will be assessed. The horse's internal and external genitalia will be examined for his size, consistency, and presence of any lesions affecting semen quality and fertility.[10] One or more ejaculates of semen will be collected and evaluated. A physical examination of the horse will be performed to identify physical limitations to breeding, such as laminitis, arthritis, incoordination or weakness, and cardiovascular problems, so that corrective measures can be instituted.

A thorough examination of the horse and his semen should assist the stallion owner in efficiently managing the breeding career of the stallion. The examination should help determine any limitations in the size of the stallion's book; acceptability for use in a cooled, shipped semen or frozen semen breeding program; and selection of appropriate semen extenders.[11]

A breeding soundness evaluation should also be performed at the start of each breeding season to determine if any changes need to be made in the breeding management of the horse to maintain maximal reproductive efficiency. However, it should be noted that novice stallions and stallions at the start of a breeding season may have been sexually rested for several months. The initial ejaculates from these stallions may not be representative of the horse's ability to produce high-quality semen. Therefore, it may be necessary to collect and evaluate numerous ejaculates until semen quality stabilizes.[11]

TRAINING THE STALLION FOR BREEDING

The most efficient and safest method of breeding the Warmblood stallion is by semen collection using an artificial vagina (AV) and the artificial insemination of the mares. Because many Warmblood stallions are in training or competition during the beginning of their performance careers, safety of the stallion during mating is a prime concern. Natural service mating information has been presented in Chapter 7 of this text.

Estrous Mare Mount

Collection of semen from the stallion while the stallion is mounted on an estrous mare is a common and acceptable method of obtaining semen from the Warmblood stallion. However, many risk factors associated with live cover are not eliminated. In addition, it will be necessary for the breeding farm to have a large selection of available, non-pregnant mares to be used as mount mares or have a trained or ovariectomized, estrogen-treated mare at the breeding farm for use as a mount mare. Maintenance of the mount mare is an added expense to the farm and still requires the stallion to mount a live horse. The more suitable option for semen collection from the Warmblood stallion is to train the stallion to mount a "phantom" or "dummy" mare (Fig. 8-1).

Phantom or "Dummy" Mare Mount

Training the novice breeding stallion to mount a phantom or dummy mare as a sexual object is usually a rewarding process. Because these stallions have not been allowed to live cover mares, they are easier to train to the phantom than most experienced stallions. The stallion handler needs to exercise a great

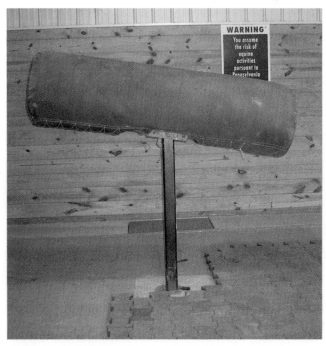

Figure 8-1. A "phantom" mare.

deal of patience toward the stallion being trained and still maintain control and discipline in the breeding shed. The training sessions should last 15–30 minutes per session. These breeding sessions should always follow a routine that begins with preparation of the tease mare in a chute, handling and rinsing of the stallion's penis with warm water, and encouragement of the horse to mount the phantom when erection has occurred. Normal breeding behaviors by the stallion (e.g., vocalizing, nipping, or striking at the phantom; false mounts of the phantom) should not be discouraged. Many novice stallions exposed to an estrous mare in a chute will achieve full erection in preparation for breeding. If these stallions are turned and immediately presented to the phantom, many will mount without reservation. A person with an appropriately prepared AV should always be ready to collect an ejaculate following successful mount. After four or five sequences of this nature, most young horses will be successfully mounting the phantom or, at least, progressing toward that endpoint. If the stallion loses interest or his erection when led away from the tease mare, it may be necessary to stand the estrous mare alongside or in front of the phantom. The stallion is allowed to "reach across" the phantom to tease the estrous mare and encouraged to mount after achieving an erection. As the stallion attempts to mount, the stallion handler tries to have the stallion land on the phantom. Again, a person should be prepared to collect semen if the horse is properly mounted. If the stallion is quite aggressive and anxious to tease and mount an estrous mare, he may repeatedly attempt to mount the mare after initially landing on the phantom. For this reason, it is usually more productive to have the mare a short distance away from the phantom. If the mount mare is positioned in close proximity to the phantom, the mare handler should have a clear and safe escape route in case the stallion does attempt to mount the mare. Once semen has been successfully collected from the Warmblood stallion while he is mounted on the phantom, this behavior pattern needs to be reinforced within 1 or 2 days and repeated four or five times within a 1- to 2-week period. These follow-up semen collections should be conducted in the same manner to reinforce the association of penile washing, the phantom, and exposure to an estrous mare with semen collection while mounted on the phantom. If the stallion is trained for semen collection while mounting a phantom at one clinic or breeding farm but moved to a different farm for the breeding season, some additional training is frequently necessary at the new facility. The change in environment for the stallion presents a new set of breeding circumstances, such as a different phantom, handler, collection technician, breeding shed, tease mare, and AV.

Some stallions that have a dual career as show horses and breeding stallions may have suppressed libido or interest in estrous mares or be reluctant to mount a phantom or a mare. To some extent, normal, stallion-like breeding behaviors have been conditionally suppressed by trainers, owners, and handlers during the course of the show careers of these stallions. In such cases, it is best to collect semen from the stallion in an area not associated with "show" training of the stallion. A stallion handler—someone who is not involved in training or riding the horse—should be selected for the express purpose of handling the horse for breeding. Some stallions may even have suppressed breeding behaviors in response to the voice or sight of their usual trainers. A common practice at small show stables is to trailer the stallion to a neighboring breeding farm for semen collection. These stallions behave like breeding stallions at one farm but are quiet and content at their home farm. Other cues the stallion

may associate with the breeding process include use of a chain lead shank passed through the mouth or over the bridge of the nose, twitching the nose of a restrained mare, or wearing a muzzle.

The phantom should be of sturdy construction and well padded. The total diameter of the body of the phantom should be 20–24 inches. The covering of the phantom should be durable and free of creases or wrinkles. If stallions repeatedly mount and dismount the phantom during training and breeding, they may abrade the medial aspects of the knees or fetlocks. Protective wrapping of the legs may be necessary for some stallions. The phantom should have only one or two legs for support, but the supports should be recessed away from the ends of the phantom. It is preferable to have the height of the phantom adjustable to accommodate individual stallions. Usually, the most appropriate height for the phantom will allow the stallion to "grasp" the phantom with his front legs, have good ventral abdomen contact with the phantom, and allow the horse to have fully extended hocks. When the stallion is in this position, he will not be able to crawl from one end of the phantom to the other end seeking a more comfortable position for him. The stallion should be trained to dismount the phantom by backing off the phantom instead of dismounting across the side of the phantom.

Training the experienced breeding stallion to mount a phantom is frequently more difficult than training the novice horse. A few helpful tips follow. The stallion handler should be patient but firm with these stallions. These experienced live-cover breeding stallions are familiar with the breeding procedure and may become aggressive or anxious when presented to a phantom instead of a mare. It may be necessary to attach a muzzle to the stallion's halter. At times, these stallions may perform best without a mare in the breeding shed or with a mare kept at some distance from the phantom. Again, once semen is successfully collected from the stallion while he is mounted on a phantom, this process should be repeated, under the same circumstances, within 1–2 days. If a longer interval is allowed, the entire training process may need to start over. Caution should be used in allowing the phantom-trained stallion to also breed mares by live cover. These stallions usually refuse to repeatedly accept the phantom. However, stallions used for live-cover breeding readily accept semen collection while they are mounted on a mare.

Training the Stallion for Ground Collection of Semen

The collection of semen from stallions while they remain standing on the ground has become commonplace at some breeding farms. With minimal training, many stallions readily accept this method of semen collection. This method may be preferred in horses with laminitis, tarsitis, or hind limb incoordination. In addition, ground collection of semen may be preferred at smaller farms with limited access to mount mares, limited facilities, and lack of adequate horse handlers necessary for other methods of semen collection.

The stallion is brought to the breeding shed or barn aisle that is free of equipment, or he is left in his stall. The "tease" animal may be free in a stall or 5–10 meters away, being held on a lead shank. For many stallions, it is not necessary for the tease mare to be in estrus when the stallion does not have direct access to the mare. The stallion's penis is washed with clear, very warm water following erection. With the stallion positioned against a smooth wall to prevent lateral movement, or in front of a solid wall to prevent his forward movement, the warm, lubricated

AV is placed on the horse's erect penis. The stallion is encouraged to search and thrust into the AV. Once the stallion has engaged in the AV, the collection person's right hand is used to stimulate additional urethral pulsations while the AV is held against the stallion's abdomen with the left hand. The stallion handler may help support the stallion by pushing against the stallion's shoulder with the right hand.

Stallions respond in one of three ways: standing up while ejaculating; wanting to walk forward while ejaculating; or continuing to stand with all four feet on the ground. The handler should not discourage the horse from walking forward or standing up. Once horses are trained to the procedure, they usually stand flat-footed with arched back and a head-down posture. At first application of the AV to the standing stallion, a few stallions may kick out or want to nip or bite at the handler. The veterinarian should inform the stallion handler and mare handler of how the process works as well as likely responses by the stallion before the initiation of this method of semen collection. After a successful collection, the procedure should be repeated in 1–2 days, preferably in the same location with the same handler and collection person.

BREEDING SEASON CONSIDERATIONS

The owner, breeding farm manager, and veterinarian should develop a coordinated plan for the sporthorse breeding stallion that takes into consideration the horse's show and training schedule, availability of the stallion for semen collection, site of semen collection, number of mares to be bred, quality of the stallion's semen, and other factors. These factors will be important for the farm manager or owner to relay to individual mare owners wishing to breed to the stallion. Mare owners need to be informed of the availability and quality of stallion semen when they commit to a fresh, cooled semen breeding program. The informed mare owner can help optimize the chances for successful pregnancy despite certain limitations on semen availability or quality. For example, if the stallion's sperm longevity drops rapidly 24 hours after semen collection, it may be necessary to inseminate the mare as soon as possible after receiving the semen and not rely on sperm survival in shipping containers 36–72 hours after semen collection.

Cooled Semen Evaluation

Each collection (or at least periodic collections) of stallion semen used in a fresh, cooled semen shipment program should be monitored by the breeding farm for sperm longevity and semen quality throughout the breeding season. The results of these tests should be compared with replies by mare owners concerning the semen quality of shipments they receive. Farm management may be able to make adjustments in their semen collection and shipping protocol, such as extender selection, dilution ratio, or semen collection frequency to improve the overall quality of semen sent to mare owners.

Semen Collection Frequency

Many sporthorse stallions breed a very limited book of mares each breeding season. The interval between successive semen collections may be too long to maintain optimal semen quality for a fresh, cooled semen shipment program. The effect of infrequent semen collection in some stallions is so dramatic

that sperm longevity is reduced to zero within 12 to 24 hours of semen collection and extension. Stallions affected in this manner may need to be put on a collection schedule even if no mares are to be bred. Maintenance of optimal semen quality in most stallions can be achieved with a semen collection frequency of two to three semen collections per week.

If a stallion is scheduled to breed a large book of mares and semen is collected each day, the stallion's sperm concentration may be so low that inadequate sperm numbers are shipped to mare owners after further dilution of the semen in an extender. In most cases this situation can be rectified by putting the stallion on a more strict semen collection schedule, or extended semen can be centrifuged in order to concentrate the semen sample by decanting seminal plasma.[12] After centrifugation and removal of adequate seminal plasma, the more concentrated semen sample can be diluted with the extender for semen shipment.

Records of Collections

The breeding farm should maintain a record of the semen collection dates for the stallion. The record should include the volume of semen collection, total sperm collected, initial sperm motility, extender used, and mares bred with each ejaculate. Periodically, the longevity of sperm motility in extender, sperm morphology, and bacterial culture of extended semen should also be evaluated and recorded. This information may help identify the early onset of semen quality problems.

Semen Freezing

Another breeding management consideration for the sporthorse stallion owner is the feasibility of freezing semen from the horse. Frozen semen may be useful for the stallion with a busy competition schedule, for international use of the stallion's semen, and for those stallions not able to compete and train successfully while actively breeding mares. In addition, freezing high-quality semen allows the owner some degree of insurance should the stallion be lost to breeding via injury, advancing age, or death. Freezing of semen from sporthorse stallions is frequently done during the non-breeding season or when the stallion is temporarily out of training or competition. Once semen has been frozen from a given sire, it is wise for the horse owner to proceed with test breedings using the frozen semen. There are numerous cases in which frozen stallion semen has very good post-thaw characteristics but has been unable to establish pregnancies in mares. The fertilizing capacity of the frozen semen should be established before the product is sold to mare owners unless mare owners are fully aware that the frozen semen has not been tested or has not resulted in pregnancies.

REFERENCES

1. National Research Council: *Nutrient Requirements of Horses*. Washington, DC: National Academy of Sciences, National Research Council, 1989.
2. Brinsko SP, Varner DD, Love CC et al: Effect of feeding a DHA-enriched nutriceutical on the quality of fresh, cooled and frozen stallion semen. *Theriogenology* 63(15):1519-1527, 2005.
3. Pearson H, Weaver BMQ: Priapism after sedation, neuroleptanalgesia and anaesthesia in the horse. *Equine Vet J* 10:85, 1978.
4. Wheat JD: Penile paralysis in stallions given propriopromazine. *JAVMA* 148:405, 1966.
5. Timoney P, McCollum WH: Equine viral arteritis: essential facts about the disease. Proc AAEP 43:199, 1997.

6. Timoney PJ, McCollum WH, Murph TW, et al: The carrier state in equine arteritis virus infection in the stallion with specific emphasis on the venereal mode of virus transmission. *J Reprod Fertil Suppl* 35:95, 1987.

7. Varner DD, Blanchard TL: Current perspectives on handling and storage of equine semen. Proceedings AAEP 1994, pp, 39-40.

8. Blanchard TL, Kenney RM, Timoney PJ: Venereal disease. In Blanchard TL, Varner DD eds: *The Veterinary Clinics of North America: Equine Practice*. Philadelphia: WB Saunders, 1992, pp 191-203.

9. Hoyumpa AH, McIntosh AL, Varner DD, et al: Normal bacterial flora of equine semen: antibacterial effects of amikacin, penicillin, and an amikacin-penicillin combination in a seminal extenders. Proc 12th Int Cong Anim Reprod 1992, pp 1427-1429.

10. Weber JA, Woods GL: Transrectal ultrasonography for the evaluation of stallion accessory sex glands. In Blanchard TL, Varner DD, eds: *The Veterinary Clinics of North America: Equine Practice*. Philadelphia: WB Saunders, 1992, pp 183-190.

11. Hurtgen JP: Evaluation of the stallion for breeding soundness. In Blanchard TL, Varner DD eds: *The Veterinary Clinics of North America: Equine Practice*. Philadelphia: WB Saunders, 1992, pp 149-165.

12. Jasko DJ, Moran DM, Farlin ME, et al: Effect of seminal plasma dilution or removal on spermatozoal motion characteristics of cooled stallion semen. *Theriogenology* 35:1059, 1992.

HORMONE THERAPY IN THE MARE

CLAIRE CARD

There is an increasing trend in the equine industry to engage in managed natural breeding and assisted reproductive techniques that require the regulation of estrus and ovulation.

Hormonal therapy in the mare is used primarily for inducing and managing the onset of the breeding season, programming natural matings by induction of estrus and ovulation, implementing assisted reproductive procedures, and delaying or suppressing estrus and its behavior.

The current hormonal options and methods of hastening the onset of the breeding season, estrous regulation, estrous synchronization, and ovulation induction are discussed.

MANAGEMENT/MANIPULATION OF WINTER ANESTRUS

Artificial Lights

The use of a stimulatory artificial photoperiod remains the main means of controlling the onset of the breeding season in mares. Once mares enter winter anestrus, approximately 60 days of a stimulatory artificial photoperiod, mimicking the long summer days, are required before the onset of the transitional period and the first ovulation occurs.[1,2] Typically 16 hours of total light are used, beginning in November or December, with the additional light added at the end of the day. However, the photosensitive window of the mare is approximately 10 hours after the onset of darkness. A single hour of light beginning 9.5 hours after the onset of darkness may also be used in what is called a "flash" lighting protocol. The energy of the light is also important; 100 lux is recommended, but there is a dose-dependent response, with as little as 10 lux having some effect in mares.

Dopamine Antagonists

Dopamine antagonists result in increased secretion of prolactin. The mechanism of action of dopamine antagonists is unknown but may relate to a decrease in dopamine-receptor binding on the ovary or indirect effects of increased prolactin concentrations on ovarian function that have a positive influence on follicular development. Protocols describe the use of increased photoperiod beginning in anestrus/early transition for 2 weeks and then continuing the increased photoperiod while adding a dopamine antagonist such as sulpiride (1 mg/kg IM BID) or domperidone (1.1 mg/kg PO SID) daily for 3 weeks or until ovulation. There is some information that combining 2 months of artificial photoperiod with a 10-day pretreatment with estradiol benzoate (11 mg IM SID/mare) may help prime mares to respond to sulpiride (250 mg SQ SID/mare) therapy.[3-5]

Gonadotropin-Releasing Hormone

The physiologic mechanism behind gonadotropin-releasing hormone (GnRH) therapy in seasonally anestrous mares is the stimulation of follicle-stimulating hormone (FSH) and luteinizing hormone (LH) synthesis and release from the anterior pituitary, which in turn induces follicular development and ovulation, respectively. Several recent studies have demonstrated that GnRH can be used successfully to induce ovulations in seasonally anestrous mares when administered as hourly pulses of native hormone, twice-daily boluses of a potent agonist or serial insertion of slow-release implants. Products such as deslorelin implants have been used in anestrous/transitional mares. The mares receive a new implant every 3 days for up to 3 weeks or until they ovulate. Injectable deslorelin has been used twice daily (63 μg IM BID) to induce follicular activity in anestrous/transitional mares. Ovulations occur in approximately 50%–70% of anestrous mares treated. The duration from the onset of treatment to ovulation is approximately 2 weeks. Because of the insensitivity of the anestrous/transitional mares to GnRH, implants are not typically removed in anestrous mares. Deslorelin implants have been associated with a delayed return to estrus in some mares during the breeding season when the implants were not removed.[6]

Overall, however, progesterone concentrations and duration of the luteal phase following GnRH-induced ovulations are similar to those following ovulations that occur during the physiological breeding season. Mares in deep anestrus at the onset of any GnRH treatment may return to anestrus following the end of treatment, even if ovulation was induced. The failure of some non-pregnant mares to continue cyclic ovarian activity after GnRH treatment in anestrus makes it imperative that the mare be monitored carefully for follicular development and ovulation and bred to a stallion of normal fertility. Pregnancy rates following ovulations induced by GnRH in seasonally anestrous mares range from 51% to 80% and are not significantly different than pregnancy rates following the first spontaneous ovulation of the year.[6,7] Injectable superagonists, such as buserelin, are more potent and are similar to deslorelin in activity. They are not commercially available in North America at this time, but they appear to have reduced efficacy in the mare.[8]

Equine Follicle-Stimulating Hormone

Equine follicle-stimulating hormone (eFSH) has been used with good success in mares in early transition. Mares with a 20- to 25-mm follicle are treated with twice daily injections of eFSH (12.5 mg IM) until one or more follicles reaches 35 mm. The eFSH treatment is discontinued, and 36 hours later the mare is treated with hCG and bred. With this protocol the majority of mares continue to cycle following treatment, and ovulation rates are enhanced.[9]

Human Chorionic Gonadotropin

Human chorionic gonadotropin (hCG), obtained from the urine of pregnant women, is commonly used in veterinary practice to hasten ovulation in transitional and normally cycling mares. hCG is used to shorten the transitional period by stimulating the ovulation of large dominant follicles. In the absence of hCG treatment, many of these large follicles will regress without ovulation and will be replaced by development of another follicular wave that may or may not progress to ovulation. Finally, hCG has also been reported to induce the ovulation of large follicles stimulated to develop in anestrous mares by GnRH administration.[10]

The biochemical composition of hCG is similar to equine LH but has a much longer half-life because of a high sialic acid content. All gonadotropic hormones have an alpha and a beta subunit, of which the beta subunit is species specific. Various authors have expressed concern about the antigenic nature of hCG in the mare. Antibodies to hCG have been measured in the mare, and frequent hCG treatments in the same breeding season were associated with higher titers. Some researchers have reported a decreased response to hCG following frequent hCG treatments in the same season. It was inferred without measuring antibody titers that antibodies to hCG were causally related to the reduced response. Other authors reported seasonal changes in the mare's response to the hormone. Critical studies to address the hCG antibody relationship with response to hCG remain to be performed.[11]

Seasonal factors also influence the time to ovulation from treatment and the percentage of mares ovulating in relationship to hCG administration. A response to treatment with hCG is defined as ovulation within 48 hours of injection. The range of response is variable with a low percentage (12%) of mares ovulating by 24 hours, the majority by 36 hours (50%), and then some by 48 hours (12%) or beyond. Similar to other hormonal treatments, some mares do not respond to hCG.[12] In groups of mares, a 75% response rate with ovulation within 48 hours is usually reported. Reduced efficiency of hCG is found in mares treated to end transition. Mares that fail to respond to hCG during the breeding season tend to repeat the behavior and usually ovulate later (72–96 hours after treatment). Commonly used dosages are 2000 to 2500 IU, intravenously or intramuscularly. Interestingly, most mares will ovulate with much lower dosages (500 IU) of hCG.

Progesterone/Progestagen

Late transitional mares with follicles of 25 mm may be placed on altrenogest (Regumate) for 2 weeks or a 1.9-gm progesterone-containing controlled intravaginal device (CIDR) may be inserted for 2 weeks to stop the signs of heat and increase the likelihood of fertile mating. The mare should be evaluated at the end of the progestagen treatment to assess the ovarian status. The use of the CIDR in transitional mares has been variably associated with an increase in follicular development.[13]

It has been suggested that progesterone/progestagen works through changing the hormonal isoforms or secretory patterns

---

Box 9-1 | Hormonal Options for Induction and Synchronization of Estrus

Altrenogest 10 ml (0.044 mg/kg) PO daily for 8–14 days
Progesterone-in-oil (50 mg/ml) IM daily for >8 days
Long-acting (LA) progesterone single injection IM (activity 8–10 days)
Controlled intravaginal drug release (CIDR) devices 8–14 days, 1.9 g progesterone total per device
Progesterone 150 mg/estradiol 10 mg preparations (P&E) IM daily for 8–10 days
Prostaglandin F2α 1–5 mg once >5 days after ovulation SQ 1–2 injections
Cloprostenol (Estrumate) 125 μg SQ once >5 days after ovulation

---

of the hypothalamus or pituitary, or by changing ovarian sensitivity to these hormones. Some progestagen-treated mares will come into heat quickly after the discontinuation of treatment and are ready to breed in 24 to 48 hours after withdrawal of the progestagen. Transitional mares that show estrus, have a follicle >30 mm, or that were treated with progesterone/progestagen before estrus should be treated with hCG to increase the likelihood of ovulation. The presence of endometrial edema has been variably reported to relate to response to hCG. A decline in endometrial edema from the time of administration to 24 hours was associated with an increased likelihood of ovulation. The hCG acts like LH in the mare, which is low in the transitional mare. In spontaneous ovulations final maturation of the preovulatory follicle is associated with an increased production of estrogens and a more intense estrus.

Melengestrol acetate has been used in mares in late transition at 150 mg PO/mare/day for 10 days with a mean time to ovulation after the end of treatment at 14 days. The effect of this hormone on fertility has not been examined.[14]

Circularized forms of recombinant equine LH have recently been investigated. The most effective dose appeared to be 0.75 mg IM. This is a non-antigenic product that appears to have the similar efficacy to hCG.[15]

INDUCTION AND SYNCHRONIZATION OF ESTRUS

Estrus synchronization in horses has been problematic because of the long duration of behavioral estrus and the variable time frame to ovulation during estrus. Box 9-1 shows the options for estrus synchronization. There are three methods of estrus induction for breeding: physical aspiration of follicles, induction of luteolysis (prostaglandin F2α [PGF], cloprostenol), and the prevention of estrus with exogenous progesterone (long-acting progesterone, CIDR)/progestagen (altrenogest)/progesterone and estradiol (PGE), which allows natural luteolysis to occur. It is important to remember that progesterone/progestagen administration does not prolong the lifespan of the CL, nor does it suppress luteolysis. Progesterone supplementation induces diestrous-type behavior, even in the mares that undergo natural luteolysis while being treated. The diestrous behavior is of benefit in performance mares, because they neither attract nor are attracted to stallions. Progestagen/progesterone therapy is almost always combined with an ovulation induction treatment such as hCG or GnRH analog (deslorelin).

Progesterone/Progestagen Therapy

Progesterone/progestagen, regardless of the source, needs to be administered for a minimum of 8 days if the mare's status is unknown at the start of treatment. This is because some mares will be in heat at the time the treatment starts and will ovulate within the next few days while under the influence of the progesterone. None of the currently available natural or synthetic progesterone compounds stops ovulation in mares beginning treatment during estrus; however, these ovulations usually occur in the absence of estrous behavior.

On the last day of progesterone/progestagen treatment, the mares should be given prostaglandin because most of the mares will have functional luteal tissue. They may have luteal tissue from a previous ovulation or they may have ovulated while being treated (in which case they would not show estrus). The main population of treated mares should come into heat on average in about 3 days from discontinuing the administration of the progesterone/progestagen compound, which is also 3 days after prostaglandin treatment. There is wide variability in the onset of estrus from the time the progesterone/progestagen is discontinued, with a range of 1 to 7 days. The reason is that while the progesterone suppresses estrous behavior, it does not suppress follicle development. A failure to come into heat is either behavioral or the mare ovulated late during the treatment and her CL was not sensitive to the prostaglandin.[16,17] For this reason evaluating mares for follicular size on the day PGF is given is strongly recommended to determine how fast they should come into heat. Studies show that treatments with altrenogest, long-acting progesterone, or CIDR have a similar mean time to ovulation after discontinuing treatment. Long-acting progesterone is effective for 8–10 days. The CIDRs have 14 days of progesterone-releasing activity, but they may be used for as few as 8 days. The cost and convenience factor are most important when choosing a progesterone/progestagen product. Mare temperament and intramuscular irritation may be an issue if many injections or long-acting formulations are used. It has been indicated that a sustained release injectable altrenogest product may be available in the future. Mild vaginitis has been reported in mares treated with CIDR, and these devices are not recommended for use in subfertile mares.

The most effective therapy to induce synchronous estrus and ovulation involves the administration of progesterone and estradiol 17-β (P&E). Other forms of estrogen have not been shown to be effective. The P&E is a compounded product produced as a 50-mg/ml solution of progesterone and a 3.3-mg/ml solution of estradiol 17-β. Three ml of this solution are injected every day for 8–10 days. The addition of estradiol 17-β to progesterone treatment is sufficient to cause follicular regression. Similar to the other progesterone/progestagen treatments, if the mare is in estrus when the treatment is started she may ovulate in the first few days of P&E treatment. Neither hormone is luteolytic; therefore, prostaglandin is also used on the last day of this protocol. The mean time to estrus from the last day of P&E plus PGF injection is 8–10 days. These mares are usually evaluated 6 days after the last treatment to predict the onset of estrus and planned breeding. This protocol is often effectively used by rural practitioners to reliably induce estrus in mares. For example, a mare is examined and the P&E is prescribed for 8 days. The mare is checked at the end of treatment and given prostaglandin. The mare is administered prostaglandin on the last day of P&E treatment. She is then scheduled for an examination 6 days later. At that examination follicle size is measured and, assuming follicles grow at 3 mm/day, semen is ordered to arrive when the follicle is around 35 mm. The mare is injected with hCG on the day before or at the time of the breeding.[11] The pros and cons of progesterone/progestagen therapy are summarized in Table 9-1.

In summary, all of these products are effective in synchronizing estrus. They vary in terms of price, convenience, and side effects. None of the progesterone/progestagen compounds stop follicle growth or ovulation during treatment. Because of this fact during the breeding season, all progesterone/progestagen protocols should be combined with prostaglandin administration to make sure the mare comes into heat.

Prostaglandin

Many mare owners do not have access to a stallion for teasing to determine their mare's receptivity for breeding. In addition, when using live cover, access to a stallion may be subject to availability of a booking; when using cooled transported semen, access to semen shipments may be limited to specific days or delivery dates. Therefore, many people in the equine industry routinely depend on intensive breeding management, including induction or synchronization of estrus and induced ovulation.

Table 9-1 | **Progesterone/Progestagen Therapy**

PRODUCT	COST	PRO	CON	SIDE EFFECT
Regumate (altrenogest)	++++	Given PO	Does not prevent follicle growth Combine with PGF*	None alone
Progesterone in oil	+++	Daily IM	Does not prevent follicle growth Combine with PGF*	Injection reactions
LA P4	+++	Single shot	Does not prevent follicle growth Compounded Combine with PGF*	Injection reactions
CIDR	+++	Easy to insert	Does not prevent follicle growth Extra label use Combine with PGF*	Vaginitis
P&E	+++	Effective	Causes follicle suppression Compounded, give daily Combine with PGF*	Injection reactions

*Prostaglandin has the following side effects (not observed after all treatments): extreme sweating, Flehmen, increased defecation, urination, and colic-like signs.

The clinical use of PGF includes its use to "short cycle" a mare. PGF (5 mg/mare SQ) and its analogs, such as cloprostenol (125 µg/mare SQ),[10] are one of the most affordable and most widely used products in equine practice. They are used to cause regression of a CL from days 5 to 16 of the estrous cycle (day 0 is ovulation). Prostaglandin has few ovarian effects if administered in estrus but causes some sustained uterine contractions, which is why it is sometimes administered to subfertile mares before ovulation. When repeated doses of PGF are administered prior to 5 days post-ovulation, luteolysis will occur; however, the mare will not come into heat faster unless the mare is a two-wave mare and already has a medium-sized follicle. Two low-dose injections (0.5 mg/mare IM) spaced 12 hours apart are also effective in inducing luteolysis and are associated with fewer side effects.[11,16]

The beginning of behavioral estrus starts on average 3 days after PGF administration; however, the range to the onset of estrus is 1 to 7 days later, depending on status of the ovary at the time of treatment. Mares with very large follicles (i.e., >40 mm) at the time of PGF treatment may ovulate within 24 hours of administration without showing estrus. If this happens and they are bred, a mare with a healthy uterine condition will often conceive. Therefore, it is strongly advised that mares be examined on the day they are given prostaglandin to determine the time frame for the onset of estrus. A common protocol for the synchronization of estrus and ovulation is the use of two injections of PGF 14 days apart. The problem is that this treatment takes up a substantial portion of the breeding season. Two injections of PGF are required for estrus synchronization because mares in estrus at the time of the first injection and the mares in the first 5 days from ovulation do not have a CL susceptible to prostaglandin. The product works by inducing luteolysis so two treatments are required for estrous synchronization, which brings the majority of mares into the susceptible portion of their luteal phase. A modification of this method is to examine the mares using ultrasound and treat all mares that have CLs with prostaglandin and then treat the mares without CLs 10 days later. This avoids wasting the product in mares without luteal tissue. Box 9-2 shows the forms, doses, and routes of administration of prostaglandin.

Side effects are significant and may be dramatic following PGF or cloprostenol administration. The side effects do not occur after every treatment; hence, if a horse has experienced the side effect once, it does not mean it will repeat after every treatment. The natural hormone PGF and its analogs often cause excessive sweating, Flehman, increased heart rate and respiratory rate, abdominal discomfort, locomotor incoordination, and lying down. Signs occur within 10–20 minutes of injection and will decrease in another 20–30 minutes. Caution should be taken by practitioners to avoid self-injection, inhalation, or skin contact when handling these products, especially pregnant women and asthmatics, since they may cause uterine contractions and bronchoconstriction.

The mean time from prostaglandin treatment to induced ovulation is 8 days. The variability to response is related to the size of the dominant follicle on a mare's ovary at the time of PGF treatment. Follicles grow at 3 mm/day. A mare that finishes a progesterone/progestagen treatment with her largest follicle at 20 mm will take 5 days at 3 mm/day to grow a 35-mm follicle. Most light horse mares will show heat at about a 30-35–mm follicle size if no luteal tissue is present. A mare with a follicle of 40 mm may ovulate the day after the PGF, may have a short 3-day heat, or have a normal heat but grow a large preovulatory follicle (55 mm).

Nonhormonal Methods

Follicular ablation is used to reset the follicular wave. Follicles are usually ablated through a transvaginal ultrasound-guided approach or through a flank approach. In some mares follicle ablation results in an elevation in progesterone, presumably through the formation of luteal tissue, and other mares have pre-existing luteal tissue. Therefore, prostaglandin should be used 5 days after aspiration in these mares as well. Minimal risk for adhesions or negative effects on fertility has been reported. This procedure is usually performed under heavy sedation. It requires a special ultrasound probe casing, good equipment, and operator skill.[19]

Ovulation Induction

Two hormones are commonly used to induce ovulation in the mare. These include hCG and a GnRH analogue, deslorelin. These are used in combination with induction of estrus to time ovulation.

hCG

hCG is an effective product that is moderately priced. It is administered for ovulation induction in cycling mares that are showing signs of estrus with a follicle ≥35 in diameter. The hCG (2000 IU IM or IV) will induce ovulation of that follicle within 24–48 hours. The use of hCG improves the efficiency of a breeding program by reducing the duration of estrus, decreasing the number of breedings at each estrus, and providing a means of synchronizing ovulation with a stallion's breeding schedule.

GnRH Analogues: Deslorelin

Deslorelin is a highly effective product that is available as a bioresorbable pellet or in a compounded injectable formulation. It acts like native GnRH and results in the release of FSH and LH. The LH then induces ovulation. The time frame from insertion of the pellet to ovulation is 44 hours. Fewer mares ovulate outside of the mean time when compared with hCG rates.

The delay in return to estrus in some mares was attributed to prolonged pituitary suppression by the GnRH agonist. The pellets are often inserted in the vulva in a lidocaine bleb while the insertion needle is directed down into the lidocaine-filled tissue and removed by squeezing out or using a lidocaine bleb and cutting the pellet out.

HORMONAL THERAPY FOR EMBRYO TRANSFER

Based on many studies with average mares and average stallions, we should expect the fertility (pregnancy rate) on a per cycle basis to be about 50% using natural cover or AI. Therefore, with good technique we should expect to recover half as many embryos as ovulations. When ovulation induction agents, such as hCG or deslorelin, are used, ovulation rates are usually around 1.2 ovulations per estrus. Therefore, we should recover an embryo slightly more than half the time. The embryos should be graded and the quality of the majority of the embryos (around 90%) should be good to excellent. Overall we expect about a 60% embryo survival rate per transfer. In other words, for each embryo flush we have about a 32% chance of an embryo transfer (ET) pregnancy. Mare factors such as age, uterine condition, and other medical problems influence the success rate, as does stallion fertility and management.

Prostaglandin and Progesterone and Estradiol 17β

Protocols include both the induction of estrus and ovulation. Critical to the success of an ET program is the use of recipient mares that have ovulated 2 days before or up to 3 days after the donor mare. The first task is to align the estrus and ovulation of the donor mare with the recipient.

The determination of the protocol to use for donors and recipients should consider recipient cost and maintenance, cost of rectal examinations, breeding method and expenses, and the costs of pharmaceuticals. In situations where there are plenty of recipients and their daily maintenance costs are low, the use of two prostaglandin-treated diestrous recipient mares for every donor (2:1 ratio) is common. The timing of the treatment with PGF to the donor and recipients is based on the mares having a CL that is at least 5 days old and on their follicle size. Mares with bigger follicles are treated later than mares with smaller follicles in order to align donor and recipient ovulation. As the mares come into heat, hCG or deslorelin treatments may be used to induce ovulation or natural ovulation may be used to align donor and recipient ovulation times.

If there are few recipients or recipient cost and maintenance are high, P&E (150 mg progesterone and 10 mg estradiol 17β) should be used in both donors and recipients for 8 days. A 1:1 ratio of donor to recipient can be used. The practitioner should give PGF on day 8 of P&E, check the mares 6 days later, measure follicle sizes, and follow mares into heat. Eight days after the last P&E injection, the mares should be rechecked, and usually at this point hCG or deslorelin injections are planned. The treatment to induce ovulation is usually given on days 8–10 after the last P&E. Mean time to hCG-induced ovulation is 36 hours. Mares should be checked daily to confirm ovulation times. This protocol in general requires fewer rectal examinations but requires daily injection of P&E.

Generally it is preferable to have the recipients ovulate after the donor. A range of recipient mare ovulations from 2 days before to 3 days after the donor's ovulation has been reported to be acceptable. Managing ovulation is important so that the recipient's endometrium is at a developmental stage that it may receive signals involved in the recognition of pregnancy from the transferred embryo. The physical size and morphology of the embryo to be transferred should considered when selecting a recipient; therefore a small-for-date embryo should be transferred to a recipient matched to its developmental age rather than using only the day post-ovulation of the donor.

Equine Follicle-Stimulating Hormone

A commercially prepared purified equine FSH extract preparation (eFSH, Bioniche Animal Health Inc., Athens, GA) has enabled the examination of superovulatory protocols in mares.[20] In many studies, eFSH treatment has been shown to increase the number of ovulations and embryo recovery rates in transitional and cycling mares used for embryo transfer.[21-23] However, in some studies, eFSH treatments have been associated with unwanted ovarian hyperstimulation as shown by complete ovulation failure, increased numbers of large non-ovulatory follicles, lower than expected embryo per ovulation rates, or lower than expected quality in some of the recovered embryos.[20, 24-26] Some authors indicate that around 10% of eFSH-treated mares fail to ovulate within 96 hours of ovulation induction. It has been reported that other treated donor mares experience a delayed return to estrus. There was also variability noted in the superovulatory response among eFSH-treated mares.[22] Particularly in mares, some of these negative hyperstimulation effects could be related to the unique anatomic structure of the mare ovary, in which follicles develop in the interior cortex of the ovary and ovulate only through the limited area of the ovulation fossa. This anatomic arrangement may be relevant in superstimulated mares because it may restrict the number of ovulations.[24]

Recent studies have shown that treatment of mares with eFSH may disturb oocyte maturation and transport, which in part could be related to the large amount of clotted blood observed in the ovulation fossa in superovulated mares.[25] In several other studies conducted in our laboratory, we found that mares treated with eFSH had higher estrogen levels for a longer duration before and around the time of ovulation and also had alterations in uterine and cervical parameters (edema and tone), compared with control mares (Raz and Card, unpublished data).[26] These alterations in the hormonal and reproductive tract parameters during the days that oocyte maturation, ovulation, fertilization, and early embryonic development are expected to occur may contribute to the negative effects associated with eFSH treatments.

A recombinant equine FSH (reFSH) has recently been developed and was reported to stimulate the ovary and to increase the number of ovulations; however, in the single report that is available, treatment with reFSH was also associated with large follicles that failed to ovulate.[9] Further studies are required to examine the potential of reFSH as a superovulatory treatment; however, it is likely that more of the same negative hyperstimulation effects will occur in reFSH-treated mares.[26]

The basis for the use of the gonadotropin eFSH is that exogenous FSH overcomes the suppressive effects of the dominant follicle and allows the recruitment of additional follicles for ovulation. The eFSH product is expensive. Twice daily administration of 12.5 mg of eFSH/mare has provided the best ovulation rates. Recipients are administered prostaglandin based on follicle size near the time the donor gets prostaglandin, and their ovulation induction time is adjusted to align them with the donor mare. With this protocol it is advisable to have three recipients per donor. A range of ovulations per cycle has been reported, but 3.4 ovulations per cycle and 2.2 embryos per cycle have recently been reported. A higher ovulation rate should proportionately increase embryo recovery rate. Ovulations are usually synchronous but may be asynchronous. Embryo recovery is planned in relation to the day of breeding(s) and the time between the ovulations. Typically a day 8 post-ovulation recovery attempt is planned since day 8, 7, and 6 embryos may be recovered from mares with asynchronous ovulations.

Protocol 1

Donor mares are allowed to ovulate. On day 5 after ovulation (where ovulation is day 0), 12.5 mg eFSH is administered twice daily IM to the donor mare. On day 7 after ovulation the donor mare is administered PGF and allowed to come into heat. The donor mare continues to receive 12.5-mg eFSH BID until one follicle is >35 mm in diameter. At this time the eFSH treatment is discontinued and 36 hours elapse without hormonal treatment. This is called *coasting*. The donor mares, 36 hours after the last eFSH treatment, are administered 2000 IU hCG IM and bred. Ovulation should occur within 48 hours of treatment with hCG.

Protocol 2

The donor mare is followed to confirm ovulation. In early diestrus the donor mare is examined until a 20-mm follicle is detected. She is then started on 12.5 mg eFSH twice daily. The rationale is that the division in the emerging follicular wave between dominant and subordinate follicles occurs at about this time. Prior to this time the exogenous eFSH is not needed to increase the number of dominant follicles in the cohort, so it is best to administer it only when it is required since treatment is costly. Two days after eFSH is started, prostaglandin is administered. The donor continues to receive 12.5-mg eFSH BID until one follicle is >35 mm in diameter. At this time the eFSH is discontinued and 36 hours elapse without hormonal treatment (coasting). The donor mares, 36 hours after the last eFSH treatment, are administered 2000 IU hCG IM and bred.

Other Considerations

Mares that are treated with eFSH may have asynchronous ovulations. It is therefore advisable to arrange to have two breedings available per estrus, since in addition to breeding at the time of hCG administration, it may be necessary to rebreed the donor mare 2 days later. Ovulation should occur within 48 hours of treatment with hCG. In one report, hCG was found to induce more mares to ovulate than deslorelin, and therefore it is commonly used in combination with eFSH. The mares that do not ovulate in response to hCG and have had 96 hours elapse from hCG treatment are likely to have ovulation failure. The mares that fail to ovulate at ≥96 hours post-hCG and have large static follicles may be treated with a luteolytic dose of PGF, which may induce ovulation within 24 hours. Prolonged estrous behavior and a delayed return to estrus are associated with ovulation failure.

RECIPIENT MANIPULATION

Mares may be manipulated using estrus synchronization protocols to align estrus and ovulation. Ovariectomized (ovx) progesterone/progestagen-treated mares have been used as ET recipients. The ovex mare is typically started on progesterone the day the donor mare ovulates or up to 2 days later. Ovx mares are kept on exogenous progesterone through the first 100 days of pregnancy. These mares may be used again as recipient mares following foaling. Transitional mares may also be used as ET recipients by administering progesterone as mentioned previously.[27]

HORMONAL THERAPY FOR SUBFERTILITY

Prostaglandin and cloprostenol have been used at luteolytic dosages after breeding and before ovulation to induce sustained uterine contractures in subfertile mares that accumulate fluid. Post-ovulatory treatment with PGF or cloprostenol has been associated with lower luteal production, but not lower pregnancy rates in mares. Generally the use of PGF after ovulation is avoided, and it should not be used after day 3 post-ovulation because it may cause luteolysis in some mares. Similarly, oxytocin,

20 IU/mare, has been used as a uterotonic agent to evacuate post-breeding fluid in subfertile mares.[28] Steroids such as prednisone and dexamethasone have been used in subfertile mares, presumably to decrease pro-inflammatory cytokine production. Further research is required to determine the dose and application of these therapies. Mares with uterotubal obstruction have been treated via a laparoscopic approach with PGE. Old maiden mares that have a fibrotic cervix are also sometimes treated with 2–2.5 mg PGE intracervically to induce prolonged cervical softening.

HORMONAL THERAPY FOR INDUCTION OF LACTATION, ABORTION, AND PARTURITION

Induction of Lactation

A variety of protocols have been reported to induce lactation in mares that are used as surrogate dams or that have poor lactation. Lactation can be enhanced by administration of domperidone alone at 1.1 mg/kg PO. This dopamine antagonist increases prolactin secretion and lactational ability. For the induction of lactation, mares that have had a previous lactation are used. Mares are treated with progesterone (150 mg) or progestagen (0.44 mg PO), estradiol 17β 10 mg, and domperidone at 1.1 mg/kg PO the first week; in the second week they are treated daily with 150 mg progesterone, 20 mg estradiol 17β/day and 2.2 mg/kg domperidone. Domperidone is continued at 1.1 mg/kg for another 1–2 weeks (Card, personal communication, 2008). Another protocol used 150 mg progesterone and 10 mg estradiol 17β for 1 week, with 5 mg prostaglandin administered on day 7, and 500 mg sulpiride administered IM on days 1–10. It was reported that 80% of treated mares lactated. Cross-fostered foals may be introduced to the mare under supervision. It has been reported that providing vaginal stimulation along with 5–20 IU of oxytocin each time the cross-fostered foal is introduced to the mare may increase mare acceptance of the foal.[29,30]

Induction of Abortion

Abortion may be induced in mares before the 35th day of pregnancy with a single injection of prostaglandin. Some of the main applications of PGF for abortion include elimination of a twin pregnancy, medical problems in the mare requiring termination of pregnancy, and mismating. Later in pregnancy, repeated daily treatments of prostaglandin (10 mg SQ, or twice the luteolytic dose) may be required. Typically at least three daily treatments are required to induce delivery. Mares usually show side effects associated with prostaglandin treatment (profuse sweating, cramping, colic-like signs, etc.) and often have discomfort between treatments. If abortion has not been induced by the fourth treatment, oxytocin (20 IU IM) may be administered 30 minutes after prostaglandin treatment. Retained fetal membranes may be a consequence. It is not advisable to induce abortion after the seventh or eighth month of pregnancy because of the large size of the fetus.[31,32]

Induction of Parturition

Fetal maturation may be induced by administering repeated high-dose injections of dexamethasone (100 mg IM) for 4 days beginning on day 315 of pregnancy. This protocol is used in mares that are unlikely to survive to term. Delivery is expected 4 days after the last treatment. Colostrum production is typically poor.[33]

Physiologically the mare is exquisitely sensitive to oxytocin in late pregnancy, and as little as 2 IU IV may induce delivery. Following mammary secretion electrolyte changes indicating readiness for birth, daily low dose treatment with oxytocin (2–3 IU) has been reported to result in few complications.[34,35] The authors suggest that the low-dose protocol will not induce parturition if the mare is not ready to foal.

Commonly, oxytocin (5–20 IU IM) is used in mares >330 days of pregnancy with a relaxed cervix and with milk electrolyte changes indicative of readiness for birth. Parturition typically occurs within 1 hour of treatment. A higher incidence of premature placental separation has been reported in mares following induction of parturition. In mares with a non-relaxed cervix, intracervical PGE_2 (2.0–2.5 mg misoprostol) has been used before induction of parturition without deleterious effects.[36]

HORMONAL THERAPY FOR OVARIAN QUIESCENCE

Ovarian Quiescence Post-Foaling

Rates of ovarian quiescence in foaling mares or reports of ovarian failure are low. In foaling mares, lactational anestrus may be behavioral, related to fescue endophyte toxicosis or physiologic factors. Fescue endophyte toxicosis is treated by reducing exposure to the endophyte and administering domperidone at 1.1mg/kg PO daily for at least 10 days prepartum and postpartum to support lactation. Anestrus may follow foal heat in mares that foal early in the breeding season if they are not placed in a stimulatory artificial photoperiod before foaling. Although physiologic anestrus related to lactation in mares does not typically occur, and mares return quickly to foal heat estrus, mares occasionally have a failure to cycle as a result of negative energy balance or prolonged stress such as founder.

Miscellaneous Causes

Maiden mares that fail to cycle may have chromosomal abnormalities. Anabolic steroid administration may be associated with irregular patterns of ovarian activity. A failure to cycle in barren mares is often idiopathic; however, it is prudent to rule out a prolonged luteal phase by the administration of prostaglandin or measuring serum progesterone, testosterone, and inhibin levels if a granulosa theca cell tumor is a possibility. Retained endometrial cups may be demonstrated through the measurement of eCG. Anti-GnRH vaccination is also associated with a failure to return to estrous cycles in a small proportion of mares even 2 years after discontinuation of the treatment.[37] The anti-GnRH vaccine labeled for use in mares is only available in Australia.

Ovarian failure routinely occurs in aged mares; in middle-aged mares this is referred to as premature ovarian failure. Ovarian failure is associated with a loss of ovarian responsiveness to gonadotropins. The serum gonadotropins levels are very high in these mares.[38]

Treatment of Ovarian Quiescence

Treatment for lactation-related ovarian quiescence in mares that are losing weight or in poor body condition typically includes an increase in the energy density of the diet and early weaning. The combination of PMSG 5000 IU and hCG 5000 IU as a single treatment has been reported to be effective in barren and foaling mares, with 74% of mares showing estrus and 100% ovulating within 21 days of treatment.[39] It has been reported that basal LH concentrations and GnRH-induced LH release are lower in lactating than in nonlactating mares, and a lower response to exogenous GnRH has been reported in lactating mares in mid-lactation. Exogenous progesterone or altrenogest is sometimes used for 10 to 14 days in these mares and presumably influences the hypothalamo-pituitary function.[40]

HORMONAL THERAPY TO PREVENT ESTROUS BEHAVIOR

Hormonal therapy is often used in performance mares to prevent estrous behavior. A wide variety of options are currently available, including hormonal, nonhormonal, and immunologic methods to modulate estrous behavior in mares.

Induction of a Prolonged Luteal Phase

Hormonal therapy includes the induction of a diestrous ovulation using 3000 IU of hCG when a diestrous follicle reached >30 mm, which results in a prolonged luteal phase. In one study not all mares developed a diestrous follicle of that size and not all treated mares ovulated.[41] Similarly the prevention of luteolysis using twice daily treatments with 60 IU oxytocin from day 7–14 also creates a prolonged luteal phase in a high proportion of mares.[42]

Intrauterine Devices

An indirect hormonal method to prevent estrous behavior is the use of intrauterine devices. A 20 mm diameter water-filled ball introduced into the uterus on day 2–4 post-ovulation resulted in a prolonged luteal phase in 75% of mares, for a mean diestrous period of 57 days. The mares with the prolonged luteal phases did not release prostaglandin at the normal time. Glass balls (marbles) 35 mm in diameter have also been used to induce a prolonged luteal phase in 22%–40% of mares. The authors described the insertion of the glass ball during estrus. Some mares reportedly expelled the glass balls, while others retained the glass balls and continued to cycle. Insertion during early diestrus may improve the success with glass ball devices.[43,44]

Hormones, Implants, and Depot Injections

The use of oral progestagen altrenogest (0.44 mg/kg) is the common method of preventing estrous behavior. Altrenogest causes essentially no side effects in mares, and it may be used for prolonged periods. The intravaginal device (CIDR) can be used for short-term estrus suppression. Daily injections of progesterone (150 mg/mare) or a long-acting progesterone preparation may be administered once weekly. All of these treatments should be initiated at least 3 days before the time the mare is required to be out of heat, because if the mare is in estrus at the time of treatment, it takes a few days for the behavioral suppression to occur.[16] Hormonal implants such as Synovex S, which contains 25 mg of progesterone and 2.5 mg of estradiol benzoate, have been administered in mares to suppress estrous behavior. In one study 80 implants were administered to mares, and all returned to estrus on time. There is no evidence to suggest that these implants alter the expression of estrus; therefore, if there is a beneficial effect on mares, it is exerting its effect through some other means.[45] Similarly, long-acting hormonal products such as medroxyprogesterone acetate (Depo-Provera) are not effective in regulating estrous behavior.

Anti-GnRH Vaccines

Immunologic means of preventing estrous behavior include the use of anti-GnRH vaccines. The hormone GnRH is a small decapeptide and is non-antigenic, so the GnRH is conjugated to another molecule to which antibodies are produced when injected. Two vaccinations are given 2 weeks apart. This protocol resulted in 98% of vaccinated mares becoming anestrus or transitional by 4 weeks after the second vaccination. In the breeding season after vaccination, 88% of mares had estrous cycles, and in the year after that 98% had estrous cycles.[38] Behavior of the mares vaccinated with anti-GnRH is often described as passive, similar to that of anestrous mares.[46,47]

REFERENCES

1. Sharp DC: Photoperiod and artificial lighting. In Robinson NE, ed: *Current Therapy in Equine Medicine*, ed 2, Philadelphia: WB Saunders, 1987, pp 491-492.
2. Koskinen E, Kurki E, Katila T: Onset of luteal activity in foaling and seasonally anoestrous mares treated with artificial light. *Acta Vet Scanda* 32:307-312, 1991.
3. King SS, Jones KL, Mullenix BA, Heath DJ: Seasonal relationships between dopamine D1 and D2 receptor and equine FSH receptor and equine FSH receptor mRNA in equine ovarian epithelium. *Anim Reprod Sci* 108:259-266, 2008.
4. Donadeu FX, Thompson DL Jr: Administration of sulpiride to anovulatory mares in winter: effects on prolactin and gonadotropin concentration, ovarian activity, ovulation, and hair shedding. *Theriogenology* 57:963-976, 2002.
5. Kelly K, Thompson D Jr, Storer W, et al: Estradiol interactions with dopamine antagonists in mares: prolactin secretion and reproductive traits. *J Equine Vet Sci* 26:517-528, 2006.
6. Allen WR, Sanderson MW, Greenwood RE, et al: Induction of ovulation in anoestrous mares with a slow-release implant of a GnRH analogue (ICI 118 630). *J Reprod Fertil Suppl* 35:469-478, 1987.
7. Johnson AL: Gonadotropin-releasing hormone treatment induces follicular growth and ovulation in seasonally anestrous mares. *Biol Reprod* 36:1199-1206, 1987.
8. Barrier-Battut I, Poutre N, Trocherie E, et al: Use of buserelin to induce ovulation in the cyclic mare. *Theriogenology* 55:1679-1695, 2000.
9. Raz T, Carley S, Card C: Comparison of the effects of eFSH and deslorelin treatment regimes on ovarian stimulation and embryo production of donor mares in early vernal transition. *Theriogenology* 2008 (in press).
10. Grimmett JB, Perkins NR: Human chorionic gonadotropin (hCG): the effect of dose on ovulation and pregnancy rates in Thoroughbred mares experiencing their first ovulation of the breeding season. *N Zealand Vet J* 49:88-93, 2001.
11. Neely DP: Reproductive endocrinology and fertility in the mare. In Neely DP, Liu IKM, Hillman RB: *Equine Reproduction.* Nutley, NJ: Hoffman-La Roche, pp 11-22, 1983.
12. Samper J: Induction of estrus and ovulation: why some mares respond and others do not. *Theriogenology* 70:445-44, 2008.
13. Klug E, Jöchle W: Advances in synchronizing estrus and ovulations in the mare: A mini-review. *Journal of Equine Veterinary Science* 21:474-479, 2001.
14. Lopez-Bayghen C, Zozaya H, Ocampo L, Brumbaugh G, Sumano H: Melengestrol acetate as a tool for inducing early ovulation in transitional mares. *Acta Veterinaria Hungarica* 56:125-131, 2008.
15. Yoon MJ, Boime I, Colgin M, et al: The efficacy of single chain recombinant equine luteinizing hormone (reLH) in mares: Induction of ovulation, hormone profiles and inter-ovulatory intervals. *Domest Anim Endocrinol* 33:470-479, 2007.
16. Ginther OJ: *Reproductive Biology of the Mare: Basic and Applied Aspects*, ed 2. Cross Plains, WI: Equiservices, 1992.
17. Rossdale PD: Exogenous control of the breeding season. In Robinson NE, ed: *Current Therapy in Equine Medicine*, ed 2. Philadelphia: WB Saunders, 1987, pp 493-494.
18. Alcantara B, Boeta M, Porras A: Luteolysis, estrus induction, and clinical side effects in mares treated with a PGF2 alpha analog, cloprostenol (Sinocrel 11-21). *Journal of Equine Veterinary Science* 25:384-386, 2005.
19. Bergfeldt DR, Meira C, Fleury JJ, Fleury PD, Dell'Aqua JA, Adams GP: Ovulation synchronization following commercial application of ultrasound-guided follicle ablation during the estrous cycle in mares. *Theriogenology* 68:1183-1191, 2007.
20. Niswender KD, Alvarenga MA, McCue PM, Hardy QP, Squires EL: Superovulation in cycling mares using equine follicle stimulating hormone (eFSH). *Journal of Equine Veterinary Science* 23:497-500, 2003.
21. Squires EL: Superovulation in mares. *Vet Clin North Am* 22:819-830, 2006.
22. McCue P, LeBlanc M, Squires E: eFSH in clinical equine practice. *Theriogenology* 68:429-33, 2007.
23. Squires EL, Logan N, Welch S, McCue P: Factors affecting the response to administration of equine FSH. *Animal Reproduction Science* 94:408-10, 2006.
24. Alvarenga MA, Carmo MT, Landim-Alvarenga FC: Superovulation in mares: Limitations and perspectives. *Pferdeheilkunde* 24:88-91, 2008.
25. Carmo MT, Losinno L, Aquilar JJ, Araujo GHM, Alvarenga MA. Oocyte transport to the oviduct of superovulated mares. *Animal Reproduction Science* 94:337-339, 2006.
26. Raz T, Carley S, Card C. Comparison of the effects of eFSH and deslorelin treatment regimes on ovarian stimulation and embryo production of donor mares in early vernal transition. *Theriogenology* In press, 2008.
26. Niswender KD, Jennings M, Boime I, Colgin M, Roser J: In vivo activity of recombinant equine follicle stimulating hormone in cycling mares. In *Proceedings of the 52nd Annual Convention of the American Association of Equine Practitioners* 53:561-562, 2007.
27. McKinnon AO, Squires EL, Carnevale EM, Hermenet MJ: Ovariectomized steroid-treated mares as embryo transfer recipients and as a model to study the role of progestins in pregnancy maintenance. *Theriogenology* 29:1055-1063, 1988.
28. Veronisi MC, Carluccio A, Kindahl H, Faustini M, Battocchio M, Cairoli F: Oxytocin-induced PGF2alpha release in mares with and without post-breeding delayed uterine clearance. *J Vet Med A Physiol Pathol Clin Med* 53:259-262, 2006.
29. Chavatte-Palmer P, Arnaud G, Duvaux-Ponter C, Brosse L, Bougel S, Daels P, Guillaume D, Clèment F, Palmer E: Quantitative and qualitative assessment of milk production after pharmacologic induction of lactation in the mare. *J Vet Intern Med* 16:472-472, 2002.
30. Steiner JV: How to induce lactation in non-pregnant mares. *Proceedings of the 53rd Annual Convention of the American Association of Equine Practitioners.* San Antonio, Texas, USA 2-6 Dec 52:259-260, 2006.
31. Madej A, Kindahl H, Nydahl C, Edqvist L, Stewart D: Hormonal changes associated with induced late abortions in the mare. *J Reprod Fertil Suppl* 35:479-484, 1987.
32. Rathwell A, Asbury A, Hansen P, Archbald L: Reproductive function of mares given daily injections of prostaglandin F2 alpha beginning at day 42 of pregnancy. *Theriogenology* 27:621-630, 1987.
33. Alm CC, Sullivan JJ, First NL: Induction of premature parturition by parenteral administration of dexamethasone in the mare. *J Am Vet Med Assoc.* 165:721-722, 1974.
34. Villani M, Romano G: Induction of parturition with low-dose oxytocin injections in pregnant mares at term: clinical applications and limitations. *Reprod Domes An* 43:481-483, 2008.
35. Camillo F, Marmorini P, Romagnoli S, Cle M, Duchamp G, Palmer E. Clinical studies on daily low-dose oxytocin in mares at term. *Equine Vet J* 32:307-310, 2000.
36. Rigby S, Love C, carpenter K, Varner D, Blanchard T: Use of prostaglandin E2 to ripen the cervix of the mare prior to induction of parturition. *Theriogenology* 50:897-904, 2002.
37. Card C, Raz T, LeHeiget R, Sibert G: GnRF immunization in mares: ovarian function, return to cycling, and fertility. *Proceedings of the 53rd Annual Convention of the American Association of Equine Practitioners,* Orlando, Florida, USA, 1-5 December 53:576-577, 2007.
38. Carnevale E: The mare model for follicular maturation and reproductive aging in the woman. *Theriogenology* 69:23-30, 2008.
39. Deichsel K, Aurich J: Lactation and lactational effects on metabolism and reproduction in the horse mare. *Livestock Production Science* 98:25-30, 2005.

40. Tsukada T, Sato K, Moriyoshi M, Koyago M, Sawamukai Y: Treatment with a high dose combination of PMSG/hCG preparation of mares clinically diagnosed with ovarian quiescence during the breeding season (investigation from 1975 to 2000). *Journal of Equine Science* 19:35-38, 2008.

41. Hedberg Y, Dalin AM, Santesson M, Kindahl H: A preliminary study on the induction of dioestrous ovulation in the mare–a possible method for inducing prolonged luteal phase. *Acta Vet Scanda* 48:12, 2006.

42. Vanderwall D, Rasmussen DM, Woods GL: Effect of repeated administration of oxytocin during diestrus on duration of function of corpora lutea in mares. *J Am Vet Med Assoc.* 231:1864-1867, 2007.

43. Nie G, Johnason K, Braden T, Wenzel J: Use of an intra-uterine glass ball protocol to extend luteal function in mares. *J Equine Vet Sci* 23:266-273, 2003.

44. Rivera del Alamo M, Reilas T, Kindahl H, Katila T: Mechanisms behind intrauterine device-induced luteal persistence in mares. *Anim Reprod Sci* 107:94-106, 2008.

45. McCue P, Lemons S, Squires E, Vanderwall D: Efficacy of Synovex-S(R) implants in suppression of estrus in the mare. *Journal of Equine Veterinary Science* 17:327-329, 1997.

46. Elhay M, Newbold A, Britton A, Turley P, Dowsett K, Walker J: Suppression of behavioural and physiological oestrus in the mare by vaccination against GnRH. *Australian Veterinary Journal* 85:39-45, 2007.

47. Imboden I, Janett F, Burger D, Crowe M, Hassig M, Thun R: Influence of immunization against GnRH on reproductive cyclicity and estrous behavior in the mare. *Theriogenology* 66:1866-1875, 2006.

Microbiology and Diseases of Semen

Ahmed Tibary, Jacobo Rodriguez, and Juan C. Samper

The acceptance of artificial insemination (AI) by some of the major equine breed registries has had a tremendous impact on the total population of mares that can be booked to a stallion in his lifetime. International movement of semen in a cooled or frozen state has made disease transmission across countries a real threat.[1,2] Traditionally, the stallion has always been considered an important epidemiological risk factor in spreading venereal diseases. In Europe, North Africa, and some Asian countries, strict regulation of equine breeding through institutions such as national stud farms and remount stations has been implemented since before World War I in order to limit risk of disease outbreak, particularly Dourine.[3] Today, with advanced technology and ease of transport of stallions, the same risk still exists. The high risk that the stallion poses to the mare population to which his semen is exposed becomes a more serious threat when we realize that the stallion is an asymptomatic carrier of most diseases.[1,4]

Although natural mating poses the highest risk for venereal transmission of disease, other risk factors will increase the threat of contaminating a population of mares or a stallion. Managerial and hygienic procedures in the housing and bedding of a stallion are important factors that must not be overlooked because of the possibility of the colonization of the penis by certain bacteria. In breeds that permit AI, it is not uncommon for the stallion to alternate between natural cover and AI under no veterinary supervision. This inconsistency of breeding method can increase the risk of contaminating a stallion or of spreading microorganisms to several mares. The 2006 U.S. breeding season outbreak of equine viral arteritis (EVA) in several states caused by use of infected shipped semen from shedder stallions is a perfect example of this danger. AI has been used as a managerial technique to increase reproductive efficiency and reduce the risk of spreading disease. This technique allows stallions to be booked to over 300 mares during a year. This rapid multiplication and ease of access to a large population of mares requires extreme vigilance and testing for the presence of venereal diseases. In addition to biosecurity measures at the level of the stallion and mare herd, factors such as the cleanliness of the semen collection equipment and lubricants should be examined.

This chapter reviews the main epidemiological and clinical features as well as preventive measures for sexually transmitted infections in the equine. It draws primarily from a recent review by the authors.[1,5] In addition, some of the most important diseases of semen (hemospermia and urospermia) are discussed.

BACTERIAL CONTAMINATION

Breeding stallions should be routinely examined for bacterial infections as part of breeding soundness examination before and after each breeding season. The most appropriate approach to investigating the microbial flora of the stallion reproductive system is to take samples from the surface of the erect non-washed penis, the pre-ejaculate fluid, the urethra (pre- and post- ejaculation) and the semen. Specific venereal disease such as contagious equine metritis (CEM) also requires swabbing the urethral fossa.

Contaminant of the Surface of the Penis or Urethra

Many commensal bacteria (Box 10-1) including *Escherichia coli*, *Streptococcus zooepidemicus*, *Streptococcus equisimilis*, *Staphylococcus aureus*, *Bacillus* spp., *Klebsiella* spp., and *Pseudomonas* spp. are part of the exterior of the stallion penis, are not regarded as pathogenic, and may be cultured from an ejaculate or mare uterus.[6] Alterations of the normal bacterial flora on the exterior genitalia may cause the growth of opportunistic bacteria such as *Klebsiella pneumoniae*, *Pseudomonas aeruginosa*, and *Streptococcus equi* ssp. *zooepidemicus*, which, if inseminated, may cause infertility in susceptible mares. *P. aeruginosa* has been isolated from penile swab with frequencies ranging from 20% to 40%.[7-9]

S. equi ssp. *zooepidemicus*, *E. coli*, *P. aeruginosa*, and *K pneumoniae* are the most common isolates in cases of endometritis in the mare.[5,6,10] Infections caused by *P. aeruginosa* or *K. pneumoniae* are often considered venereal because of the mode of transmission of these organisms (e.g., coitus, insemination with infected semen, genital manipulations).[11-14] The capsule type of *Klebsiella* seems to be a determinant in which organism is involved in equine metritis. Capsule types K1, K2, and K5 are the most frequently associated with equine metritis. Capsule type K7 is thought to be part of the stallion's normal preputial flora.[15]

The majority of stallions with disrupted microbial flora of the genital tract can shed pathogenic bacteria and are often asymptomatic carriers. The most common manifestation of this infection transmission is persistent mating-induced endometritis or infectious endometritis leading to reduction in fertility in susceptible mares. The factors that contribute to the colonization of the penis by pathogenic bacteria are not well understood. The intact penile skin and the normal desquamation of its cells help combat the proliferation of pathogenic bacteria. However, frequent washing of the penis with soaps, detergents, and some

Box 10-1 | Common Organisms Isolated from Stallions and Mares

Pathogenic Bacteria

Pseudomonas fluorescens
Pseudomonas aeruginosa
Klebsiella pneumoniae

Questionable Pathogenicity

Beta-hemolytic streptococci
S. zooepidemicus
S. equisimilis
E. coli

Potential Pathogens

Bordetella bronchiseptica
Citrobacter spp.
Enterobacter spp.
Proteus mirabilis
Proteus morganii
Proteus rettgeri
Proteus vulgaris
Providencia spp.
Pseudomonas spp. (excluding *P. aeruginosa*)
Staphylococcus aureus

Nonpathogenic Bacteria

Alpha-hemolytic streptococcus
Lactobacillus spp.
Micrococcus spp.
Bacillus spp.
Alcalgenes spp.
Flavobacterium spp.
Serratia spp.
Coagulase-negative *Staphylococci* (*Staphylococcus lentinus*, *Staphylococcus coptis*, *St. haemolyticus*, *St. xylous*)
Non-hemolytic *Klebsiella*

Other Bacteria Isolated from Mare's Uterus

Bacillus cerus
Bacillus licheniformis
Bacillus spp.
Enterobacter aerogenes
Enterococcus spp.
Pant. Agglomerans
Proteus mirabilis
Pseudomonas pseudoalcaligenes
Pseudomonas spp.
Staphylococcus equorum
Staphylococcus gallinarum
Staphylococcus hominis
Staphylococcus hyicus
Staphylococcus kloosii
Staphylococcus lentus
Staphylococcus sciuri
Staphylococcus vitulinus
Staphylococcus warneri
Staphylococcus xylosus

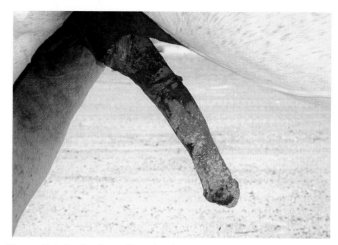

Figure 10-1. Penis of a stallion showing severe overgrowth of bacteria and fungus following aggressive use of antiseptics.

the type of organisms harbored on the external genitalia. These organisms can also be acquired at the time of coitus with a mare that has a genital infection.

Careful evaluation of breeding records with a sudden and unexplained drop in early pregnancy rates or an increase in early embryonic death should warn the stallion manager about a possible problem. Definitive diagnosis is based on isolation in a pure culture of the suspected microorganism from the stallion's reproductive tract. In addition, isolation of the same microorganism with a similar sensitivity pattern from the non-pregnant mares will help confirm the diagnosis. Bacteriological molecular genetics techniques can provide solid proof of presence of shedding in a stallion by comparing the strains isolated from the mares with endometritis and those isolated from the stallion's reproductive system.

Treatment of stallions depends on the type of bacteria and method of breeding. For stallions breeding by AI, a thorough penile wash before semen collection is recommended. The filtered semen is then diluted with an extender containing the antibiotic for which the bacterial is sensitive and incubated for 20–30 minutes before use for insemination. Minimum contamination breeding technique (MCBT) is very helpful when natural cover is the only method of breeding.[19] The mare's uterus is infused with an antibiotic-containing semen extender just before mating. Stallions breeding by natural cover should be washed and scrubbed thoroughly. After washing, the penis is dried. Alternatively, the mare may be covered and then a uterine lavage performed followed by uterine infusion with appropriate antibiotic between 4 and 6 hours after breeding. However, it should be kept in mind that misguided or improper use of antimicrobials as uterine infusion or additive may pose a serious concern regarding multiresistant bacteria and development of fungal and yeast infection. Stallions with penile colonization by *Klebsiella* or *Pseudomonas* can be washed with a weak solution of HCl (0.2%) or sodium hypochlorite (bleach 5.25%), respectively.[14,19] Systemic treatment with antibiotics should be avoided since it has proved unrewarding in most cases. Stallions with *Pseudomonas* infection have been reportedly treated with iodine-based surgical scrub followed by the application of 1% silver sulfadiazine cream daily for 2 weeks. Field observations from practitioners suggest that inoculation of penile surface with bacteria (smegma) from a normal stallion may be helpful in re-establishing the normal flora of the penis.

antiseptics change the texture of the skin and will increase the susceptibility of the penis and prepuce to colonization by pathogenic organisms.[16-18] Excessive cleansing of the stallion's penis with detergents and antiseptics may also be responsible for severe balanitis and colonization by bacteria or fungus (Fig. 10-1). The environment in which a stallion is housed may influence

Bacterial Infection from the Accessory Sex Glands

Bacterial seminal vesiculitis is the most common infection of the accessory sex gland in the stallion.[20-23] Although not very common, this disease often results in serious economic losses because of its persistent nature, possibility for venereal transmission, and detrimental effect on fertility of both the stallion and mare. The most common isolates from cases of infectious seminal vesiculitis in the stallion are *P. aeruginosa, K. pneumoniae, Streptococcus* spp., *Staphylococcus* spp., *Proteus vulgaris* and *Brucella abortus*.[13,14,20,22-26] A case of seminal vesiculitis due to *Acinetobacter calcoaceticus* has been described.[27] The infected stallions are usually identified initially by the presence of neutrophils in their ejaculates, pyospermia, hemospermia, sperm agglutination/precipitation, and poor motility along with a history of infertility or subfertility.[12,20,23,28] Confirmation as well as treatment may be achieved by direct culture and infusion of the vesicular glands using endoscopy (Fig. 10-2).[3,29] Direct sampling from the seminal vesicles can be obtained by videoscopy and catheterization of the ejaculatory duct.[3,29-31] Treatment of seminal vesiculitis is often very difficult because the majority of antimicrobials cannot reach the gland in sufficient concentration.[20,27,28] Broad-spectrum antimicrobials such as trimethoprim sulfa may be used systemically.[28] Enrofloxacin has been reported to reach sufficient concentration in the seminal vesicles following parenteral administration.[27] Direct flushing of and in situ infusion of the antimicrobial into the glands is the preferred method of treatment.[3,21,22,29] Direct lavage of the vesicular gland with amikacin combined with oral treatment with trimethoprim sulfa for 8 days has been successful for treatment in a case of seminal vesiculitis caused by *P. vulgaris*.[22] Infusion of an extender containing a specific antimicrobial in the uterus of a mare before breeding combined with post-breeding lavage helps prolong the survival of semen and control bacterial growth.[13,20,27,32-36]

Contagious Equine Metritis

The causative agent of CEM is a fastidious growing, microaerophilic, non-motile, gram-negative rod or pleomorphic coccobacillus known as *Taylorella equigenitalis,* which is not present in North America but is endemic in Europe. Efforts for eradicating the disease from the breeding industry have been successful, but CEM still occurs sporadically in some countries.[15,37,38]

All breeding stallions in countries with no surveillance system or stallions that are imported from countries where CEM is present should be tested prior to breeding during the quarantine. CEM-infected stallions are asymptomatic carriers and harbor the organism in the urethral fossa, the urethra, or the sheath. Diagnosis of CEM is made by culturing the organism from these sites as well as from semen.[39,40] Transport medium is Amies supplemented with charcoal. Swabs are plated on Columbia blood-chocolate agar at 37°C and 7% carbon dioxide. Because of the slow growth of *T. equigenitalis,* the possibility of false-negative results is relatively high. It is estimated that a single clitoral swab would detect 95% of the carrier mares if infected more that 8 weeks earlier. Cervical swabs detect about 85% of the acutely infected mares and only 30% of chronically infected mares.

Another test that is commonly used is the polymerase chain reaction (PCR) assay, which appears to be very sensitive. However, because of the sensitivity of this test, an increase in the number of false positives may be present.[41-45] There is also a risk that the test may reveal non-pathogenic strains.

Mares bred to infected stallions will develop a severe purulent vaginitis, cervicitis, and catarrhal endometritis, resulting in infertility and, rarely, abortion. These mares will appear to clean up but will remain infected, and the organism can be cultured from the clitoral fossa.[39]

Positive stallions must be removed from breeding, and treatment consists of daily washing of the penis and urethral fossa with 2% chlorhexidine gluconate followed by packing the areas with nitrofurazone (0.2%) ointment daily for 7 consecutive days.[39,46] In countries where nitrofurazone cannot be used, a suitable alternative is enrofloxacin. Association of the local antiseptic treatment to systemic treatment with sulfamethizole trimethoprim (30 mg/kg) every 12 hours for 10 days.[40] Treated stallions should be tested several times within 6 weeks after treatment before breeding. Two swabs must be obtained no sooner than 7 days after completing treatment with at least 2 days between cultures. Regular washing with chlorhexidine is not 100% efficacious for the prevention of CEM in stallions.[47]

In countries where mule production is important, veterinarians should be aware of a risk of CEM organisms in the jackass. A species of *Taylorella* has been isolated from donkey jacks in Kentucky and California.[48-50] These asinine strains named *T. asinigenitalis* did not cause a CEM syndrome in mares bred naturally (Kentucky) or with shipped semen (California). However, experimental infection with the Kentucky isolate resulted in infection. *T. asinigenitalis* has been isolated recently from the genital tract of a 3-year-old Ardennes stallion with a natural infection.

Other Potentially Harmful Microorganisms

Other microorganisms that can be potentially transmitted venereally include *Chlamydia* spp. and *Mycoplasma* spp. *Mycoplasma* spp. have been isolated from the external genitalia and semen of clinically normal and infertile stallions, but their exact role in uterine infection is not well established.[51-53] *M. equigenitalium, M. subdolum,* and *Acholeplasma* spp. have been associated with infertility, endometritis, vulvitis, and abortions in mares and with reduced fertility and balanoposthitis in stallions.[51,54,55] *M. equigenitalium* and *M. subdolum* were isolated from the genital tract of mares (5%–34%) and aborted equine fetuses (7%); however, the occurrence of *Mycoplasma* spp. was not always correlated with reduced fertility.[51,54-56]

Genital chlamydiosis of horses has been reported to result in mild chronic salpingitis,[57] reduced reproductive rates,[58,59] low ejaculate quality,[60] and occasionally abortion.[61-64]

Detection of chlamydial organisms from aborted equine fetuses ranges from 20% to 55%.[64,65] However, these reported rates may be too high because other infections were present and it is difficult to culture this organism. Chlamydial organisms that have been found in the horse include *Chlamydophila pneumoniae,* equine biovar associated with respiratory diseases, and *C. abortus* and *C. psittaci,* which were both detected in equine abortion cases.[63]

It is important to be aware of the possibility of these agents causing infertility both in mares and stallions. Although not commonly present in semen or the genital tract of the stallion, *Candida* spp. and *Aspergillus* spp. can be potential pathogens, particularly in AI programs where the hygiene of the collection and processing equipment is not well monitored.

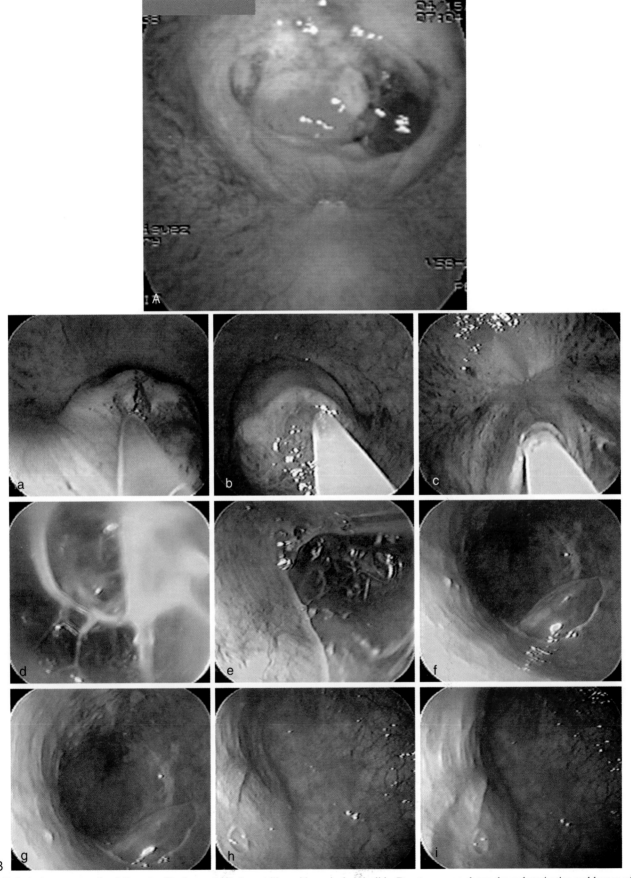

Figure 10-2. A, Appearance of an inflamed colliculus seminalis in a stallion with seminal vesiculitis. **B,** *a-i* sequence shows the catheterization and lavage of the seminal vesicle.

VIRAL CONTAMINANTS

Although many viruses have the potential to be found in semen during the viremic phase of the disease, only equine arteritis virus (EAV) responsible for EVA and equine herpes virus III, the etiologic agent for equine coital exanthema are considered as sexually transmissible.[66] The potential for the equine infectious anemia virus to be transmitted through semen has been suspected and is still a subject of debate.

Equine Arteritis Virus

EAV is a small RNA virus of the genus Arterivirus belonging to the family of Arteriviridae. EVA has a worldwide distribution except for Iceland and Japan.[67-71] The virus is non-arthropod–borne and primarily transmitted from stallion to mare.[72,73] Horizontal transmission from stallion to another via fomites or contaminated bedding is possible.[74] Presently EAV is responsible for major restrictions in the international movement of horses and semen. Prevalence of seropositive stallions in some countries reaches 60%–80% of all stallions.[15,72,75-77]

The virus targets primarily the endothelium of the small blood vessels and macrophages. The incubation period is 3 to 14 days. The acute phase of the disease is characterized by fever (up to 41°C) and panvasculitis resulting in limb and ventral edema, depression, rhinitis, conjunctivitis, serous nasal discharge, palpebral periorbital and supraorbital edema, and edema of the ventral abdomen.[39,68,69,78,79] The virus may cause abortion and has caused mortality in neonates. Stallions may show severe preputial and scrotal edema with variable effects on spermatogenesis and sperm quality.[80,81] Experimentally infected stallions experience a necrotizing vasculitis in the testicles, epididymis, and accessory sex glands. Natural EAV exposure results in long-term immunity to disease. Mares and geldings eliminate virus within 60 days, but 30%–60% of acutely infected stallions will become persistently infected, temporarily or permanently shedding virus in the semen.[68,69] Mares infected venereally may not show any clinical signs, but they shed large amounts of virus in nasopharyngeal secretions and in urine, which may result in the lateral spread of infection by the aerosol route.

Venereal infection does not affect fertility, but mares infected at later stages of gestation may abort. Identification of carrier stallions is crucial to control the dissemination of EAV. These animals can be identified by serological screening using virus neutralization test. If positive at a titer of 1:4, the stallion should be tested for persistent infection by virus isolation from the sperm-rich fraction of the ejaculate or by test mating. Shedding stallions should not be used for breeding or should be bred only to seropositive mares through natural infection or vaccination technique.[68,78,82-86] Total spontaneous elimination of viral shedding has been reported in some stallions.[87]

Abortion is one of the greatest risks of EAV infection. In cases of natural exposure, the abortion rate has varied from less than 10% to more than 60% and can occur between 3 and 10 months of gestation.[76,88,89] Abortion is due to a severe edema and necrosis of the endometrium leading to placental detachment.[68,69] The abortions appear to result from the direct impairment of maternal-fetal support and not from fetal infection.

Although mares and geldings are able to eliminate virus from all body tissues by 60 days after infection, 30%–60% of stallions become persistently infected. In these animals, virus is maintained in the accessory organs of the reproductive tract, principally the ampullae or the vas deferens, and is shed constantly in the semen. The development and maintenance of virus persistence is dependent on the presence of testosterone.[90] Persistently infected stallions that were castrated but were given testosterone continued to shed virus, whereas those administered a placebo ceased virus shedding. Furthermore, stallions treated with an anti-GnRH product stopped shedding the virus during the treatment period but resumed within a few weeks after treatment ceased.[87] Three carrier states are known in the stallion: (1) short-term during convalescence, (2) medium-term (lasting for 3–9 months), and (3) chronic shedder, which may persist for years after the initial infection. Virus shedding in mares and geldings is limited to the convalescence state.

After clinical recovery from initial infection, there is no significant decrease in the fertility of shedding stallions. Mares infected after service by a carrier stallion do not appear to have any related fertility problems during the same or subsequent years, and there are no reports of mares becoming EAV carriers or chronic shedders, nor of virus passage by the venereal route from a seropositive mare causing clinical disease or seroconversion in a stallion.

EAV is transmitted mostly through aerosols generated from respiratory or urinary secretions from acutely infected animals or from secretions from recent abortions. The other route of transmission is by the venereal route through semen from a shedding stallion. Close contact between animals is generally required for efficient virus spread in aerosol transmission. Personnel and fomites may play a minor role in virus dissemination. Virus is viable in fresh, chilled, and frozen semen, and venereal transmission is efficient, with 85%–100% of seronegative mares seroconverting after being bred to stallions shedding virus. In several cases, outbreaks of clinical disease have been traced to a persistently infected stallion.

Diagnosis requires laboratory confirmation with acute infections having a four-fold or greater increase in neutralizing antibodies between acute and convalescent serum samples. Definitive diagnosis is reached by the cytopathic effect of the virus on monolayers of rabbit kidney cells. In the case of abortion, virus isolation can be attempted from fetal and placental tissues. Persistent infection in stallions can be diagnosed by first screening serum for antibody in serum neutralization (SN) test. If seropositive at a titer of 1:4, virus isolation should be performed, and the untreated, sperm-rich fraction of the ejaculate or the stallion should be test-mated to seronegative mares who are monitored for seroconversion. Some countries require testing all stallions for viral shedding by culture and isolation or PCR technique in semen.[2,69,75,76]

On suspect animals several samples can be submitted for diagnosis of EVA. In abortions, both fetus and placenta contain large amounts of virus. Samples of fresh placenta, spleen, lung, and kidney along with fetal and placental fluids should be collected and submitted for virus isolation. Blood should be obtained from the mare at the time of the abortion and 3 weeks later for testing by SN.

Sample submissions from stallions include serum and semen. Semen should be collected using an artificial vagina or a condom. Although less satisfactory, a dismount sample can be collected at the time of breeding. The sample should be from the sperm-rich fraction of the full ejaculate and should be chilled immediately and shipped at 4°C to arrive at the diagnostic facility within 24 hours. If this is not possible, the sample should be frozen in dry ice and shipped to the diagnostic facility under these conditions. Washing of the penis with antiseptics or disinfectants before collection of the samples should be avoided. Samples of commercial frozen semen could also be tested, but it is necessary to have at least 2 billion sperm cells for the sample to be representative. False negatives have been reported because of the lack of seminal plasma in cryopreserved semen.

Prevention and control are implemented by rigorous vaccination schemes with a modified live vaccine.[69,81,91-93] The vaccine does not appear to produce any side effects in vaccinated stallions apart from a possible short-term abnormality of sperm morphology, and a mild fever with no overt clinical signs.[39,94,95] However, live virus can be isolated sporadically from the nasopharynx and blood after MLV vaccination.[96,97] Vaccinated horses should not be mixed with naïve pregnant mares for at least 1 month. Neutralizing antibody titers are induced within 5–8 days and persist for at least 2 years. The vaccine strain was isolated from an aborted fetus of a mare that was vaccinated with the live attenuated vaccine. An inactivated vaccine is commercially available in some countries, but data on its efficacy and duration of immunity remain limited. Stallions should not be vaccinated unless they are proven to be seronegative by an accredited laboratory. Most states in the United States require testing of stallions whose semen is shipped into the state. A recent study on natural shedders as well as on semen spiked with viral particles has shown that a double semen processing protocol based on density gradient centrifugation followed by swim-up technique could be beneficial for removal of the virus from semen of shedder stallions.[98] However, further research is needed before these techniques could be applied to commercial semen.

Equine Herpes Virus-3; Coital Exanthema

Coital exanthema, equine genital herpes, is caused by equine herpes virus type III (EHV-3). The disease can be transmitted by the stallion to the mare or from the mare to the stallion at the time of coitus. The incubation period varies from 2 to 10 days. The disease may also be transmitted by infected AI equipment or gynecological examination instruments.[99-102] It is characterized by the formation of small (0.5–1.5 cm) blister-like or scabby nodular lesions on the penis and prepuce of stallions or on the perineal area of the mare[103-105] (Fig. 10-3). These lesions may become confluent and will eventually rupture, forming irregular erosions. The lesions usually resolve completely in 2–4 weeks, leaving round white scars in the area where the lesions were. Sometimes mild fever and slight depression can be observed. Diagnosis can be obtained from the typical clinical signs or definitive diagnosis can be made by the inclusion bodies observed on histopathology.

The effect on fertility is thought to be minimal, but stallions and mares during the acute phase of the disease should be sexually rested to avoid further spread. Abortion has been induced experimentally following intrauterine inoculation. Stallions may remain asymptomatic carriers for a long period. The penis can be treated with a 2% chlorhexidine solution for 3 consecutive days to prevent secondary bacterial contamination. Prevention includes good hygiene and sexual rest of affected animals or the use of AI in breeds that allow the procedure.[15]

PARASITIC CONTAMINANTS

Dourine

Dourine, caused by *Trypanosoma equiperdum*, is a venereal disease found in Africa, South and Central America, and the Middle East.[3,5] Dourine had a global distribution during World War I and has been eradicated from North America and most of Europe. It is still reported in Africa (Botswana, Ethiopia, Namibia, and South Africa) and Asia (Kyrgyzstan, Mongolia, Pakistan, Russia, Turkmenistan, and Uzbehkistan). Suspected cases have been reported in other areas (Germany, the Middle East).[106-109] It is perhaps the only protozoal organism that can be transmitted

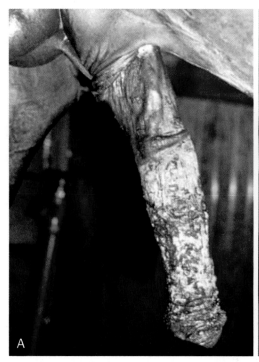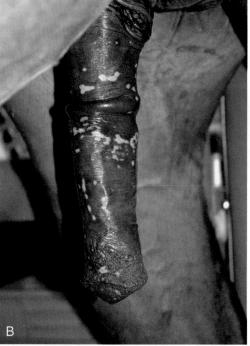

Figure 10-3. Coital exanthema lesions in stallions. **A,** Active lesions; **B,** healed (scared) surface of the penis.

venereally. Tentative diagnosis is made based on the clinical signs, which include intermittent fever, depression, progressive loss of body condition, and severe purulent discharge from the urethra. Characteristic cutaneous lesions from which the disease derives its name "dourine" have been described as circular elevated plaques of thickened skin ranging in size from 1 to 10 cm in diameter resembling money or "douros." These plaques are observed mostly on the neck, hip, and ventral abdomen. Terminal stages of the disease are characterized by severe anemia and nervous signs, progressive ataxia, hind limb paralysis, or paraplegia followed by death. Diagnosis is performed by complement fixation. However, recent studies have shown that this test cannot distinguish between *T. equiperdum*, *T. evansi*, and *T. b. brucei*.[106,107,110,111]

Piroplasmosis

Piroplasmosis has recently gained attention because of the increase of movement of horses from infected areas. The disease is caused by the hemoparasite *Babesia equi* or by a less severe strain, *Babesia caballi*. It is considered to be enzootic in many areas of the southern United States and is found throughout the world. The protozoal agent is most often spread by ticks, but mechanical transmission has also been documented; therefore, there is concern for venereal transmission if blood from an infected horse contaminates the semen.

Habronemiasis

Habronemiasis, also known as "summer sores," consists of granulomatous parasitic lesions caused by larvae of worms belonging to the *Habronema* genus (*H. muscae* and *H. microstoma*) and *Draschia* genus (*D. megastoma*). The larvae are deposited by flies that act as intermediate hosts.[3,29] This is not a venereally transmitted or semen-transmitted disease. However, it is a good indicator of poor management and dirty conditions. The diagnosis is based on epidemiology (appearance during the hot, wet season) and characteristic lesions (Fig. 10-4). Definitive diagnosis can be achieved by histopathological evaluation of biopsies (visualization of the larvae and characteristics lesions). Ivermectin (twice a month *per os*) is very efficacious against these parasites. Ivermectin-resistant cases require cryosurgical removal of the granulomatous lesions.[3,5] Topical corticosteroids or intralesional triamcinolone injection help to control the inflammation. Many of these lesions may recur despite treatment. Surgical debridement of large lesions is often necessary.

PREVENTION OF TRANSMISSION OF PATHOGENS

To prevent the spread of any disease to susceptible populations through breeding, correct identification of infected animals as well as the implementation of biosecurity measures is critical. A carrier stallion of a bacterial disease should not be used for breeding through natural service, and his semen should be treated with proper antibiotics before insemination. Stallions shedding arteritis virus can still be used, provided that the mare owners are informed of the stallion status. The option to use a particular stallion in a breeding facility may depend on the value of the stallion as a breeding animal and individual regional regulations. Regardless, all stallions should have a diagnosed status before each breeding season.

Stallions should undergo complete semen evaluation and microbiological examination from pre- and post-ejaculation urethral swabs as well as semen. Vaccination status as well as previous exposure to specific disease agents should be determined.

Quarantine of recently introduced animals should be considered, particularly in regions with high risk of contagious diseases. Animals returning from events where commingling has occurred (breeding farms, shows, etc.) should be placed in quarantine for a minimum of 3 weeks. Animals in quarantine should be monitored on a daily basis, and proper veterinary care should be provided promptly if abnormal demeanor or clinical signs of illness are seen. Personnel attending quarantined animals should always don protective clothing (coveralls, etc.) and boots or shoe covers that are devoted solely to the quarantine facility. Clothing and boots should be washable and boots or shoe covers should be made of rubber or other impervious materials. All other equipment and supplies used in a quarantine facility (halters, ropes, blankets, feeders, buckets, etc.) must be solely devoted to the facility.[1,5]

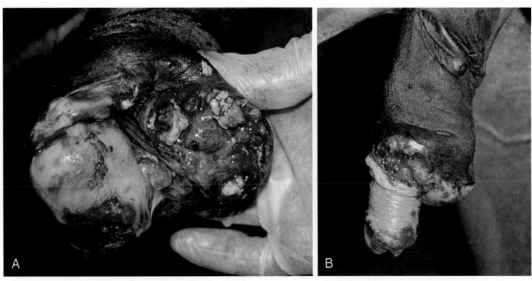

Figure 10-4. A and **B,** Case of severe granulomatous lesions caused by habronemiasis.

Prevention of introduction of diseases into the herd should also take into account other vector animals (insects, birds, and rodents) as well as proximity with other species (e.g., donkeys). Pest control may be difficult but should not be overlooked. Regular cleaning and disinfection of the barns and common areas is critical to breaking transmission cycles of disease agents that contaminate housing, feeding, and treatment equipment, or other vectors or fomites.

Breeding hygiene should be strictly observed to avoid transmission of contaminants to mares. The surface of the penis may harbor several organisms that may be pathogenic.[7-9,112,113] If AI is used, particular attention should be paid to the origin of semen and health certificate of stallions at the time of collection.[11, 114-116] Antibiotic-containing extenders do not eliminate risk of transmission of organisms.[7,117] Unfortunately, in many areas of the world there is a complete lack of quality control of semen processing, particularly shipped cooled semen.[114] Original bacterial load and type of organism within semen can greatly affect the efficacy of the antibiotic within the extender. Method of

semen collection has also been shown to affect the bacteriological quality of semen.[116] Veterinarians and horse breeders should be aware that antibiotics within the extender do not guarantee bacteriological quality of semen and in fact may be harmful to semen and to the industry if used abusively.[6-8] Health importation requirements for frozen semen should be verified for each country of origin and strictly followed.[2,15] The stallion status with regard to EVA and CEM are of particular importance. Guidelines are available for use of stallions that are EAV shedders.[118]

DISEASES OF SEMEN

Hemospermia

Hemospermia is the contamination of the ejaculate with blood. The color of the ejaculate may vary from pinkish to red depending on the amount of bloody discharge. In some extreme cases, the ejaculate presents frank blood or even blood clots (Fig. 10-5). The consequence of this contamination of the ejaculate is poor fertility or complete infertility.[23,28,119-125] One retrospective study

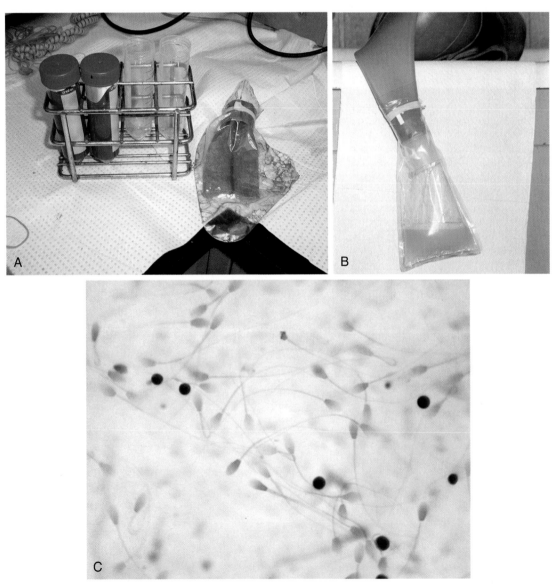

Figure 10-5. Hemospermia. **A,** Severe case showing frank blood and blood clots in the collection tube. **B,** Moderate hemospermia. **C,** Discrete hemospermia detected only by microscopic evaluation (presence of red blood cells).

of cases of hemospermia showed that the age of affected stallion varies from 3 to 18 years (mean 7.1 years) and is not influenced by the number of years in breeding, as previously thought (0–13 breeding seasons, mean 3.1 seasons).[122] Quarter Horses and Thoroughbreds may be over-represented in the prevalence of this syndrome.

The most common causes of hemospermia include infectious urethritis primarily caused by *Streptococcus* spp., *E. coli* and *P. aeruginosa*,[120] urethral defects and lesions of the surface of the penis and urethral process. The inflamed urethral mucosa bleeds easily under the pressure of the erectile tissue and muscular contractions. Cases of viral urethritis have been suspected as a cause of hemospermia.

Urethral defects (or rents) are generally located at the level of the ischial arch or slightly cranial to it and range in size from 5 to 10 mm (Fig. 10-6).[3,29] Hemospermia that appears or increases after belling of the glans penis suggests an ulcer or rent in the urethral mucosa that communicates with the erectile layer (stratum cavernosum).[121,122] These rents may be single or multiple and range in size from 3 to 10 mm. They are generally linear and appear on the convex surface of the urethra near the level of the ischial arch. These defects are thought to extend to the corpus spongiosum penis (CSP) and are believed to be due to an inherent wall weakness on the convex surface of the urethra at the level of the ischial arch.[121] Urethral rents have been reportedly resolved with subischial urethrostomy as well as laser surgery combined with supportive care and sexual rest.

Urethral strictures, growths, ulcers, fissures, and prolapsed subepithelial vessels have also been reported as visible urethral abnormalities.[120-122]

Contamination of the ejaculate with blood may also occur from lesions on the surface of the penis, such as in the case of trauma, habronemiasis, or presence of squamous cell carcinoma lesions on the urethral process (Fig. 10-7).[23,121,122,126] Hemospermia has also been reported in cases of seminal vesiculitis and sperm-occluded ampullae (blocked ampullae).[127]

Diagnosis of hemospermia is often obvious upon dismount of the stallion after ejaculation (presence of bloody discharge from the mare or at the tip of the penis) or after examination of the color of the ejaculate.[23,128] The origin of the bleeding can be determined by examination of the surface of the penis, urethral orifice, and serial collection of fractionated ejaculate using an open-ended artificial vagina. Videoendoscopic evaluation of the urethra, colliculus seminalis, and vesicular glands remains the best technique for the evaluation of the stallion with hemospermia.[23,29,121,122]

In a retrospective study on 18 cases, hemospermia was attributed to urethritis, varicose urethral veins, urethral rents, and lymphosarcoma.[122] Lesions were located at the level of the pelvic portion of the penis (44%), the free portion of the penis (16.7%), or both (33,3%). Over half of the case of urethritis (55.6%) yielded positive bacteriological culture (*E. coli*, *P. aeruginosa*, *S. alpha hemolyticus*, *S. equisimilis*, *Proteus* spp.).[122]

Treatment of hemospermia may be very challenging and requires a definitive diagnosis of the cause. In mild cases direct collection of semen into an appropriate extender or infusion of extender into the mare's uterus prior to breeding (MCBT), if AI is not allowed, may improve fertility. Treatment of urethritis or vesiculitis requires sexual rest and antimicrobial therapy.[23,120]

Sexual rest (week to months) alone may be sufficient to resolve hemospermia caused by urethral defects. However, the hemospermia may reappear after return of the stallion to breeding activity. Temporary (6–10 weeks) subischial urethrotomy (Fig. 10-8) combined with daily topical treatment with antimicrobials and anti-inflammatories has been advocated as the method of choice in stallions with hemospermia caused by urethral defects.[121,123] This technique allows urine to bypass the distal aspect of the urethra[120] and reduce the pressure in the CSP at the end of urination.[121] Post-surgical management includes antimicrobial therapy (Procaine penicillin-G, 22.000 U/kg IM, BID for 5 days, or sulfonamide, 16 mg/kg *per os* BID for 14 days; or Trimethoprim-sulfa) and sexual rest for 6 weeks.[121]

Suture of the laceration or laser ablation of the urethral defect has been reported by some authors; information on the efficacy of these techniques remains limited.[127,129]

Urospermia

Urospermia is defined as the contamination of the ejaculate with various quantities of urine. This suggests a failure in the normal synchronization of emission/ejaculation and bladder neck closure, which occurs in normal ejaculation. Urospermia may be observed as an intermittent or permanent phenomenon in some stallions. Urine contamination may occur at any moment during the ejaculatory process and the quantity of urine varies from a few milliliters to more than 250 ml.[3,130-135] The first few jets of the ejaculate may be completely normal followed by urine contamination at the end of the ejaculation.[132] The presence of urine causes a decrease in viability and motility of the spermatozoa, probably caused by changes in pH and osmolarity of the ejaculate.[136]

The etiology and pathophysiology of urospermia remain rather speculative. Urospermia may be due to failure of the alpha-adrenergic sympathetic system, which controls bladder neck sphincter closure and sperm emission. Neurological disorders reported in cases of urospermia include bladder paralysis, cauda equine neuritis, EHV-1 infection, and sorghum and Sudan grass intoxication.[3,127,134] Urospermia may also be the result of complications of urogenital surgeries or a manifestation of generalized neoplasia or severe painful conditions.[3]

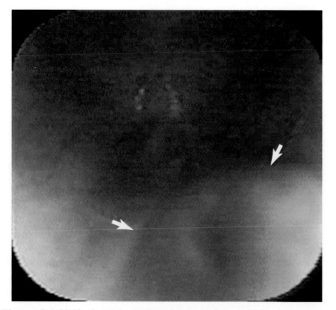

Figure 10-6. Urethral rent *(arrows)* at the level of the ischial arch in stallion with hemospermia.

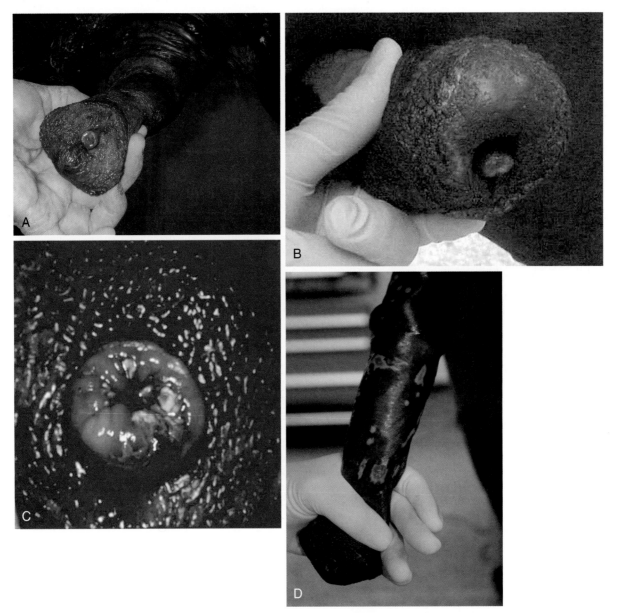

Figure 10-7. External causes of hemospermia. **A,** Urethritis. **B,** Laceration of the glans penis. **C,** Squamous cell carcinoma of the urethral process. **D,** Ulcerated lesions on the surface of the penis.

A case of urospermia has been described following surgical treatment of urolithiasis (bladder stones) in a stallion.[137] The authors have seen a case of urospermia in a stallion with generalized osteosarcoma. Urospermia may be the consequence of other disorders, including osteomyelitis and hyperkalemic periodic paralysis.[127]

The presence of urine in the ejaculate may be obvious (amber or yellow and typical urine odor) or very discrete (Fig. 10-9). The timing of contamination with urine during the ejaculatory process may be determined by separate collection of each fractionation of the ejaculate.[130,135] This technique requires the use of an open-ended artificial vagina[138,139] or, even better, the use of phantoms such as the Equidam that can separate the ejaculate into its different fractions.[3,116] Urine presence may be detected by determination of the concentration of urea (>25–30 mg/dl) or creatinine (>2 g/dl).[131] Under field condition, urine contamination may be detected using a strip test for detection

of urea (Azostix, Miles Laboratories, Pittsburgh, PA) or nitrites (Multistix, Miles Laboratories). These tests allow detection of a contamination of as little as 10% of the total volume.[130] In one case of a 10-year-old stallion, the first fraction of the ejaculate contained 16.4 nmol/l of urea and 584 μmol/l of creatinine.[131]

Treatment options for urospermia remain limited given the complexity of its etiology and pathophysiology. Management of the stallions with urospermia centers around the following points aimed at reducing the contamination by emptying the bladder, enhancing bladder neck function or fractionated ejaculate collection, or reducing the effect of urine on sperm viability (collection into an extender) or a combination of the following:

1. Allowing urine voiding by stimulating the stallion to urinate before semen collection or natural cover. This can be accomplished by introducing the stallion into a freshly bedded stall or placing fresh feces from another stallion in his stall.

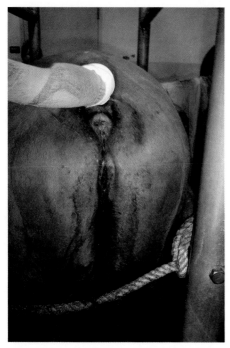

Figure 10-8. Urethrotomy site to relieve hemospermia.

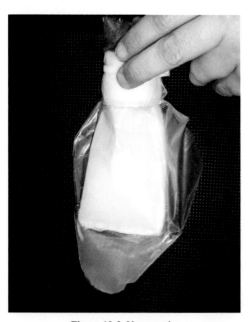

Figure 10-9. Urospermia.

2. Administration of diuretics (furosemide 250 mg IV) before collection[132]
3. Catheterization of the bladder before mating or semen collection. However, excessive use of this technique may predispose the stallion to urethritis or cystitis.[127,132]
4. Catheterization and lavage of the bladder with sterile physiologic saline before semen collection or mating[127]
5. Collection of fractionated ejaculate[135]
6. Collection into a semen extender; filtration and resuspension in a new extender. We have successfully managed a stallion with mild urospermia using this technique.

7. Improve bladder neck tone using alpha-adrenergic agents (imipramine hydrochloride 0.8 mg/kg per os 2–4 hours before collection or phenylpropanolamine 0.35 mg/kg PO BID) and noradrenaline.[133,140,141] However, pharmacological management of stallions with urospermia is not always successful. In a report on three cases, no improvement was observed following administration of bethanechol, imipramine, or furosemide. This points to the complexity of this syndrome and the need to use various methods for the management of affected stallions.[142]

CONCLUSION

Special consideration has to be given to the microbiology and diseases of semen during the reproductive life of the stallion. Despite the danger of venereal diseases and the number of outbreaks reported every year, several stallion owners continue to practice unsafe breeding methods without veterinary supervision. Proper management of the stallion to reduce risks of transmission of diseases or poor fertility should include rigorous testing and vaccination programs, health certificate on the mares to be bred (particularly in natural service system), and regular complete evaluation of the stallion and its semen production and quality. For breeds that allow AI, the best insurance for stallion fertility is the storage of sufficient insemination doses of frozen semen.

REFERENCES

1. Samper JC, Tibary A: Disease transmission in horses. *Theriogenology* 66:551, 2006.
2. Metcalf ES: The role of international transport of equine semen on disease transmission. Anim Reprod Sci 68:229, 2001.
3. Tibary A: Pathologie genitale. In Tibary A, Bakkoury M, eds: Reproduction equine Tome II L'Etalo., Rabat, Morocco: Actes editions, 2005, pp 185-316.
4. Parlevliet JM, Samper JC: Disease transmission through semen. In Samper JC, ed: *Equine Breeding Management and Artificial Insemination*. Philadelphia: WB: Saunders, 2000.
5. Tibary A, Fite CL: Reproductive tract infections. In Sellon DC, Long MT, eds: Equine Infectious Diseases. St Louis: Saunders-Elsevier, 2007, pp 84-102.
6. Corona A, Cossu I, Bertulu A, Cherchi R: Characterization of bacteria in fresh semen of stallions during the breeding season. *Anim Reprod Sci* 94:85, 2006.
7. Aurich C, Spergser J: Influence of genitally pathogenic bacteria and gentamicin on motility and membrane integrity of cooled-stored stallion spermatozoa. *Anim Reprod Sci* 94:117, 2006.
8. Aurich C, Spergser J, Nowotny N, et al: Prevalence of venereal transmissible diseases and relevant potentially pathogenic bacteria in Austrian Noriker draught horse stallions. *Wiener Tierarztliche Monatsschrift* 90:124, 2003.
9. Malmgren L, Engvall EO, Engvall A, et al: Aerobic bacterial flora of semen and stallion reproductive tract and its relation to fertility under field conditions. *Acta Vet Scan* 39:173, 1998.
10. Ghasemzadeh-nava H, Ghasemi F, Tajik P, Shirazi A: A review of mare endometritis in Iran. *J Equine Vet Sci* 24:188, 2004.
11. Clement F, Vidament M, Guerin B: Microbial contamination of stallion semen. Proc VI International Symposium Equine Reproduction. Brazil: 1994, pp 199-200.
12. Blanchard TL, Kenny RB, Timoney PJ: Venereal disease. *Vet Clin North Am Equine Prac* 8:191, 1992.
13. Blanchard TL, Varner DD, Love CC: Use of a semen extender containing antibiotic to improve the fertility of a stallion with seminal vesiculitis due to *Pseudomonas aeruginosa*. *Theriogenology* 28:541, 1987.
14. Klug E, Sieme H: Infectious agents in equine semen. *Acta Vet Scand Suppl* 88:73, 1992.

15. Wood JL, Cardwell J, Castillo-Olivarez J, et al: Transmission of diseases through semen. In Samper JC, Pycock JF, McKinnon AO, eds: *Current Therapy in Equine Reproduction.* St Louis: Elsevier, 2007, pp 266-274.
16. Bowen JM, Tobin N, Simpson RB: Effect of washing on the bacterial flora of the stallion's penis. *J Reprod Fertil Suppl* 32:41, 1982.
17. Huthwohl H, Weiss R, Schmeer N, et al: Occurrence and significance of coagulase-negative staphylococci in the genital tract of horses. *Dtsch Tierarztl Wochenschr* 96:256-258, 1989.
18. Jones RL, Squires EL, Slade NP, et al: The effect of washing on the aerobic bacterial flora of the stallion's penis. Proc AAEP 30:90, 1984.
19. Kenny RM, Cummings MR: Potential control of stallion penile shedding of *Pseudomonas aeruginosa* and *Klebsiella pneumoniae.* Proc Symposium Voortplanting Pard. Gent, Belgium:, 1990.
20. Blanchard TL, Varner DD, Hurtgen JP, et al: Bilateral seminal vesiculitis and ampullitis in a stallion. *J Am Vet Med Assoc* 192:525, 1988.
21. Gay Y, Perrin R: Exploration des voie génitales de l'étalon par fibroscopie. *Pratique Veterinaire Equine* 31:37, 1999.
22. Gay Y, Perrin R: Deux cas d'étalons présentant une vésiculite. *Pratique Veterinaire Equine* 31:57, 1999.
23. Sojka JE, Carter GK: Hemospermia and seminal vesicle enlargement in a stallion. *Comp Cont Educ Pract Vet* 7:S587, 1985.
24. Hamm DH: Gentamicin therapy of genital tract infections in stallions. *J Eq Med Surg* 6:243, 1978.
25. Johnson TL, Kenney RM, McGee WR, et al: Pseudomonas infection in a stallion: case report. Proc AAEP 1980, pp 111-116.
26. Malmgren L, Sussemilch BI: Ultrasonography as a diagnostic tool in a stallion with seminal vesiculitis: a case report. *Theriogenology* 37:935, 1992.
27. Blanchard TL, Woods JA, Brinsko SP, et al: Theriogenology question of the month. *J Am Vet Med Assoc* 221:793, 2002.
28. Freestone JF, Paccamonti DL, Eilts BE, et al: Seminal vesiculitis as a cause of signs of colic in a stallion. *J Am Vet Med Assoc* 203:556, 1993.
29. Tibary A: Endoscopy of the reproductive tract in the stallion. In Samper JC, Pycock JF, McKinnon AO, eds: *Current Therapy in Equine Reproduction.* St Louis: Elsevier, 2007, pp 214-219.
30. Cooper WL: Methods of determining the site of bacterial infections in the stallion reproductive tract. *Proc Soc Theriogenol* 1:1-4, 1979.
31. Reifenrath H, Jensen A, Sieme H, et al: Urethroscopic catheterization of the vesicular glands in the stallion. *Reprod Domest Anim* 32:47, 1997.
32. LeBlanc MM, Asbury AC: Rationale for uterine lavage after breeding in mares. Proc Ann Mtg AAEP 1988, pp 623-628.
33. Brinsko SP: How to perform uterine lavage: indications and practical techniques. Proc AAEP 47:407, 2001.
34. Brinsko SP, Varner DD, Blanchard TL: The effect of uterine lavage performed four hours post insemination on pregnancy rate in mares. *Theriogenology* 35:1111, 1991.
35. Brinsko SP, Varner DD, Blanchard TL, et al: The effect of postbreeding uterine lavage on pregnancy rate in mares. *Theriogenology* 33:465, 1990.
36. Varner DD: External and Internal Genital Infections in Stallions, Proc Stall Reprod Symp Soc Theriogenol, Baltimore MD. 1998, pp 84-94.
37. Moore JE, Matsuda M, Anzai T, Buckley T: Molecular detection and characterization of *Taylorella equigenitalis.* *Vet Rec* 152:543, 2003.
38. Jackson G, Carson T, Heath P, et al: CEMO in a UK stallion. *Vet Rec* 151:582, 2002.
39. Timoney PJ: Contagious equine metritis. *Comp Immunol Microbiol Infect Dis* 19:199, 1996.
40. Kristula AA, Smith BI: Diagnosis and treatment of four stallions, carriers of the contagious metritis organism—case report. *Theriogenology* 61:595, 2004.
41. Anzai T, Eguchi M, Sekizaki T, et al: Development of a PCR test for rapid diagnosis of contagious equine metritis. *J Vet Med Sci* 61:1287, 1999.
42. Anzai T, Wada R, Okuda T, et al: Evaluation of the field application of PCR in the eradication of contagious equine metritis from Japan. *J Vet Med Sci* 64:999, 2002.
43. Chanter N, Vigano F, Collin NC, et al: Use of a PCR assay for *Taylorella equigenitalis* applied to samples from the United Kingdom. *Vet Rec* 143:225, 1998.
44. Parlevliet JM, Bleumink Pluym NMC, Houwers DJ, et al: Epidemiologic aspects of. *Taylorella equigenitalis. Theriogenology* 47:1169, 1997.
45. Duquesne F, Pronost S, Laugier C, et al: Identification of *Taylorella equigenitalis* responsible for contagious equine metritis in equine genital swabs by direct polymerase chain reaction. *Res Vet Sci* 82:47, 2007.
46. Schluter H, Kuller HJ, Friedrich U, et al: Epizootiology and treatment of contagious equine metritis (CEM), with particular reference to the treatment of infected stallions. *Praktische Tierarzt* 72:503, 1991.
47. Tainturier D, Fieni F, Bruyas JF, et al: Effet du trempage du penis de l'étalon, après saillie, dans une solution antiséptique, sur la transmission de la metrite contagieuse équine. *Rev Medecine Veterinaire* 139:705, 1988.
48. Katz JB, Evans LE, Hutto DL, et al: Clinical, bacteriologic, serologic, and pathologic features of infections with atypical *Taylorella equigenitalis* in mares. *J Am Vet Med Assoc* 216:1945, 2000.
49. Jang SS, Donahue JM, Arata AB et al: *Taylorella asinigenitalis* sp. *nov.,* a bacterium isolated from the genital tract of male donkeys (*Equus asinus*). *Int J Syst Evol Microbiol* 51:971, 2001.
50. Tibary A, Sghiri A, Bakkoury M, et al: Reproductive patterns in donkeys. 9th Congress of the Wold Equine Veterinary Association. Marrakech. January 22-26, 2006, pp 311-319.
51. Moorthy ARS, Spradbrow PB, Eisler MED: Isolation of mycoplasmas from the genital tract of horses. *Aust Vet J* 53:167, 1977.
52. Zgorniak-Nowesielka IN, Bredlanski W, Kosiniak K: Mycoplasmas in stallion semen. *Anim Reprod Sci* 7:343, 1984.
53. Spergser J, Aurich C, Aurich J, et al: High prevalence of mycoplasmas in the genital tract of asymptomatic stallions in Austria. *Vet Microbiol* 87:119, 2002.
54. Kirchhoff H, Naglic T, Heitmann J: Isolation of *Acholeplasma laidlawii* and *Mycoplasma equigenitalium* from stallion semen. *Vet Microbiol* 4:177, 1979.
55. Heitmann J, Kirchhoff H, Petzoldt K: Isolation of acholeplasmas and mycoplasmas from aborted horse fetuses. *Vet Rec* 104:350, 1979.
56. Bermudez V, Miller R, Johnson W, et al: The prevalence of *Mycoplasma* spp. and their relationship to reproductive performance in selected equine herds in southern Ontario. *J Reprod Fertil Suppl* 35:671, 1987.
57. Medenbach K, Aupperle H, Schoon D, et al: Pathology of the equine salpinx. *Pferdeheilkunde* 15:560, 1999.
58. Herfen K, Jager C, Wehrend A: Genital chlamydial infection in mares and their clinical significance. *Reprod Dom Anim* 34:20, 1999.
59. Wittenbrink MM: Aetiological significance of chlamydial infections in equine reproductive disorders? *Pferdeheilkunde* 15:538, 1999.
60. Veznik Z, Pospisil L, Svecova D, et al: Chlamydiae in reproductive disorders and pathology of reproductive organs in man and animals. *Reprod Dom Anim* 31:595, 1996.
61. Blanco Loizeiler A, Marcotegui Jaso MA, Delgado Casado I: Clamidiosis equina (aborto y poliartitis clamidial en equinos), Anales del Instituto Nacional de Investigatciones Agrarias. *Higiene y Saidad Animal Spain* 3:105, 1976.
62. Glavits R, Molnar T, Rady M: *Chlamydia*-induced abortion in a horse. *Acta Vet Hung* 34:55, 1988.
63. Henning K, Sachse K, Sting R: Isolation of *Chlamydia* from an aborted equine fetus. *Deutsche-Tierarztliche-Wochenschrift* 107:49, 2000.
64. Lehmann C, Elze K: Keimspektrum infektios bedingter Aborte bei Pferd, Rind, Schwein und Schaf von 1983 bis 1993 in Nordwest- und Mittelthuringen. *Tierarztliche-Umschau* 52:495, 1997.
65. Dilbeck PM, Evermann JF, Kraft S, et al: Equine chlamydial infections: comparative diagnostic aspects with bovine and ovine chlamydiosis. Proc 28th Annu Meet Am Assoc Vet Lab Diagnost 1985, pp 285-298.
66. Timoney P.J: Aspects of the Occurrence, Diagnosis and Control of Selected Venereal Diseases of the Stallion. Proc Stallion Reproduction Symposium Society for Theriogenology. Baltimore, MD: 1998, pp 76–83.
67. Larska M, Rola J: Molecular epizoology of equine arteritis isolates from Poland. *Vet Microbiol* 127:392, 2008.
68. Glaser AL, Chimside ED, Horzinek MC, et al: Equine viral arteritis. *Theriogenology* 47:1275, 1997.
69. Del Piero F: Equine viral arteritis. *Vet Pathol* 37:287, 2000.
70. Balasuriya UBR, Hedges JF, Smalley VL, et al: Genetic characterization of equine arteritis virus during persistent infection of stallions. *J Gen Virol* 85:379, 2004.
71. Balasuriya UBR, Leutenegger CM, Topol JB, et al: Detection of equine arteritis virus by real-time TaqMan (R) reverse transcription—PCR assay. *J Virol Methods* 101:21, 2002.
72. Ahlswede L, Leyk W, Zurmuhlen K: Studies on equine viral arteritis: serological investigations, virus detection in semen and aborted fetuses, and vaccination. *Praktische Tierarzt* 24:18, 1998.
73. Ahlswede L, Zurmuhlen K: What should a practitioner know about EVA? *Praktische Tierarzt* 82:1040, 2001.

74. Guthrie A, Howell PG, Hedges JF, et al: Lateral transmission of equine arteritis virus among Lipizzaner stallions in South Africa. *Eq Vet J* 35:596, 2003.

75. Balasuriya UBR, Evermann JF, Hedges JF, et al: Serologic and molecular characterization of an abortigenic strain of equine arteritis virus isolated from infective frozen semen and an aborted equine fetus. *JAVMA* 213:1586, 1998.

76. Balasuriya UBR, Hedges JF, Nadler SA, et al: Genetic stability of equine arteritis virus during horizontal and vertical transmission in an outbreak of equine viral arteritis. *J Gen Virol* 80:1949, 1999.

77. Wood JL, Chirnside ED, Mumford JA, et al: First recorded outbreak of equine viral arteritis in the United Kingdom. *Vet Rec* 136:381, 1995.

78. Chirnside ED: Equine viral arteritis: a free market threat. *Eq Vet Edu* 5:137, 1993.

79. Moore B, Balasuriya U, Watson J, et al: Virulent and avirulent strains of equine arteritis virus induce different quantities of TNF-alpha and other proinflammatory cytokines in alveolar and blood-derived equine macrophages. *Virology* 314:662, 2003.

80. Neu SM, Timoney PJ, Lowry SR: Changes in semen quality in the stallion following experimental infection with equine arteritis virus. *Theriogenology* 37:407, 1992.

81. Neu SM, Timoney PJ, McCollum WH: Persistent infection of the reproductive tract in stallions experimentally infected with equine arteritis virus. Equine infectious diseases V. Proc Fifth International Conference, Lexington, KY: 1988, pp 149–154.

82. Chirnside ED, Spaan WJM: Reverse transcription and cDNA amplification by the polymerase chain reaction of equine arteritis virus (EAV). *J Virol Meth* 30:133, 1990.

83. Fukunaga Y, Wada R, Sugita S, et al: In vitro detection of equine arteritis virus from seminal plasma for identification of carrier stallions. *J Vet Med Sci* 62:643, 2000.

84. Gilbert SA, Timoney PJ, McCollum WH, et al: Detection of equine arteritis virus in the semen of carrier stallions by using a sensitive nested PCR assay. *J Clin Microbiol* 35:2181, 1997.

85. Starick E: Rapid and sensitive detection of equine arteritis virus in semen and tissue samples by reverse transcription polymerase chain reaction, dot blot hybridisation and nested polymerase chain reaction. *Acta Virologica* 42:33, 1998.

86. Starick E, Ginter A, Coppe P: ELISA and direct immunofluorescence test to detect equine arteritis virus (EAV) using a monoclonal antibody directed to the EAV-N protein. *J Vet Med Series* B48:1, 2001.

87. Fortier G, Vidament M, DeCraene F, et al: The effect of GnRH antagonist on testosterone secretion, spermatogenesis and viral excretion in EVA-virus excreting stallions. *Theriogenology* 58:425, 2002.

88. Clayton H: 1986 outbreak of EVA in Alberta, Canada. *J Equine Vet Sci* 7:101, 1987.

89. Golnik W: The results of serological examinations of stallions for equine arteritis virus antibodies. *Medycyna Weterynaryjna* 56:573, 2000.

90. Little TV, Holyoak GR, McCollum WH, et al: Output of equine arteritis virus from persistently infected stallions is testosterone-dependent. Proc VIth Int Conf Equine Infectious Diseases. In Plowright W, Rossdale PD, Wade JF, eds. R & W Publications: Newmarket, 1992, pp 225-230.

91. Cullinane AA: Equine arteritis virus in an imported stallion. *Vet Rec* 132:395, 1993.

92. Timoney PJ, McCollum WH: Equine viral arteritis. *Can Vet J* 28:693, 1987.

93. Newton JR, Wood JL, Castillo-Olivares FJ, et al: Serological surveillance of equine viral arteritis in the United Kingdom since the outbreak in 1993. *Vet Rec* 145:511, 1999.

94. McCollum WH, Timoney PJ, Roberts AW, et al: Responses of vaccinated and non-vaccinated mares to artificial insemination with semen from stallions persistently infected with equine arteritis virus. Proc Vth Int Conf Equine Infectious Diseases. Powell DG, ed: Lexington: University Press of Kentucky, 1988, pp 13-18.

95. McCollum WH, Timoney PJ, Tengelsen LA: Clinical, virological and serological responses of donkeys to intranasal inoculation with the Ky-84 strain of equine arteritis virus. *J Comp Pathol* 112:207, 1995.

96. Fukunaga Y, Wada R, Hirasawa K et al: Effect of the modified Butyrous strain of equine arteritis virus experimentally inoculated into horses. *Bull Eq Inst* 19:97, 1982.

97. Timoney PJ, McCollum WH: Equine viral arteritis: epidemiology and control. *J Equine Vet Sci* 8:54, 1988.

98. Morrell JM, Geraghty RM: Effective removal of equine arteritis virus from stallion semen. *Eq Vet J* 38:224, 2006.

99. Jacob RJ, Cohen D, Bouchey D et al: Molecular pathogenesis of equine coital exanthema: identification of a new equine herpesvirus isolated from lesions reminiscent of coital exanthema in a donkey. Proc Equine Infect Dis V, 1988, pp 140-146.

100. Moreno PE: Clinical case report: venereal disease compatible with equine coital exanthema. *Notas Veterinarias* 2:18, 1992.

101. Pascoe RR: The effect of coital exanthema on the fertility of mares covered by stallions exhibiting the clinical disease. *Austr Vet J* 57:111, 1981.

102. Rathor SS: Equine coital exanthema in thoroughbreds. *J Equine Vet Sci* 9:34, 1989.

103. Seki Y, Seimiya YM, Yaegashi G, et al: Occurrence of equine coital exanthema in pastured draft horses and isolation of equine herpesvirus 3 from progenital lesions. *J Vet Med Sci* 66:1503, 2004.

104. Gibbs EPJ, Roberts MC, Morris JM, et al: Equine coital exanthema in the United Kingdom. *Eq Vet J* 4:74-80, 1972.

105. Uppal PK, Yadav MP, Singh BK, et al: Equine coital exanthema (EHV 3 virus) infection in India. *J Vet Med Series B* 36:786, 1989.

106. Claes F, Buscher P, Touratier L, et al: *Trypanosoma equiperdum*: master of disguise or historical mistake? *Trends Parasitol* 21:316, 2005.

107. Claes F, Ilgekbayeva GD, Verloo D, et al: Comparison of serological tests for equine trypanosomosis in naturally infected horses from Kazakhstan. *Vet Parasitol* 131:221, 2005.

108. Clausen PH, Chuluun S, Sodnomdarjaa R, et al: A field study to estimate the prevalence of *Trypanosoma equiperdum* in Mongolian horses. *Vet Parasitol* 115:9, 2003.

109. Kumba FF, Claasen B, Petrus P: Apparent prevalence of dourine in the Khomas region of Namibia. *Onderstepoort J Vet Res* 69:295, 2002.

110. Robinson EM: Serological investigations into some diseases of domesticated animals in South Africa caused by trypanosomes. *Rep Direct Vet Educ Res Dept Agr S Afr* 19:11, 1926.

111. Brun R, Hecker H, Lun ZR: *Trypanosoma evansi* and *T. equiperdum*: distribution, biology, treatment and phylogenetic relationship. *Vet Parasitol* 79:95, 1998.

112. Tischner M, Kosiniak K: Techniques for collection and storage of stallion semen with minimal secondary contamination. *Acta Vet Scand Suppl* 88:83, 1992.

113. Madsen M, Christensen P: Bacterial flora of semen collected from Danish warmblood stallions by artificial vagina. *Acta Vet Scand* 36:1, 1995.

114. Bielanski A: Disinfection procedures for controlling microorganisms in the semen and embryo of humans and farm animals. *Theriogenology* 68:1, 2007.

115. Burns SJ, Simpson RB, Snell JR: Control of microflora in stallion semen with a semen extender. *J Reprod Fert Suppl* 23:139, 1975.

116. Lindeberg H, Karjalainen H, Koskinen E, et al: Quality of stallion semen obtained by a new semen collection phantom (Equidame (R)) versus a Missouri (R) artificial vagina. *Theriogenology* 51:1157, 1999.

117. Pickett BW, Voss JL, Jones RL: Control of bacteria in stallions and their semen. *J Equine Vet Sci* 19:426, 1999.

118. Mann A: EVA guidelines for breeding a mare to an equine arteritis shedding stallion. U.S. American Horse Association. Report of the committee, 101, 1997, pp 259-264.

119. Cermak O: The haemolytic factor of bull and stallion semen and its relationship with some indices of semen quality. *Zivocisna Vyroba* 20:279, 1975.

120. McKinnon AO, Voss JL, Trotter GW, et al: Hemospermia of the stallion. *Eq Pract* 10:17, 1988.

121. Schumacher J, Varner DD, Schmitz DG, et al: Urethral defects in geldings with hematuria and stallions with hemospermia. *Vet Surg* 24:250, 1995.

122. Sullins KE, Bertone JJ, Voss JL, et al: Treatment of hemospermia in stallions: a discussion of 18 cases. *Comp Cont Edu Pract Vet* 10:1396, 1988.

123. Voss JL, Pickett BW: Diagnosis and treatment of haemospermia in the stallion. *J Reprod Fert Suppl* 23:151, 1975.

124. Voss JL, Pickett BW, Schideler RK: The effect of hemospermia on fertility in horses. 8th ICAR 1:271, 1976.

125. Voss JL, Wotowey JL: Hemospermia. Proc AAEP 1972, pp 103-112.

126. Bedford SJ, McDonnell SM, Tulleners E, et al: Squamous cell carcinoma of the urethral process in a horse with hemospermia and self-mutilation behavior. *JAVMA* 216:551, 2000.

127. Turner RMO: Urospermia and hemospermia. In Samper JC, Pycock JF, McKinnon AO, eds: *Current Therapy in Equine Reproduction*. St Louis: Elsevier, 2007, pp 258-265.

128. Scoggins RD: Hemaspermia: a case report. *J Equine Vet Sci* 6: 176, 1987.
129. Palmer SE: Use of lasers in urogenital surgery. In Wolfe DF, Moll HD, eds: *Large Animal Urogenital Surgery*. Philadelphia: Williams & Wilkins, 2000, pp 165-178.
130. Althouse GC, Seager SWJ, Varner DD, et al: Diagnostic aids for the detection of urine in the equine ejaculate. *Theriogenology* 31:1141, 1989.
131. Danek J, Wisniewski E, Krumrych W: A case of urospermia in a stallion. *Medycyna Weterynaryjna* 50:129, 1994.
132. Lowe JN: Diagnosis and management of urospermia in a commercial Thoroughbred stallion. *Eq Vet J* 13:4, 2001.
133. Leendertse IP, Asbury AC, Boening KJ, et al: Successful management of persistent urination during ejaculation in a Thoroughbred stallion. *Eq Vet Edu* 2:62, 1990.
134. Mayhew IG: Neurological aspects of urospermia in the horse. *Eq Vet Edu* 2:68, 1990.
135. Nash JGJ, Voss JL, Squires EL: Urination during ejaculation in a stallion. *JAVMA* 176:224, 1980.
136. Griggers S, Paccamonti DL, Thompson RA, et al: The effects of pH, osmolarity and urine contamination on equine spermatozoal motility. *Theriogenology* 56:613, 2001.
137. Sertich PL, Pozor MA, Meyers SA, et al: Medical management of urinary calculi in a stallion with breeding dysfunction. *JAVMA* 213:843, 1998.
138. Tischner M, Kosiniak K: Bacterial contamination of stallion semen collected by open artificial vaginas. *Vlaams Diegeneesk* 55:90, 1986.
139. Tischner M, Kosiniak K, Bielanski W: Analysis of the pattern of ejaculation in stallions. *J Reprod Fert* 41:329, 1974.
140. Turner ORM, McDonnell SM, Hawkins JF: Use of pharmacologically induced ejaculation to obtain semen from a stallion with a fractured radius. *JAVMA* 206:1906, 1995.
141. McDonnell SM: Ejaculation physiology and dysfunction. *Vet Clin North Am Equine Pract* 8:57, 1992.
142. Hoyos Sepulveda ML, Quiroz Rocha GF, Brumbaugh GW, et al: Lack of beneficial effects of bethanechol, imipramine or furosemide on seminal plasma of three stallions with urospermia. *Reprod Dom Anim* 34:489, 1999

ANATOMY AND PHYSIOLOGY
OF THE MARE

DON R. BERGFELT

Fundamentally, the inherent goals of all species are (1) to survive and (2) to reproduce. In regard to the latter, it is presumed that equine veterinary clinicians and breeding managers are well aware of the major roles that the environment and animal husbandry play in determining the success of any reproductive management program in horses. Hence, this and subsequent chapters are focused on the mares' innate capacity to reproduce beginning with the anatomical and physiological relationships among the female reproductive organs, especially the role that the endocrine system plays within and among the various organs involved in reproduction.

Major female reproductive organs include the ovaries (follicles, corpora lutea, and oocytes), internal (oviducts, uterus, cervix, and vagina) and external (vulva and labia) tubular genitalia, and mammary glands or udder, which are functionally dependent, in part, on hormones and hormone-receptor interactions, especially the neuroendocrine hormones produced and secreted by the hypothalamus and pituitary gland. In addition to the systemic, long-loop hormonal feedback mechanisms between the central nervous system and reproductive organs, certain organs (e.g., ovary and uterus) can communicate within and among themselves through the local production and secretion of hormones via short-loop hormonal feedback mechanisms. Thus, the endocrine system serves a communicative role within and among organs of the reproductive system to regulate, modulate, and coordinate the timely, rhythmic events that occur throughout the reproductive life of the mare.

Comprehension of the anatomy and physiology associated with reproduction in the mare is essential for optimizing breeding management practices. This chapter provides an overview of structural and functional relationships associated with the reproductive system in mares compiled from previous and more recent reference texts and publications[1-8] that is expected to serve as the foundation when considering the basis for various reproductive management regimens discussed in subsequent chapters.

The chapter begins with a presentation of the general arrangement of the reproductive system with focus on the reproductive tract and support structures. Thereafter, structural anatomy is discussed with respect to gross morphological aspects of the ovaries, tubular genitalia, and mammary glands *in situ* and *ex situ*. Functional anatomy is discussed from a practical perspective with respect to the hormonal regulation of the reproductive organs in fillies during the prepubertal and peripubertal periods and in adult mares during the estrous cycle and fall and spring transitional periods. Functional anatomy during other reproductive states (e.g., pregnancy and parturition) is discussed in subsequent chapters in context with various management practices.

TOPOGRAPHIC ANATOMY

The anatomy and relationships among various reproductive organs and supporting structures presented herein were compiled from several texts on veterinary anatomy in animals and the horse[9,10] and reproductive biology in mares.[1-4,8] Beginning with the central nervous system, the diencephalon of the forebrain is made up of three regions or glands (hypothalamus, hypophysis or pituitary gland, and epiphysis or pineal gland) that produce neural and endocrine signals to regulate development and maintenance of reproductive events. The hypothalamus is medially located and is the most ventral region of the diencephalon forming the lower parts of the lateral walls of the third ventricle; gonadotropin-releasing hormone (GnRH) is produced in this region of the brain. The pituitary gland is suspended below the hypothalamus by the infundibulum and lies in a recess on the floor of the cranium. The pituitary gland is composed of anterior, intermediate, and posterior lobes. The anterior lobe is associated with production of the gonadotropins, follicle-stimulating hormone (FSH), and luteinizing hormone (LH), which stimulate morphological (e.g., follicle and luteal development) and physiological (e.g., steroidogenesis) events within the ovaries, and prolactin, which is thought to primarily affect the mammary glands but may also be involved in seasonal reproductive changes. Thyroid-stimulating hormone (TSH) and adrenal corticotropic hormone (ACTH) are also produced by the anterior portion of the pituitary, in which the latter may also be produced to some extent by the intermediate lobe. Both hormones can have direct and indirect effects on reproduction, but they are primarily involved in growth, development of the central nervous system, and homeostasis. The posterior pituitary produces oxytocin, which is involved in morphological (e.g., smooth-muscle contractions) and physiological (e.g., endometrial prostaglandin production) events that affect the reproductive tract and mammary glands. Structural and functional abnormalities of the pituitary gland in horses (e.g., neoplasm or tumor) not only affect the reproductive organs directly but can commonly affect the adrenal glands (e.g., pituitary pars intermedia dysfunction, previously called Cushing's disease) and thyroid and, therefore, affect reproduction indirectly.[5,7] Finally, the pineal gland is a small, median body projecting dorsally from the brain stem behind an invagination of the roof of the third ventricle and is responsible for the production of melatonin that is also thought to play a role in seasonality.

Thus, the production and transport of neural and endocrine signals between the central nervous system and reproductive organs, especially the gonads, form a long-loop communicative link or feedback mechanism often called the hypothalamic-hypophyseal (or pituitary)-ovarian axis that is facilitated by the hypothalamic-pituitary portal and peripheral vascular systems.

The arrangement of the mare's reproductive tract has been depicted and illustrated in several reference texts.[1,2,8,10] The arrangement presented in Fig. 11-1 has been adopted from one of those texts[1] to facilitate the following discussion. Overall, the reproductive tract is composed of the ovaries and tubular genitalia, associated vascular, lymphatic and nervous tissue, and suspensory ligaments. Most of the reproductive tract lies within the abdominal cavity and the remainder lies within the pelvic cavity. The bony architecture around the pelvic cavity is enclosed by symmetric halves of the hip bones (ilium, ischium, pubis), sacrum, and the last few tail vertebrae. Internally, the entrance to the pelvic cavity is represented by an inlet and outlet that can be demarcated by the position of the intravaginal transverse fold separating the vagina proper (cranial) from the vestibule (caudal). The cavity outlet may be smaller than the inlet, but the former expands during parturition as the wide sacrosciatic ligaments that border the outlet begin to relax in response to the placental hormone relaxin, especially as parturition approaches. Despite the distensible effect of relaxin on the pelvis, either the cavity inlet or outlet can represent major impediments during parturition as reviewed[2,5,7,8] and discussed in Chapter 22.

Developmentally, the cranial portion of the reproductive tract is of mesodermal origin and the caudal portion is of ectodermal origin. The intravaginal transverse fold marks the convergence of these tissues from different origins (see Fig. 11-1, *A*). Thus, the cranial portion of the reproductive tract includes the ovaries, oviducts, uterus, cervix, and vagina proper, and the caudal portion includes the vulva, which is often subdivided to include the vestibule, labia, and clitoris.

In situ size, shape, and placement changes of the reproductive tract are influenced by breed or type of horse (riding, draft, pony, miniature), season (ovulatory, anovulatory, transitional), age, reproductive status (puberty, nonpregnant, pregnant, postpartum, parity), body condition (weight), and health as well as whether the mare is in a standing position or sternal or lateral recumbency. More immediate changes are influenced by the extent of distention and activity of the colon, rectum, and urinary bladder. The ovaries and uterus are in intimate contact with the abdominal viscera and, therefore, may be suspended among the intestinal loops and appear Y-shaped or ride upon the viscera and appear T-shaped when viewed dorsally (see Fig. 11-1, *A*). Depending on the extent of suspension, the uterus may appear V-shaped when viewed from the side (see Fig. 11-1, *B*). The ventral aspect of the rectum and the dorsal aspect of the urinary bladder are in close contact with the uterine body. Consequently, the body of the uterus may be positioned laterally, away from midline, as a result of fullness of either the rectum or bladder. Thus, consideration of the physical relationships of the ovaries

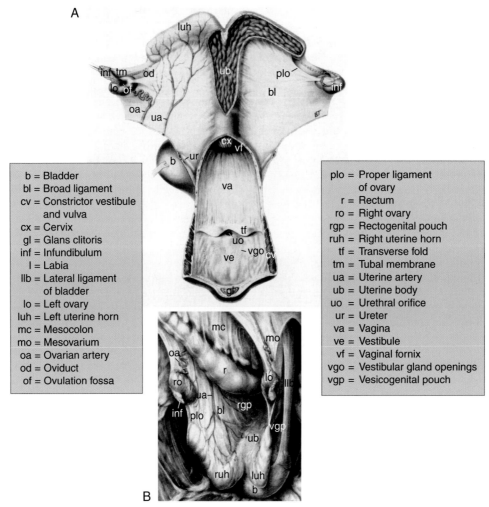

b = Bladder	plo = Proper ligament
bl = Broad ligament	of ovary
cv = Constrictor vestibule	r = Rectum
and vulva	ro = Right ovary
cx = Cervix	rgp = Rectogenital pouch
gl = Glans clitoris	ruh = Right uterine horn
inf = Infundibulum	tf = Transverse fold
l = Labia	tm = Tubal membrane
llb = Lateral ligament	ua = Uterine artery
of bladder	ub = Uterine body
lo = Left ovary	uo = Urethral orifice
luh = Left uterine horn	ur = Ureter
mc = Mesocolon	va = Vagina
mo = Mesovarium	ve = Vestibule
oa = Ovarian artery	vf = Vaginal fornix
od = Oviduct	vgo = Vestibular gland openings
of = Ovulation fossa	vgp = Vesicogenital pouch

Figure 11-1. Dorsal **(A)** and lateral **(B)** views of the reproductive tract in the mare. (From Ginther OJ: *Reproductive Biology of the Mare: Basic and Applied Aspects,* 2nd ed. Cross Plains, WI: Equiservices Publishing, 1992.)

and uterus with the abdominal viscera and bladder is important when examining the reproductive tract using transrectal palpation or ultrasonic imaging techniques.[11,12]

STRUCTURAL ANATOMY

Suspensory Ligaments and Related Structures

The cranial portion of the reproductive tract, which is mostly in the abdominal cavity, is relatively fixed to the body wall by the broad ligaments.[1-4,8,10] The broad ligaments are bilayers of serous membranes of the peritoneum that originate from the sublumbar region (approximately the third or fourth lumbar vertebra to the fourth sacral vertebra). The caudal portion of the reproductive tract in the pelvic cavity is retroperitoneal and lies within loose fascia and adipose tissue. Apart from their physical role, the broad ligaments have a functional role as corridors for blood and lymphatic vessels as well as nerves serving the reproductive organs. The broad ligaments are divided into areas with respect to the reproductive organs that they support. The mesometrium represents the majority of the broad ligament because it is supportive of the relatively large uterine horns and uterine body. The mesosalpinx is supportive of the oviducts, and the mesovarium is supportive of the ovaries. Portions of the mesosalpinx and mesovarium contribute to the ovarian bursa, an enclosed pouch into which the ovary can project. The lateral wall of the bursa is formed by the mesosalpinx, and the medial wall is formed by a fold of broad ligament with the proper ligament of the ovary on the free border of the fold. The proper ligament of each ovary attaches the caudal or uterine pole of the ovary to the cranial aspect of the respective uterine horn. Attachments of the various divisions of the broad ligaments are on the dorsal to lateral aspects of the tubular genitalia (see Fig. 11-1, *B*). Thus, for orientation purpose during transrectal palpation, the free surface of the uterine horns and body is ventral. To ensure proper assessment of the ovaries by transrectal palpation or ultrasonic imaging, it may be necessary to digitally manipulate the ovaries and position them medial to the broad ligament and free them from the mesovarium that extends over the medial and lateral surfaces.

Migration of portions of the digestive, urinary, and reproductive tract into the abdominal cavity and toward the pelvic cavity during embryonic and fetal development is associated with movement of respective peritoneal folds in which pouches form between suspending ligaments of respective organs. The rectum is dorsal and the bladder is ventral to the reproductive tract (see Fig. 11-1). Thus, the rectogenital pouch forms between the rectum and the genital organs, and the vesicogenital pouch forms between the bladder and the genital organs; both pouches project caudally into the pelvic cavity. These pouches are of clinical importance because they are entered surgically during colpotomy[2,7,8] or during ultrasound-guided transvaginal manipulation of the ovaries[7,8,11,12] and uterus[13] as discussed in Chapter and 18. The bladder is suspended by two lateral ligaments and a ventral ligament that attaches to the pelvic floor. Transrectally, the lateral ligaments are readily palpable and are convenient for distinguishing the bladder from an advanced gravid uterus; the two lateral ligaments become extremely taut when the bladder is full.

Although the suspensory ligaments of the reproductive organs are the primary support for a gravid uterus, the ventral abdomen (i.e., linea alba and prepubic tendon) provides secondary support, especially during the later stages of pregnancy.

Although the linea alba is mainly formed from the aponeuroses of the flank muscles, its caudal aspect combines with insertion tendons of the right and left rectus abdominis muscles to form a broad transverse plate, the prepubic tendon, which attaches to the pubis at the iliopubic eminence.[9,10] With branching of the prepubic tendon, a relatively weak region exists cranial to the pubic brim between the two branches that connect to the pubis. Diagnosis, management, and prognosis associated with rupture of the prepubic tendon and other ventral abdominal ruptures or hernias, especially during advanced pregnancy, have been described.[2,5]

Blood Vessels, Lymphatics, and Nerves

The ovarian artery branches from the abdominal aorta and courses ventrolaterally along the cranial portion of the broad ligament (see Fig. 11-1). The artery eventually divides into uterine and ovarian branches; the uterine branch of the ovarian artery (cranial uterine artery) supplies blood to the oviduct and anterior portion of the uterine horn. The ovarian branch takes a more tortuous course within the mesovarium before dividing into several branches that spread out over the periphery of the ovary. The middle uterine artery branches and descends from the external iliac artery and is the main arterial blood supply to the uterus because of its large diameter, which expands even more during pregnancy. The uterine artery branches cranially and caudally as it approaches the dorsal mesometrial border of the caudal portion of the uterine horn and cranial portion of the uterine body. The vaginal artery (caudal uterine artery) originates from the internal pudendal artery and courses through the retroperitoneal tissue to supply blood to the caudal portion of the uterine body, cervix, and vagina. The vestibular branch of the internal pudendal artery supplies blood to the vagina proper, vestibule, and vulva. Essentially, veins draining the genital organs are satellites to the arteries, but the main venous drainage of the uterus is via the uterine branch of the ovarian vein. Unlike other species (e.g., bovids), the ovarian veins and arteries are not as closely opposed in the mare, which reflects the systemic route and uniqueness of how this species regulates the life span of the corpus luteum, especially during the mare's first luteal response to pregnancy.[1,14]

In pregnant mares, there is a progressive increase in uterine weight and blood flow as gestation advances, stretching uterine arteries and making them susceptible to rupture or hemorrhage, especially during maternal strain and fetal movement and positioning associated with parturition, as discussed in more detail in Chapter 22. The right middle uterine artery is the most common site of vascular rupture, but the external iliacs and utero-ovarian (cranial uterine) arteries have also been known to rupture. Hemorrhage of a uterine artery may occur directly into the abdominal cavity or may be contained within the layers of the broad ligament; either condition is life threatening. Although blood emanating from the vulva may be a sign of uterine hemorrhage, it is more likely caused by rupture of varicose veins in the vagina since bleeding is not usually excessive and occurs during the latter part of gestation. Varicosities of the vaginal wall are most common in older mares, developing during estrus as well as pregnancy. Diagnosis, management, and prognosis associated with uterine hemorrhage and vaginal varicosities have been described.[2,5,7,8]

Lymph from the ovaries and cranial portion of the tubular genitalia passes to the lumbar aortic lymph nodes, whereas lymph from the caudal portion of the reproductive tract passes to the medial iliac lymph nodes and other lymph nodes in the pelvic cavity, all of which eventually reach the thoracic duct and empty into the venous system near the heart. The lymphatic system is a principal component of the uterine clearance mechanism for removing accumulated fluid in the uterine wall after estrus and particulate matter from the uterine lumen after insemination, embryo/fetal loss, and parturition. Blockage or damage of lymphatic vessels can alter optimal uterine clearance of fluid and debris; consequently, a hostile intra-uterine environment may ensue and jeopardize fertilization and pregnancy maintenance. Hence, oxytocin and/or low-dose administration of prostaglandin-$F_{2\alpha}$ ($PGF_{2\alpha}$) are sometimes used in conjunction with or immediately after ovulation following insemination in mares with a history of subfertility that may be due to dysfunctional uterine clearance mechanism, as reviewed[5,7,8] and discussed in Chapter 13.

Innervation of the reproductive tract is primarily autonomic, with sympathetic and parasympathetic fibers of the renal, aortic, uterine, and pelvic plexuses innervating the ovaries, oviducts, uterus, and vagina. Pudendal and caudal rectal nerves derived from the third and fourth sacral nerves innervate the vestibule and the vulva.

Caudal Reproductive Tract (Perineum, Vulva, Clitoris, Vestibule)

The caudal portion of the reproductive tract is relatively stable within the pelvic cavity; therefore, gross shape and positional changes are minimal compared with the cranial reproductive tract that lies mostly within the abdominal cavity. The dimensions ascribed to the reproductive organs in this chapter relate primarily to excised organs taken from riding-type horse mares

at necropsy and, therefore, may not be precisely representative of organ dimensions *in situ*.[1,2,3,4,9]

Perineum

The perineum or perineal region is broadly defined to include the external portions of the vulva and anus and surrounding area such that it may extend from the base of the tail to the ventral commissure of the vulva and, in some instances, to the dorsocaudal aspect of the udder. Any deviation from optimal conformation of the perineum (area surrounding the anus and vulva) may compromise the vulvar seal and result in the influx of air into the vagina (i.e., pneumovagina, or "wind-sucking"). Malconformation of the perineum may also result in the pooling of urine in the vagina (urovagina). Any of these conformational disfigurements of the perineum predispose the mare to acute or chronic inflammation of the vagina, cervix, and endometrium, thus affecting fertility. The degree of malconformation of the perineum and management (e.g., Caslick's vulvoplasty operation) have been described.[2,5,7,8]

Vulva

The vulva, which usually includes the labia (vulvar lips) and clitoris, is the most caudal portion of the reproductive tract and is considered the first line of defense to protect against contamination of the uterus. The vulvar cleft is represented by a vertical slit (approximately 12–15 cm in length), with pointed dorsal and rounded ventral commissures, and marks the external orifice of the urogenital tract, which is controlled by the striated vulvar constrictor muscle that runs along either side of the length of the vulvar lips. The mucocutaneous junction of the labia demarcates the aglandular mucous membrane from the glandular pigmented skin. The gross appearance of the vulva/labia can be influenced by the stage of the estrous cycle as presented in Table 11-1. Approximately two thirds of the vulva extends caudoventrally over

Table 11-1 | Tactile and Visual Changes of the Tubular Genitalia Using Various Instrumentation and Direct Sensation and Observation During the Estrous Cycle in the Mare

METHOD OF EXAMINATION	GENITALIA	MID-DIESTRUS	ESTRUS EARLY	ESTRUS MIDDLE	ESTRUS LATE
Transrectal palpation	Uterus	Maximal tone and thickness	Decreasing turgidity and thickness ⟶		
	Cervix	Firm and distinct	Beginning to flatten	Flatter, shorter, and wider	Indiscernible, very flat
			Decreasing turgidity and thickness ⟶		
Transrectal ultrasonic imaging	Uterus	Minimal edema	Increasing endometrial folding ⟶ (nonechoic areas indicating edema)		
	Cervix	Echogenic	Increasing nonechoic areas ⟶		
Transvaginal palpation	Vagina	Dry	Increasing wetness ⟶		
	Cervix	Firm, protruding	Decreasing turgidity and thickness ⟶		
	Cervical orifice	Difficult to dilate	Easier to dilate ⟶		
			1 Finger	2 Fingers	≥3 Fingers
Speculum or endoscope	Vagina and cervix	Viscous fluids, vaginal walls sticky	Increasing fluid with decreasing viscosity ⟶		
		Dull, yellow-gray	Pink	Bright pink	Glistening red
		Minimal vascularity	Increasing vascularity ⟶		
	Cervical orifice	Protruding, central location, tight	Drooping and opening	Drooped below center, open	Near floor of vagina
Direct	Vulva/labia	Wrinkled, pale, dry	Increasing redness, moisture, smoothness ⟶		

Adapted and summarized from Ginther OJ: *Reproductive Biology of the Mare: Basic and Applied Aspects,* 2nd ed. Cross Plains, WI: Equiservices Publishing, 1992.

the ischial arch; therefore, safe passage of the forearm, pipette, or other instruments into the vestibule and vagina is at an upward angle.

Clitoris

The clitoral glans appears wrinkled and creased and is located in a protective cavity or pouch (clitoral prepuce) at the ventral commissure of the vulva (see Fig. 11-1, *A*). The clitoral retractor muscle and the vulvar constrictor muscle are responsible for the natural inversion of the labia and exposure of the clitoris ("clitoral wink") during urination or during behavioral estrus. It can be exposed manually for examination and swabbing of its various sinuses (three to five) to test for harmful and contagious bacteria such as *Taylorella equigenitalis* responsible for equine metritis and *Klebsiella pneumoniae* and *Pseudomonas aeruginosa* as reviewed.[2,5,7,8]

Vestibule

The vestibule generally occupies a median position in the pelvic outlet and extends from the external vulvar lips to the transverse fold (approximately 10–12 cm in length) that often lies over the urethral orifice, caudal to the fold (see Fig. 11-1, *A*). In young, maiden mares, the fold may be partial or complete, forming the hymen, which may temporarily restrict entrance into the vagina until broken by the penis or manually by palpation. The mucous membrane of the vestibule has rows of papilla in the ventral and lateral walls that mark the opening of minor vestibular glands (see Fig. 11-1, *A*); striated muscles and the vestibular bulb (mass of erectile tissue) are associated with the lateral walls only.

Cranial Reproductive Tract (Vagina, Cervix, Uterus, Oviducts, Ovaries)

The caudal (ectodermal origin) and cranial (mesodermal origin) portions of the urogenital system converge at the juncture between the vestibule and vagina proper and are demarcated by the transverse fold. In this regard, the fold is often referred to as the vestibular or vaginal (vestibulovaginal) seal and is considered the second line of defense to protect against contamination of the uterus.

Vagina

The vagina proper (approximately 20–35 cm in length) in non-pregnant mares generally occupies a median position in the pelvic inlet while the remainder of the cranial portion of the reproductive tract lies in the abdominal cavity. The vagina usually exists as a collapsed lumen that is highly distensible in length and width to accommodate the penis or forearm during natural or artificial insemination and foal at parturition. The vagina proper is thin walled and aglandular but does receive secretions from the cervix, and, therefore, its gross appearance can be influenced by the stage of the estrous cycle (see Table 11-1). The vaginal fornix at the cranial aspect of the vagina represents an annular cavity in which the caudal portion of the cervix projects (see Fig. 11-1, *A* and Fig. 11-2). The mucosa is normally pale pink but darkens with prolonged exposure to air during vaginoscopy (see Fig. 11-2). During transvaginal ultrasonic imaging of the reproductive tract, it is the cranial wall of the vaginal fornix that is in contact with the face of the ultrasound transducer as well as the surface that is penetrated to enter the rectogenital pouch during an ultrasound-guided needle approach to the ovaries or uterus and that is incised during colpotomy.

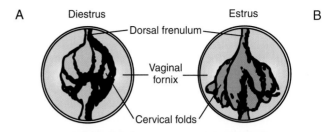

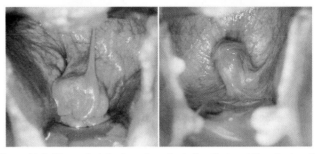

Figure 11-2. The vaginal fornix and cervix during diestrus **(A)** and estrus **(B)** in the mare. The gross morphology of the cervix as viewed with a speculum appears tight during diestrus (progesterone dominance) and flaccid during estrus (estrogen dominance).

Cervix

The cervix is a sphincter-like muscle (5–8 cm in length and 2–5 cm in diameter) that protrudes caudally into the vaginal fornix (2–4 cm in length) and is the third and final line of defense to protect against contamination of the uterus (see Figs. 11-1 and 11-2). It has a thick wall of smooth muscle that is rich in elastic fibers and that changes in tone (turgid vs. flaccid), size, color, and secretions depending on whether the hormonal milieu is dominated by progesterone during diestrus and pregnancy (see Fig. 11-2, *A*) or estrogen during estrus (see Fig. 11-2, *B*) as indicated in Table 11-1. The cervix is arranged in longitudinal mucosal or cervical folds that are continuous with endometrial folds of the uterine body and horns (see Fig. 11-1, *A*). The intravaginal portion has a lobed appearance as a result of extension of the cervical folds into the vaginal fornix (see Figs. 11-1, *A,* and 11-2). A dorsal or ventral fold may continue onto the floor of the fornix as a distinct frenulum. A unique clinical feature of the longitudinal folds of the cervix is that they allow relatively easy access to the uterine lumen by digital or tactile dilation, especially during estrus, compared with domestic species with cervical rings (e.g., bovids). Unlike the aglandular vagina, mucus-producing cells of the cervix secrete copious amounts of mucus. The hormonally timed changes in cervical tone and its secretions are essential physical and physiological barriers to protect the uterus and facilitate uterine clearance, delivery, and transport of semen, fertilization, pregnancy development and maintenance, and parturition. Physical examination of the cervix can be done by using ultrasonography, palpation, a speculum, or endoscopy. Cervical dysfunction attributed to congenital defects or physical trauma and consequential effects on fertility have been reviewed.[2,5,7,8]

Uterus

The uterus consists of a uterine body and two uterine horns and is classified as a simplex bipartitus uterus (see Fig. 11-1). General dimensions in non-pregnant mares are that the length and diameter of the uterine body are relatively shorter (~18–20 cm in length) and larger (~8–12 cm in diameter) compared with longer (~20–25 cm in length) and smaller (~1–6 cm in diameter) uterine horns. The uterine body is continuous with the cervix and lies mostly in the pelvic inlet and abdominal cavity. Two uterine horns diverge from the uterine body and are joined by the intercornual ligament at the corpus-corneal junction; a short uterine septum marks the internal bifurcation (see Fig. 11-1, *A*). The corpus-corneal junction is important clinically because it represents a structural and functional region within each uterine horn where the early embryonic vesicle becomes "fixed" and readily detected by ultrasonic imaging to evaluate its status. Structurally, the degree of curvature or flexure of the uterine horns near the corpus-corneal junction (see Fig. 11-1, *B*), the increase in uterine tone (i.e., turgidity), and the expansion of the conceptus act in concert as physical impediments to trap the previous mobile vesicle in the caudal aspect of either the left or right uterine horn. The cessation of embryonic mobility that occurs 15–16 days after ovulation, defined as "fixation," has been reviewed,[1,2,11,12] and is discussed in Chapter 19.

Peripherally, the uterus is enclosed by visceral peritoneum—the perimetrium—and is continuous with the suspending portion of the broad ligament—the mesometrium. As discussed earlier, the mesometrium of the broad ligament attaches to the dorsal border of the uterine horns and the lateral aspects of the body and cervix (see Fig. 11-1, *B*).

The uterine wall consists of longitudinal (outer) and circular (inner) smooth muscle layers with a vascular layer in between, which makes up the myometrium (Fig. 11-3, *A*). The outer muscle layer and vasculature are continuous with the mesometrium.

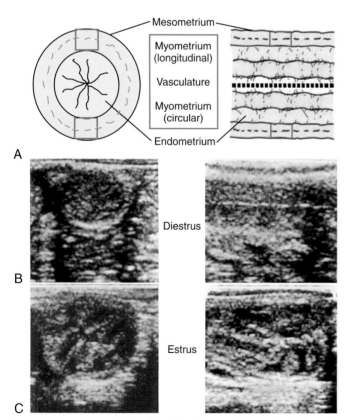

Figure 11-3. The cross and longitudinal sections of the uterus **(A)** during diestrus **(B)** and estrus **(C)** in the mare. The gross morphology of the endometrium is relatively homogenous during diestrus (progesterone dominance) and heterogeneous during estrus (estrogen dominance).

The myometrium is, in part, responsible for mobility of the early embryonic vesicle around the extent of the uterus and the force to expel the fetus at parturition.

The intrauterine environment consists of a gland-free core of connective tissue arranged in longitudinal folds (12–15) and covered by a reddish-brown mucosa, the highly glandular endometrium. The lumen of the uterus is essentially collapsed, in which the endometrial folds are in close apposition but can be easily dilated by air or fluid. Ultrasonic morphology of the endometrium appears relatively homogeneous during diestrus (see Fig. 11-3, *B*) compared with heterogeneous during estrus (see Fig. 11-3, *C*). Changes in the ultrasonic echogenicity of the endometrium during the luteal and follicular phases are due to the degree of edema associated with the endometrial folds during progesterone and estrogen dominance (see Table 11-1), respectively, which has clinical importance in the timing of ovulation and insemination discussed in Chapter 12.

The endometrium is highly glandular with prominent openings on the surface toward the lumen; extreme branching and coiling of the tubular structures exist below the surface. Glandular changes are considered a prime indicator of uterine health when assessing uterine tissue biopsy specimens.[2,5,7,8] Typically, histological assessment of glandular changes of an endometrial biopsy includes periglandular fibrosis, cystic dilation of glands, and glandular necrosis. In addition to biopsy score, microscopic evaluation of the endometrium may include characterization of lymphatic lacunae, endometrial atrophy, and cellular infiltration. Clinically, endometritis—acute or chronic inflammation involving the endometrium—is generally considered a major cause of reduced fertility in mares as reviewed[2,5,7,8] and discussed in Chapter 13.

Oviducts

The tortuous oviducts (~20–30 cm in length) extending beyond the cranial tips of beach uterine horn are sometimes called uterine tubes or salpinges (see Fig. 11-1). There are three divisions extending from the ovary to the tip of the uterine horn: (1) funnel-shaped infundibulum with finger-like fimbriae, (2) expanded ampulla, and (3) narrow isthmus. Irregular fimbriae are present along the margin of the infundibulum, in which a portion of them are attached to the cranial pole of the ovary to form the cranial edge of the ovulation fossa. Remaining fimbriae and the infundibulum are free to spread over the ventral aspect of the ovary and cover the ovulation fossa.

The abdominal opening of the oviduct (~6 mm in diameter) is at the approximate center of the infundibulum and marks the beginning of the ampulla. The ampulla (10–15 cm in length and about 6 mm in width) gradually narrows into the isthmus (10–15 cm in length and about 3 mm in width) and opens (2–3 mm in diameter) eccentrically into the cranial portion of the uterine horn through a small papilla that projects into the uterine lumen (uterotubal junction).

The uterotubal junction marks the convergence of the oviduct and the uterine horn and, clinically, is sometimes the deposition site for sperm during low-dose intrauterine insemination as discussed in Chapters 14 and 15. Oviductal morphology is similar to the uterus (see Fig. 11-3, *A*), with a peripheral, serosal layer; two layers of smooth muscle (outer longitudinal and inner circular divided by a vascular layer); and a mucosal layer. However, extending from the uterine horns to the ovaries, the musculature of the isthmus is apparently more developed than the ampulla, and the mucosa of the ampulla more plicated than the isthmus.

The plicated nature of the ampulla is highly complex, with primary, secondary, and even tertiary folds, thus providing a relatively quiet and nourishing environment for fertilization, whereas the isthmus, being dominated by muscle and ciliated epithelial cells, provides a relatively active environment for propelling sperm to the site of fertilization and subsequently the fertilized egg to the uterus. Unlike other large domestic animals (e.g., cattle) in which unfertilized ova eventually reach the uterus, the mare is unique in that unfertilized ova are typically retained in the isthmus and, therefore, are not usually observed in the uterine-flush media associated with embryo transfer procedures.

The oviducts are often associated with various forms of fluid-filled embryonic vestiges that may involve the ovary and affect fertility. Structural and functional anatomy as well as diagnosis and treatment of these various cysts and nodules have been described.[2,5,7,8]

Ovaries (Follicles, Ovum, Corpora Lutea)

In the neonate and during the prepubertal period, the ovaries of the filly appear oval and the cortical zone with the germinal epithelium is superficial. As the filly approaches puberty, or as early as 5–7 months of age, there is an anatomical transformation such that the ovarian cortex invaginates into the medulla so that the ovary appears kidney-bean–shaped in adult mares (Figs. 11-4 and 11-7).

In the adult mare, the ovaries (~4–8 cm in length × 3–6 cm in width × 3–5 cm in height) have migrated only slightly from the site where they originated embryologically near the kidneys and commonly lie in the dorsal part of the abdomen, cranioventral to the iliac wings of the hip in the plane of the third to fifth lumbar vertebrae. The left ovary is usually more caudal than the right as a result of the more caudal position of the left kidney during development. The length of the mesovarium allows considerable leeway for positional changes of the ovaries as they move above or intermingle with the intestines. In this regard, it may be difficult to identify poles (cranial/caudal or tubal/uterine) and surfaces (lateral/medial) of the ovary by transrectal palpation. The border regions (dorsal/ventral or attached/free), however, are more easily identified because of their characteristic shape as a result of the morphological transformation during the peripubertal period. The dorsal or attached ovarian border is convex and is structurally called the greater curvature, which is also the hilus of the ovary—the point at which blood and lymphatic vessels and nerves reach the ovary through its attachment with the mesovarium and enter and disperse into the ovarian medullary (see Figs. 11-1, 11-4, A, and 11-5). The ventral or free border is concave as a result of formation of the ovulation fossa. Thus, the adult equine ovary is unique among domestic species with a peripheral medullary zone of connective, neural, and vascular tissue and an internal cortical zone with germinal tissue that is externalized only at the ovulation fossa.

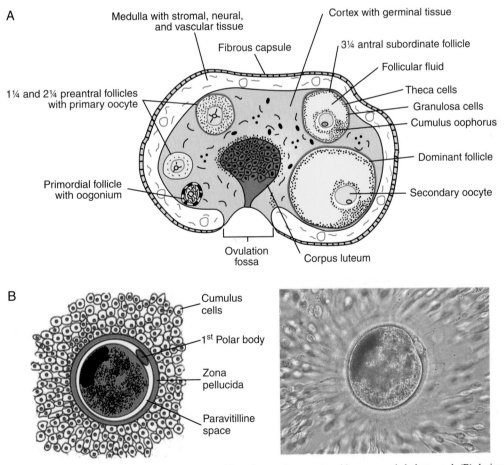

Figure 11-4. The morphological characteristics of the adult equine ovary **(A)** and secondary oocyte with accompanied photograph **(B)** during the ovulatory season. Note the sequential transformation of a primordial follicle to a dominant follicle and corpus luteum following ovulation and first polar body characteristic of a secondary oocyte ready for fertilization.

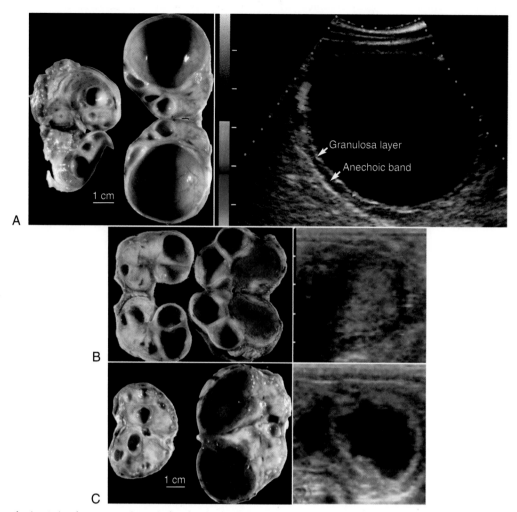

Figure 11-5. Photographs *(ex situ)* and sonograms *(in situ)* of equine ovaries during the ovulatory season depicting gross structural characteristics of the preovulatory follicle and associated small follicles **(A)**, a mature corpus luteum without an intraluteal cavity and associated small to medium-sized follicles **(B)** and a corpus luteum with an intraluteal, blood-filled cavity (corpus hemorrhagicum) and associated small follicles **(C)**. Note the ultrasonic detection of the granulosa cell layer and potential site of ovulation (apical region in upper left) associated with the preovulatory follicle **(A)** and the demarcation between luteal tissue and blood clot associated with a corpus hemorrhagicum **(C)**.

FOLLICLES. Follicular development within the ovary involves growing, ovulating, and anovulatory hemorrhagic or regressing follicles (see Figs. 11-4, *A.* and 11-5). In general, primordial follicles are sometimes referred to as *resting follicles* while developing follicles are represented by early-stage, pre-antral follicles and later-stage, antral follicles. The latter are the more mature stage of follicles and are of clinical importance because they are the main source of reproductive steroids (estrogens, progestogens, and androgens) that influence follicle growth and regression, uterine and cervical structural and functional changes, estrous behavior, oocyte development, and ovulation. Antral follicles exist as fluid-filled cavities composed of blood transudate and follicle cell secretions; single to multiple layers of granulosa cells encircle the inner follicle wall, and theca (interna and externa) cells encircle the outer follicle wall, as illustrated in Fig. 11-4. To support the two-cell theory of ovarian steroidogenesis (i.e., androgens aromatized to estrogens), follicle theca cells have the specific capacity to acquire LH receptors necessary for androgen production, whereas follicle granulosa cells have the capacity to acquire both FSH and LH receptors necessary for estrogen production.[1] The vascularized theca cell layer is separated from the avascular granulosa cell layer by a basal lamina, connective tissue that allows for the transport and exchange of steroidal substrates, nutrients, and metabolic waste between the systemic circulation and follicle.

Ovarian follicular development occurs in a wave-like fashion during the equine estrous cycle, pregnancy, and seasonal transition (fall and spring) between the ovulatory and anovulatory seasons.[1,11,15,16] Follicular waves have been categorized as major (primary and secondary) and minor waves depending on whether the largest follicle of a wave reaches ≥30 mm in association with follicle selection (major wave) or <30 mm without selection (minor wave) as summarized and illustrated during the estrous cycle in Fig. 11-6. Both types of wave patterns exhibit a common growth phase associated with a group of antral follicles at the beginning of a wave, but only major waves exhibit a dominance phase after selection for the largest follicle (dominant) and selection against the next largest follicles (subordinates) at the end of the common growth phase. Minor waves lack dominance since there is no selection process for or against follicles other than the eventual regression of all follicles of the wave.

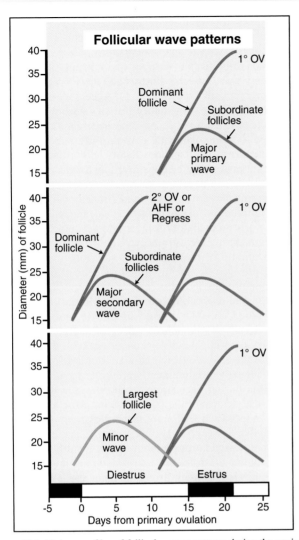

Figure 11-6. Various profiles of follicular wave patterns during the equine estrous cycle depicting ovulation (OV) of the dominant follicle (≥30 mm) of a primary major wave at the end of estrus and OV or anovulation and formation of a hemorrhagic follicle (AHF) or regression of the dominant follicle of a secondary major wave during diestrus. Alternatively, either minimal follicular growth (<15 mm) or a minor follicular wave (largest follicle, <30 mm) precedes the primary major wave.

The pattern of follicular waves varies with reproductive status as follows:

1. A combination of sequential major (anovulatory) and minor follicular waves is associated with the transitional seasons (fall and spring)
2. Major primary (ovulatory) waves are associated with estrus (follicular phase) and either major secondary (ovulatory or anovulatory) or minor waves are associated with diestrus (luteal phase) during the estrous cycle
3. A combination of sequential major secondary (ovulatory or anovulatory) and minor follicular waves is associated with early pregnancy.

In general, follicular wave emergence during the estrous cycle is associated with the growth of a group of 5–10 antral follicles (4–6 mm) within 2–3 days of one another. During the common growth phase, most follicles increase in diameter 2–4 mm/day until the largest follicle reaches 20–25 mm near the end of the common growth phase. Afterwards, either all follicles (minor wave) or all

but the largest follicle (major wave) begin to gradually regress. The differential change in growth rates between dominant and subordinate follicles associated with major (primary and secondary) waves is defined morphologically as follicle deviation and marks the time of follicle selection. Subordinate follicles decrease in diameter while the dominant follicle increases in diameter until it ovulates, becomes anovulatory and hemorrhagic, or regresses (see Fig. 11-6), which depends, in part, on season and reproductive status of the mare.

A random section through an ovary may contain antral follicles of various sizes at different stages of growth and regression, as depicted grossly in Fig. 11-5, where follicles ranged from <2 to >30 mm in diameter. Small, medium, and large antral follicles are usually spherical and firm; however, a high percentage of preovulatory follicles (85%–90% of follicles ≥35 mm) become less turgid and non-spherical, forming an apical area that becomes the site of follicle rupture at ovulation, as depicted in the ultrasound image in Fig. 11-5, A.[1,2,7,11,12,17]

In general, spontaneous ovulation of a single preovulatory follicle of a major wave occurs when the dominant follicle reaches about 40 mm in diameter; however, maximum diameter of the preovulatory follicle is related, in part, to season, breed, type of mare (draft or miniature), and number of preovulatory follicles.[2] Although transrectal palpation can be used as a general approach to determine the degree of follicular activity, presence of dominant follicle (≥30 mm), status of preovulatory-sized follicles, and transrectal ultrasonic imaging are a more precise and accurate approach to determine follicle numbers, size, shape, and structural and functional characteristics.[2,12,16] In regard to the latter, ultrasonography can be used to determine the thickness of the follicle wall (theca and granulosa cell layer and basal lamina), degree of separation of the granulosa cell layer, and prominence of an anechoic area between the granulosa and basal lamina (see Fig. 11-5, A), which may be used as a diagnostic aid in estimating the time of spontaneous or induced ovulation for synchronization or insemination purposes.[7,16]

OVUM. Depending on the stage of follicle development, each ovarian follicle contains either a primary or secondary oocyte that is surrounded by a group of granulosa cells called cumulus cells (see Fig. 11-4). The area of the internal follicle wall where the cumulus-oocyte complex is attached to mural granulosa cells via the cumulus oophorus is referred to as the hillock. Near the time of ovulation, the oocyte detaches from the hillock, severing its communicative link with mural granulosa cells of the follicle but still maintains its intimate layer of cumulus cells known as the corona radiata (see Fig. 11-4). Functionally, outside the follicle and apart from the ovary, these cells are thought to be important for oocyte pickup by fimbriae of the infundibulum and ciliary transport to the ampulla of the oviduct after ovulation.

Dislodgement of the cumulus-oocyte complex from the follicle wall near the time of ovulation is associated with development of the oocyte from the primary (diploid; 2N) to the secondary (haploid; 1N) stage, an event necessary for proper fertilization and embryo development.[1,2] Microscopically, a secondary oocyte can be differentiated from a primary oocyte by extrusion of the first polar body located in the perivitelline space as shown in Fig. 11-4, B. The oocyte is discussed in more detail in Chapter 18 and elsewhere.[1,2,5,7]

CORPORA LUTEA. Ovulation is a process by which the wall of the follicle ruptures in the vicinity of the ovulation fossa, thus allowing follicular fluid, granulosa cells, and the oocyte to be evacuated. Two types of follicle evacuation have been identified: abrupt and gradual.[1,2,7,11,12] For the abrupt type, about 82% of the antral area is evacuated in less than 1 minute and, for the gradual type, there is a slow loss of follicular fluid that takes about 4 minutes for about 83% of the antral area to be lost. Eventually, with the complete loss of follicular fluid, the follicle wall collapses into the antrum, which can be readily palpated as a depression on the ovarian surface or viewed as a hyperechoic area using ultrasonic imaging.[1,2,7,11,12] If more than 24 hours has elapsed between examinations when a large follicle was present at one examination and not the next, the antrum of the ovulated follicle may refill with blood (see Fig. 11-5, C) and be confused with an unovulated follicle when using transrectal palpation. Alternatively, ultrasonic imaging can readily differentiate between ovulated follicles that have refilled with blood to form a corpus hemorrhagicum and unovulated follicles that have filled with blood without rupture of the follicle wall to form a hemorrhagic anovulatory follicle.[1,2,7,11,12,18]

Two types of luteal gland morphologies are distinctly apparent after ovulation[1,2,7,11,12]: those that develop an intraluteal blood clot (see Fig. 11-5, C), and those that do not (see Fig. 11-5, B). An intraluteal blood-filled cavity develops at the site of ovulation with luteal tissue around the periphery 50%–70% of the time and has been termed a *corpus hemorrhagicum*, as described in Table 11-2. Although corpora lutea that develop an intraluteal cavity during early diestrus are about 17% larger than corpora lutea without a blood-filled cavity, the luteal tissue area is comparable between the two morphologies. Ultrasonic imaging can readily differentiate luteal tissue from non-luteal tissue of a corpus hemorrhagicum, as shown in Fig. 11-5, C. The intraluteal cavity of a corpus hemorrhagicum eventually decreases in size as the blood clot becomes more organized during luteal maturation. Although irregularities associated with ovulation have been well documented,[1,2,7,8,11,12] it appears that the main characteristics that distinguish a corpus hemorrhagicum resulting from ovulation and an anovulatory hemorrhagic follicle is that the latter initially has numerous free-floating echoic specks in the antrum, increases in size beyond that which usually occurs at the time of ovulation (e.g., >80 mm in diameter), and is relatively more spherical. More recent research[18] has indicated that an anovulatory follicle is associated with higher plasma concentrations of estradiol a few days before expected ovulation and increased vascularity as determined by color Doppler ultrasonography on the day before ovulation than an ovulatory follicle. The use of color Doppler ultrasonography to assess the status of a preovulatory follicle is depicted in Fig. 11-7.[17]

Regardless of luteal gland morphology, primary corpora lutea result from ovulations of dominant follicles (≥30 mm) of major primary waves at or near the end of estrus when estrogen prevails, which can include single or double synchronous or double asynchronous (<3 days apart) ovulations, whereas secondary corpora lutea result from ovulations of dominant follicles of major secondary waves during diestrus and early pregnancy when progesterone prevails (see Fig. 11-6). Accessory corpora lutea result from dominant anovulatory follicles during diestrus and early pregnancy. Both secondary and accessory corpora lutea are referred to as supplemental corpora lutea (see Table 11-2). Notably, the formation of an anovulatory hemorrhagic follicle in non-pregnant mares may be considered an accessory corpus luteum, especially if it develops during a progestational state (i.e., diestrus) during the estrous cycle or fall transitional period. Nevertheless, morphological and physiological characteristics of the conversion of a preovulatory follicle into a hemorrhagic anovulatory follicle during the estrous cycle have been described.[17,18]

Luteinization involves structural and functional morphogenesis of estrogen-producing granulosa cells of the follicle to progesterone-producing luteal cells of the corpus luteum.[1] Disorganization and restructuring of the follicle wall allows fibroblasts and blood vessels to invade the follicle antrum in concert with hypertrophy of granulosa cells. Structural transition of granulosa cells to luteal cells is concurrent with the functional transition of the steroidogenic pathway from predominantly estrogen producing to predominantly progesterone producing.

Luteolysis during the estrous cycle involves the structural and functional demise of the corpus luteum, whether it is spontaneously induced via $PGF_{2\alpha}$ from the uterus or artificially induced with $PGF_{2\alpha}$ treatment as discussed in Chapter 9. The scar tissue of a regressed corpus luteum can be identified within the ovary during late diestrus/early estrus and later in pregnancy as a hyperechoic area using ultrasonic imaging and is referred to as a *corpus albicans* (see Table 11-2).

Detecting the presence of a corpus luteum using transrectal palpation is impractical in the mare, in part because the unique anatomy of the equine ovary prohibits an accurate tactile determination. Alternatively, ultrasonic imaging is a readily available and superior approach to detect and monitor luteal gland development from ovulation to regression.[11,12] Structural attributes of the corpus luteum that can be determined by using ultrasonic imaging and, subsequently, aid in diagnosing the developmental stage (early, mature, regressed) and functional status (progesterone output) are diameter and volume or area of the gland and degree of luteal tissue echogenicity (brightness) in which the latter appears to reflect the degree of luteal cell hypertrophy and vascularization associated with luteogenesis. In regard to the latter, color Doppler ultrasonography has been used to assess the degree of vascularity of the corpus luteum as depicted in Fig. 11-7, B.[17]

Table 11-2 | Luteal Gland Terminology Used During the Estrous Cycle and Pregnancy in the Mare

LUTEAL STRUCTURE	DEFINITION
Primary corpora lutea phase	Result from single or multiple ovulations during the follicular stage (*estrogen dominance*)
Secondary corpora lutea	Result from ovulations (>2 days from the primary ovulation) during diestrus and early pregnancy (*progesterone dominance*)
Corpora hemorrhagica	Primary or secondary corpora lutea that develop an intraluteal blood-filled cavity subsequent to ovulation
Accessory corpora lutea	Result from luteinization of anovulatory follicles during diestrus and early pregnancy (*progesterone dominance*)
Supplemental corpora lutea	Includes secondary and accessory corpora lutea that develop early pregnancy
Corpora albicantia	Regressed corpora lutea regardless of reproductive status

Adapted and summarized from Ginther OJ: *Reproductive Biology of the Mare: Basic and Applied Aspects,* 2nd ed. Cross Plains, WI: Equiservices Publishing, 1992.

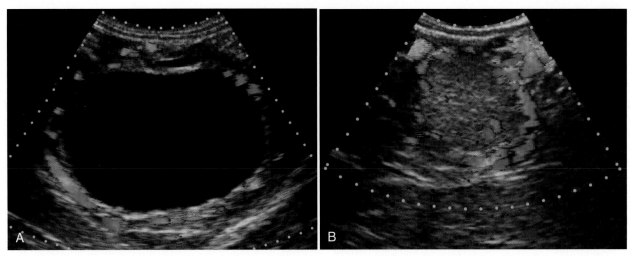

Figure 11-7. Sonograms of B-mode and color Doppler characteristics of a preovulatory follicle **(A)** and corpus luteum **(B)**. Notice the color signals indicative of blood flow encompassing the follicle in association with the vascular thecal cell layer of the follicle wall **(A)** and the higher intensity of the signals encompassing the luteal gland, especially at the upper right in the area of the hilus of the ovary **(B)**.

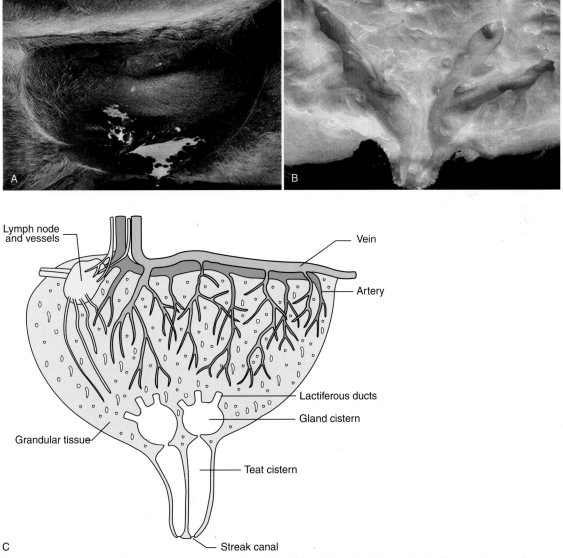

Figure 11-8. The equine mammary glands depicting gross structural characteristics of the udder before **(A)** and after **(B, C)** sectioning one of the mammae.

Mammary Glands (Udder)

The mammary glands (mammae) are enclosed in the udder located high in the inguinal region below the caudal aspect of the abdominal floor and cranial aspect of the pelvis between the hind legs (Fig. 11-8, *A*). The udder is covered by thin, highly pigmented skin with numerous sweat and sebaceous glands and is mostly devoid of hair except for the cranial portion. The position and gross characteristics of the udder reduces the risk of physical trauma, sunburn, and infections.

Mammogenesis from birth to puberty (i.e., first ovulation) occurs isometrically or at the same rate as body growth, primarily as a result of an increase in fat and connective tissue. At puberty and thereafter, mammae development occurs allometrically or at a different rate than body growth, primarily as a result of changes in the glandular tissue associated with various stages of the estrous cycle, pregnancy, and post-partum. Grossly, the udder is relatively small in dry, non-lactating mares, especially in nulliparous mares compared with lactating, multiparous mares where the skin may be more wrinkled and teats longer.

The mammae (left and right) are internally separated by a facial sheet of connective tissue running along the midline and supported by a medial suspensory ligament. Hence, on either side of the midline there is an independent left and right mamma that is grossly visible by the external longitudinal intermammary groove (see Fig. 11-8, *A*). Each mamma is further supported primarily by respective lateral suspensory ligaments running under the skin.

Within the glandular tissue of the mammae are numerous secretory alveoli (milk-producing cells) that are grouped together to form multiple lobules that compose a single lobe. Multiple lobes are joined together by the lactiferous duct system that leads to the gland cistern and into the teat cistern and streak canal of each teat of each mamma (see Fig. 11-8, *B* and *C*). According to the number of independent lactiferous duct systems within each mamma (typically two, but sometimes three), two or three ostia or openings perforate the apex of each teat (see Fig. 11-8, *A*). From a clinical perspective, the size of the lactiferous ducts (cranial is typically larger than the caudal) and number of openings per teat have implications concerning mammary disease and intramammary therapy.[7,8] A sphincter associated with each teat opening prevents the leakage of milk prior to parturition and between sucklings; however, ostia may be breached, resulting in a loss of copious amounts of milk during late pregnancy and during post-partum lactation. During late pregnancy, a slight secretion of colostrum and buildup of sebum and small amounts of cellular debris occur at the teat openings. This event has been called *waxing* and is often considered a sign of impending parturition.

Physiologically, each mamma is structurally and functionally supported by the vascular, lymphatic, and nervous systems. On each side of the midline, arterial blood enters each mammary gland via the external pudendal arteries that descend through respective inguinal canals and into the caudal part of each gland, subsequently branching into cranial and caudal mammary arteries (see Fig. 11-8, *C*). Unlike the arterial blood supply, venous blood leaving the mammary glands occurs, first, through a venous plexus at the base of each gland and, second, via the external pudendal veins ascending through the inguinal canals or a superficial vein of the thoracic wall. The latter apparently develop during the first pregnancy and are prominent on the abdomen (ventrolateral) of lactating mares; hence, they are often referred to as the *subcutaneous abdominal milk veins*.

Lymphatic drainage of the mammary glands occurs via superficial inguinal lymph nodes at the base of each gland and associated vessels that connect with the main circulatory lymph system (see Fig. 11-8, *C*). Innervation of the glandular tissue of the udder is mainly provided for by the genitofemoral nerves that reach the mammary glands through the inguinal canals, whereas cutaneous innervation is supplied by nerves of the flank and a descending branch of the pudendal nerve.

FUNCTIONAL ANATOMY

Puberty

There is a paucity of documented information on the hormonal and ovarian relationships in fillies compared with adult mares. Nevertheless, a synopsis of available information is presented according to a previous review[1] and more recent publications.[19-22] Puberty is defined as the first ovulation in the reproductive life of the mare, which is thought to occur as a result of maturation of the hypothalamic-pituitary-ovarian axis. Generally, puberty in fillies is reached between 12 and 24 months of age. Spring-born fillies (January to May in the Northern Hemisphere) of the first year with good nutrition and health throughout the prepubertal period may be expected to reach puberty during the following spring of the second year. Conversely, summer- to fall-born fillies (June to November) may be expected to reach puberty slightly later (e.g., summer) during the second year. In a study done with pasture-raised Thoroughbreds in the Southern Hemisphere (New Zealand), fall-born foals reached puberty about the same time as spring-born foals during the spring of the second year.[21] Hence, fall-born colts and fillies were younger and weighed less than spring-born colts and fillies at puberty. Regardless of the season of birth, stress associated with poor nutrition and health during the prepubertal period can alter the endocrine environment and, consequently, suppress maturation of the hypothalamic-pituitary-ovarian axis in fillies and, therefore, delay the first ovulation (i.e., puberty).

Circulating concentrations of pituitary FSH are relatively high throughout the first year in fillies born during the spring or summer, whereas circulating concentrations of pituitary LH are relatively low. In the fall and winter, FSH concentrations may decrease slightly while LH concentrations remain low and constant. In the spring of the second year, concentrations of FSH may increase slightly as LH gradually begins to increase. At puberty (first ovulation), FSH concentrations are relatively low and LH concentrations are relatively high in response to the negative and positive hormonal feedback effects between the ovaries and hypothalamus/pituitary, similar to what occurs in adult mares (see the following section). Despite relatively high concentrations of FSH during the first year, ovarian follicular development is minimal such that follicles rarely exceed 10 mm in diameter. However, between the first winter and second spring, there is a dramatic increase in the number of antral follicles >10 mm in diameter. The changing pattern of circulating gonadotropin concentrations and ovarian activity in spring-born fillies during the spring of the second year is likely related to maturation of the hypothalamic-pituitary-ovarian axis, especially with respect to the strong link between hypothalamic GnRH and pituitary LH. Thus, the peripubertal period beginning during the second year of life in spring-born fillies appears similar to what occurs in adult mares during transition from the anovulatory to the ovulatory season (spring transition) (see section on seasonality). It is suspected that morphologic changes in the ovaries and tubular genitalia in young maiden mares during the estrous cycle are similar to that in more mature mares (see the following section).

In most instances there is no reason to hasten puberty in fillies. It is generally accepted to allow puberty to occur spontaneously, with breeding starting at about 3 years of age. Giving the young mare an additional 1.5 years on average to develop before breeding may be necessary for some animals to complete maturation of stature and reproductive capacity. Alternatively, breeding before 3 years of age may jeopardize pregnancy and, perhaps, the life of the dam. When a total of 137 yearling fillies were pastured with separate stallions in small groups, 69%–95% of the fillies became pregnant; however, approximately 45% of the pregnancies were lost by 160 days of gestation.[23] If it is decided to breed mares <3 years old, pregnancy loss may be circumvented by using embryo transfer technologies. In 2-year-old donor mares, a mean embryo collection rate of 78% was reported with a mean 33% pregnancy rate after embryo transfer to older recipient mares; all pregnancies were maintained until parturition.[20,24]

Estrous Cycle

Transition from the anovulatory to the ovulatory season (resurging phase) is discussed in more detail in the next section on seasonality; however, briefly, the beginning of the ovulatory season occurs primarily in response to an increase in day length, in which the increasing ratio of light to dark is initially interpreted by the mare through the central nervous system. Photoreceptors in the eye recognize the increase in day length, which is neurologically relayed to the pineal gland where apparent changes in melatonin secretion alter appropriate changes at the hypothalamus, resulting in an increase in GnRH synthesis and secretion. GnRH reaches the anterior pituitary gland via a portal circulatory system stimulating primarily LH but also FSH synthesis and secretion into the peripheral circulatory system. Upon reaching the ovaries, the gonadotropins stimulate resurgence in follicular growth (i.e., spring transition) involving minor and major anovulatory waves. Follicle selection eventually occurs, resulting in development of a dominant follicle and ovulation. The increase in ovarian steroids produced by the growing follicles (estradiol) and corpus luteum (progesterone) subsequent to the first ovulation of the year not only affects sexual behavior, but also subsequently modulates GnRH and gonadotropin synthesis and secretion during the estrous cycle in a rhythmic fashion that repeats approximately every 22 days unless the sequence is interrupted by pregnancy, season, or a pathological condition. The hypothalamic-pituitary-ovarian axis and the endocrinological and morphological events associated with the estrous cycle are summarized and illustrated in Fig. 11-9, which was adapted from several previous reviews[1,2] and more recent reviews[7,11] and publications.[25-27]

Behaviorally, the estrous cycle is divided into periods of estrus and diestrus, which correspond physiologically to the follicular and luteal phases, respectively (see Fig. 11-9, B). Although the duration of estrus is highly variable within and among mares and is a major impediment when attempting to synchronize ovulations among mares for breeding and embryo transfer purposes, it typically ranges from 5 to 9 days in which the mare exhibits overt signs of receptivity toward the stallion. Behavioral estrus is

attributed to the effects of increasing circulating concentrations of estrogen, primarily estradiol, in association with selection of the dominant follicle of the primary follicular wave. Usually, the intensity of estrous behavior is stronger as ovulation approaches, which corresponds with maximum diameter of the dominant follicle, endometrial heterogeneity, and peak concentrations of estradiol 1–3 days before ovulation; thereafter, estradiol concentrations decrease and estrous behavior and endometrial heterogeneity wane. In some instances, however, estrous behavior may continue for 1–2 days after ovulation. The gradual increase in circulating concentrations of progesterone associated with development of the corpus luteum after ovulation during the luteal phase is responsible for the suppression of estrous behavior and elicitation of diestrous behavior. Diestrus is usually less variable. lasting 14–16 days in which the mare typically has a negative response toward the presence or advance of a stallion.

The end of one estrous cycle and the beginning of another is marked by ovulation. The day of ovulation is defined as Day 0 and is often used as a point of reference to more precisely describe events and prescribe the time of treatments during the estrous cycle as well as during pregnancy. The period between ovulation associated with estrus and ovulation associated with the next estrus is termed an *interovulatory interval*.

In general, follicular wave development during the estrous cycle is dependent on surges in circulating concentrations of FSH preceding the emergence of major secondary or minor waves during early diestrus and major primary waves during mid-diestrus (see Figs. 11-6 and 11-9, B). Subsequent to emergence of a primary wave and, at the end of the common growth phase during late diestrus/early estrus, the selection process is for a dominant follicle resulting in continued growth and, against subordinate follicles, resulting in regression. Follicle selection and subsequent dominance are temporally associated with a decrease in FSH and an increase in LH concentrations. The decrease in systemic FSH concentrations is attributed, first, to the negative feedback effect of increasing systemic concentrations of inhibin emanating from the group of growing antral follicles of the wave and, second, to the negative feedback effect of increasing systemic concentrations of estradiol, emanating primarily from the dominant follicle after selection. The negative synergistic effect of inhibin and estradiol at the hypothalamic-pituitary level (see Fig. 11-9, A) depresses FSH to basal concentrations several days before ovulation. The gradual increase in LH during late diestrus/early estrus is attributed to regression of the corpus luteum and a decrease in the negative feedback effect of progesterone (see Fig. 11-9, A). Recent research suggests that the increase in LH is held at an intermediate level (see Fig. 11-9, B) by the attenuating effect of increasing but intermediate concentrations of estradiol until late estrus.[28] Acquisition and abundance of granulosa cell LH receptors along with existent FSH receptors in combination with intrafollicular regulatory factors (e.g., insulin-like growth factors) allow the dominant follicle to continue growth after selection despite decreasing FSH concentrations. In contrast, subordinate follicles lack sufficient granulosa cell LH receptors and intrafollicular regulatory factors and, therefore, are not capable of responding to declining FSH concentrations; hence, they regress. Notably, the selective regression of subordinate follicles can be overridden by administering a gonadotropin preparation rich in FSH to stimulate and maintain the growth of subordinate follicles, resulting in multiple dominant follicles and ovulations as reviewed[5,7,8] and discussed in Chapter 9.

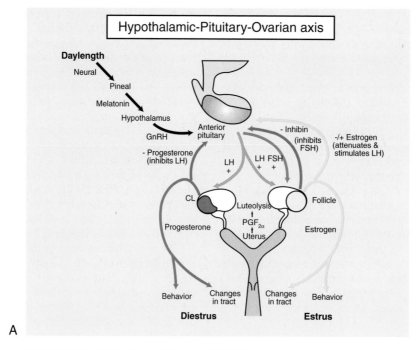

A

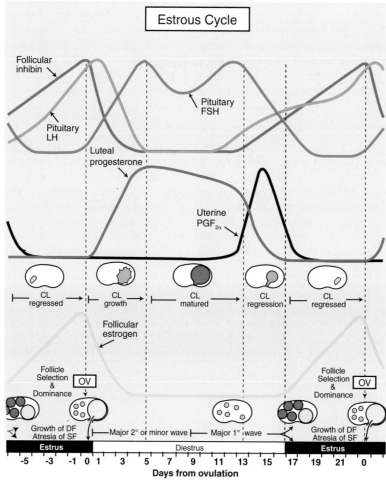

B

Figure 11-9. The positive and negative feedback relationships among various reproductive organs involved in the hypothalamic-pituitary-ovarian axis (**A**) and hormonal profiles depicting the endocrinological and morphological relationships during the estrous cycle in mares (**B**).

Continued growth and maintenance of the dominant follicle after selection is dependent on the intermediate concentrations of LH. Follicular and systemic estradiol concentrations continue to increase in parallel with the increase in size of the dominant follicle and reach peak concentrations about 1–2 days before ovulation near the time that maximum diameter of the ovulatory follicle is reached (see Figs. 11-6 and 11-9, B). High concentrations of estradiol that typically peak before ovulation have a positive feedback effect at the hypothalamic-pituitary level (see Fig. 11-9, A), resulting in a marked increase in LH during late estrus such that peak concentrations occur after ovulation. The decrease in estradiol beginning before ovulation corresponds with a slight increase in FSH prior to ovulation despite high concentrations of inhibin. Subsequent to ovulation, there is a marked decrease in ovarian hormones, especially inhibin, allowing for a further increase in FSH concentrations during early diestrus (see Fig. 11-9, B). In the mare, ovulation is spontaneous at the end of estrus in response to endogenous LH but can be readily induced with exogenous GnRH or LH or LH-like preparations to hasten or control the time to ovulation as described in Chapter 9 and other reviews.[1,2,5,7,8]

The use of B-mode ultrasonic imaging is a readily available clinical approach to detect and monitor structural aspects of the dominant follicle (e.g., size, shape, thickness of the follicle wall and degree of separation of the granulosa cell layer, and prominence of an anechoic area between the granulosa and basal lamina) that can aid in estimating the time of spontaneous or induced ovulation.[7,11,12] More recently, color Doppler ultrasonography has been used to identify functional aspects of the dominant follicle that can provide additional clinical information for estimating the time of spontaneous or induced ovulation as well as aid in determining whether a follicle is destined to be ovulatory or anovulatory.

The feasibility of color-flow Doppler ultrasonography in equine reproduction was first demonstrated in 1997[12] when it was shown that color signals (indicative of blood flow) associated with the ovary (follicle and corpus luteum) and early pregnancy (embryo/fetus) could be generated and recorded from the mare. Since then, color Doppler technology has advanced such that many ultrasound machines for veterinary use have the option to combine real-time, B-mode ultrasonography with color Doppler imaging as described in a reference text[17] on the basic and applied aspects of color Doppler ultrasonography in domestic animal reproduction, which includes the mare. As a practical example taken from the text, the percentage of circumference of the preovulatory follicle with color-flow signals decreased approximately 4 hours before ovulation (see Fig. 11-7, A) concurrent with a decrease in circumference of the anechoic area associated with the apical area of the follicle where follicle rupture and ovulation occurred (see Fig. 11-5, A). Potentially, therefore, the combined use of color Doppler and B-mode ultrasonography can provide additional clinical functional and structural information of preovulatory-sized follicles to make a more accurate estimate of the time to ovulation for synchronization and insemination purposes.

Failure of ovulation of the dominant follicle at the end of estrus has been reported to range from 5% to 20% during the early and late ovulatory season (i.e., fall transition period), respectively. In general, persistent anovulatory follicles, anovulatory hemorrhagic follicles, and hemorrhagic anovulatory follicles as well as the colloquial term *autumn follicles* may be descriptively similar structures associated with the failure of a dominant

follicle to ovulate; however, physiological and morphological events encompassing their development may be different, especially those that form during the estrous cycle compared with the fall transitional period and early pregnancy. Although there are no apparent studies that have directly compared anovulatory hemorrhagic follicle formation among cycling, transitional, and pregnant mares in the same experiment, structural and functional development of anovulatory hemorrhagic follicles have been compared to ovulatory follicles during the estrous cycle.[18] The repeatability of formation of an anovulatory hemorrhagic follicle in individual mares was confirmed such that 31% to 54% of the mares had anovulatory hemorrhagic follicles in the year preceding the study. With B-mode ultrasonography, it was found that there were no significant structural differences (e.g., decrease in follicle turgidity, loss of spherical shape, excess echoic specks in the antrum, serration of the granulosum, and formation of an apical area) between ovulatory and anovulatory mares. Conversely, color Doppler ultrasonography indicated that the percentage of follicle circumference with color-flow signals (i.e., vascularity) was greater preceding anovulatory hemorrhagic follicle formation than that associated with ovulation (see Fig. 11-7, A). Despite the novelty of these results, it was concluded that the apparent increase in vascularity preceding the formation of an anovulatory hemorrhagic follicle was not a reliable indicator of impending anovulation. Retrospectively, however, an anovulatory follicle can be diagnosed around the expected time of spontaneous or induced (e.g., hCG) ovulation by the presence of numerous free-floating echoic specks within the follicle antrum.[11,17] Nonetheless, the combined use of B-mode and color Doppler ultrasonography provides structural and functional information of the dominant follicle and, when used together with age and history of the mare and time of year, veterinary clinicians and breeding managers will be more informed to judge or predict the outcome of preovulatory-sized follicles, which may be especially useful during the transitional seasons.

Functional development and maintenance of the corpus luteum immediately after ovulation involves the luteotropic effect of periodic, low-magnitude surges of LH that result in the increase in circulating concentrations of progesterone (see Fig. 11-9, B). The LH-dependent growth and maturation of the corpus luteum during early diestrus results in progesterone reaching maximum concentrations by about Day 6, around the time postovulatory LH reaches basal concentrations as a result of the negative feedback effect of progesterone (see Fig. 11-9, A). Although progesterone concentrations decrease slightly as the positive effect of LH on the luteal gland gradually wanes, moderate concentrations are maintained throughout mid to late diestrus. Despite distinct morphological differences between a corpus hemorrhagicum and a corpus luteum with and without an intraluteal cavity (see Fig. 11-5, B and C), respectively, there appear to be no functional differences. That is, circulating concentrations of progesterone and length of the interovulatory interval are comparable in mares with either type of luteal gland morphology.[1] Daily profiles of structural and functional changes of the corpus luteum are similar in non-pregnant and pregnant mares until about Day 14 when luteolysis is initiated in non-pregnant mares.[7,12]

Spontaneous termination of the luteal phase in the absence of an embryonic vesicle to block the luteolytic mechanism involves a cascade of hormonal events that includes an effect of pituitary oxytocin on the uterus leading to endometrial $PGF_{2\alpha}$ production. The luteolytic effect of $PGF_{2\alpha}$ reaches the corpus luteum via a systemic route to initiate functional and structural demise of the luteal gland.[1] After Day 14, there is a precipitous decrease in progesterone concentrations that is immediately preceded by the pulsatile release of uterine $PGF_{2\alpha}$. The rapid frequency of pulses results in a surge of $PGF_{2\alpha}$ that completes luteolysis by about Day 17 when progesterone concentrations decrease <2 ng/ml. The timely production of uterine $PGF_{2\alpha}$ at late diestrus may be naturally interrupted as a result of the first luteal response to pregnancy or uterine pathology or artificially interrupted by the early administration of $PGF_{2\alpha}$. In regard to the latter, native or analogues of $PGF_{2\alpha}$ are commonly used in equine reproductive management practices as discussed in Chapter 9 and other reviews.[1,2,5,7,8]

The use of B-mode and color Doppler ultrasonography to detect and monitor structural and functional attributes of the corpus luteum (see Figs. 11-5, B and C and 11-7, B) can aid in determining the functional status of the luteal gland.[7,11,12,17] The daily profile of progesterone concentrations throughout the estrous cycle is positively related to the diameter and luteal tissue area profiles, negatively related to the luteal tissue echogenicity profile based on gray-scale scores, and positively related to luteal tissue vascularity based on color Doppler signals. Hence, the combined clinical use of B-mode and color Doppler ultrasonography provides structural and functional information that can aid in determining the morphological and physiological status of the corpus luteum during the estrous cycle as well as during early pregnancy.

The ratio of circulating concentrations of estradiol to progesterone emanating from the ovaries controls the extent of morphological changes associated with the tubular genitalia.[1,2] The prevalence of relatively high systemic concentrations of estradiol during the follicular phase and progesterone during the luteal phase results in gross structural changes of the vagina, cervix, and uterus that can be used for clinical diagnosis of diestrus, estrus, and impending ovulation. Table 11-1 summarizes major changes of the tubular genitalia during the estrous cycle. The vulva and labia can be inspected directly; however, the appearance of either structure during estrus or diestrus is not dramatic and, apparently, the variation is too great for reliable diagnosis of the stage of the estrous cycle. Conversely, the vagina, cervix, and uterus undergo dramatic visual (speculum and ultrasound assisted) and palpable changes during estrus and diestrus.

Inspection of the vagina and cervix can be made with the assistance of a speculum, endoscope, or palpation per vagina (see Fig. 11-2). It is important that visual inspection of the vagina and cervix be made immediately upon insertion of the viewing instruments, because exposure of the mucosa to air may alter interior characteristics. Probably more important than determining the stage of the estrous cycle, speculum and endoscopic examinations of the vagina and cervix are done to assess any pathological condition or physical trauma to these organs.[5,7,8]

Volume, viscosity, pH, and cytological changes of cervical/vaginal secretions have been reported and may be used as additional information for determining reproductive status or pathological condition. Specifically, fluids derived from the cervix/vagina during estrus are voluminous, thin, and clear, with high lubricating properties (i.e., low viscosity). Conversely, fluid characteristics during diestrus are minimal in volume and maximal in viscosity, imparting an adhesive quality to the mucosa of the vagina. The pH of cervical/vaginal secretions is relatively low, or alkaline, during estrus compared with a more neutral pH during diestrus. Changes in viscosity and pH of cervical/vaginal secretions have been the basis for development of devices (e.g., transvaginal probes) to detect the onset of estrus or impending ovulation. The reliability of these devices in the mare, however, is equivocal. Cytological evaluation may be more informative but may not be practical considering other more advanced technologies (e.g., ultrasonography).

Transvaginal inspection, transrectal palpation, and ultrasonic imaging of the reproductive organs are the most common and reliable clinical approaches used for determining the stage of the estrous cycle. Palpation of the tubular genitalia is often done to support findings found during gross visual inspection or ultrasonic imaging. Tactile assessment of the uterus and cervix is primarily done to determine the extent of tone or the turgidity or flaccidity of the organ. Physiologically, tone is, in part, a reflection of the degree of vascularity and amount of intracellular or extracellular fluids, which is influenced by the ratio of circulating concentrations of estrogen to progesterone. Cervical and uterine tone is minimal during estrus (see Figs. 11-2, B and 11-3, C), when estradiol predominates, and maximal at mid-diestrus (see Figs. 11-2, A and 11-3, B), when progesterone predominates. At estrus, the relaxed and flaccid cervix and uterine horns are easily flattened and compressed during palpation. In addition, the predominant endometrial folds can be felt slipping through the fingers when the hand is moved across the horns and body of the uterus. The extent of cervical relaxation during estrus can also be assessed transvaginally by the number of fingers that can be inserted into the cervical os. At diestrus, the firm and turgid cervix and uterine horns are more resistant to compression and dilation; thus, the organs have a more tubular feel or shape.

Transrectal ultrasonic imaging of the uterus has been used to characterize changes in endometrial echotexture, horn diameters, and myometrial contractility during the estrous cycle and early pregnancy.[11,12] The clinical importance of uterine edema is discussed in Chapter 12. Briefly, however, the degree of development of endometrial folds during the estrous cycle is reflected in changes in uterine echotexture and cross-sectional diameter of the uterine horns (see Fig. 11-3, B and C). The alternating echogenic and non-echogenic areas of the ultrasound image during estrus (see Fig. 11-3, C) are attributable to the dense walls and fluid-filled central regions of the endometrial folds; endometrial folds are less discernible during diestrus (see Fig. 11-3, B), in part because there is less edema. The degree of prominence or heterogeneity of the endometrial folds during estrus is positively related to increasing concentrations of estradiol and estrus-like behavior, whereas relative homogeneity of the endometrium during diestrus is positively related to increasing concentrations of progesterone. Although myometrial contractions are present throughout the estrous cycle and pregnancy, the stage of the cycle and pregnancy determines the degree of smooth muscle contractility. In cyclic and non-pregnant mares, increased uterine contractions occur in association with luteolysis (i.e., increased $PGF_{2\alpha}$). The increased to-and-fro movement of the intrauterine walls during estrus facilitates the expulsion of debris and transport of sperm.

Seasonality

Reproductive seasonality in the mare refers to morphological and physiological changes of the reproductive organs primarily as a result of the changing ratio of light-hours to dark-hours within a day throughout the year. The estrous cycle during the period of long days (ovulatory season) was discussed in the

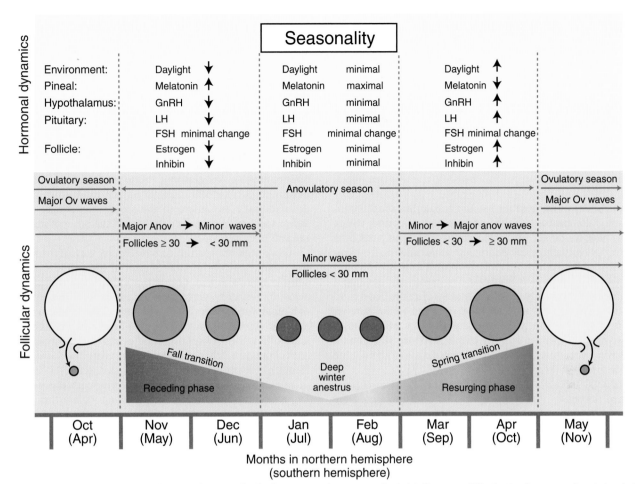

Figure 11-10. The effects of season (daylight) on various reproductive hormones and, consequently, their influence on follicular development and ovulation during the fall and spring transitional periods and winter anestrus in mares.

previous sections; therefore, this section focuses on transition and acyclicity during the period of short days (anovulatory season) based on the results from previous publications[1,2] and more recent reviews.[5,8,15,16]

The general seasonal pattern is that the incidence of ovulation is transitionally decreasing in the fall, minimal or absent during the winter (anovulatory season), transitionally increasing during the spring, and maximal during the summer (ovulatory season), as summarized and illustrated in Fig. 11-10. Regardless of latitude, the mare is ingrained to a distinct ovulatory and anovulatory season even in latitudes where the difference in length between the longest and shortest day is only a couple of hours long (e.g., Venezuela and southern Mexico). Despite seasonality in the mare, approximately 20% of animals will continue to cycle throughout the year with more mares at the equatorial region than at more northern and southern regions.

The nature of seasonality generally involves photoreceptors in the eye that relay changes in the length of daylight to the pineal gland (see Fig. 11-9, *A*). Although the role that melatonin plays in seasonality is not thoroughly known, it is generally accepted that melatonin synthesis and secretion from the pineal gland increases as day-length decreases (higher during dark hours) in the spring and decreases as day-length increases (lower during light hours) in the fall. Regardless of the precise role of melatonin in seasonality, the hormonal signal appears to initiate a chain of events that directly and indirectly affects the hypothalamus and

GnRH production, pituitary gland and FSH and LH production and, consequently, the ovary and follicular development, steroidogenesis, and ovulation. Apart from melatonin, experiments with naloxone and sulpiride have indicated that opioids and catecholamines, respectively, may also be involved with seasonal changes associated with the hypothalamus and pituitary.[5,8,16]

Although sunlight may be the primary factor influencing seasonality, body condition, age, and mare type may be secondary factors interacting with day length to influence seasonality. Mares with high body weight and percentage of body fat or high body-condition scores were observed to have greater reproductive activity (i.e., follicular growth and ovulation) during the winter and that mares placed on green pasture in the spring with a 30-mm follicle ovulated sooner.[15] In contrast, mares that lost weight and the greater the weight loss, the later the ovulations occurred during spring transition. In mares 2 to 5 and >15 years of age, the ovulatory season was shorter because of an earlier onset of the anovulatory season during the fall in younger mares and later onset of the ovulatory season in older mares in spring compared to mares 6 to 15 years of age. In regard to mare type, the ovulatory season begins earlier and ends later in horses compared with ponies.

For discussion purposes, the anovulatory season is divided into three phases primarily with respect to the degree of ovarian structural and functional activities (see Fig. 11-10). In its simplest form, the receding phase is defined as a gradual progression toward a decrease in follicular growth and anovulation as the daylight hours, hypothalamic GnRH, pituitary LH, and ovarian steroids decrease during the fall (fall transition), whereas the re-surging phase is the opposite, with a gradual progression toward an increase in follicular growth and ovulation as daylight hours, hypothalamic GnRH, pituitary LH, and ovarian steroids increase during the spring (spring transition). The period between the re-ceding and resurging phases (winter anestrus) represents mini-mal follicular activity in terms of number and size of follicles, reduced hypothalamic GnRH and pituitary LH content, and de-creased ovarian steroid production.

Fall Transition

There is a paucity of information available regarding the fall tran-sition period compared with the spring transition period, which is due, in part, to greater practical importance of the latter than the former. Nevertheless, the beginning of the anovulatory sea-son can be recognized by failure of a dominant follicle (≥30 mm) of a major wave to ovulate at the end of estrus and develop a corpus luteum. Reportedly,[15] within 60 days after the last ovula-tion of the year, there is a progressive decrease in the number of mares (100% to 0%) with major anovulatory waves and a progressive increase in the number of mares (0% to 100%) with minor waves. Thereafter, minor waves continued throughout the anovulatory season (see Fig. 11-10).

Hormonally, circulating concentrations of FSH are essentially unchanged during the fall transition period and throughout the anovulatory season, whereas LH concentrations progressively decrease. Considering that elevated concentrations of LH are necessary for continued growth of the dominant follicle after se-lection and final growth and development prior to ovulation, the gradual decrease in LH concentrations that occurs initially dur-ing fall transition becomes insufficient to sustain final growth and development of the dominant follicle. Therefore, ovulation fails. As LH concentrations continue to decrease, there are insufficient concentrations to support follicle selection and dominance of major waves (largest follicle ≥30 mm in diameter). Hence, during late transition, only minor waves (largest follicle <30 mm in dia-meter) occur that continue into the winter anovulatory period such that the largest follicle of minor waves is minimal (e.g., 10–15 mm in diameter) as illustrated in Fig. 11-10. Thus, the onset of the anovulatory season is attributable to an inadequate surge of LH and final growth and development of the preovulatory follicle.

Failure of the dominant follicle to ovulate at the beginning of the anovulatory season is usually followed by gradual regression of the follicle; however, in some instances, the follicle becomes hemorrhagic. The frequency and morphological and physiologi-cal characteristics of development of anovulatory hemorrhagic follicles, or *autumn follicles*, was discussed in the previous sec-tion during the estrous cycle. It appears that during the estrous cycle, the preovulatory LH surge was not different between ovu-latory and anovulatory mares; however, preovulatory estradiol concentrations were higher in mares that formed anovulatory hemorrhagic follicles. Although it seems that the physiologi-cal basis for the formation of anovulatory hemorrhagic follicles during the fall transitional period versus the estrous cycle may be different, gross morphological changes (e.g., numerous free-floating echoic specks in the antrum >80 mm in diameter and maintenance of sphericity) may be similar.

As estradiol production declines in association with decreas-ing follicular activity during the fall transitional period, behav-ioral signs of estrus may be shallow, erratic, or absent relative to signs during the ovulatory season. The lull of winter anestrus can be diagnosed morphologically using palpation and ultra-sonic imaging to characterize ovaries that are relatively small and firm with minimal or no follicular and luteal activity and a uterus that is flat or flaccid and irregular or non-tubular with homogeneous echotexture.[11]

Spring Transition

The spring transitional period is one of the most challeng-ing times of year for equine veterinary clinicians and breed-ing managers, in part because of the periodic development of dominant-sized follicles that fail to ovulate. In this regard, and because of its practical importance, numerous studies have been done to study the nature of the spring transitional period and various regimens to artificially control the onset of the ovulatory season.[1,2,5,8,15,16]

There is extreme variation in follicular wave dynamics among individual mares prior to the onset of the ovulatory season. In some mares there may be a period of minor waves followed by a major ovulatory wave or a period of one or two major an-ovulatory waves before the ovulatory wave. Apparently, growth rates of dominant anovulatory follicles are similar to ovula-tory follicles. In some instances, estrus-like behavior and uter-ine echotextural changes may be associated with major waves. Hence, these observations are not considered reliable predictors of impending ovulation. More recently, with the use of color Doppler ultrasonography,[17] it has been shown that color-flow signals were less for dominant-sized anovulatory follicles than ovulatory follicles during the spring transition period (see Fig. 11-7, A). Although not critically determined, the status of domi-nant follicles during spring transition may be determined by de-gree of vascularity, as discussed in the previous section during the estrous cycle. Regardless, practical techniques or regimens (e.g., hormones, lighting, housing, nutrition) for controlling and managing reproduction during the transitional seasons have been reviewed[1,2,5,7,8] and are discussed in Chapter 9.

In general, the onset of the ovulatory season involves a chain of events associated with increasing day length, the pineal, hy-pothalamus and pituitary leads to a gradual increase in circulat-ing concentrations of LH. Correspondingly, the diameter of the largest follicle associated with the periodic emergence of minor waves gradually increases in the presence of FSH surges un-til it reaches 25–30 mm. Thereafter, LH-supported growth of the dominant follicle (≥30 mm) associated with the periodic emergence of major anovulatory waves gradually increases un-til emergence of the ovulatory wave when there is decrease in circulating concentrations of FSH and preovulatory LH surge. Thus, as the FSH-follicle feedback relationship is reestablished in association with follicle selection, there is a marked increase in circulating concentrations of estradiol, LH, and final growth and development of the dominant follicle leading to ovulation.

REFERENCES

1. Ginther OJ: *Reproductive Biology of the Mare: Basic and Applied Aspects*, 2nd ed. Cross Plains, WI: Equiservices Publishing, 1992, p 642.
2. McKinnon AO, Voss JL: *Equine Reproduction*. Philadelphia: Lea & Febiger, 1993, p 1137.
3. Davies Morel MCG: *Equine Reproductive Physiology, Breeding and Stud Management*. Oxford: CABI Publishing, 2003, p 384.
4. Knottenbelt DC, Pascoe RR, Leblanc M, Lopate C: *Equine Stud Farm Medicine and Surgery*. St Louis: Saunders, 2003, p 368.

5. Robinson NE: *Current Therapy in Equine Medicine*, 5th ed. Philadelphia: Saunders, 2003, p 930.
6. England G: *Fertility and Obstetrics in the Horse*. Oxford: Blackwell Publishing, 2005, p 307.
7. Samper JC, Pycock JF, McKinnon AO: *Current Therapy in Equine Reproduction*. St Louis: Saunders, 2007, p 492.
8. Youngquist RS, Threlfall WR: *Current Therapy in Large Animal Theriogenology*. St Louis: Saunders, 2007, pp 3-218.
9. Dyce KM, Sack WO, Wensing CIG: *Textbook of Veterinary Anatomy*. Philadelphia: WB Saunders, 1987, p 820.
10. Clayton HM, Flood PF, Rosenstein DS: *Clinical Anatomy of the Horse*. St Louis: Saunders, 2005, p 118.
11. Ginther OJ: Ultrasonic Imaging and Animal Reproduction: Horses, 2nd ed. Cross Plains, WI: Equiservices Publishing, 1995, p 394.
12. Rantanen NW, McKinnon AO: *Equine Diagnostic Ultrasonography*. Philadelphia: Lea & Febiger, 1997, p 677.
13. Silva LA, Gastal EL, Gastal MO, et al: A new alternative for embryo transfer and artificial insemination in mares: ultrasound-guided intrauterine injection. *J Equine Vet Sci* 24(8):324-332, 2004.
14. Samper JC: *Equine Breeding Management and Artificial Insemination*, 1st ed. Philadelphia: WB Saunders, 2000, p 306.
15. Ginther OJ, Gastal EL, Gastal MO, Beg MA: Seasonal influence on equine follicle dynamics. *Anim Reprod* 1:31-44, 2004.
16. Donadeu FX, Watson ED: Seasonal changes in ovarian activity: lessons learnt from the horse. *Anim Reprod Sci* 100:225-242, 2007.
17. Ginther OJ: *Ultrasonic Imaging and Animal Reproduction: Color-Doppler Ultrasonography*. Book 4. Cross Plains, WI: Equiservices Publishing, 2007, p 258.
18. Ginther OJ, Gastal EL, Gastal MO, Beg MA: Conversion of a viable preovulatory follicle into a hemorrhagic anovulatory follicle in mares. *Anim Reprod* 3:29-40, 2006.
19. Nogueira GP, Barnabe RC, Verreschi ITN: Puberty and growth rate in Thoroughbred fillies. *Theriogenology* 48:581-588, 1997.
20. Camillo F, Vannozzi I, Rota A, et al: Age at puberty, cyclicity, clinical response to PGF2 alpha, hCG and GnRH and embryo recovery rate in yearling mares. *Theriogenology* 58:627-630, 2002.
21. Brown-Douglas CG, Firth EC, Parkinson TJ, Fennessy PF: Onset of puberty in pasture-raised Thoroughbreds born in southern hemisphere spring and autumn. *Equine Vet J* 36:499-504, 2004.
22. Nogueira GP: Follicle profile and plasma gonadotropin concentration in pubertal female ponies. *Brazilian J Med Biol Res* 37:1-10, 2004.
23. Mitchell D, Allen WR: Observation on reproductive performance in the yearling mare. *J Reprod Fertil Suppl* 23:531, 1975.
24. Savage NC, Woodcock LA: Use of two-year-old mares as embryo donors in a commercial embryo transfer programme. *Equine Vet J Suppl* 8:68, 1989.
25. Ginther OJ, Beg MA, Bergfelt DR, et al: Follicle selection in monovular species. *Biol Reprod* 65:638-647, 2001.
26. Ginther OJ, Beg MA, Gastal MO, Gastal EL: Follicle dynamics and selection in mares. *Anim Reprod* 1:45-63, 2004.
27. Beg MA, Ginther OJ: Follicle selection in cattle and horses: role of intrafollicular factors. *Reproduction* 132:365-377, 2006.
28. Ginther OJ, Utt MD, Beg MA, et al: Negative effect of estradiol on luteinizing hormone throughout the ovulatory luteinizing hormone surge in mares. *Bio Reprod* 77:543-550, 2007.

UTERINE EDEMA IN THE MARE

JUAN C. SAMPER

Although evaluation of uterus is done by rectal palpation, a more detailed examination as well as the observation of otherwise non-palpable structures and artifacts is done ultrasonographically. Ultrasonographic evaluation of the uterus is done in order to determine pathological or physiological conditions and uterine contents.[1] Because the mare is a seasonal polyestric animal, there are physiological changes that must be taken into account when examining the mare. The cervix, uterus, and ovaries change significantly between anestrus, transition, and regular cyclicity (estrus and diestrus).[2]

ANESTRUS

Rectal palpation of the physiologically anestrous mare during the late fall and winter results in a very typical thin uterus with very poor or no tone. The cervix can be difficult to identify both on rectal and ultrasonographic examination. On ultrasound the uterus is small and uniformly echogenic unless the mare has endometrial cysts, and sometimes identification of the uterus can be difficult, particularly in young mares with small uteri. Furthermore, if too much pressure is placed on the rectum during the examination, the flaccid uterus will flatten and will be even more difficult to identify.

SPRING TRANSITION

In contrast to the poorly identifiable cervix of the anestrus mare, the mare in mid to late transition will have a slight increase in uterine tone and is easier to palpate per rectum. The cervix of mares that have previously had foals will be easier to palpate and identify whereas the cervix of maiden mares will not be as obvious. The cervix in late transition will be edematous in most mares, but the degree of edema will vary significantly between mares.[3]

The uterus of the transitional mare will be characteristic because of the presence of endometrial edema, which is characterized by the visualization of the endometrial folds giving the characteristic appearance of a "cart wheel" or "sliced orange"[1,2] The hallmark of the uterus of transitional mares particularly in mid to late transition is the persistence of the endometrial edema for several days or even weeks with no significant change. In many instances a small amount of fluid accumulation in the uterus can be detected. Because the uterine folds increase in thickness, there is also a significant increase of the surface area of the uterus, and small fluid accumulations can easily dissipate within the uterus. The presence of multiple medium to large follicles 25–35 mm or larger is typical of the transitional period.[2]

THE CYCLING MARE

Once the mare has had the first ovulation of the year, the interovulatory interval is on the average 20–22 days. Ovulation is preceded by a follicular phase that typically lasts 5–7 days during which the mare shows behavioral estrus, and followed by a luteal phase that lasts 14–16 days and the mare is not receptive. However, unlike other domestic animals, the mare has an LH peak after ovulation and often displays strong signs of heat for up to 48 hours after ovulation has taken place. Although mares can be bred as far as 6 days prior to ovulation with acceptable pregnancy results, in order to maximize their fertility mares should be mated within 48 hours prior and up to 6 hours after ovulation.[4] A single mating as many as 5 or 6 days before ovulation with a fertile stallion will often result in pregnancy, but pregnancy rates increase when mares are bred closer to ovulation.

Accurate prediction of ovulation timing becomes a critical component of breeding management in order to maximize the efficiency of a breeding operation and ultimately the pregnancy rates.[5] Reducing the number of breedings or inseminations per cycle maximizes stallion or semen usage and reduces mare contamination and farm labor with the associated costs. The ideal number of covers or inseminations per cycle when a healthy mare is bred using a fertile stallion or good quality semen is one. However, well-managed breeding operations can allow up to 10% rebreeds in the same cycle. Current systems to determine the timing of breeding rely on several of the following: (1) teasing by a stallion, (2) cervical relaxation determined by rectal palpation or vaginal speculum examination, (3) the presence of a "large" follicle detected by rectal palpation and ultrasonography, (4) appearance of the follicle on ultrasound examination, (5) timing from treatment with an inducing agent, and (6) the presence and pattern uterine edema.[6-8]

Teasing

Routine teasing is done mostly in operations that breed by natural cover and requires the presence of a stallion, appropriate facilities, and knowledgeable personnel. Because of the infrastructure and labor required, mares bred by artificial insemination are seldom teased. Estrus detection done by teasing is helpful to determine stage of the cycle (estrus vs. diestrus); however, predicting the time of ovulation is not reliable. It is also important to realize that although the estrogen-dominated phase of the cycle lasts for 5–7 days, mares do not necessarily show estrus for the same period.

Cervical Relaxation

When in heat the normal mare has a relaxed cervix that drops down to the vaginal floor. The degree of relaxation depends on the age of the mare as well as her reproductive status and can be determined by rectal palpation as well as a vaginal examination through a speculum. Lack of cervical relaxation when in heat is often seen in mares with long-standing uterine infections, in older maiden mares, and in some young maiden mares that have not yet had a foal .The ultrasonographic image of the cervix is commonly observed as a fishbone appearance (Fig. 12-1).

Presence of a Large Follicle

Follicular growth in the mare is a dynamic process that does not appear to be related to the presence of progesterone and is well described in Chapter 11. As stated previously, it is not uncommon to have mares develop follicles >35 mm in diameter during diestrus. During estrus the follicular phase is characterized by the growth of follicles at about 3 mm per day until it reaches its pre-ovulatory size of 40–45 mm on the average mare but often 50–55 mm in larger breeds. Mares that are in estrus will have a dominant follicle, but not all mares with a large follicle are in heat. Inexperienced veterinarians that do not have access to a teasing stallion can often be confused by the presence of such a follicle and breed mares during diestrus because of the presence of a large follicle. Mares with diestrus follicles, regardless of size, will not respond to ovulatory-inducing agents.

Ultrasonographic Appearance of the Pre-ovulatory Follicle

The ultrasonographic appearance of the follicle as the mare approaches ovulation will vary depending on the position of the follicle within the ovary or the proximity to the ovulation fossa. Follicles that are close to the ovulation fossa will not have a significant change in shape; however, follicles that are at one of the ovarian poles will have a "pear-like" appearance and will become more flaccid at palpation and the mare will often show varying degrees of discomfort or pain when the follicle is touched. When using power Doppler ultrasonography, one can detect an increase in blood flow to the follicular wall area, as shown in Chapter 11.

Ovulatory-Inducing Agents

Because of the advantages of having ovulations at a predictable time as well as the increase in pregnancy rates when mares are bred close to ovulation, many veterinarians are relying on pharmacological agents to induce ovulation. Maximal effectiveness of these agents occurs in mares with obvious endometrial edema, a relaxed cervix, and a large pre-ovulatory follicle. There are several products commercially available to induce ovulation in mares: (1) human chorionic gonadotropin (hCG) and the GnRH analogue, deslorelin (Ovuplant), (2) Injectable compounded deslorelin, and (4) recombinant LH (rLH). All of these products are highly effective (>80%) when given to mares at the appropriate time in their estrous period. The resulting ovulations occur at around 36–44 hours after treatment. However, if the hormone is given too early the mare will have a delayed ovulation, and if the mare's endogenous LH is already high, the mare will ovulate before the expected time.[2,9,10]

Presence and Pattern of Uterine Edema

The mare under the influence of estrogen will have increased edema of the reproductive tract. This includes mild hyperemia of the vulvar lips and vagina with a concomitant relaxation of the vaginal vault and cervix. In addition there is a typical estrogenic appearance of the uterus that has been described as a cartwheel pattern (Fig. 12-2).

The appearance and disappearance of endometrial edema is a progressive phenomenon that is related to the levels of estrogen and progesterone.[6,11-14] Fig. 12-3 shows the uterine edema pattern of a normal mare during the estrous period. Once the estrogens reach the maximal level, and as the mares approach ovulation, the intensity of the edema starts to decrease. Most mares will ovulate with endometrial edema that is almost undetectable. It is important to use some kind of scoring system to be able to reduce the subjectivity, record and identify changes, and determine patterns of endometrial edema. Therefore, a grading system using plus signs (e.g., +, ++, +++) or a numeric system is often used. In the author's practice, a numeric subjective score from 0 to 5 to grade the degree of endometrial edema is used,

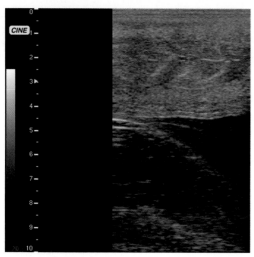

Figure 12-1. Normal cervical edema with the characteristic fishbone appearance.

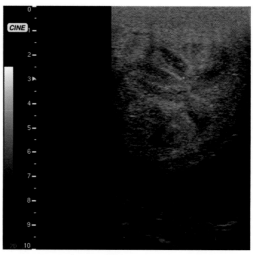

Figure 12-2. Normal uterine endometrial edema with the typical cartwheel pattern. Mares with this type of uterine echotexture will have a dominant size follicle and a relaxed cervix.

with 0 being no edema and 5 being maximal edema. A typical mare would have 0 edema during diestrus, and 4 for maximal degree of normal edema. A uterine edema score of 5 is used for what the author considers an abnormal edema, which is referred to as *hyperedema* and is shown in Fig. 12-9.

Normal Uterine Edema

On or around day 15 of diestrus, the non-pregnant mare releases prostaglandin from the endometrium, which causes luteolysis. Progesterone levels reach basal levels between 12 and 24 hours of this release.[15] Concomitantly, the estrogen that is present in the dominant follicle or follicles starts to show its effect first by a slight relaxation of the cervix and second by a change in receptivity toward a stallion. Since the stallion is not always present, veterinarians are often saddled with the task of determining whether the mare is in heat or not, or whether the mare is starting or finishing her heat period. Following the pattern of uterine edema is a key managerial tool to follow and manage the breeding cycle of the mare.[3]

UTERINE EDEMA 0 (UE-0). Uterine edema 0 is characterized by homogeneity. A corpus luteum and a closed cervix are typical features of this grade (Fig. 12-4).

UTERINE EDEMA 1 (UE-1). A mare that is just starting to come into heat will be characterized by a moderately soft cervix at palpation and the presence of a 25–35 mm follicle depending on breed and size of the mare. Uterine folds of a uterus with UE-1 can be difficult to identify; unless the practitioner has previous examinations, it could be undetectable (Fig. 12-5). Rectal palpation might give more information. Following this, the uterine edema and the follicle size will increase gradually.

UTERINE EDEMA 2 (UE-2). The first real sign of uterine edema in the mare most often will be detected at the cervix and is visualized ultrasonographically as a fishbone appearance. Follicles can be >35 mm and the practitioner can often easily identify some of the endometrial folds on ultrasonography (Fig. 12-6).

UTERINE EDEMA 3 (UE-3). Follicles are 38 mm and the endometrial folds can be easily observed throughout the uterus. Oftentimes the edema in the uterine body can be one grade

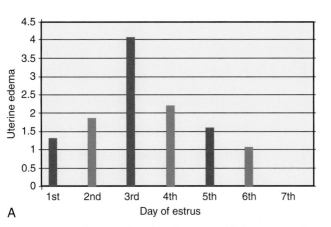

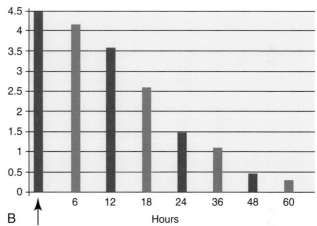

Figure 12-3. A, Normal pattern of uterine edema detectable in most normal mares. Although there is a significant variation among mares, most mares will have a gradual increase in the degree of edema and a dissipation as they approach ovulation. **B,** Significant reduction of the degree of uterine edema in the normal mare is evident only 12–24 hours after treatment with an ovulatory-inducing agent *(arrow).*

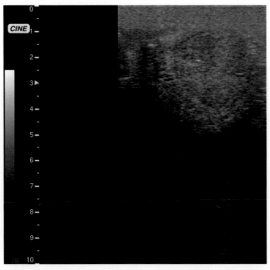

Figure 12-4. Uterine edema grade 0 (UE-0). Typical endometrial echotexture of a progesterone-dominated uterus. Note the homogeneity of the uterus. Presence of a corpus luteum and a closed cervix accompanies this edema grade.

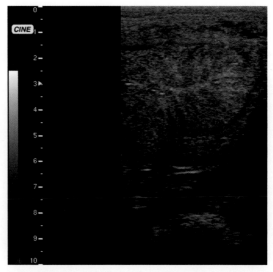

Figure 12-5. Uterine edema grade 1 (UE-1). Although there is no visualization of individual endometrial folds, there is a distinct heterogeneity compared with the image in Fig. 12-4.

higher. The endometrial folds will be slightly thicker than in UE-2 (Fig. 12-7).

UTERINE EDEMA 4 (UE-4). Follicles will be >40 mm, and there is an increase in the width of the endometrial folds. Ultrasonographically the folds have hyperechoic borders and a hypoechoic center. However, the ultrasonographic uterine architecture (cartwheel) is still maintained (Fig. 12-8).

At this point in a normal mare the uterine edema will start to decrease as the mare approaches ovulation, reaching its nadir immediately before or after ovulation. Follicle size will remain the same (40–55 mm) as the edema decreases or can decrease slightly as it changes shape during its migration toward the ovulation fossa.

In most normal mares the variation in endometrial edema from estrus to diestrus is very pronounced (ranging from 1 to 4). However, not all mares will have this pronounced variation in uterine edema, but well over 90% of the mares will have detectable uterine edema when in estrus. Mares that do not display uterine edema while progesterone levels are basal should be considered abnormal. Even though the mare has a heavy inflammatory reaction shortly after insemination because of the presence of sperm (post-breeding–induced endometritis), this reaction is seldom detected as an increase in the degree of endometrial edema in the normal mare at 24 hours after breeding.

Abnormal Uterine Edema

There are several instances when the veterinarian performing an ultrasonographic examination of the uterus should suspect the possibility of uterine problems when assessing the degree of edema.

UTERINE EDEMA 5 (UE-5) OR HYPEREDEMA. This type of edema has several characteristics shown on Fig. 12-9. The endometrial folds are abnormally thick, making the uterus lose the

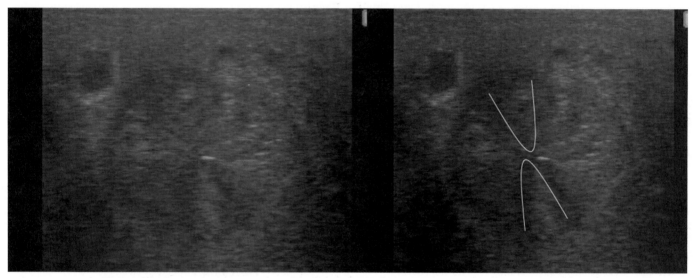

Figure 12-6. Uterine edema grade 2 (UE-2). This edema grade is characterized by the appearance of distinct endometrial folds, although they are not visible throughout the uterus.

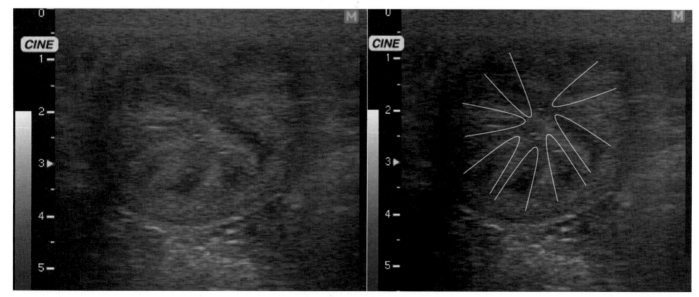

Figure 12-7. Uterine edema grade 3 (UE-3). Cartwheel pattern with folds visible through the uterus. However, the folds are slightly hypoechoic in the center.

normal architecture of the cartwheel pattern. It is persistent even after the mare ovulates and therefore follicles, although mostly large and of pre-ovulatory size, can be of any size. In addition, abnormal edema can be evident by premature presence of endometrial edema and a large follicle 14–15 days after ovulation. Failure to reduce the edema as the mare approaches ovulation, persistence of marked endometrial edema 24 hours after ovulation, significant increase in the degree of uterine edema after insemination, and lack of uterine edema during the estrous period.

In most normal mares the variation in endometrial edema from estrus to diestrus is very pronounced (ranging from 0 to 4). Although not all mares will have this pronounced variation in uterine edema, more than 90% of the mares will have detectable uterine edema when in estrus. Mares that do not display uterine edema while progesterone levels are basal and estrogen is high should be considered abnormal.[6]

Even though the mare has a heavy inflammatory reaction shortly after insemination because of the presence of sperm (post-breeding–induced endometritis), this reaction is seldom detected as an increase in the degree of endometrial edema in the normal mare at 24–48 hours after breeding.

Uterine edema can be indicative of uterine pathology when there is one or more of the following: (1) Presence of obvious endometrial edema and a large follicle 14–15 days after ovulation, (2) presence of hyperedema during the normal estrous period, (3) failure to reduce the edema as the mare approaches ovulation and the presence of marked uterine edema 24 hours after ovulation, (4) significant increase in the degree of uterine edema 12–24 hours after breeding, and (5) lack of uterine edema during the estrous period.[1,5,6]

In a recent study,[9] the pregnancy rate was significantly higher for mares with uterine edema grades of 1, 2, or 3 at ovulation, but it was 10%–14% lower for mares that ovulated with edema

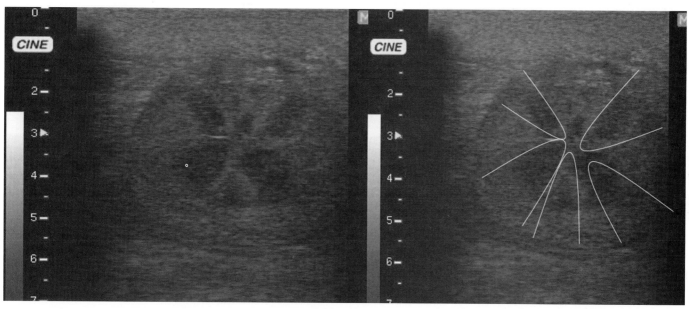

Figure 12-8. Uterine edema grade 4 (UE-4). Folds are prominent with a distinct hyperechoic border and an increase in the endometrial fold thickness.

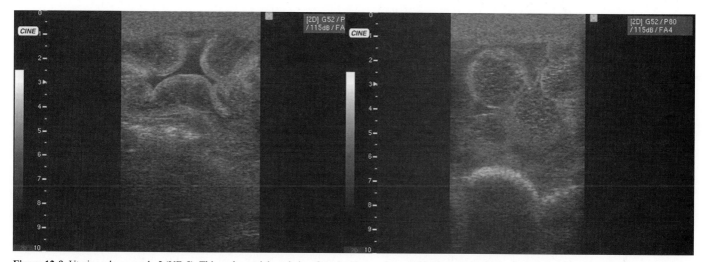

Figure 12-9. Uterine edema grade 5 (UE-5). This endometrial grade is referred as *hyperedema* and is characterized by a disruption of the normal uterine architecture. Folds are significantly thickened, with hyperechoic borders and hypoechoic centers. Free fluid can often be detected in some areas of the uterus, particularly in the uterine body and the cervix.

scores of 4 or 5. The presence of uterine fluid at the time of ovulation was significantly lower ($P <.05$) for mares with edema grades 1 and 2 at the time of ovulation (12.6% and 24.4%, respectively), compared with mares ovulating with edema 3 (32.4%), edema 4 (38.8%), or edema 5 (58.4%). All mares that were considered to have hyperedema, or mares whose edema did not decrease at the time of ovulation were cultured and an endometrial cytology performed. Of these mares 56.9% had a positive culture and/or cytology. The seasonal pregnancy rate for mares bred with hyperedema was 73.8% but the average number of cycles per pregnancy was increased compared with the mares in the other groups.

THE POST-PARTUM MARE

The ultrasonographic appearance of the normal post-partum mare in the foal heat is fairly consistent across mares. Although the cervix is difficult to visualize because of its wide diameter, the uterus will have a low but constant degree of edema that does not follow the normal pattern described previously. Fluid accumulations are frequently observed, particularly in the uterine body because of the presence of lochia. The diameter of the uterine horns is obviously increased, with the previously gravid horn being much bigger. Ovarian activity will resume at about days 3–4 with ovulation occurring between days 7–12.

Involution of the uterus in the mare after foaling is a rapid process. Normalcy of parturition and day of ovulation will determine the suitability of the mare to be mated in the foal heat. A detailed description of management of the mare for foal heat breeding can be found in Chapter 24.

Interpretation of endometrial edema requires a good-quality ultrasound and evaluation of the mare on a regular basis during the late diestrus and the estrus period until ovulation is detected. If used critically and consistently, the pattern of uterine edema can aid the practitioner in determining uterine health and guide the veterinarian for possible diagnostic or therapeutic procedures that may help increase the fertility of mares.[8] Following the pattern of endometrial edema is a key tool to help veterinarians manage mares reproductively and can help in giving a prognosis with respect to the breeding cycle.

REFERENCES

1. McKinnon AO, Squires EL, Carnevale EM, et al: Diagnostic ultrasonography of uterine pathology in the mare. Proc 33rd AAEP. 1988: pp 605-622.
2. Daels PF, Hughes JP: The normal oestrous cycle. In McKinnon AO, Voss JL, eds: *Equine Reproduction.* Philadelphia: Lea & Febiger, 1993, pp 121-133.
3. Samper JC: Ultrasonographic appearance and the pattern of uterine edema to time ovulation in mares. Proc 43rd Annu AAEP Conv.1997, pp 189-191.
4. Woods J, Bergfelt DR, Ginther OJ: Effect of time of insemination relative to ovulation on pregnancy rate and embryonic loss in mares. *Eq Vet J* 22:410-415, 1990.
5. Squires EL, McKinnon AO, Shideler RK: Use of ultrasonography in reproductive management of mares. *Theriogenology* 29:55-70, 1988
6. Pelehach LM, Greaves HE, Porter MB, et al: The role of estrogen and progesterone in the induction and dissipation of uterine edema in mares. *Theriogenology* 58:441-444, 2002.
7. Ginther OJ, Pierson RA: Ultrasonic anatomy and pathology of the equine uterus. *Theriogenology* 2:505-516, 1994.
8. Watson ED, Thomassen R, Nikolakopoulos E: Association of uterine edema with follicle waves around the onset of the breeding season. *Theriogenology* 59:1181-1187, 2003.
9. Samper JC: Fertility of mares with different grades of endometrial edema. Proc 53rd Annu AAEP Conv. 2007, pp 571-573.
10. Samper JC: Induction of estrus and ovulation: Why some mares respond and some do not. *Theriogenology* 70:445-447, 2008.
11. Pycock JF, Dieleman S, Drijfhout P, et al: Correlation of plasma concentrations of progesterone and estradiol with ultrasound characteristics of the uterus and duration of estrous behavior in the cycling mare. *Reprod Dom Anim* 30:224, 1995.
12. Hayes KEN, Pierson RA, Scraba ST, Ginther OJ: Effects of oestrous cycle and season on ultrasonic uterine anatomy in mares. *Theriogenology* 24:465-477, 1985.
13. Plata-Madrid H, Youngquist RS, Murphy CN, et al: Ultrasonographic characteristics of the follicular and uterine dynamics in Belgian mares. *J Eq Vet Sci* 14:421-423, 1994.
14. Griffin PG, Ginther OJ: Dynamics of uterine diameter and endometrial morphology during the estrous cycle and early pregnancy in mares. *Ann. Reprod Sci* 25:133-142, 1991.
15. Bragg Wever ND, Pierson RA, Card CE Assessment of endometrial edema and echotexture in naturally and hormonally manipulated estrus in mares. *Theriogenology* 58:507-510, 2002.

Chapter 13

BREEDING MANAGEMENT OF THE PROBLEM MARE

JONATHAN F. PYCOCK

The objective of the veterinarian, farm manager, and owner working in any type of horse-breeding enterprise, regardless of size, should be to produce the maximum number of live, healthy foals from the mares bred during the previous season; in many breeding programs, "as early as possible" could be added to that objective. Perhaps the biggest obstacle to achieving this aim is the "problem breeding mare." Very few mares are permanently and completely infertile, but subfertility of varying degrees is a major problem. There are many causes of subfertility that warrant a mare to be categorized as a problem breeding mare, and although it is important to recognize the underlying cause, the implementation of a successful treatment strategy is equally important. Veterinarians and managers must be able to help maximize the chance of breeding problem mares whenever possible. It might take several cycles to establish a pregnancy in these mares, and even then an increased possibility of pregnancy failure exists. Commitment from all concerned is needed, and the mare owner should be advised accordingly and be given a realistic expectation as to the chance of success. This chapter considers the problem breeding mare and how to provide an effective management policy that can be applied in daily clinical practice. Particular emphasis is placed on the mare susceptible to persistent post-breeding endometritis.

To understand subfertility, some understanding of normal expectations of fertility is useful. For a breeding operation, regardless of size, it is essential to measure reproductive efficiency.

MARE REPRODUCTIVE EFFICIENCY

The following are some of the parameters used to measure reproductive efficiency:

1. Fertilization rate
2. Per cycle pregnancy rate
3. End of season pregnancy rate
4. Live foal rate
5. Pregnancy loss rate
6. Early embryonic death (EED)

Chapter 26 has a detailed description of the goals for reproductive efficiency for which breeders and veterinarians should strive and the major factors that affect these parameters.

The clinician should be aware of how to investigate the problem breeding mare. Box 13-1 outlines a suggested approach for the examination of a problem breeding mare.

Many causes of subfertility can act either alone or in combination with one another. Subfertility causes can be broadly categorized into infectious or noninfectious factors, with the latter being further divided into anatomic abnormalities and functional

| Box 13-1 | Outline of a Protocol for the Clinical Examination of a Problem Breeding Mare |

1. The mare's previous breeding history
2. Assessment of her physical condition, general health, and perineal conformation
3. Culture swab samples collected from the vestibule, clitoral fossa, and sinuses
4. Examination per vaginam using a speculum, and collection of endometrial swabs for bacterial culture and cytological smear
5. Manual vaginal examination
6. Examination of the reproductive tract by rectal palpation
7. Transrectal real-time ultrasound examination of the reproductive tract
8. Endometrial biopsy
9. Endoscopic examination of the endometrium
10. Peripheral venous blood sample for hormone analysis
11. Peripheral venous blood sample or hair follicle for chromosome analysis

aberrations. This format, as shown in Box 13-2, is used to discuss the various causes of subfertility and infertility in this chapter.

ANATOMIC ABNORMALITIES OF THE FEMALE REPRODUCTIVE TRACT

Defective Vulva

In the normal mare, the vulva provides the first effective barrier to protect the uterus from ascending infection. The vulvar lips are full and firm and meet evenly in the midline, and 80% or more of the vulvar opening is below the brim of the pelvis. If the vulvar seal is incompetent, aspiration of air and contamination into the vagina can occur. The initial vaginitis may lead to cervicitis and acute endometritis, resulting in subfertility. Caslick[1] first pointed out the importance of this condition in relation to genital infection, which is very prevalent in breeds such as the Thoroughbreds or Saddlebreds and is almost unknown in others such as Shires and ponies. Defective vulvar conformation can be congenital, which is very rare, or acquired, which is due to (1) vulvar stretching following repeated foalings, (2) injury to perineal tissue, or (3) poor body condition (old, thin mares).

Older, pluriparous mares are more commonly affected with pneumovagina (aspiration of air into the vagina, also called *wind sucking*). However, pneumovagina can also develop in young mares that are in work and have little body fat or poor vulvar conformation. In some mares, pneumovagina may occur only during estrus when the perineal tissues are more relaxed. Some mares make an obvious noise while walking, but the diagnosis may be

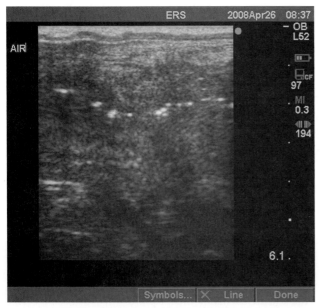

Figure 13-1. Hyperechogenic reflections appearing as a line at the opposed luminal surfaces of the uterine body. The reflections are caused by air in the uterine body.

more difficult in other mares. The presence of hyperemia and a frothy exudate in the anterior vagina on examination with a speculum is pathognomonic. Rectal palpation of a ballooned vagina or uterus from which air can be expelled confirms the diagnosis. Real-time ultrasound examination of the uterus may reveal the presence of air as hyperechogenic (white) foci sometimes seen as a line at the opposed luminal surfaces (Fig. 13-1). Cytologic and histologic examination of the endometrium may demonstrate significant numbers of neutrophils indicative of an endometritis. Rarely, eosinophils are also found in association with pneumovagina.

Treatment should be directed at correcting the cause of pneumovagina and concurrently treating the resulting acute endometritis. The former can be done surgically by performing a Caslick's procedure, although in some cases increasing the physical condition and fat status of the mare may be sufficient. When the angle of the vulvar surface relative to the vertical is the primary defect, the Caslick's procedure is ineffective, and perineal resection should be used to achieve a satisfactory vulvar conformation.[2] Many mares are subjected to a Caslick's procedure unnecessarily; the operation should be reserved for mares with a true vulvar defect rather than be performed merely because the mare has failed to become pregnant.

Defects of the Vestibule and Vagina

Immediately in front of the external urethral opening is the vulvovaginal constriction or vestibular seal. In mares with healthy genitalia, this forms the second line of defense against aspirated air and fecal material. Poor perineal muscular tone results in inadequate vestibular seal function.

Persistent Hymen

Manual vaginal examination of maiden mares often reveals the presence of hymen tissue, which generally breaks down with pressure. A complete persistent hymen can also occur, which can result in the accumulation of fluid within the vagina and uterus because of impaired natural drainage. Sometimes the hymen may be so tough that it can be ruptured only by using a guarded scalpel blade or scissors. In some cases a whitish band can be observed when mares are laying down. The small incision can then be enlarged using the fingers and hand. Rarely, failure of proper fusion of the Müllerian ducts may result in the presence of dorsoventral bands of fibrous tissue in the anterior vagina and fornix. They do not interfere with fertility and are easily broken down manually.

Vesicovaginal Reflux

Also known as *urovagina* or *urine pooling,* vesicovaginal reflux is the retention of incompletely voided urine in the cranial vagina as a result of an exaggerated downward cranial slope of the reproductive tract. Pneumovagina from a defective vulvar conformation also predisposes to the condition. Transient urine pooling, which is sometimes found in postpartum mares, usually resolves after uterine involution has occurred. Clinical signs can include urine dripping from the vulva, urine scalding, and a history of failure to conceive. Diagnosis is made using a speculum examination during estrus to detect urine in the cranial vagina. Uterine infection with an accumulation of exudate in the vagina can be confused with the condition and urine sediment can sometimes be observed in the uterine lumen without fluid accumulation. In severe cases, urine pooling should be corrected surgically.

Vaginal Bleeding

Vaginal bleeding from varicose veins in the remnants of the hymen at the dorsal vestibulovaginal junction is occasionally seen in older mares, particularly during estrus and the second half of pregnancy. Although diathermy can be used, treatment is not usually necessary because the varicose veins normally shrink spontaneously.

Abnormal Cervix

The cervix, although forming an important protective physical barrier to protect the uterus, must also relax during estrus to allow intrauterine ejaculation or insemination of semen and drainage of uterine fluid. An inflammation of the cervix is usually associated with endometritis or vaginitis.

Fibrosis of the cervix often occurs, particularly in old maiden mares because of the loss of muscle. Artificial insemination has been used successfully in mares with an abnormally narrow cervix. However, the impaired cervical drainage of uterine fluid can predispose to persistent endometritis. Mares with a fibrosed cervix and that become pregnant do not normally have any difficulties at foaling.

Cervical Adhesions

Adhesions of the cervix arise from trauma at mating or parturition, or because of long-standing chronic infections. These adhesions can be broken down manually, but this must be done daily to prevent recurrence. If severe, adhesions may contribute to the development of pyometra.

Uterine Cysts

Uterine cysts are the most common type of uterine lesion identified in the mare. They can be diagnosed easily with the use of ultrasonography and it has been shown that the incidence is much greater than originally suspected based on rectal palpation alone. One detailed study found an overall prevalence of uterine cysts of 26.8%, with mares older than 11 years being 4.2 times more likely to have cysts.[3]

There are two types of uterine cysts recognized in mares: endometrial glandular cysts and lymphatic lacunar cysts. Endometrial cysts are usually smaller (5–10 mm) compared with lymphatic cysts, which are the coalescence of the smaller glandular cysts. Cysts are normally luminal pedunculated or not pedunculated. However, mural cysts are also observed but do not protrude into the uterine lumen.

The relationship between subfertility and uterine cysts is not clear. Some authors suggest that uterine cysts can reduce pregnancy rates.[4] However, a large field study concluded that there was no evidence to suggest that uterine cysts adversely affect the establishment or maintenance of pregnancy.[3] Their effect on fertility could be by restricting early conceptus mobility and later in pregnancy by interfering with nutrient absorption by contact between the cyst wall and yolk sac or allantois. However, it is difficult to substantiate their primary role because they are a common sign of uterine disease in general, including senility and previous endometritis. In my experience, only mares with multiple large lymphatic cysts have a reduced pregnancy rate.

Cysts can be confused with an early conceptus and give rise to false early pregnancy diagnosis or the incorrect diagnosis of twin pregnancies during ultrasound scanning. Differentiation is based on previous cyst mapping, but also the early mobility of the conceptus, the presence of specular reflections, the spheric appearance of the conceptus, and growth rate. Although some cysts can be easily confused with an early pregnancy, there is often an opportunity to scan the mare before or immediately after breeding. In the illustrated case, it is impossible to be certain whether there are twin unilateral vesicles of approximately 20 and 16 days, a single pregnancy and a 19-mm cyst, a cyst with adjacent free fluid, or a 19-mm conceptus with adjacent free fluid. In these cases, it is vital to study the ultrasonographic image carefully. A close look at the wall between the two structures in Fig. 13-2, *A,* shows a relatively thick and hyperechogenic wall compared with the twin vesicle shown in Fig. 13-2, *B.* This would confirm that at least one structure is a cyst. Reassessment of the irregular structure confirms that the fluid is contained and does not extend up or down the horn, as would be found with free fluid. The appearance of an embryo proper at around 22 days and a heartbeat at around 25 days of pregnancy provides a definitive diagnosis. Thorough identification of cysts at the beginning of the breeding season minimizes the chance of false pregnancy diagnosis.

Larger lymphatic cysts may interfere with the mobility phase of the early conceptus, resulting in failure of the mare to recognize the presence of a pregnancy and failure to prevent luteolysis. Later in pregnancy, the absorption of nutrients and the development of chorionic villi may be diminished in places of contact between cysts and fetal membranes, leading to an increased risk of embryonic death.

The need for endometrial cyst therapy is uncertain. If at the beginning of the breeding season a mare is found to have a large number of cysts, it is generally best to continue to attempt to get the mare pregnant that season. If she fails to become pregnant,

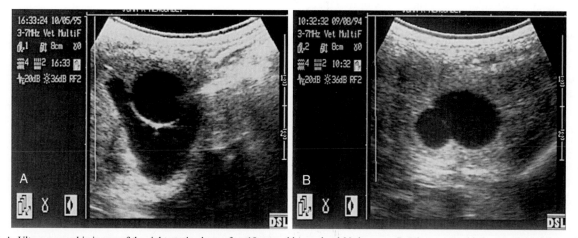

Figure 13-2. A, Ultrasonographic image of the right uterine horn of an 18-year-old mare bred 20 days ago. **B,** Ultrasonographic image of the right uterine horn of a mare with unilateral twins of 14 and 17 days of gestation.

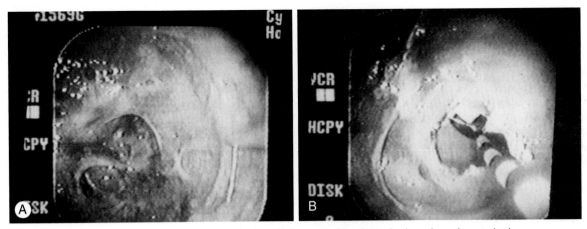

Figure 13-3. A, Adhesion almost completely obstructing the left uterine horn. **B,** Removal of the obstruction by endoscopic cauterization.

some form of therapy should be attempted and an endometrial biopsy should be done to help determine the likelihood of her carrying a foal to term. Because of risks such as uterine hemorrhage, mechanical uterine curettage is rarely used. Larger cysts can be punctured using an endometrial biopsy apparatus or manually if the cervix allows passage of one hand. Chemical curettage has equivocal results: the cysts may disappear but scar tissue may form. An endoscope and laser ablation or a thermocautery method involving looping and subsequent burning of cysts is possible. Wounds after cautery appear to heal quickly, usually within 4–6 weeks. Because the endoscopy should take place while the mare is in diestrus when the cervix is relatively closed, prostaglandin-$F_{2\alpha}$ ($PGF_{2\alpha}$) should be given after cauterization and the uterus should be lavaged with 2–3 L of sterile lactated Ringer's solution to clear any debris.

Most uterine cysts involve the endometrium, but occasionally an extraluminal uterine cyst lying external to the endometrium can be identified on ultrasound examination. Its location should be verified by identification of the uterine lumen. Extraluminal or mural cysts usually have no significance on breeding potential.

Partial Dilation of the Uterus

The discrete collection of fluid in permanent ventral dilations at the base of one or rarely both horns of the uterus, which can be palpated per rectum, was first reported by Knudsen.[5] Ventral uterine enlargements have subsequently been discussed by Kenney and Ganjam,[6] who suggested that they originate by one of four mechanisms: mucosal atrophy, myometrial atony, lymphatic lacunae, or endometrial cysts. Their precise relationship to subfertility is not clear, but mares that fail to eliminate the fluid and debris that accumulate in these sacculations after mating are susceptible to the establishment of chronic endometritis; treatment for mares with defective uterine clearance is discussed later in this chapter.

Uterine Adhesions

Uterine adhesions are most frequently suspected when mares have had a long-standing uterine infection and cervical tags are detected when performing uterine procedures such as artificial insemination or uterine cultures. The extent of the adhesions in the uterus is diagnosed by endoscopic examination of the uterus.[7] Multiple adhesions adversely affect fertility by causing fluid accumulation or by affecting the mobility of the conceptus. Severe adhesions can completely obstruct one or both

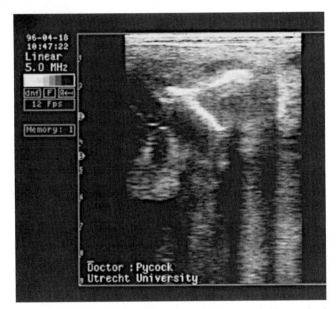

Figure 13-4. Hyperechoic fetal bone visible on ultrasonographic examination of the uterine body.

of the uterine horns. It is possible to remove the obstruction endoscopically by either cauterization or laser techniques, starting at the thin membranous parts of the obstruction (Fig. 13-3, *A*). It is important not to "burn" too deeply into the uterine wall because more severe damage to the uterine wall might occur. After removing the obstruction, the uterus should be flushed to remove any debris and the mare given $PGF_{2\alpha}$. In addition to an assessment of an endometrial biopsy, the prognosis for future breeding also depends on the severity of the obstruction and to what extent the obstruction could be removed. Severe adhesions can be too thick to safely treat with cautery or laser techniques (Fig. 13-3, *B*), and the mare needs to be retired from breeding or placed in an in vitro fertilization (IVF) program.

Uterine Foreign Bodies

Uterine foreign bodies, which may act as a nidus for the establishment of chronic endometritis or pyometra, have been documented but are uncommon.[8] In one case, seen by the author, the mare had a history of failure to conceive and short interestrus intervals following a dystocia. Ultrasound examination revealed hyperechogenic fetal bone (part of the scapula) (Fig. 13-4), which was removed manually via the cervix. The mare conceived after appropriate intrauterine lavage and antibiotic treatment to correct the endometritis. Other foreign bodies that have been reported include straws following insemination with frozen semen and the tips of uterine swabs.

Oviductal Abnormalities

Oviductal abnormalities are rarely reported in the mare, and although evidence of salpingitis can be detected in problem-breeding mares, the incidence is not different than that noted in normal, fertile mares.[9] However, a recent a study by Fiala et al.[10] suggested that salpingitis is more frequent in aged mares than previously thought. They studied oviducts from Brazilian mares collected at an abattoir and determined that bilateral salpingitis was present in 43.7% whereas unilateral salpingitis was present in 28.1%. Fiala et al. also determined that slight, moderate, and severe inflammation of the oviducts was 74.3%, 17.6%, and 8.0%, respectively, and they speculated that this could be a cause of subfertility in mares.

The presence of collagenous masses within the oviduct that might occlude its lumen has been documented.[11] Dye tests are used in cattle to test the patency of the oviducts, but this is difficult in the mare because of the tightness of the uterotubal junction. Case studies have shown that blocked oviducts in the mare are rare. In a study by Allen et al.,[12] 15 mares 10-21 years of age with unexplained infertility were treated with 0.5 ml of gel containing 0.2 mg of $PGE_{2\alpha}$. The solution was dripped onto the oviducts through a laparoscope, and 14 of 15 mares were pregnant in that or the next breeding season. The authors concluded that older mares suffering repeated conception failure over several breeding seasons in the absence of identifiable pathology may benefit from $PGE_{2\alpha}$ gel treatment. These authors also concluded that oviductal blockage does occur sporadically within any population of aging brood mares, and this results from a moveable accumulation of intraluminal debris rather than any permanent physical obstruction.

Surgical techniques for the diagnosis and treatment of oviductal pathology have been described elsewhere.

Periovarian Cysts

Cysts lying within the ovarian stroma near the ovulation fossa of the ovary arise from the surface epithelium and are often seen in older mares during examination of the ovary. They are known as retention, inclusion, or fossa cysts and generally have no adverse effect on fertility (Fig.13-5, *A*).

Fossa cysts, normally only a few millimeters in diameter, are not usually seen as large as in Fig. 13-5, *B*. Care must be taken not to confuse them with a normal ovary with several small follicles (see Fig. 13-5, *C*) or conceptus. Careful examination allows accurate identification of their position; if they are

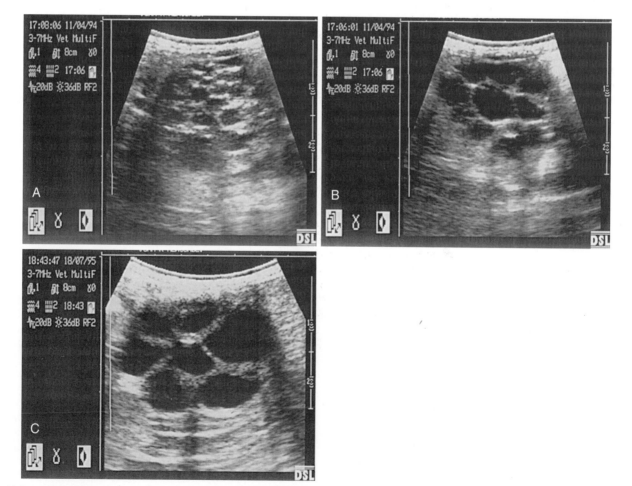

Figure 13-5. A, Ultrasonographic image of the ovary of a 15-year-old mare showing retention cysts, each a few millimeters in diameter. **B,** Ultrasonographic image of the ovary of a 17-year-old mare showing large retention cysts. **C,** Ultrasonographic image of the normal ovary of a 16-year-old mare with seven small follicles.

particularly large and/or numerous, as can occur in older mares, they could impede the release of the oocyte from the ovulation fossa. Small nodules located within the loose connective tissue covering of the ovary known as adrenocortical nodules have also been identified.

Periovarian cysts, which are fairly common, especially in Shires and Clydesdales, are not endocrinologically active and do not usually interfere with the process of ovulation nor do they affect fertility. Occasionally, large cysts associated with the oviduct may be palpated or imaged with ultrasonography and may cause confusion with follicular structures. However, the lack of change in size or appearance of these structures is usually diagnostic. These structures are believed to be remnants of the Müllerian duct system during embryologic differentiation.

Pituitary Abnormalities

Rarely, Cushing's syndrome caused by adenomatous hyperplasia of the intermediate pituitary has been associated with anestrus in aged mares. This is presumably due to destruction of the cells secreting luteinizing hormone (LH) and follicle-stimulating hormone (FSH). Reproductive clinical signs in mares with Cushing's syndrome include failure to cycle properly and failure to conceive.

FUNCTIONAL SUBFERTILITY

There are two major reasons why fertility in the equine population is less efficient compared with other farm animals. First, reproductive efficiency has not been a criterion used to select breeding animals. Second, since January 1 was declared the official birth date for Thoroughbred foals in the early nineteenth century, regardless of their actual birth dates within that year, there has been a plague of problems in attempting to breed mares in the winter and early spring outside their most fertile period. The promotion of yearlings in the autumn sales also contributes to the pressure for early breeding, because well-grown older yearlings tend to sell for higher prices.

Irregularities of the Estrous Cycle

Mares are seasonally polyestrous, and environmental and other factors can exert a profound effect on reproductive function, particularly during the transitional period between winter anestrus and the onset of cyclic activity in the spring. Although irregularities of follicular development, ovulation, and behavioral patterns are also observed during the normal breeding season, they are not as common. However, endometritis can also cause cyclic irregularities.

Anestrus, which refers to the failure of a mare to cycle, is due to several physiological and pathological conditions.

Chromosomal Abnormalities

The normal chromosome complement for the domestic horse is 2n = 64. Various sex chromosome anomalies have been described in the horse. The incidence of chromosomal abnormalities is difficult to assess but must be suspected in maiden mares with small, inactive ovaries and an immature tubular genital tract once winter anestrus has been eliminated as a cause of acyclicity. However, some genetically normal young fillies in training can be acyclic. They must be given more time to mature

reproductively, and karyotyping must be performed before a final diagnosis is made.

The main karyotypic abnormality of such mares is the 63, XO (Turner's syndrome) genotype. Examination detects very small ovaries (<1 cm in diameter) and a poorly developed tubular genital tract, which is difficult to palpate. These mares are usually small for their age and do not cycle, although occasionally they may show passive estrous signs. Definitive diagnosis requires cytogenetic analysis of a blood sample. There is no treatment and the mare is sterile.

Other chromosome abnormalities include ovarian hypoplasia and testicular feminization. These are also rare but must be considered in female horses with irregular cycles and small ovaries during the breeding season.

Pregnancy and Pseudopregnancy

Pseudopregnancy is a term used to describe a syndrome in which non-pregnant mares that have been bred do not return to estrus. It occurs if there is EED after 15 days of gestation with persistence of the corpus luteum resulting in a prolonged luteal phase. The cervix remains tightly closed and the uterus is tense and tubular. It is differentiated from pregnancy by the absence of a conceptus on ultrasound examination. If early fetal death occurs after endometrial cup formation at 36 days, mares either become anestrus or show estrus with irregular follicular patterns. In the latter case, follicular luteinization without ovulation is thought to occur and, therefore, the estrus is not fertile. This failure of ovulation lasts until the endometrial cups regress spontaneously at 90–150 days. There is currently no practical way of destroying endometrial cups prematurely. It has also been reported recently that endometrial cups can be retained after abortion, fetal death, or parturition. These mares will have irregular follicular activity and a high incidence of follicular luteinization. It has recently been reported that in a small number of mares, endometrial cups may persist for many months following pregnancy loss.[14] This may explain the failure of some mares to show regular behavioral estrus during the breeding season.

Silent Estrus

Silent estrus is the condition in which some mares either do not show estrus or are slow to show detectable signs using standard teasing methods despite the fact that ovulation occurs. The degree of reduced expression of estrus varies from partial (subestrus) to complete (anestrus). Estrus has a higher incidence in maiden mares early in the breeding season and in mares with a young foal "at foot." Other factors that affect estrous behavior include being turned out with very dominant mares and stallion preferences. Fillies that are in training and that have been given anabolic steroids may be more likely to have the condition as a result of "androgenization."

The diagnosis is based on repeated rectal and vaginal examinations, which confirm that the mare is in estrus and has follicles of an ovulatory size. It is essential to distinguish the condition from a prolonged luteal phase in which there is also follicular development.

The treatment is based on thorough and careful teasing. Frequent and persistent teasing may get the mare to show estrous signs. Alternatively, placing the mare in a stable next to a stallion may be helpful. If permissible, artificial insemination can be used. To naturally breed mares during a silent estrus, some form of restraint may be necessary; many mares approaching ovulation accept the stallion when twitched and hobbled. An intramuscular injection of estradiol benzoate (10–20 mg) 6 hours before breeding can be tried as a last resort. The veterinarian must ensure that the mare is physiologically ready to be bred. In some cases when the mare is not psychologically prepared for breeding, estrogens are of little value and tranquilizers may be more appropriate. In many cases, it is a failure of the estrus detection system rather than a true reproductive disorder of individual mares. Veterinarians must be aware of the possibility of the presence of large diestrus follicles where mares, despite the presence of a large follicle, are still under progesterone influence. In these cases, the therapy of choice is a luteolytic dose of prostaglandin.

Irregular or Prolonged Estrus

True persistent estrus appears to be rare in mares other than during the transitional period from winter anestrus or in association with steroid hormone–producing ovarian tumors. Some mares that are thought to have persistent estrus may actually have normal behavior, or other types of behavior may be misinterpreted as being persistent estrus. Mares that are anestrus because of disease, or old mares whose ovaries have ceased to function normally, may be receptive to a stallion. Frequent urination as a result of hind limb or back pain, or a urogenital problem may be mistaken for persistent estrus.

Transitional "Spring" Estrus

During the transitional period before the first ovulation of the year, mares demonstrate erratic estrous behavior of varying intensity. The presence of multiple large follicles, possibly as large as 30 mm, makes detection of ovulation difficult by palpation alone.

Pressure to breed mares early in the year before the onset of their natural breeding season can cause problems for the veterinarian. Because of the considerable variation in the duration of estrus during the transitional period, efficient breeding of the mare can be difficult. During the transitional period, the behavior is variable, ranging from total rejection of the stallion, to interest but resistance to his mounting, to normal acceptance. These behavioral signs can be consistent or inconsistent. Practitioners traditionally recommend that the interval between matings should not exceed 3 days if a normal fertile stallion is being used; however, the optimal interval between breeding and ovulation is not accurately defined. Few critical studies exist on survival time of sperm in the oviduct of the mare. No significant difference between day of insemination in pregnancy rate for mares inseminated from 1–6 days before ovulation has been reported.[15] It is important not to begin breeding too early or the mare will be mated too many times. A recent study found that intervals between mating and ovulation of >2 days significantly lowered pregnancy rates.[16] The optimum interval may depend on susceptibility of the mare to delayed uterine clearance (DUC) (see later). In mares with DUC, a longer interval from mating to ovulation >48 hours resulted in higher pregnancy rates.[17] The appearance of uterine edema (Fig. 13-6) is an indication that the follicles present gain steroidogenic competence, leading to an increase in circulating estrogen concentrations, which cause the release of LH from the pituitary as a result of a positive feedback mechanism. Estrogen, in the absence of progesterone, is responsible for the appearance of uterine edema, so this may

be why the detection of uterine edema is clinically important in signaling the emergence of the mare from the transitional period into the ovulatory period.

Visualization of uterine edema is done by thorough ultrasonic examination and rectal palpation, which reveals transitional follicles reaching preovulatory size (>35 mm). A detailed description of uterine edema patterns is discussed in Chapter 12. Visual identification of a corpus luteum with progesterone levels >4 ng/ml confirms that the first ovulation has occurred and, hence, normal ovarian cyclic activity.

Several hormonal regimens are available to reduce the length of the transitional period and induce a fertile ovulation The most widely used treatment of mares in transitional stage is based on progesterone or progestogens, with or without the addition of estradiol, involving several parenteral routes of administration. Progesterone can be administered as an oil-based intramuscular injection, orally as the synthetic progestogen (altrenogest), or intravaginally by using a progesterone-releasing device of which three types are currently available: PRID, CIDR, and Cue-Mate.

Progesterone exerts a negative feedback on gonadotropin secretion, which is followed by an increased release of FSH and LH. When the source of progesterone is withdrawn or its effect wanes, there is follicular growth, maturation, and ovulation. Progesterone treatment is more effective in mares that are in late transitional stage and is ineffective in mares with minimal follicular activity, particularly during deep anestrus. Currently, the most effective treatment is the use of in-feed medication with the potent progestogen altrenogest (Equine Regumate). This liquid, which contains 2.2 mg/ml of the active substance, should be added to the food once per day at a dose rate of 0.044 mg/kg body weight for approximately 10 consecutive days; estrus should occur within 6 days and ovulation between 7 and 13 days after the last treatment. It is useful to examine the ovaries after 7 days and, if a large follicle (>35 mm) has already developed, the progestogen can be stopped (or the coil removed) and the mare monitored for ovulation. If the follicles are <35 mm, supplementation is continued for 5 further days at which time the treatment is stopped or the

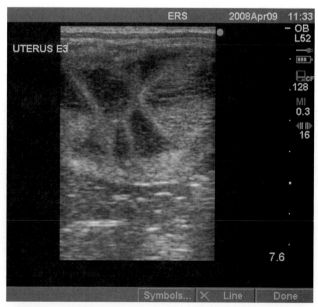

Figure 13-6. Ultrasonographic image of the uterine body of a mare showing a marked edema pattern.

coil removed. By examining the mare while under treatment, the possibility of an unexpected ovulation can be minimized. Use of hCG or deslorelin will advance ovulation by 1–2 days and reduce the percentage of mares that fail to ovulate. The use of intramuscular injections of progesterone and estradiol-17β in oil for 10 days produces a similar response to altrenogest, but the interval to estrus is longer because there is suppression of follicular development by the estradiol. The use of dopamine antagonists such as domperidone or sulpiride is also commonly used, but results have been equivocal, and nutritional status and environmental conditions seem to affect the response of the mares.

Regardless of the hormones used, mares undergoing treatment early in the season need 16 hours of adequate light and good housing and nutrition to ensure success.

Cystic Ovarian Disease

Cystic ovarian disease comparable with the condition described in the cow where anovulatory follicles remain hormonally active for extended periods does not occur in the mare. The presence of persistent follicles that occur during the transitional phase, the presence of anovulatory follicles, or the presence of cystic structures on the ovary accompanied by other pathological conditions such as ovarian tumors may explain why this condition has been diagnosed in the past.

OVULATORY DYSFUNCTION

Anovulatory Hemorrhagic Follicles

A form of ovulatory failure has been described in the mare in which the preovulatory follicle grows to an unusually large size, fails to rupture and ovulate, typically fills with blood and fibrin (Fig. 13-7), and then gradually regresses. These structures can be as large as 8–10 cm and occasionally much larger and may develop an outer wall of luteal tissue. These structures if undisturbed can persist for a variable period ranging from 3 to 7 weeks, but prostaglandin administration will accelerate their regression when luteal tissue is present. The condition is known as hemorrhagic anovulatory follicle syndrome (AHF) and is initially recognized, using transrectal ultrasound, by the presence of scattered free-floating echogenic spots within the follicular antrum (Fig. 13-8). As the blood coagulates and the fibrin deposits, the ultrasonic appearance varies from honeycomb, or net-like, to a uniformly echogenic mass (Fig. 13-9). The palpation features of these structures are smooth, with varying degrees of firmness. This can be confusing in that they may feel like preovulatory follicles or corpora hemorrhagica, or they may become very large. The most obvious difference in their appearance is when they are examined ultrasonographically. The structures may have a similar appearance to that of a granulosa thecal cell tumor (GTCT): the anechoic areas are separated by trabeculae and are similar to those of a multicystic GTCT. The diagnosis of a hemorrhagic follicle may be made on the basis of clinical signs, namely maintenance of cyclicity, a normal contralateral ovary, the presence of an ovulation fossa, and speed of enlargement and regression of the ovary with time.

Hemorrhagic follicles may be difficult to predict before the appearance of the first signs. The cause of these hemorrhagic follicles is not known but is likely to be possible hormonal pituitary insufficiency to induce ovulation. Similar structures are seen under continued equine chorionic gonadotropin (eCG)

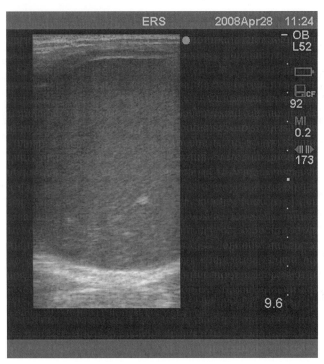

Figure 13-7. Ultrasonographic image of an anovulatory hemorrhagic follicle measuring 90 × 70 mm in the right ovary of a mare.

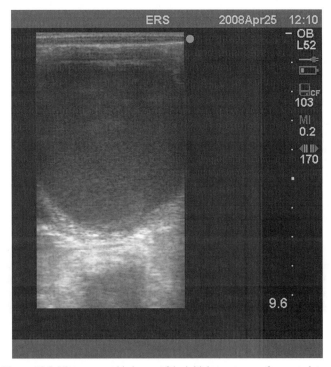

Figure 13-8. Ultrasonographic image of the initial appearance of an anovulatory follicle measuring 55 × 40 mm in the ovary of a mare.

stimulation during days 40–50 of pregnancy. However, in a study by Gastal et al.,[18] the only abnormality found in AHFs compared with normal ovulatory follicles was an elevated estrogen level and an increase in vascularity of the follicular wall of the AHF.

Anovulatory follicles were reported by McCue and Squires[19] to occur in approximately 8.2% of estrous cycles. These authors also reported an increased incidence associated with age and make a distinction between the majority of anovulatory follicles

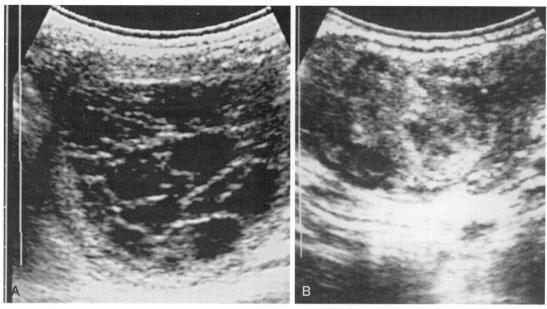

Figure 13-9. A, Ultrasonographic image of an anovulatory hemorrhagic follicle with a net-like appearance within the follicular fluid. **B,** Ultrasonographic image of an anovulatory hemorrhagic follicle with a more echogenic, uniform appearance.

that become luteinized (86%) and those that remain as follicular structures (14%), with the latter ones not responding to prostaglandin.

The hallmark of AHF is that the follicle does not evacuate the follicular fluid, hence the oocyte is not released and remains within the large unruptured hemorrhagic follicle. Therefore, pregnancies are never established from a true AHF. The abrupt decrease in follicle diameter normally associated with ovulation is not noted but, rather, a steady increase in size can be detected. It is important to differentiate, however, between a hemorrhagic follicle and a hemorrhagic CL since these two structures can be difficult to separate, particularly when examinations are performed at long intervals.

Anovulatory Follicles in Aged Mares

Even though there is no documented menopause in mares, an age-related ovulation failure has been documented.[20] Some aged mares, particularly those >20 years of age, fail to ovulate, despite showing estrous behavior, and hence anovulation may not be detected. On ultrasound examination, their ovaries resemble those of seasonally anovulatory mares with a few small (<10 mm) follicles. Endometrial biopsy shows evidence of gland atrophy. Treatments for these conditions, although not consistent, include eFSH or GnRH therapy. On the other hand, it is important to recognize that some mares ovulate smaller follicles (20–25 mm) and ovulation might go undetected. In these instances progesterone detectable in blood and uterine and cervical tone are present and endometrial biopsy shows evidence of glandular branching.

Ovarian Neoplasia

There are several conditions that cause unilateral or bilateral large ovaries in mares. As stated previously, large bilateral ovaries are commonly found in transitional ovaries, large follicles during the breeding season, and ovaries of pregnant mares past day 35. Other conditions that can cause large ovaries include ovarian hematomas, ovarian abscesses, hemorrhagic and luteinized follicles, and neoplastic conditions such as GTCT, teratoma, dysgerminoma, cystadenoma, and carcinoma.

Although many types of tumors have been described, ovarian neoplasia is uncommon in the mare, with GTCTs being by far the most common.[21] GTCTs arise from the sex cord stromal tissue within the ovary and may be hormonally active, producing variable amounts of steroids that cause behavioral changes and alteration in normal cyclic activity. Mares can exhibit nymphomania, anestrus, or aggressiveness with signs of virilism (clitoral enlargement, stallion-like conformation). There appears to be no breed predisposition for GTCTs, and there is a wide range of age distribution. The tumors are often large before they are diagnosed. The presence of one grossly enlarged ovary (>10 cm diameter) (Fig. 13-10, *A)* with the opposite ovary being small and firm on palpation with no visible follicles of >1 cm (resembling an ovary of a mare in deep anestrus) is indicative but not diagnostic of a GTCT. In mares with GTCTs, behavioral changes alone can be misleading because many affected mares do not show virilism or any other behavioral changes, and tumors other than GTCTs can also result in elevated plasma testosterone values. Owners sometimes express the opinion that their mare is "awkward" when in estrus, and they request veterinary treatment. Frequently such mares are required to perform to a high level (e.g., advanced dressage). If examination during a reported period of abnormal behavior reveals marked follicular development, it is tempting to diagnose cystic ovaries as the cause of the behavioral changes. On other occasions, the mare may even be in diestrus when examined. In any case, owner pressure to perform an ovariectomy on suspicion of a GTCT should be resisted, at least until the mare has been monitored throughout several cycles to determine whether her behavioral problems are related to estrus.

When the behavioral problems are thought to be truly linked to estrus, daily supplementation with progesterone or a synthetic progestagen should prevent the mare from showing estrous behavior. Although rare in an unbred mare, there is a possibility of an increased risk for endometritis in a mare on long-term progesterone supplementation, and she should be monitored.

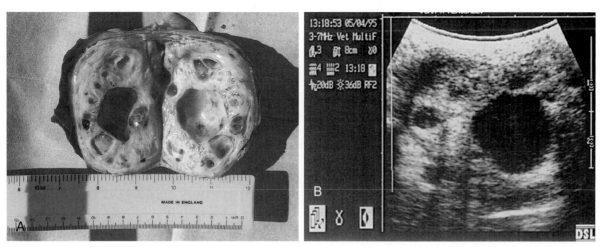

Figure 13-10. A, Gross appearance of a granulosa thecal cell tumor (GTCT) of the left ovary of a 7-year-old mare. **B,** Ultrasonographic image of the left ovary of the mare.

In addition, the problems may well recur following cessation of treatment. Abnormal behavior related to estrus can be solved with pregnancy. Potential disadvantages of getting the mare pregnant are that she cannot be shown or compete in the later stages of pregnancy and the problems may recur after birth. Veterinarians dealing with mares exhibiting abnormal behavior should also be aware that refractory visceral pain can be induced in mares with severe pneumovagina and that a simple Caslick operation can sometimes solve the problem.[22]

The presence of a large ovary is not necessarily indicative of a tumor, and removal of an ovary should be done only after thorough client education and discussion and consent. It is important to accurately diagnose the reason for the enlarged ovary. For example, in one report, 39% (11 of 28) of surgically excised enlarged ovaries did not warrant removal.[23] Cases of GTCT may be found at routine examination of mares, maybe even after foaling, and rarely have these mares shown any behavioral changes. Larger tumors that have been present for some time are more likely to cause erratic behavior and colic signs.

It is important not to presume that a large ovary in a mare with behavioral problems is caused by a GTCT. A peripheral blood sample for a GCTC panel (testosterone, estrogen, progesterone, and inhibin levels) is useful. Increased concentrations of testosterone occur in approximately 50% of cases, estradiol concentrations may be raised, and progesterone concentrations are usually low (<1 ng/ml) because these mares are mostly not cycling. Identification of elevated concentrations of the hormone inhibin is more reliable than testosterone in confirming the presence of a GTCT. In a single blood sample of a mare with a granulosa cell tumor, inhibin is elevated in approximately 90% of cases.[24, 25]

The secretion of high amounts of inhibin by the neoplastic granulosa cells inhibits FSH secretion and is thought to be the reason for atrophy of the contralateral ovary—a sign that is present in well over 90% of the mares with a GTCT.[12] A GTCT often appears ultrasonographically as a large (7–40 cm), spheric mass, with a multicystic or "honeycomb" appearance (Fig. 13-10, *B*). However, there is no typical appearance of a GTCT on ultrasound. Some are uniformly dense and others have a single, large, fluid-filled cyst or even several large cysts. The echogenicity of the cyst wall differentiates it from persistent, large anovulatory follicles. However, the ultrasonic appearance of some GTCTs can be similar to that of luteinized, unruptured ("hemorrhagic") follicles. Histopathologic examination is the only method of obtaining a definitive diagnosis.

Unilateral ovariectomy is the only satisfactory treatment for GTCTs, because the prospect of breeding from the mare is extremely poor unless the neoplastic ovary is removed. It is important not to be too hasty in removing the ovary, and a mare should always be scheduled for a second examination some weeks later. In the case of a tumor, the ultrasonic appearance would change little in the short term and would certainly appear similar if reexamined several weeks later. The reproductive prognosis of the mare is generally good, depending on the state of inhibition of the other ovary and provided that no uterine tissue had to be removed. Most mares return to normal cyclic ovarian activity, although this often takes as long as one breeding season, especially in cases of severe suppression of the remaining ovary. Most GTCTs are unilateral, although a bilateral case has been reported. Metastasis of the tumor is rare but does occur.[21]

Multiple Ovulation

Double ovulations occur during 8%–35% of estrous cycles, the frequency depending on the breed and type of the mare with Thoroughbreds and Warmbloods having the highest rate and ponies the lowest rate. Accurate detection of such ovulations is important because twinning is highly undesirable. Rectal palpation alone can be misleading in detecting a double ovulation, particularly when the two follicles are on the same ovary. The use of ultrasound examination of the ovaries, which should routinely be performed in conjunction with a thorough rectal examination, usually allows detection of twin follicles and double ovulations. Sometimes, the ovulatory area can appear indistinct for the first 24 hours; in these cases, the mare should be checked again 2 days later, when it can be seen more easily whether there is more than one corpus luteum (Fig. 13-11).

Management of Twin Ovulation

Multiple ovulation in the mare should not be regarded as a reason for withholding breeding. Instead, pregnancy rates are improved after twin ovulation. Although accurate interpretation of the ultrasound image of early pregnancies in the mare and the technique of crushing a conceptus are skills that require experience, the advent of B-mode ultrasound imaging has provided a method to more readily diagnose and manage twin pregnancies in the mare.

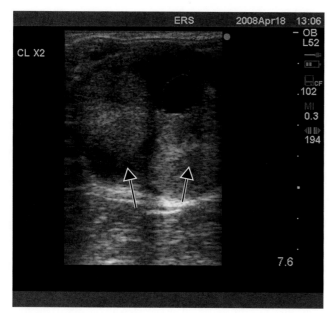

Figure 13-11. Ultrasonographic image of an ovary with a double ovulation at 48 hours after ovulation.

There are two approaches to dealing with twins:

1. If the initial examination of the mare is done before fixation (day 15–16), the twin embryos are reduced to a singleton by the manual destruction of one, either by pressure with the transducer or the use of the hand. I prefer to gently separate the embryonic vesicles using the transducer to enable the procedure to be imaged. When the conceptual vesicles are of dissimilar sizes, the smaller one should be ruptured. This is easier before day 16 after ovulation when they are 14–20 mm in diameter rather than on days 11–13, when they are 6–11 mm in diameter. The disadvantage of this method is that it is more expensive, in that all mares are scanned before the time of return to estrus. In addition, if ovulations that occur more than 3 days apart have not been detected, a mistaken diagnosis of a single pregnancy may be made if the second vesicle is too small to detect. With experience, however, this technique is highly effective. Analysis of data over several breeding seasons has shown that there is no increased incidence of mid- to late-term abortion in mares that have had one of twin vesicles crushed.

2. If initial examination is done after fixation but before day 35, and if both conceptuses are in one horn (unilaterally fixed), one option is to terminate a pregnancy using PGF$_{2\alpha}$. Alternatively, transvaginal ultrasound-guided puncture of one conceptus can be attempted. If the pregnancies are in separate horns (bilaterally fixed), they can be reduced by crushing one conceptus. Management of twin pregnancies after this period (day 35) is complicated by the formation of endometrial cups, and if twin pregnancies are not successfully managed before the cups are formed, the mare usually will not return to a fertile estrus for a prolonged period.

As twin pregnancy is allowed to progress further in gestation, after endometrial cup formation the management options are reduced and success rates become lower. Management options include dietary energy restriction, surgical removal of one vesicle, intracardiac injection of one fetus, transvaginal ultrasound–guided needle puncture, and craniocervical dislocation. Transvaginal ultrasound–guided needle puncture is successful in approximately one third of cases, whereas craniocervical dislocation is successful approximately two thirds of the time. Craniocervical dislocation is performed via a standing flank laparotomy at 70–90 days of gestation. The neck of one of the fetuses is dislocated manually after identification by direct palpation of the uterus through the flank incision.[26]

PREGNANCY FAILURE

Pregnancy failure is a source of major economic loss to the horse industry. Embryonic death occurs before 40 days of gestation when organogenesis is complete, with EED occurring before maternal recognition of pregnancy. Early fetal death occurs before 150 days of gestation and late fetal death occurs after that. Abortion is defined as expulsion of the fetus and its membranes before 300 days, whereas a stillbirth is expulsion of the fetus and its membranes from day 300 onward (expulsion of a dead fetus that would have been capable of life outside the uterus).

Embryonic Death

In normal fertile mares, the fertilization rate is more than 90%, which is comparable with other domestic species, with estimates of the EED rate at 5%–24%. In subfertile mares, the rate is higher. The differences in the estimates are due to varying methods of pregnancy detection and differences in the animals studied. The period of greatest embryonic death in subfertile mares occurs in the interval before pregnancy and can be detected with ultrasound (day 11), particularly at the time the embryo enters the uterus. Between days 14 and 40, the rate of embryonic death varies between 10% and 17%. EED is multifactorial; external factors such as the environment and management as well as pathophysiologic factors are involved. However, the evidence for many of these associations is anecdotal and frequently contradictory.

External Factors

External factors involved in embryonic death include stress, nutrition, season of the year, climate, sire effects, and rectal palpation. Maternal stress caused by severe pain, malnutrition, and transport has been implicated as a cause of EED. Frequently, mares at stud are transported at various stages of pregnancy; there are no reports of any difference in pregnancy rates between transported and non-transported mares. Transporting pregnant mares home from stud a distance of 300 miles (500 km) in <9 hours of traveling time can be stressful but should not result in embryonic death. If a longer journey is necessary, the journey should be broken after 8 hours. Waiting until the fifth week of pregnancy or later to transport brood mares may be advisable when critical events such as descent of the embryo into the uterus and transition from the yolk sac to the chorioallantoic placentation have occurred. The common practice of transporting mares to stud for mating and returning home the same day should not be detrimental to their fertility as long as the transport is safe and comfortable.

Regular exercise is important during pregnancy, although during the latter half of pregnancy, forced exercise should be decreased. Rectal palpation and ultrasound examinations should be considered safe procedures when performed correctly, and recent evidence gives no indication that ultrasound examination is detrimental to the embryo.[27]

Maternal Factors

A number of abnormal maternal factors including hormone deficiencies and imbalances, uterine environment, age, and lactation have been implicated in fetal death.

Hormonal Deficiencies and Imbalances

Progesterone is critical for the maintenance of pregnancy in mares. The only source of progesterone during the embryonic period is the primary corpus luteum. On the assumption that luteal insufficiency is important in EED, many mares are given exogenous progesterone or progestogens to prevent it from occurring. However, the rationale for this widespread practice is highly questionable, although primary luteal insufficiency as a cause of EED has been reported.[28] Progesterone supplementation has been reviewed by Allen,[29] who is skeptical of any benefit. Many dosage regimens do not effectively elevate or maintain plasma progesterone levels. Withdrawal of supplementary progesterone therapy during midgestation may leave the clinician open to criticism if the mare subsequently aborts. I believe that progesterone therapy is most appropriate in mares that have uterine edema and an indistinct corpus luteum at the time of first examination for pregnancy (15 days). These pregnancies are usually lost within a few days, but some can be successfully "saved" by exogenous progesterone, and the pregnancy can be carried normally through to term. Progesterone in oil (100 mg) or altrenogest (35 mg; Regumate) is given daily until a corpus luteum is obvious on ultrasound examination and all uterine edema has disappeared. A single injection of 40 µg of the GnRH agonist buserelin has also been shown to reduce the incidence of EED when given 10 days after ovulation.[30] However, when the same dosage was tested on a larger group of mares, the significance of GnRH treatment to EED was not detected.

Uterine Environment

An abnormal uterine environment is detrimental to embryonic survival. Acute endometritis may result in EED by inducing premature luteolysis or because of its direct effect on the embryo. Severe periglandular fibrosis of the uterine glands appears to be associated with uterine inactivity and advanced age. This is one of the reasons for the reduced fertility of mares older than 12 years of age.

FOAL HEAT BREEDING AND LACTATION. Mares normally resume cyclic ovarian activity shortly after parturition, so that they are sometimes bred as early as 7–10 days post partum (at the foal heat). There is conflicting evidence about the level of embryonic death when fertilization occurs at this time, with some studies showing a higher rate and others no effect. An advantage of breeding at the first estrus post partum is that the foaling-to-conception interval is significantly shorter. Mares bred in foal heat may have reduced fertility because of the hostile uterine environment caused by delayed uterine involution or persistent endometritis. However, pregnancy rates are clearly influenced by the strictness of the selection criteria for mating at the foal heat. Traditionally, such factors as a normal foaling, placental expulsion, minimal vaginal bruising, and absence of infection have been used. Endometrial cytology and ultrasonic scanning of the genital tract of each mare may be more reliable methods on which to base a decision. More pregnancy failures are detected in lactating than non-lactating (maiden or barren) mares; this phenomenon also increases with the age of the mare. The combination of estrus cycle irregularities, uterine contamination, and energy demands influence embryo survival.

Embryonic Factors

Embryonic abnormalities are also important to consider in relation to embryonic death. Embryos recovered from subfertile mares are smaller and have more morphologic defects than embryos from fertile mares; however, this may be due to an abnormal uterine environment. Certain morphologic features detected with ultrasound are typical of mares in which embryonic death is occurring. Some of the consistent features include (1) presence of fluid within the uterine lumen, (2) prominent endometrial edema, (3) decreased or prolonged conceptus mobility, (4) undersized or irregularly shaped conceptus, (5) cessation of embryonic heartbeat, (6) reduced volume of placental fluids (Fig. 13-12, *A*), (7) disorganization of placental membranes (Fig. 13-12, *B*), and (8) hyperechogenic areas in the

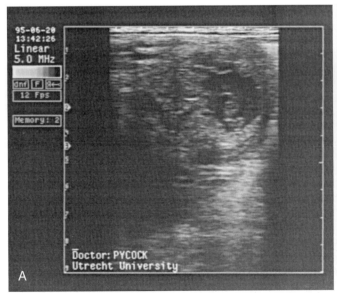
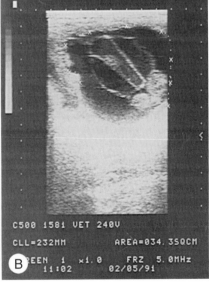

Figure 13-12. A, Ultrasonographic image illustrating gestational failure in a 36-day pregnancy. Note the reduction of expected volume of embryonic fluid. **B,** Ultrasonographic image illustrating gestational failure in a 42-day pregnancy. Note the disruption of the fetal membranes (amnion and allantochorion).

embryo and membranes. A detailed discussion on early pregnancy can be found in Chapter 19.

Fetal Death and Abortion

An overall abortion rate after 60 days of gestation of 10% is usually cited for the horse. The causes of equine abortion can be broadly divided into non-infectious (70%), infectious (15%), and unknown (15%). In practice, it is important to distinguish infectious from non-infectious causes. Vaginal discharge, premature lactation, and colic in pregnant mares may indicate an impending or recent abortion. When abortion occurs, the mare should be isolated, a history obtained, and the fetus sent to an approved laboratory for autopsy. If a veterinarian wishes to perform a postmortem examination, small but representative samples of liver, lung, thymus, spleen, and chorioallantois (two samples, one of which is from the cervical star, which is the irregular, star-shaped avillous area of the chorion that lies over the internal os of the cervix) should be sent in formalin saline for histologic examination. In addition, frozen samples of fresh fetal liver and lung should be stored in a deep freeze in case viral isolation investigation is required at a later stage. Paired serum samples from the mare and close companions should also be obtained for serologic investigation. Swabs from fetal heart or liver and the cervical pole of the chorion are used to screen for bacterial infection. The fetus and fetal membranes (amnion, chorioallantois, and umbilical cord) must be examined carefully for the presence of abnormalities and areas of discoloration. Placental evaluation in the field has been described by Cottrill[31] and is addressed in Chapter 22. Detailed description of abortion in mares can be found in Acland[32] and is discussed in Chapter 21.

Mare Reproductive Loss Syndrome

In 2001 and 2002, large numbers of first and last trimester fetal losses occurred in mares in Kentucky. In addition to the reproductive losses, other systemic problems such as pericarditis were observed in the mares. The term *mare reproductive loss syndrome (MRLS)* was given to the condition. Although much remains to be learned about the syndrome, ingestion of the eastern tent caterpillar otitis feces seems to be directly associated with the syndrome.[33]

Endometritis

The local inflammatory process in the lumen of the uterus, endometritis, is a physiological process, but it is also a major cause of fertility reduction. Both acute and chronic endometritis have been recognized for many years in brood mares. This subfertility is due to an unsuitable environment within the uterus for the developing conceptus. Endometritis can be an acute or a chronic inflammatory process and in general develops because of the establishment of microbial contamination. However, there are also non-infectious causes of endometritis. Infectious endometritis is one of the main obstacles limiting reproductive efficiency in horses. The ability of mares to "fight" bacterial contaminants or inflammatory products from the uterus has resulted in the classification of susceptible or resistant mares with persistent acute endometritis following breeding.

Cause and Pathogenesis

The underlying cause of endometritis determines the type of treatment to be used, and the following classification system for equine endometritis is useful:
1. Acute infectious endometritis
2. Chronic infectious endometritis
3. Endometrosis (chronic degenerative endometritis)
4. Persistent mating-induced endometritis (PMIE; also referred to as delayed uterine clearance)

It is generally assumed that the uterine lumen of the normal fertile mare is bacteriologically sterile or may have a temporary, non-resident microflora, despite the fact that the mare's reproductive tract is often contaminated with bacteria from the act of coitus, foaling, and/or veterinary procedures. Mares with defective vulvar conformation can also aspirate air and bacteria into the vagina, which can develop into endometritis. The bacteria can gain access into the uterus either as (1) contaminants and commensals, (2) opportunist, causing an acute endometritis, and (3) venereally transmitted. Normally, the vestibular and clitoral areas have a harmless and constantly fluctuating bacterial population. In association with benign saprophytic organisms, opportunistic organisms such as *Streptococcus zooepidemicus*, *Escherichia coli*, and *Staphylococcus* spp. can be found. The stallion's penis is colonized by similar organisms. *Str. zooepidemicus* is the most commonly isolated bacterial species from acute endometritis, particularly in the initial stages. *E. coli* is the next most common isolate. When the uterus is contaminated with bacteria, there is a rapid influx of neutrophils.[34] Normally, these neutrophils phagocytose and kill the bacteria rapidly (within 24 hours). These inflammatory by-products are then mechanically removed from the endometrium by rhythmical and frequent uterine contractions. Susceptible mares have a DUC and the inflammatory by-products accumulate as uterine fluid. Such mares have a reduced pregnancy rate because of an unsuitable environment for the early developing conceptus. In addition to opportunist pathogens, three bacteria are venereally transmitted: *Taylorella equigenitalis* (contagious equine metritis organism [CEMO]), *Klebsiella pneumoniae* (capsular types 1, 2, and 5), and *Pseudomonas aeruginosa* (some strains).

Asymptomatic carriers of both sexes allow persistence within the horse population. Mares can harbor the organisms in the vestibular area, particularly the clitoral fossa and sinuses and, at the time of mating or of gynecologic examination, may transfer the organisms into the uterus.[35] Stallions may harbor the organisms over the entire surface of the penis and in the distal urethra. Control is performed by routine screening of swabs obtained before mating in laboratories experienced in the isolation and identification of these organisms.

Anaerobic bacteria have been isolated from the mare's uterus, with *Bacterioides fragilis* being the most frequent.[36] Further work is needed to assess the importance of anaerobes in endometritis.

Venereal Disease Screening

It is customary in the United Kingdom, before the breeding season, to swab the clitoral fossa and clitoral sinuses (only the central sinus may be obvious) and the vestibule. The perineal area of the mare should not be cleaned except for wiping with a dry paper towel to remove gross contamination of the vulva with feces. The veterinary surgeon should wear a protective disposable glove on the hand used to evert the ventral commissure of the vulva and to expose the clitoris. The swabs should be placed in transport medium, clearly labeled with the mare's name, and sent to an approved laboratory. It is important to penetrate the clitoral sinus; therefore, a large swab tip should not be used. Swabs are cultured aerobically on blood and MacConkey agar to screen for the presence of *K. pneumoniae* and *P. aeruginosa*. Microaerophilic culture on chocolate blood agar (with and without streptomycin) each must also be performed for the detection of *T. equigenitalis*. In addition, in stallions, two sets of swabs each must be obtained from the pre-ejaculatory fluid (if possible), penile sheath, urethra, and urethral fossa.

The code of practice described previously for Thoroughbred mares does not apply to North America.

Endometrial Culture and Cytology

A diagnosis of endometritis can be made by collection of concurrent endometrial swab and smear samples during early estrus for bacteriologic culture and cytologic examination, respectively. This allows time for resolution before mating and maximizes the chances of pregnancy. The ideal technique should ensure that the swab enters the uterus and collects bacteria from only the uterine lumen. It is important to ensure that the method of swabbing does not introduce bacteria into a previously normal uterus. Two methods can be used:

1. A non-guarded endometrial swab on a sterile extension rod is carefully passed via a sterile speculum through the cervix into the uterine body and, after withdrawal, is placed in transport medium. A second swab culture is obtained immediately afterward for the endometrial smear.
2. A guarded swab is passed into the uterine lumen using a sterile speculum or enclosed in a disposable plastic arm-length glove. The swab tip is exposed only when it is in the uterine lumen. A swab specimen for cytologic examination should again be obtained. To reduce the risk of contamination, the use of guarded swabs is advised.

Swabs for culture should be plated on blood and MacConkey agar and incubated at 37°C for 48 hours. Cultures should be examined at 24 and 48 hours. An air-dried smear is made by gently rolling the second swab either on a Testsimplet (Minitube, Verona, WI), which is a pre-stained slide, or on a clean dry microscope slide. The smear can be differentially stained with a rapid stain such as Diff-Quick (EV-Vet, Shropshire, UK). The stained smear should then be examined for the presence of inflammatory and endometrial cells (Fig. 13-13), the latter confirming contact of the swab with the endometrium.

The veterinarian must ensure that the mare is not pregnant before passing a swab through the cervix.

INTERPRETATION. A positive culture result, with no evidence of inflammatory cells in the smear (usually neutrophils), could be considered the result of a contaminant during collection. Diagnosis of acute endometritis is based on the presence or absence of significant numbers of neutrophils in the smear. Mares that have more than five neutrophils per high-power field (×40) on a cytology smear should be considered to have active endometritis.

If a pathogen is present in the uterus, the mare's immune system will usually, but not always, mount a response and neutrophils will be observed in a cytology sample. However, some bacteria will elicit a very low or no inflammatory reaction. Therefore, veterinarians must be aware that if bacteria are cultured from the uterus with proper techniques, the result should be considered significant since there is no "normal flora" in the uterus.[37] It has recently been reported that in some cases a positive culture with a negative cytology warrants treatment.[38] In cases where a mare

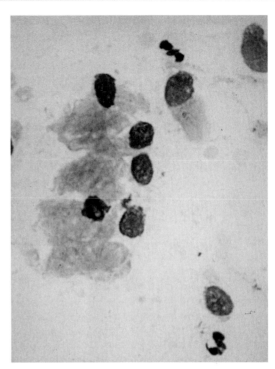

Figure 13-13. Stained endometrial smear showing inflammatory and endometrial cells.

is showing clinical evidence of endometritis, but no evidence can be detected using traditional swab and smear techniques, culture of an endometrial biopsy or a low-volume endometrial flush can provide useful diagnostic information.

Endometrial Histology

In some cases, endometrial biopsy may be a useful diagnostic aid. For detailed reviews of the clinical application and pathologic findings, see Kenney[39] and Ricketts.[40] The technique involves the insertion of a biopsy instrument through the cervix and into the uterus. With the biopsy instrument in the uterine lumen, a gloved hand is inserted into the rectum to allow manipulation of the instrument into the desired position. The sample is obtained by closing the jaws of the instrument and tugging sharply. To avoid damage, the tissue is carefully transferred into a fixative solution by dislodging it from the jaws of the punch with a fine hypodermic needle. The instrument most commonly used is the Yeoman (basket-jawed) biopsy forceps, ideally 60–70 cm in length, with which tissue specimens 2 × 3 × 1 cm (about 0.2% of the whole endometrial surface) are obtained. If the uterus appears normal on palpation, the sample should be obtained from one of the areas of embryo fixation—that is, the uterine hom-body junction on either side. Single samples are usually representative of the entire endometrium. If the uterus is abnormal on palpation per rectum, biopsy samples should be obtained from both the affected area and a normal area. Biopsy specimens should be fixed in Bouin's solution, followed by sectioning and staining with hematoxylin and eosin. The endometrial biopsy sample should be sent to a laboratory that is experienced in evaluating such samples.

Uterine Luminal Fluid

Since the first description of the identification, through the use of ultrasound of small volumes of intrauterine fluid that could not be palpated per rectum,[8] general awareness of the frequency of this abnormality has increased. The detection of uterine fluid during both estrus and diestrus has been reported.[41] Endometrial secretions and the formation of the small volume of free fluid may be associated with the same mechanism that causes normal estral edema. In many cases, the uterine luminal fluid that accumulates before mating is sterile and contains no neutrophils.[42] The importance of these sterile fluid accumulations is that, although initially sterile, the fluid may act as a culture medium for bacteria that gain entry to the uterus at mating to multiply and may be spermicidal.[43] The amount of fluid that should be considered significant is not clear, and it may be that the *quantity* of fluid is more important than *nature* of the fluid. This is particularly true of fluid appearing during estrus. The significance depends to some extent on when during estrus the fluid is observed; fluid detected early in estrus may have disappeared when the mare is further advanced in estrus and the cervix relaxes more. Small volumes of intrauterine fluid during estrus do not affect pregnancy rates, in contrast to mares with larger (>2-cm depth) collections of fluid.[42] In mares that are susceptible to endometritis, there is an accumulation of more fluid than in resistant mares.

Generally, if there is >1 cm of fluid during estrus, some attempt should be made to remove this before breeding using oxytocin. If the volume is >2 cm, the fluid may need to be drained and investigated for the presence of inflammatory cells and bacteria. The mare may then need to have a large-volume uterine lavage. Intrauterine fluid during diestrus indicates inflammation and is associated with subfertility as a result of EED and a shortened luteal phase.[44]

Intraluminal uterine fluid can be graded I to IV according to the degree of echogenicity (Fig. 13-14). The more echogenic the fluid, the more likely the fluid is contaminated with debris, including white blood cells. However, cellular fluid can appear relatively anechogenic, so care is needed in interpretation. Inspissated pus can be so echogenic that it is overlooked. The actual appearance of the fluid and the ultrasonographic appearance might not be as closely linked as was once thought. Ultrasonographic appearance may be proportional to the size and concentration of particulate matter within the fluid, rather than the viscosity of the fluid (e.g., purulent exudates can appear non-echogenic). Air has hyperechogenic foci, and fluid with air bubbles appears cellular. Urine in the bladder can appear echogenic, despite being a watery liquid (Fig. 13-15).

Detection of Intraluminal Uterine Fluid Using Transrectal Ultrasound Imaging.

Transrectal ultrasonography provides a rapid, non-invasive method of assessing the uterus. In a study involving the ultrasonic examination, cytologic and bacteriologic sampling of the uterus in 380 brood mares before mating, Pycock and Newcombe[42] concluded the following:

1. If no free fluid is detected during estrus, acute endometritis as detected in cytologic study is absent in 99% of cases.
2. Free fluid does not always indicate inflammation.
3. Endometrial cytologic study and culture fail to detect sterile fluid accumulations.

Therefore, in mares that are particularly susceptible to endometritis and in which vaginal contact should be minimized,

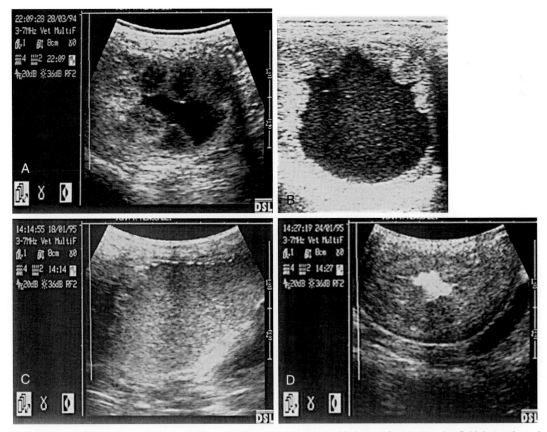

Figure 13-14. A, Ultrasonographic image of grade I uterine fluid: anechogenic. **B,** Ultrasonographic image of grade II uterine fluid: hypoechogenic with hyperechogenic particles. **C,** Ultrasonographic image of grade III uterine fluid: moderately echogenic. **D,** Image of hyperechogenic fluid in the uterus of an infected mare.

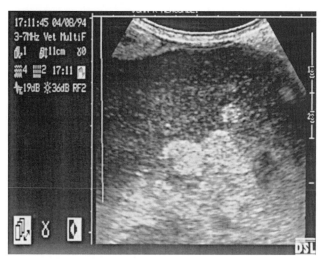

Figure 13-15. Ultrasonographic image of a full urinary bladder.

endometritis can often be diagnosed on the basis of intrauterine fluid accumulation. This is more meaningful when the mare has already been swabbed and cleared of potential venereal diseases. If fluid is present in the uterus, there is vulvar discharge, or the mare has abnormally short luteal phases, uterine swabs should be taken to determine the cause of these symptoms.

MUCOCILIARY ACTIVITY

Recently, Causey[45] speculated on the influence of mucociliary activity on the uterine defense mechanism. This author indicated that mucus plays a mechanical role in the defense mechanism of organ systems such as the respiratory system. Mucus traps particles and carries them long distances. However, for mucus to have the proper activity, it must be a continuum with adequate elasticity and viscosity. Mucus overhydration will disrupt the elasticity and viscosity, breaking that continuum. Since the endometrium has mucoid-producing cells, it is not inconceivable that that mucus could be involved in the mechanism of uterine defense. So a speculative pathogenesis of the disruption in mucociliary defense mechanism could start with a poor perineal conformation, disturbance of myoelectrical contractility, and/or cervical incompetence. These anatomical problems would lead to fluid accumulation, uterine dilation, and mucus overhydration. Furthermore, it is known that mucus elasticity and viscosity can be affected by the type of bacteria. For example, *Str. zooepidemicus* decreases mucus viscosity, thus breaking the continuum, whereas *K. pneumoniae* increases mucus viscosity, thereby decreasing the ability of cilia to move the mucus.

Venereal Infections and Chronic Infectious Endometritis

Any mare suspected of having a venereal infection must not be bred. In the case of clitoral or vestibular infections, topical treatment is used. This involves thorough cleaning with chlorhexidine surgical scrub (for *T. equigenitalis*) or a non-antiseptic soap (for *K. pneumoniae* and *P. aeruginosa*) followed by the application of nitrofurazone ointment for *T. equigenitalis*, 1% aqueous solution of hypochlorite and gentamicin cream for *K. pneumoniae*, or silver nitrate and gentamicin cream for *P. aeruginosa*. Treatment should be for at least 5 days and up

to 10 days. These pathogens, particularly *K. pneumoniae* and *P. aeruginosa*, are difficult to eliminate from the clitoris; hence, clitoral sinusectomy or clitorectomy, followed by daily medical treatment as outlined previously, may be a more appropriate first line of treatment. A broth culture containing a mixture of growing organisms prepared from the normal clitoral flora can suppress venereal pathogens in some cases. Evidence for the successful elimination of infection is based on three negative sets of clitoral and endometrial swabs, taken at weekly intervals. Swabbing should start 7 days after the end of treatment.

Mares with uterine infections are treated with 5–7 days of intrauterine irrigation with an appropriate antibiotic based on the infecting organism's *in vitro* antibiotic sensitivity pattern.

Chronic infectious endometritis is found most frequently in older mares that have had several foals. Such mares have a breakdown in uterine defense mechanisms that allows the normal genital flora to contaminate the uterus and develop into persistent endometritis. The approach to treatment most favored by practitioners has been the infusion of various antibiotics, dissolved or suspended in water or saline, into the uterine lumen during estrus. The intrauterine route is preferable to systemic therapy because most acute endometritis cases are localized. Systemic treatment alone or in combination with local application is suitable in a few circumstances. Ideally, the choice of antibiotic for local treatment should be based on *in vitro* antibiotic sensitivity tests. However, in many cases, this is not possible and a broad-spectrum combination, which is effective against the mixed aerobic and anaerobic infections that commonly occur, should be used. A buffered, water-soluble antibiotic combination dissolved in 30 ml of sterile water and then instilled through the cervix into the uterus via a sterile irrigation catheter is a sufficient volume to cover the entire endometrial surface in most mares. A larger volume (up to 80 ml) may be better in older, pluriparous mares to ensure distribution throughout the uterus. Larger volumes will flow back out through the cervix and be lost. The use of broad-spectrum, non-irritant, soluble preparations has not resulted in superinfection with *Pseudomonas* spp., *Klebsiella* spp., yeasts, or fungi. The number of treatments required depends on individual circumstances, but daily infusions for 3–5 days during estrus works well in most cases. The success of this treatment can be monitored using ultrasonography to identify the presence of intrauterine fluid. When antibiotics are combined with oxytocin, a single daily treatment for 3 days has been successful in many cases. Repeated endometrial swab and smear examinations may be used to monitor the response to therapy; however, every time the cervix is breached, there is the risk of introducing more bacteria. An indwelling intrauterine device that can retain a narrow-diameter infusion catheter within the cervix has been used; however, there is a risk of ascending infection.

In addition to the antibiotic therapy, repeated treatment with $PGF_{2\alpha}$ increases the frequency of the follicular phases, thus allowing intrauterine therapy to be used more readily. It also reduces the duration of the luteal phase when progesterone increases the susceptibility to infection.

Recently, immunomodulators have been suggested as useful adjunct therapy in treatment of endometritis in the broodmare.[46-48] Available products use *Propionibacterium acnes* or a *Mycobacterium* cell wall extract. The mechanism by which fertility may be improved is not clear.

Predisposing causes to the persistent endometritis, such as defective vulval conformation, also deserve attention.

Fungal Infections

Mycotic endometritis is not as common as that of bacteriologic origin, but recognition of a fungus as the causal agent is important in that commonly used intrauterine antibiotic therapy is ineffective. In cases of fungal endometritis, mares may have a history of normal or abnormal estrous cycles, they may be anestrus or barren, and they may have had a recent abortion or a fetal membrane retention; there may be a history of repeated intrauterine antibiotic therapy. Yeasts more frequently cause endometritis than molds; *Candida albicans* is the most common isolate.

The diagnosis is based on the presence of fungal elements and inflammatory cells in endometrial smears. In addition, yeasts can also be identified following staining with Diff-Quick, using a magnification of ×400. Fungal elements are more readily identified in endometrial biopsy specimens following staining with Gomori's methenamine silver or periodic acid–Schiff (PAS). Successful culture of endometrial smears for fungi can be difficult because the organisms may be present in low numbers; furthermore, they require a long incubation period.

These infections are difficult to treat, particularly if they are chronic or deep-seated infections and tend to recur. Intrauterine lavage with 2 to 3 L of warm saline, followed by antimycotic preparations such as tamed povidone-iodine (1%–2% solution daily for 5 days), nystatin (200,000–500,000 U daily for 5 days), or clotrimazole (400–600 mg every other day for 12 days), has been used with limited success. Selection of the correct treatment should be based on sensitivity results. Uterine irrigation with vinegar or dilute acetic acid has shown anecdotal success, presumably by altering the uterine pH. Most fungi have a plasma membrane surrounded by a cell wall made of chitin. Chitin inhibitors such as lufenuron have been reportedly used with some success.[49] However, recent studies have suggested that lufenuron does not appear to have good antifungal properties.[50] This author suggests that Nikkomycin Z, another chitin inhibitor, may be useful, particularly in conjunction with itraconazole, but cautions against recommending intrauterine chitin inhibitors until further research is done.

The prognosis for the subsequent fertility of mares with mycotic endometritis is guarded to poor for future fertility. If there is no success in eliminating the yeast or fungal infection after three attempts, the owner must be advised of the unlikely chance of success. It is suggested that a normal healthy uterus can eliminate mycotic infection; this means that even if the mycotic infection is successfully treated, the mare must be treated as a susceptible mare.

Endometrosis

At the First International Symposium on Equine Endometritis, Kenney[51] suggested that the term *endometrosis* should not be applied to the degenerative changes within the endometrium often associated with age and parity. The old term *chronic degenerative endometritis* should be replaced by *endometrosis*. Endometrosis can, therefore, be defined as the collective term to describe the wide range of degenerative changes (fibrosis and glandular degenerative changes), and the condition is diagnosed by endometrial biopsy.

Successful treatment of endometrosis is difficult. Improved fertility after endometrial curettage has been reported. This has involved the use of mechanical and chemical agents (namely povidone-iodine and kerosene) that cause endometrial necrosis.

This treatment, apart from being of questionable efficacy, can cause irreversible damage (e.g., adhesions). Repeated daily lavage with 2–3 L of hot (50°C), sterile, isotonic saline has been suggested as a method of reducing the size of the lymphatics and thereby the whole uterus. The prognosis for fertility remains poor regardless of the treatment used.

Persistent Mating-Induced Endometritis

PMIE is the most common cause of reproductive failure in mares, particularly older mares and mares being bred for the first time in their teenage years.

Uterine Defense Mechanisms

At coitus, the mare's uterine lumen becomes contaminated with microorganisms and debris. Even if mares are bred by artificial insemination, semen is deposited directly into the uterus. In addition, studies have shown that spermatozoa without bacterial contamination induce a uterine inflammatory response.[52,53] These authors showed that the intensity of the reaction was dependent on the concentration and/or volume of the inseminate—that is, concentrated semen (e.g., frozen semen) induced a stronger inflammatory reaction in the uterus than fresh or extended semen. Parlevliet and co-workers,[54] who measured the inflammatory response following insemination with raw semen, extended semen, and various extenders, concluded that the intensity of the inflammatory response following insemination depends on the sperm themselves rather than any extender. The inflammatory reaction of the uterus is not different for live or dead spermatozoa.[55] Seminal plasma is known to modulate the endometrial immune response either beneficially[56] or adversely.[57] Recently it has been suggested that the time pattern of the endometrial immune response depends on the stimulus.[58]

In most mares, this transient endometritis resolves spontaneously within 24–72 hours so that the environment of the uterine lumen is compatible with embryonic and fetal life. It is important not to regard this endometritis as a pathologic condition. Rather, it is a physiological reaction to clear excess sperm, seminal plasma, and inflammatory debris from the uterus before the embryo descends from the oviduct into the uterine lumen 5.5 days after fertilization.

However, if the endometritis persists after day 4 or 5 of diestrus, in addition to being incompatible with embryonic survival, the premature release of $PGF_{2\alpha}$ results in luteolysis and a rapid decline of progesterone and an early return to estrus. These mares are referred to as susceptible, and a persistent endometritis persists.[41]

The concept of susceptibility to endometritis was first suggested by Farrelly and Mullaney,[59] who stated that infective endometritis is essentially the failure of an individual mare to limit the uterine and cervical microflora to a nonresident type. Hughes and Loy[60] developed this concept and confirmed that resistant mares could eliminate induced infection without treatment, whereas susceptible mares could not. In general, reduced resistance to endometritis is associated with advancing age and multiparity. Susceptibility to endometritis is not an absolute state because failure of uterine defense mechanisms need only slow the process of eliminating infection. In practice, a wide range of susceptibility to endometritis is seen, and it must not be thought that mares can be neatly packaged into "resistant" or "susceptible" categories.[61] Studies on immunoglobulins, opsonins, and the functional ability of neutrophils in the uterus of susceptible mares have not confirmed the presence of an impaired immune response (see the review by Allen and Pycock[62]). Evans and co-workers[63] first suggested that reduced physical drainage may contribute to an increased susceptibility to uterine infection. The physical ability of the uterus to eliminate bacteria, inflammatory debris, and fluid has come to be known as the critical factor in uterine defense. It is a logical conclusion that any impairment of this function (i.e., defective myometrial contractility) renders a mare susceptible to persistent endometritis.[64-66]

The reason susceptible mares have this defective contractility is not known. It has been suggested that the regulation of muscle contraction by the nervous system may be impaired.[67] The resulting fluid accumulation could be due to failure to drain via the cervix or decreased reabsorption by lymphatic vessels. Lymphatic drainage could play an important role in the persistence of post-breeding inflammation, and it is interesting that lymphatic lacunae (lymph stasis) is a common finding in endometrial biopsy specimens obtained from susceptible mares.[39,68]

The difference between resistant and susceptible mares has recently been reviewed by Causey.[69]

Detection of the Susceptible Mare

Detection of the susceptible mare is essential for successful breeding, but it can be difficult because there may only be subtle changes in the uterine environment, not readily detected by current diagnostic procedures. Many mares show no signs of inflammation before mating but fail to resolve the inevitable endometritis that follows mating.

Response to bacterial challenge has been used in a research setting. History is perhaps the most useful indicator of a susceptible mare in practice. Demonstration of clearance failure using scintigraphy and other methods based on charcoal clearance has been used to make an accurate diagnosis that a mare has a clearance problem,[66] but such methods are difficult to apply in practice. Use of ultrasonography to detect uterine luminal fluid has also proved useful to identify mares with a clearance problem and appears to be the most useful technique in practice. The presence of free intraluminal fluid before breeding strongly suggests susceptibility to persistent endometritis.[42] It has been suggested that excessive production of fluid resulting from glandular alterations may cause intrauterine fluid accumulation rather than a failure of lymphatic drainage.[70] However, it is currently not known whether the fluid accumulates because of an excess production, a delay in physical clearance via the open cervix, or a decrease in reabsorption by lymphatic vessels. It may well involve a combination of all three.

Treatment Options for the Susceptible Mare

The aim of the treatment should be to assist the uterus to physically clear the debris, contaminants, and excess sperm as well as the normal inflammatory by-products of the response to breeding. Because the spermatozoa necessary for fertilization are present within the oviduct within 4 hours of mating and because the embryo does not descend into the uterus for about 5.5 days, mares may safely undergo treatment from 4 hours after mating until 2 days from ovulation, as long as isotonic solutions are used. Progesterone concentrations increase rapidly after ovulation in the mare and it is preferable to avoid treatment involving uterine interference beyond 2 days after ovulation. Both coitus

and artificial insemination can be a source of uterine contamination; it is well known that spermatozoa themselves are responsible for initiating a marked inflammatory response. The successful management of susceptible mares should logically require some form of post-mating therapy such as intrauterine antibiotic infusion, uterine lavage, and intravenous oxytocin; these may be used alone or in combination. The emphasis should be on treatment in relation to breeding and not ovulation. Too often in the past veterinarians have waited until ovulation before treating these mares. By then, there has usually been a large accumulation of fluid and the bacteria are in a logarithmic phase of growth.

Uterine Lavage

Recognition of the importance of the mechanical evacuation of uterine contents accounted for the introduction of large-volume uterine lavage. The technique involves the mechanical suction or siphonage of 2–3 L of previously warmed (to 42°C) sterile physiologic (buffered) saline or lactated Ringer's solution infused into the uterus via a catheter that has been retained within the cervix via a cuff. The most convenient is a large-bore (30 French, 80 cm) autoclavable equine embryo flushing catheter (EUF-80, Bivona, IN) (Fig. 13-16). The cuff is useful because it effectively seals the internal cervical os. The catheter should be inserted only after thorough cleansing of the perineum. Such an approach accomplishes the following:

1. Removes accumulated uterine fluid and inflammatory debris, which may interfere with neutrophil function and the efficacy of antibiotics
2. Stimulates uterine contractility
3. Recruits fresh neutrophils through mechanical irritation of the endometrium

The fluid is infused by gravity flow 1 L at a time and the washings inspected to provide immediate information concerning the nature of the uterine contents. The lavage should be repeated until the fluid recovered is clear. In most cases, the fluid evenly distributes in both horns, making transrectal massage of the uterus unnecessary. If a rectal examination is performed while the catheter is in the uterus, the veterinarian should be very careful to avoid contaminating the catheter. The fluid should be recovered into the same container in which it was infused, thereby preventing air from being aspirated into the uterus via the catheter. Measurement of the recovered fluid and ultrasonographic examination of the uterus should be performed after flushing to ensure that all the fluid has been recovered. This is necessary because the mare has an impaired ability to spontaneously drain the uterus. For this reason, the process is usually combined with oxytocin injection. Ideally, these mares are bred only once, but if repeated matings are necessary, uterine lavage should be performed after each mating. Previous uterine lavage does not adversely affect a second breeding.[71]

Large volume lavage is beneficial in many cases, particularly in the mare with a relatively large accumulation of fluid (>2 cm depth) after breeding. The process is time consuming, and there is the possibility of further contamination of the uterus by passage of a drainage tube. Nonetheless, when there is >2 cm of uterine fluid or a mare is known to be highly susceptible, the risks are outweighed by the benefit of treatment.[72]

Studies have shown that saline lavage and uterotonic drugs such as $PGF_{2\alpha}$ are as effective as antibiotics in eliminating bacteria from the uterus.[73] However, this was a controlled experimental type situation in which a single bacterial species was infused

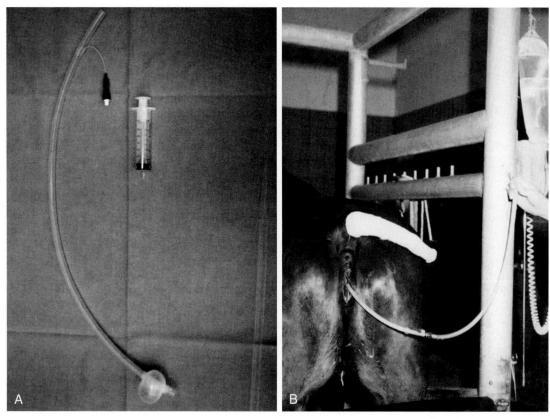

Figure 13-16. A, Large-bore (30-French) embryo flushing catheter, 80 cm in length. Note the inflated cuff. **B,** Performing large-volume uterine lavage with a large-bore catheter in position.

into the uterus and lavage was within 12 hours of mating. Under normal clinical conditions, there is a mixed bacterial contamination, and lavage cannot always be performed within 12 hours. I prefer to continue to use intrauterine antibiotics as part of the therapeutic protocol.

Oxytocin

The ideal method of treatment involves the use of a non-invasive technique with early and complete elimination of any intrauterine fluid. Oxytocin stimulates uterine contractions in the cyclic, pregnant, and postpartum mare and was first suggested to promote uterine drainage in mares with defective uterine clearance by Allen.[74] Until then, oxytocin was not considered to be an appropriate treatment for endometritis, probably because it was thought by many that oxytocin-induced uterine contractions occur only in the first 48 hours after foaling. Also, use of oxytocin was discouraged because of the worry that it would cause severe colic.

However, after the pioneering study of Allen,[74] subsequent clinical experience[70,75-78] has allayed early fears that oxytocin would cause colic when given as an intravenous bolus. All these workers reported improved pregnancy rates in susceptible mares after oxytocin administration. Oxytocin therapy should be used wherever free uterine fluid is detected before or after breeding. I give a dose of oxytocin of 25 international units (IU) for large mares (>600 kg) and 20 IU for average size Thoroughbred, Standardbred, Quarterhorse, and Warmblood mares and all pony mares either intravenously (IV) or intramuscularly (IM). There is no advantage in using more than 25 IU, and it may even be that the same effect can be obtained by use of 10 IU as long as treatment is occurring during the preovulatory

period.[79] Although the initial change in intrauterine pressure appeared more pronounced with a larger (25 IU) dose of oxytocin at 5 and 10 minutes after treatment, the change in pressure at subsequent time intervals was similar between the two doses (25 IU and 10 IU). These authors also found a significant effect of day of administration of oxytocin on the uterine response, with a weaker response when oxytocin was administered after ovulation. Later work by these authors confirmed that myometrial activity and the increase in intrauterine pressure after exogenous oxytocin are inversely related to the concentration of progesterone.[80] Although it is preferable to treat mares with uterine clearance problems before ovulation, when oxytocin is used after ovulation the larger dose of 25 IU should be used for all mares.

No untoward effects have been noted except for rare mild and transient discomfort. Any possible adverse effect on gamete transport seems to be outweighed by the ability to improve uterine fluid clearance. The half-life of oxytocin has been reported for the mare as 6.8 minutes.[81] In most mares, the response is rapid, with fluid being voided almost immediately.

Oxytocin is known to stimulate prostaglandin release,[66] although the precise mechanism that controls myometrial contraction remains unclear. The uterine response to oxytocin is due in part to direct effect of oxytocin on the myometrium and in part to the indirect effect of oxytocin causing $PGF_{2\alpha}$ release.[81,82]

Support for this dual mode of action comes from the fact that oxytocin has been shown to override the inhibitory effect of phenylbutazone on uterine clearance.[83] Phenylbutazone inhibits prostaglandin synthesis and has been shown to slow uterine clearance in reproductively normal mares.[82] Phenylbutazone is a commonly used drug in brood mares for conditions such as laminitis, and oxytocin would be preferable to $PGF_{2\alpha}$ analogues to improve uterine clearance in mares on phenylbutazone therapy. Even reproductively normal mares receiving phenylbutazone because of lameness should be given oxytocin after breeding.

Prostaglandin Analogues

Because of the relatively short half-life of oxytocin, ecbolic drugs with a longer duration of action have been investigated. Endogenous prostaglandins are released very early in mares with endometritis.[34] The useful role of prostaglandin in increasing myometrial activity and assisting uterine clearance has subsequently been shown.[73,81,84] These latter authors showed that the prostaglandin analogue cloprostenol given at a dose rate of 500 μg IM caused increased clearance of radiocolloid in susceptible mares, but at a significantly slower rate and with a delayed increase in uterine activity than that caused by oxytocin. However, the uterus did contract for a longer time—5 hours vs. 45 minutes. Of the prostaglandins administered ($PGF_{2\alpha}$, cloprostenol, and fenprostalene), cloprostenol produced the most consistent response. Cloprostenol seems to be indicated in mares with lymphatic stasis as shown by excessive fluid within the endometrium or large lymphatic cysts.[83] Uterine edema often persists after ovulation in these mares. The suggested dose of cloprostenol is 250 μg given at 12 and 24 hours after breeding.[85]

When using prostaglandin analogues for the treatment of PMIE, the time of administration relative to ovulation must be considered. It is accepted that the equine corpus luteum is resistant to the luteolytic effect of prostaglandin until 5 or 6 days after ovulation, but this resistance is not absolute. Progesterone concentrations have been reported to be lower in mares for 5–7 days following administration of cloprostenol in the post-ovulatory period compared with mares receiving oxytocin, saline, or sterile water.[86,87] However another study found that cloprostenol could be used to treat post-breeding mares through the second day following ovulation without decreasing pregnancy outcome.[88] This was despite finding an impaired luteal function as evidenced by lower circulating progesterone concentrations. These latter authors only used a dose of 250 μg cloprostenol. Despite this, prostaglandin analogues are best avoided after ovulation.

Long-Acting Oxytocin

Recently a long-acting synthetic analogue of oxytocin, carbetocin, has become commercially available in Europe, Canada, and Mexico. This drug may have an indication in situations where a more prolonged uterine contraction is desired. In a recent study, carbetocin was well tolerated following IV administration of 175 μg to a group of horses.[89] These authors reported the half-life of carbetocin to be 17 minutes, only some 2.5 times that of oxytocin. An earlier study had shown a more prolonged action when compared with oxytocin.[90] Maximum concentrations of carbetocin in plasma were obtained almost 20 minutes later after IM administration of 280 μg compared with 10 IU IV oxytocin. Preliminary clinical work by the author has shown carbetocin to be safe and effective at inducing uterine clearance. Two IM injections of 175 μg carbetocin are given 12 and 24 hours after breeding in mares with marked uterine edema or free fluid before breeding or in mares with uterine fluid >2 cm in depth when examined 12 hours after breeding.

Oxytocin remains the drug of choice in mares that accumulate free intraluminal uterine fluid and is my "first choice" uterotonic drug.

Intrauterine Plasma Infusions

Based on the research findings of the 1970s and 1980s, which emphasized the immunological aspects of the uterine defense mechanisms, intrauterine plasma has been used in the susceptible mare. Studies following its use have indicated an improvement of fertility.[91,92] Both authors suggested that the plasma had an enhancing effect on phagocytosis by uterine neutrophils. Adams and Ginther,[93] in a study that included control groups of mares, found that intrauterine plasma was not efficacious in treating endometritis because there was no improvement in pregnancy rates. In addition, transfer of infectious agents is also possible. Troedsson and colleagues[94] suggested that plasma treatment might only benefit certain susceptible mares. This latter point was also alluded to recently by Pascoe,[92] who, while remaining enthusiastic about the use of plasma in the management of immunoincompetent mares, conceded that this may apply only to mares without a mechanical clearance problem. Consequently, plasma is best used in mares that repeatedly fail to become pregnant but have no history of fluid accumulation. Because mares that are susceptible to endometritis do not possess a quantitative deficiency of immunoglobulins, it is questionable whether such treatment is truly effective.

Intrauterine Antibiotics

The infusion of broad-spectrum antibiotics after breeding is controversial.[42,53,75] At least one scientific experiment in which an endometritis model was used showed that saline lavage and uterotonic drugs such as prostaglandin $F2_\alpha$ are as effective as antibiotics in eliminating bacteria from the uterus.[53] In this controlled experiment-type situation, however, a single bacterial species (usually streptococci) was infused into the uterus and lavage treatment was performed at a fixed time (within 12 hours of mating).

Under normal clinical conditions there is a mixed bacterial contamination and lavage cannot always be performed within 12 hours. This is why the author prefers to continue to use intra- uterine antibiotics as part of the therapeutic protocol. The treatments have entirely different modes of action on the uterus, often resulting in an additive benefit. The uterine lavage provides mechanical evacuation of intraluminal fluid and inflammatory products, whereas the single infusion of broad-spectrum antibiotics should prevent any growth of bacteria introduced during insemination or uterine lavage. Furthermore, mares susceptible to post-breeding endometritis have, according to their history, a reduced capacity of uterine clearance and defense mechanisms. Therefore, they cannot be compared with healthy mares used in experiments. Routine administration of intrauterine antibiotics has no negative effect on pregnancy rate of treated mares.[42,75]

Systemic Antibiotics

There is a paucity of information in the literature about the use of systemic antibiotics in the management of the mare susceptible to PMIE, and their use is not widespread. In certain situations, systemic administration of antibiotics may be useful. Such situations include where it is desired to continue administration after ovulation into the luteal phase because of fluid accumulation persisting or recent urogenital surgery making intrauterine administration of antibiotics difficult. Through the use of usually systemic doses, antibiotics that have been used systemically include the following: procaine penicillin, gentamicin, amikacin, ampicillin, and trimethoprim sulpha.[95]

Corticosteroids

The antigenic nature of spermatozoa in the uterus is well established, and the post-breeding reaction is inflammatory in nature, making it logical that corticosteroids may play a role in modulating the response. The precise nature of the damage caused by this inflammatory response is unknown. It has been reported that seminal plasma has a suppressive effect on complement activation and PMN chemotaxis.[96] Perhaps this is the reason this subject has only been written about recently in the literature, with a group from Brazil describing how the corticosteroid prednisolone modified the uterine response to insemination.[97] The corticosteroid therapy (prednisolone acetate at a dose rate of 0.1mg/kg) was given every 12 hours for a total of five treatments. Four treatments were given before insemination and one treatment at the time of insemination. They concluded that prednisolone treatment led to a reduction in neutrophil function and decreased uterine fluid content. Further work by Papa and colleagues[98] in Brazil indicated corticosteroid therapy to be safe and an option for mares with a history of PMIE, but they concluded further clinical research was necessary. One protocol is to use 200 mg prednisone (not prednisolone) orally once a day starting when ovulation is detected and continuing until pregnancy is determined and then continue until 30 days gestation when the dose is gradually decreased over a period of 4 weeks (K. Wolfsdorf, personal communication, 2007). Recently, Bucca et al.[98a] reported that dexamethasone modulated the inflammatory reaction of the uterus.

The Old Maiden Mare Syndrome

It is particularly important to recognize and manage appropriately the older maiden mare because, in many cases, these mares are susceptible to post-breeding endometritis even though they have never been bred before. Often, sport or Warmblood mares may not be presented to be bred until they are in their teens, and these older maiden mares can be difficult to get pregnant.

Many of these mares have some common characteristics that resemble a syndrome. Endometrial biopsy samples reveal glandular degenerative changes and stromal fibrosis (endometrosis) as an inevitable consequence of aging, despite the fact that these mares have not been bred.[99] Another of the most common characteristics of these mares is the presence of uterine fluid. Often, an older maiden mare has an abnormally tight cervix, which fails to relax properly during estrus so that fluid is unable to drain and accumulates in the uterine lumen.[100] In many cases, this fluid is negative for bacterial growth and presence of neutrophils. Once the mare is bred, the fluid accumulation is aggravated because of poor lymphatic drainage and impaired myometrial contraction compounded by the tight cervix. The amount of intrauterine fluid varies in individual mares, ranging from a few milliliters to more than a liter in extreme cases.

To maximize the fertility of these mares, it is vital that the veterinarian be aware of the possibility of this type of uterine and cervical condition. All too often owners assume that the fertility of these mares is comparable with that of young maiden mares; one of the most important aspects of breeding the old maiden mare is to make the owner aware that there is an increased possibility that she will be a problem. These mares must be considered highly susceptible and managed accordingly.

Management Protocol Useful in the Highly Susceptible Mare

A mare that is known to produce a large amount (several centimeters depth) of luminal fluid after mating should be managed using the following protocol. Overall management of such mares must be excellent before breeding.

Hygiene

Good hygiene at foaling is essential, and all mares should be thoroughly examined post-partum for the presence of trauma that might compromise the physical barriers to uterine contamination. Gynecologic examinations, particularly of the vagina, should be performed as aseptically as possible. Thorough digital examination of the cervix can identify fibrosis, lacerations, or adhesions that may need treatment before breeding. Because air in the vagina can cause irritation of the mucosa, it should be expelled by applying downward pressure with the hand through the rectal wall. Attention to hygiene at mating by using a tail bandage and washing the mare's vulva and perineal area with clean water (ideally from a spray nozzle that avoids the need for buckets) is important.

Correction of Any External Conformation Defects

The mare should be evaluated for any conformational defects, and such defects should be corrected.

Correct Timing of Breeding

Breeding should occur at the optimal time and the number of breedings should be minimized. This means that these mares need very close monitoring of the estrous period by rectal palpation and ultrasonography. Prediction of ovulation is made easier by not breeding these mares too early in the year before they have begun to cycle regularly. The use of ovulation induction agents is strongly recommended in such mares in an attempt to ensure that they are bred only once. If feasible, the use of artificial insemination with fresh semen can be helpful to reduce (but not eliminate) the inevitable post-breeding endometritis.

Ultrasound Evaluation of the Uterus

The uterus should be examined by ultrasound examination to detect intraluminal fluid, in addition to conventional endometrial cytological and bacteriological techniques, before mating. Even if cytological and bacteriological studies have yielded negative results before breeding, mares susceptible to PMIE usually accumulate fluid in the uterine lumen for more than 12 hours after mating. Ultrasound examination of the uterus 3–12 hours after mating is performed to assess the amount and echogenicity of any intrauterine fluid. This examination of mares and treatment given very soon after mating, before the bacteria have been long in a logarithmic growth phase, are important for the susceptible mare.

Tailoring of the Treatment Regimen to the Individual Mares

No standard approach can be given. Susceptibility to endometritis is not an absolute state[61]: failure of the defense mechanisms only needs to be of the degree necessary to slow the process of clearance past a critical point. Because many stud farms are visited on an every-other-day basis for routine reproductive work, treatment schedules should be based around a visit. Most multiparous mares are at risk for either clinical or subclinical endometritis following insemination, whether it is natural or artificial. The treatment adopted should be based on history and clinical findings, including ultrasonographic evaluation of the uterus after breeding.

BEFORE BREEDING. Work has shown that, although initially sterile and free of neutrophils, mares with uterine fluid accumulation before mating have a reduced pregnancy rate when no treatment is performed.[42,75] If >0.5 cm fluid is detected, give 20 IU oxytocin as an intravenous bolus. Confirm that the fluid has gone at the next ultrasound examination. If intraluminal fluid is still visible, repeat the dose of oxytocin and, possibly, digitally dilate the cervix also. If >2 cm of fluid was present, the uterus was lavaged as described earlier. In general, antibiotics before breeding should be avoided because of possible irritant and/or spermicidal action.

A single breeding must be arranged 1–2 (or even 3) days before the anticipated time of ovulation (if natural covering or fresh semen is to be used). It is my experience that most stallion spermatozoa are viable at least 48–72 hours after mating, as supported by the findings of Umphenour et al.[101] In any case, records based on previous early pregnancy examinations will soon indicate if the semen from a particular stallion is not viable after 48 hours. This early mating allows more time for drainage of fluid via an open estrous cervix and uses the natural resistance of the tract to inflammation during estrus. It allows sufficient time to flush the mares more than once before ovulation if necessary. Although uterine lavage is possible after ovulation, it is more complicated since the cervix starts closing. Moreover, the resistance of the tract is reduced and the uterotonic effect of oxytocin is reduced because of the increasing amount of circulating progesterone.[102]

Treatment for endometritis is ideally performed before ovulation. Progesterone concentrations rise rapidly in the mare and any post-ovulation treatment carries an increased risk of uterine contamination. In addition, uterine fluid is less likely to drain if the cervix is beginning to close.

AFTER BREEDING. Doses of 20 IU of oxytocin are given every 4–6 hours, intramuscularly, after breeding by the stud farm personnel. Ultrasound examination of the uterus the following day after mating, or earlier, is performed to assess the amount and echogenicity of any intrauterine fluid. If >2.0 cm of fluid is present in the uterine lumen, lavage of the uterus with warmed, lactated Ringer's solution or buffered, sterile physiological saline via a uterine flushing catheter is performed. This process is repeated two, three, or four times until the effluent is clear. Treatment has been successful as early as 2 hours after mating. The optimum time for uterine lavage therapy in highly susceptible mares was found to be between 4 and 6 hours in a study by Knutti et al.[103] During lavage, intravenous administration of 20 IU oxytocin is given.

When the cervix fails to relax adequately, digital dilation of the cervix, with scrupulous attention to cleanliness, should be performed. This is one reason for ideally giving treatment to the susceptible mare before ovulation; a second reason is that oxytocin is less effective at increasing uterine pressure once the mare has ovulated.[79]

After 20 minutes, the mare should be reexamined and any fluid pooling in the vagina removed. This is followed by infusion of a low volume (25 ml) of water-soluble, broad-spectrum antibiotic such as ceftiofur sodium (1 g) (Excenel, Pfizer) instilled through the cervix into the uterus via a sterile irrigation catheter. Use a low volume of antibiotic solution since, if these mares

have a drainage problem, it seems logical to use the minimum effective volume. Older, pluriparous mares may need larger volumes (up to 50 ml). It is my experience that with larger volumes (>100 ml), some of the solution is lost via cervical reflux. It is vital that the antibiotic used does not irritate the endometrium or predispose to overgrowth with fungal organisms. Neither of these problems has been observed using the antibiotic described here.

Further doses of 20 IU of oxytocin are given every 4–6 hours, intramuscularly, by the stud farm personnel. In mares with lymphatic stasis, the slower release of carbetocin (0.175 mg IM) or prostaglandin (cloprostenol 250 µg IM) may be useful in addition to oxytocin. The carbetocin or prostaglandin should be given some 6–8 hours after the first oxytocin injection.

The mare is reexamined the following day and oxytocin treatment repeated if fluid is still present. Only rarely will a second infusion of antibiotics or lavage procedure be performed because of the risk of uterine contamination. The day after mating is a crucial time to assess all mares, but too many clinicians fail to perform post-breeding evaluation of the uterus. Another important concept is to treat in relation to breeding and not wait for ovulation.

Conclusions

A problem mare, once inseminated or mated, should not only be checked for ovulation, but also for fluid accumulation in the uterus, one of the most reliable clinical signs of susceptibility to post-breeding endometritis. If a mare is recognized as being susceptible to PMIE, intensive post-breeding monitoring and, eventually, treatment are necessary in order to improve the chances of conception. The early post-breeding lavage supported by oxytocin and the infusion of broad-spectrum antibiotics have proved to be an effective management for mares susceptible to mating-induced endometritis.

Some questions remain unanswered. Hearn[104] voiced the concern that the early embryonic or fetal loss rate in susceptible mares with endometritis who receive aggressive post-mating therapy will be much higher despite the temporary improvement in uterine environment. Undoubtedly, the live foal rate in the mares that receive such therapy after breeding is less than in young, genitally healthy mares. Often, however, susceptible mares are old, and uterine biopsy results, when available, frequently confirm degenerative changes within the endometrium. Consequently, live foal rates can be expected to be lower in these mares in any case.

This consideration does not constitute a reason to avoid post-mating treatment, however. Of course the practitioner should optimize the chances for conception by the foregoing methods, but the susceptible mare still requires treatment after mating.

In my daily routine, I assume that most multiparous mares are at risk for either clinical or subclinical endometritis following insemination, be it natural or artificial. Routine post-mating treatment of mares believed to be at risk of persistent acute endometritis is dependent on balancing cost and time against benefits to the breeder. This view is also held by Australian colleagues (e.g., DR Pascoe, personal communication, 1995) who claim increased pregnancy rates and subsequent foaling rates through adoption of a routine post-mating treatment.[92] The results of published clinical studies[42,76,78,92] and field experience with large numbers of mares over several breeding seasons have demonstrated the effectiveness of a single post-mating treatment to combat endometritis. This has certainly been the case in the mares with which I have been involved.

Against this demonstrable improvement in pregnancy rate, a point of concern is whether, apart from economic considerations, routine treatment of all mares after mating is indicated. Certainly management standards must not fall. Post-mating treatment should not be seen as a means of getting away with poor management practices.

No bacterial resistance problems or increase in fungal endometritis must be apparent with the intrauterine antibiotics used. At the first International Symposium on Equine Endometritis, Zent[105] reported that, of 4000 broodmares under the care of members of his Kentucky veterinary practice, all those except maiden mares were routinely given at least one post-mating intrauterine antibiotic infusion. He believed that this treatment had improved pregnancy rates, without the development of a resistance problem or an increased incidence of fungal endometritis.

It is difficult to be dogmatic about determining at what point the susceptible mare should be bred and when she should be treated and either short cycled or bred at the next natural estrus. This must be a matter of clinical experience based on history and findings of clinical and laboratory examinations.

Viral Infectious Disease—Equine Coital Exanthema

In addition to EHV-1, EHV-4, and equine viral arteritis infection, which cause abortion, EHV3 causes a relatively benign venereal disease referred to as coital exanthema; it affects both sexes. There have been reports of its transfer during gynecologic examination.

The virus can remain dormant until conditions favor its proliferation with the development of the characteristic clinical signs. Normally, following coitus, signs develop after an incubation period of 4–7 days. Multiple vesicles appear on the vulval mucosa and perineum, resulting in a short period of local irritation. These rupture, leaving small ulcers 3–10 mm in diameter, which are painful to touch. In the absence of infection with opportunist pathogens, healing occurs in 10–14 days, when the virus ceases to be contagious. There is permanent loss of pigmentation at the site of the healed lesions. Pregnancy rates are not reduced. In the stallion, the vesicles develop on the shaft of the penis and the prepuce; if severe, the stallion may be reluctant to breed.

Treatment consists of immediate sexual rest and the application of an antiseptic powder or spray to prevent secondary bacterial infection; this allows the ulcers to heal. The disease is controlled by withholding breeding of all affected stallions and mares and taking hygienic precautions when handling these animals.

Metritis

Metritis is the inflammation of the entire thickness of the uterine wall. It occurs when there is massive contamination of the uterus, frequently in association with trauma or retained placenta during foaling. It has a grave prognosis, particularly in heavy horses, because the absorption of toxins from the uterine lumen into the general circulation results in systemic signs including pyrexia, depression, loss of appetite, and laminitis. Toxin production is associated with rapid bacterial growth, frequently involving gram-negative organisms. Treatment involves repeated lavage of the uterus with warm sterile saline (2–3 L) several times

per day until it is free of inflammatory exudates and placental debris. Bacterial growth should be controlled to limit toxin production; a broad-spectrum antibiotic effective against *E. coli*, which is invariably present, should be used. Supportive therapy with parenteral antibiotics, antihistamines (in cases of retained placenta), oxytocin, and intravenous fluid therapy is indicated in many cases.

Systemic signs such as pulse rate and mucous membrane color are used to monitor the response to therapy in conjunction with examination of the uterine fluid.

Despite all efforts, some mares die of toxemia or irreversible changes in the foot following laminitis such as pedal-bone rotation.

Pyometra

Pyometra is the accumulation of large quantities of inflammatory exudate in the uterus, causing its distention.[106] It must be distinguished from the smaller, intermittent accumulations of fluid that can be detected by ultrasonography in acute endometritis. Pyometra occurs because of interference with natural drainage of fluid from the uterus, which may be due to cervical adhesions or an abnormally constricted, tortuous, or irregular cervix. In some cases, the fluid accumulates in the absence of cervical lesions, presumably as a result of an impaired ability to eliminate the exudate. Other predisposing factors are chronic infection with *P. aeruginosa* or fungi.

When the endometrium is severely damaged, there is extensive loss of surface epithelium, severe endometrial fibrosis, and glandular atrophy causing a prolonged luteal phase, presumably resulting from interference with the synthesis or release of $PGF_{2\alpha}$. This is in contrast to mild endometritis with collection of small amounts of intraluminal uterine fluid, which is more likely to cause premature release of $PGF_{2\alpha}$ and luteolysis.

Some clinicians restrict the term *pyometra* to cases in which, in addition to the accumulation of exudate within the uterine lumen, the corpus luteum persists beyond its normal life span. Some mares with pyometra have normal, regular cyclic ovarian activity. Persistence of the corpus luteum is probably due to the failure of the synthesis or release of prostaglandins from the uterus. Mares that have prolonged luteal activity have the greatest endometrial damage.

The mare with pyometra seldom shows overt signs of systemic disease, even when there is up to 60 L of exudate in the uterine lumen. Occasionally, there is weight loss, depression, and anorexia. Pyometra has been classified into two categories in mares: open and closed.[107] In a case of closed pyometra, the fluid accumulates because the cervix is closed. In open pyometra, the cervix remains open, but purulent material accumulates because there is impaired uterine clearance. A vulval discharge is often observed in open pyometra, especially at estrus, which may vary in consistency from watery to creamlike. Although the culture of endometrial swabs can sometimes result in the growth of mixed organisms or sometimes no bacterial growth at all, in most cases, the organism isolated is *Str. zooepidemicus*.

The diagnosis of pyometra is based on rectal palpation, ultrasonic examination of an enlarged fluid-filled uterus (Fig. 13-17), and analysis of the uterine fluid. Pregnancy must be ruled out, as should rare conditions such as mucometra and pneumouterus.

Because there is no systemic illness, cases of pyometra have often become chronic before treatment is sought. In such cases, the prognosis is poor because there is severe endometrial

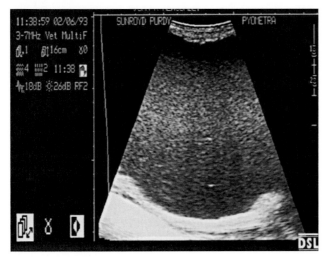

Figure 13-17. Ultrasonographic image of pyometra.

damage, which is unlikely to be able to sustain a normal pregnancy. The aim of treating pyometra is to expel the purulent material from the uterus.

In the absence of systemic illness or an unsightly vulvar discharge, treatment of chronic pyometra may not be indicated, although some mares can show signs of discomfort during exercise.

Many cases can be significantly improved by repeated large-volume lavage with several liters of warm saline via a wide-bore tube, such as a nasogastric tube. Initially, $PGF_{2\alpha}$ can be used to induce luteolysis of the corpus luteum, if present, which should allow the cervix to relax sufficiently for digital exploration for the presence of any adhesions. Estradiol or PGE_2 may also help relax the cervix. A broad-spectrum antibiotic (e.g., Excenel) should be infused after repeated large-volume lavage and oxytocin to achieve drainage of exudate, and an endometrial biopsy is useful in assessing the degree of endometrial damage. Monitoring the uterus by a combination of rectal palpation and ultrasound provides information on the response to treatment. Even if treatment is successful, the mare must be considered a susceptible mare if she is to be bred and managed accordingly.

In non-responsive cases, hysterectomy can be performed following aspiration of the exudate from the uterus, although great care must be taken to prevent contamination of the peritoneal cavity.

REFERENCES

1. Caslick EA: The sexual cycle and its relation to ovulation with breeding records of the Thoroughbred mare. *Cornell Vet* 27:187, 1937.
2. Pouret EJ: Surgical technique for the correction of pneumo and urovagina. *Equine Vet J* 14:249, 1982.
3. Eilts BE, Scholl DT, Paccamonti DL, et al: Prevalence of endometrial cysts and their effect on fertility. *Biol Reprod Monogr* 1:527, 1995.
4. Adams GP, Kastelic JP, Bergfelt DR, et al: Effect of uterine inflammation and ultrasonically-detected uterine pathology on fertility in the mare. *J Reprod Fertil Suppl* 35:445, 1987.
5. Knudsen O: Partial dilatation of the uterus as a cause of sterility in the mare. *Cornell Vet* 54:423, 1964.
6. Kenney RM, Ganjam VK: Selected pathological changes of the mare's uterus and ovary. *J Reprod Fertil Suppl* 23:335, 1975.
7. Stone R, Bracher V, Mathias S: Severe intralumenal uterine adhesions in an eight-year-old barren maiden mare. *Equine Vet Educ* 3:181, 1991.
8. Ginther OJ, Pierson RA: Ultrasonic anatomy and pathology of the equine uterus. *Theriogenology* 21:505, 1984.
9. Ball BA, Brinsko SP, Schlafer DH: Histopathologic examination of the oviduct and endometrium of fertile and subfertile mares. *Pferdeheilkunde* 13:548, 1997.
10. Fiala SM, Amaral MG, Pimentel CA, et al: Inflammatory lesions in the mare's oviducts. *Anim Reprod Sci* 94:265, 2006.
11. Liu IKM, Lantz KC, Schlafke S, et al: Clinical observations of oviductal masses. Proc 36th Annu AAEP Convention. Lexington, KY: 1990, p 41.
12. Allen WR, Wilsher S, Morris L, et al: Re-establishment of oviductal patency and fertility in infertile mares. *Anim Reprod Sci* 94:242, 2006.
13. Bennett SD. Diagnosis of oviductal disorders and diagnostic techniques. In: Samper JC, Pycock JF, McKinnon AO, eds: *Current Therapy in Equine Reproduction.* St Louis: Elsevier, 2007.
14. Steiner J, Antczak DF, Wolfsdorf K, et al: Persistent endometrial cups. *Anim Reprod Sci* 94:274, 2006.
15. Woods J, Bergfelt DR, Ginther OJ: Effect of time of insemination relative to ovulation on pregnancy rate and embryonic loss rate in mares. *Equine Vet J* 22:378, 1990.
16. Blanchard TL, Thompson JA, Brinsko S, et al: Effects of breeding to ovulation interval and repeat service during the same estrus on pregnancy rates in Thoroughbred mares. Proc 53rd Annu AAEP Convention. Orlando: 2007, p 568.
17. Newcombe JR, Cuervo-Aranga J: The effect of interval from mating to ovulation on pregnancy rates and incidence of intra-uterine fluid in the mare. 2008 Poster at ICAR meeting, Budapest. *Reprod Domest Anim* 43:109, 2008.
18. Gastal EL, Gastal MO, Donadeu FX, et al: Temporal relationships among LH, estradiol, and follicle vascularization preceding the first compared with later ovulations during the year in mares. *Anim Reprod Sci* 102:314, 2007.
19. McCue PM, Squires EL: Persistent anovulatory follicles in the mare. *Theriogenology* 58:541, 2002.
20. Vanderwall DK, Woods GL, Freeman DA, et al: Ovarian follicles, ovulations and progesterone concentrations in aged versus young mares. *Theriogenology* 40:21, 1993.
21. Meagher DM, Wheat JD, Hughes JP, et al: Granulosa cell tumours in mares: a review of 78 cases. Proc 23rd Annu AAEP Convention. Vancouver, BC: 1977, p 133.
22. Christoffersen M, Lehn-Jensen H, Bogh IB: Referred vaginal pain: cause of hypersensitivity and performance problems in mares? A clinical case study. *J Equine Vet Sci* 27:32, 2007.
23. Bosu WTK, Van Camp SC, Miller RB, et al: Ovarian disorders: clinical and morphological observations in 30 mares. *Can Vet J* 23:6, 1982.
24. McCue PM: Equine Granulosa Cell Tumors. Proc 38th Annu AAEP Convention. Orlando, FL: 1992, p 587.
25. Piquette GN, Kenney RM, Sertich PL, et al: Equine granulosa-theca cell tumors express inhibin α and β A-subunit messenger ribonucleic acids and proteins. *Biol Reprod* 43:1050, 1990.
26. Wolfsdorf KE, Rodgerson D, Holder R: How to manually reduce twins between 60 and 120 days gestation using craniocervical dislocation. *Proc Am Assoc Eq Pract* 51:284, 2005.
27. Vogelsang MM, Vogelsang SG, Lindsey BR, et al: Reproductive performance in mares subjected to examination by diagnostic ultrasound. *Theriogenology* 32:95, 1989.
28. Bergfelt DR, Woods JA, Ginther OJ: Role of the embryonic vesicle and progesterone in embryonic loss in mares. *J Reprod Fertil* 95:339, 1992.
29. Allen WR: Progesterone and the pregnant mare: unanswered chestnuts. *Equine Vet J* 25(Suppl):90, 1993.
30. Pycock JF, Newcombe JR: The effect of the gonadotrophin-releasing hormone analog, buserelin, administered in diestrus on pregnancy rates and pregnancy failure in mares. *Theriogenology* 46:1097, 1996.
31. Cottrill CM: Placental evaluation in the field. *Equine Vet Educ* 3:204, 1991.
32. Acland HM: Abortion in mares. In McKinnon AO, Voss JL, eds; *Equine Reproduction.* Philadelphia: Lea & Febiger, 1993, pp 554-562.
33. Riddle WT, LeBlanc MM: Mare reproductive loss syndrome. In Samper JC, Pycock JF, McKinnon AO, eds: *Current Therapy in Equine Reproduction.* St Louis: Saunders, 2007, p 384.
34. Pycock JF, Allen WE: Inflammatory components in uterine fluid from mares with experimentally induced bacterial endometritis. *Equine Vet J* 22:422, 1990.
35. Hinrichs K: The role of endometrial swabs in the diagnosis (and pathogenesis?) of endometritis. *Cornell Vet* 81:233, 1991.
36. Ricketts SW, Mackintosh ME: Role of anaerobic bacteria in equine endometritis. *J Reprod Fertil Suppl* 35:343, 1987.

37. Riddle WT, LeBlanc MM, Stromberg AJ: Relationships between uterine culture, cytology and pregnancy rates in a Thoroughbred practice. *Theriogenology* 68:395, 2007.

38. LeBlanc MM, Magsig J, Stromberg AJ: Use of a low-volume uterine flush for diagnosing endometritis in chronically infertile mares. *Theriogenology* 68:403, 2007.

39. Kenney RM: Cyclic and pathologic changes of the mare endometrium as detected by biopsy; with a note on early embryonic death. *J Am Vet Med Assoc* 172:241, 1978.

40. Ricketts SW: Histological and histopathological studies on the endometrium of the mare. Fellowship Thesis, London: Royal Col Vet Surg, 1978.

41. Allen WE: Pycock JF: Cyclical accumulation of uterine fluid in mares with lowered resistance to endometritis. *Vet Rec* 122:489, 1988.

42. Pycock JF, Newcombe JR: The relationship between intraluminal uterine fluid, endometritis and pregnancy rate in the mare. *Equine Pract* 18:19, 1996.

43. McKinnon AO, Voss JL, Squires EL, et al: Diagnostic ultrasonography. In McKinnon AO, Voss JL, eds: *Equine Reproduction*. Philadelphia: Lea & Febiger, 1993, pp 266-302.

44. Newcombe JR: The effect of the incidence and depth of intra-uterine fluid in early dioestrus on pregnancy rates in mares (abstract). *Pferdeheilkunde* 13:545, 1997.

45. Causey RC: Mucus and the mare: How little do we know. *Theriogenology* 68:386, 2007.

46. Rohrbach B, Sheerin P, Steiner J, et al: Use of *Propionibacterium acnes* as adjunct therapy in treatment of persistent endometritis in the broodmare (abstract). *Anim Reprod Sci* 94:259, 2006.

47. Rohrbach B, Sheerin P, Cantrell C, et al: Effect of adjunctive treatment with intravenously administered *Propionibacterium acnes* on reproductive performance in mares with persistent endometritis. *J Am Vet Med Assoc* 231:107, 2007.

48. Rogan D, Fumoso E, Rodriguez E, et al: Use of a mycobacterial cell wall extract (MCWE) in susceptible mares to clear experimentally induced endometritis with *Streptococcus zooepidemicus*. *J Equine Vet Sci* 27:112, 2007.

49. Hess MB, Parker NA, Purswell BJ, Dascanio JJ: Use of lufenuron as a treatment for fungal endometritis in four mares. *J Am Vet Med Assoc* 221:266, 2002.

50. Dascanio JJ: Treatment of fungal endometritis. In Samper JC, Pycock JF, McKinnon AO, eds: *Current Therapy in Equine Reproduction*. St Louis: Saunders, 2007, p 116.

51. Kenney RM: The aetiology, diagnosis and classification of chronic degenerative endometritis (CDE) (endometrosis). Proceedings of JP Hughes International Workshop on Equine Endometritis summarized by WR Allen (abstract). *Equine Vet J* 25:186, 1993.

52. Kotilainen T, Huhtinen M, Katila T: Sperm induced leukocytosis in the equine uterus. *Theriogenology* 41:629, 1994.

53. Troedsson MHT: Uterine response to semen deposition in the mare. Proc Soc Theriogenology San Antonio, TX: 1995, p 130.

54. Parlevliet JM, Tremoleda IM, Cheng FP, et al: Influence of semen, extender and seminal plasma on the defence mechanism of the mare's uterus (abstract). *Pferdeheilkunde* 13:540, 1997.

55. Katila T: Interactions of the uterus and semen. *Pferdeheilkunde* 13:508, 1997.

56. Troedsson MHT, Lee CS, Franklin RD, Crabo BG: The role of seminal plasma in post-breeding uterine inflammation. *J Reprod Fert Suppl* 56:341, 2000.

57. Portus BJ, Reilas R, Katila T: Effect of seminal plasma on uterine inflammation, contractility and pregnancy rates in mares. *Equine Vet J* 37:515, 2005.

58. Palm F, Walter I, Budik S, Aurich C: Influence of different semen extenders and seminal plasma on the inflammatory response of the endometrium in estrous mares. *Anim Reprod Sci* 94:286, 2006.

59. Farrelly BY, Mullaney PE: Cervical and uterine infections in Thoroughbred mares. *Irish Vet J* 18:210, 1964.

60. Hughes JP, Loy RG: Investigations on the effect of intrauterine inoculations of *Streptococcus zooepidemicus* in the mare. Proc 15th Annu AAEP Conv. Houston, TX: 1969, p 289.

61. Pycock JF, Paccamonti D, Jonker H, et al: Can mares be classified as resistant or susceptible to recurrent endometritis? *Pferdeheilkunde* 13:431, 1997.

62. Allen WE, Pycock JF: Current views on the pathogenesis of bacterial endometritis in mares with lowered resistance to endometritis. *Vet Rec* 125:298, 1989.

63. Evans MI, Hamer JM, Gason LM, et al: Clearance of bacteria and non-antigenic markers following intrauterine inoculation into maiden mares: effect of steroid hormone environment. *Theriogenology* 26:37, 1986.

64. Troedsson MHT, Liu IKM: Uterine clearance of non-antigenic markers (51-Cr) in response to a bacterial challenge in mares potentially susceptible and resistant to chronic uterine infections. *J Reprod Fertil Suppl* 44:283, 1991.

65. Troedsson MHT, Liu IKM, Ing M: Multiple site electromyography recordings of uterine activity following an intrauterine bacterial challenge in mares susceptible and resistant to chronic uterine infection. *J Reprod Fertil* 99:307, 1993.

66. LeBlanc MM, Neuwirth L, Mauragis D, et al: Oxytocin enhances clearance of radiocolloid from the uterine lumen of reproductively normal mares and mares susceptible to endometritis. *Equine Vet J* 26:279, 1994.

67. Liu IK, Rakestraw P, Coit C, et al: An *in vitro* investigation of the mechanism of neuromuscular regulation in myometrial contractility (abstract). *Pferdeheilkunde* 13:557, 1997.

68. LeBlanc MM, Johnson RD, Calderwood Mays MB, et al: Lymphatic clearance of India ink in reproductively normal mares and mares susceptible to endometritis. *Biol Reprod Monograph* 1:501, 1995.

69. Causey RC: Making sense of equine uterine infections: the many faces of physical clearance. *Vet J* 172:405, 2006.

70. Rasch K, Schoon HA, Sieme H, et al: Histomorphological endometrial status and influence of oxytocin on the uterine drainage and pregnancy rate in mares. *Equine Vet J* 28:455, 1996.

71. Vanderwall DK, Woods GL: Effect of fertility of uterine lavage performed immediately prior to insemination in mares. *JAVMA* 222:1108, 2003.

72. Knutti B, Pycock JF, van der Weijden GC, Kupfer U: The influence of early postbreeding uterine lavage on pregnancy rates in mares with intrauterine fluid accumulations after breeding. *Equine Vet Educ* 12:267, 2000.

73. Troedsson MHT, Scott MA, Liu IKM: Comparative treatment of mares susceptible to chronic uterine infection. *Am J Vet Res* 56:468, 1995.

74. Allen WE: Investigations into the use of oxytocin for promoting uterine drainage in mares susceptible to endometritis. *Vet Rec* 128:593, 1991.

75. Pycock JF, Newcombe JR: Assessment of the effect of three treatments to remove intrauterine fluid on pregnancy rate in the mare. *Vet Rec* 138:320, 1996.

76. Pycock JF: A new approach to treatment of endometritis. *Equine Vet Educ* 6:36, 1994.

77. LeBlanc MM: Oxytocin: the new wonder drug for treatment of endometritis? *Equine Vet Educ* 6:39, 1994.

78. Pycock JF: Assessment of oxytocin and intrauterine antibiotics on intrauterine fluid and pregnancy rates in the mare. Proc 40th Annu AAEP Convention. Vancouver, BC: 1994, p 19.

79. Paccamonti DL, Gutjahr S, Pycock JF, et al: Does the effect of oxytocin on intrauterine pressure vary with dose or day of treatment (abstract). *Pferdeheilkunde* 13:553, 1997.

80. Gutjahr S, Paccamonti DL, Pycock JF, et al: Effect of dose and day of treatment on uterine response to oxytocin in mares. *Theriogenology* 54:447, 2000.

81. Paccamonti DL, Pycock JF, Taverne MAM, et al: PGFM response to exogenous oxytocin and determination of the half-life of oxytocin in nonpregnant mares. *Equine Vet J* 31:285, 1999.

82. Cadario ME, Thatcher MJD, LeBlanc MM: Relationship between prostaglandin and uterine clearance of radiocolloid in the mare. *Biol Reprod Monogr* 1:495, 1995.

83. LeBlanc MM: Effects of oxytocin, prostaglandin and phenylbutazone on uterine clearance of radiocolloid. *Pferdeheilkunde* 13:483, 1997.

84. Combs GB, LeBlanc MM, Neuwirth L, et al: Effects of prostaglandin F2α, cloprostenol and fenprostalene on uterine clearance of radiocolloid in the mare. *Theriogenology* 45:1449, 1996.

85. Leblanc MM: Persistent mating induced endometritis in the mare: pathogenesis, diagnosis and treatment. In Ball BA, ed: *Recent Advances in Equine Reproduction*. Ithaca, NY: International Veterinary Information Service, 2003.

86. Brendemuehl JP: Influence of cloprostenol, PGF2alpha and oxytocin on luteal formation, function and pregnancy rate in the mare. In Proc 46th Annu Convention Am Assoc Equine Pract. San Antonio, TX: 2000, p 267.

87. Troedsson MHT, Ababneh MM, Ohlgren AF, et al: Effect of periovulatory prostaglandin F2alpha on pregnancy rates and luteal function in the mare. *Theriogenology* 55:1891, 2001.

88. Nie GJ, Johnson KE, Wenzel JG, Braden TD: Effect of administering oxytocin or cloprostenol in the periovulatory period on pregnancy outcome and luteal function in mares. *Theriogenology* 60:1111, 2002.

89. Schramme AR, Pinto CR, Davis JL, et al: Pharmacokinetics of carbetocin, a long-acting oxytocin analogue, following intravenous administration in horses. *Theriogenology* 68:517, 2007.

90. Handler J, Hoffmann D. Weber F, et al: Oxytocin does not contribute to the effects of cervical dilation on progesterone secretion and embryonic development in mares. *Theriogenology* 66:1397, 2006.

91. Asbury AC: Uterine defence mechanisms in the mare: The use of intrauterine plasma in the management of endometritis. *Theriogenology* 21:387, 1984.

92. Pascoe DR: Effect of adding autologous plasma to an intrauterine antibiotic therapy after breeding on pregnancy rates in mares. *Biol Reprod Monogr* 1:137, 1995.

93. Adams GP, Ginther OJ: Efficacy of intrauterine infusion of plasma for treatment of infertility and endometritis in mares. *J Am Vet Med Assoc* 194:372, 1989.

94. Troedsson MHT, Scott MA, Liu IKM: Pathogenesis and treatment of chronic uterine infection. Proc 38th Annu AAEP Convention. Orlando, FL: 1992, p 595.

95. Asbury AC, Lyle SK: Infectious causes of infertility. In McKinnon AO, Voss JL, eds: *Equine Reproduction.* Philadelphia: Lea & Febiger, 1993, p 381.

96. Troedsson MHT, Lee CS, Franklin RD, Crabo BG: The role of seminal plasma in post-breeding uterine inflammation. *J Reprod Fertil Suppl* 56:341, 2000.

97. Dell'Aqua JA Jr, Papa FO, Lopes MD, et al: Modulation of acute uterine inflammatory response after artificial insemination with equine frozen semen. *Anim Reprod Sci* 94:270, 2006.

98. Papa FO, Dell'Aqua JA Jr, Alvarenga MA, et al: Use of corticosteroid therapy on the modulation of uterine inflammatory response in mares after artificial insemination with frozen semen. *Pferdeheilkunde* 24:79, 2008.

98a. Bucca S, Carli A, Buckley T, et al: The use of dexamethasone administered to mares at breeding time in the modulation of persistent mating-induced endometritis. *Theriogenology* 70:1093-1100, 2008.

99. Ricketts SW, Alonso S: The effect of age and parity on the development of equine chronic endometrial disease. *Equine Vet J* 23:189, 1991.

100. Pycock JF: Cervical function and uterine fluid accumulation in mares. Proceedings of JP Hughes International Workshop on Equine Endometritis, summarized by WR Allen. *Equine Vet J* 25(Suppl):191, 1993.

101. Umphenour NW, Sprinkle TA, Murphy HQ: Natural service. In McKinnon AO, Voss JL, eds: *Equine Reproduction.* Philadelphia: Lea & Febiger, 1993, pp: 798-808.

102. Gutjahr S, Paccamonti D, Pycock JF, et al: Intrauterine pressure changes in response to oxytocin application in mares. *Reprod Anim Suppl* 5:118, 1998.

103. Knutti B, Pycock JF, Van der Weijden GC, et al: The influence of early postbreeding uterine lavage on pregnancy rates in mares with intrauterine fluid accumulations after breeding. *Equine Vet Educ* 12:267, 2000.

104. Hearn P: The relationship of uterine inflammation to fertility. *Proc Soc Theriogenol* 39, 1993.

105. Zent W: Post-ovulation intrauterine antibiotics. Proceedings of JP Hughes International Workshop on Equine Endometritis summarized by WR Allen (abstract). *Equine Vet J* 25:192, 1993.

106. Hughes JP, Loy RG, Asbury AC, et al: The occurrence of *Pseudomonas* in the reproductive tract of mares and its effect on fertility. *Comell Vet* 56:595, 1966.

107. Hughes JP, Stabenfeldt GH, Kindahl H, et al: Pyometra in the mare. *J Reprod Fertil Suppl* 27:321, 1979.

ARTIFICIAL INSEMINATION WITH FRESH AND COOLED SEMEN

JUAN C. SAMPER

Even though the mare's fertility and her reproductive management are key factors in the establishment of pregnancies, supplying semen of optimal quality for artificial insemination (AI) is imperative. All semen collection procedures described in Chapter 3 can result in samples that are adequate for AI. However, semen must be collected, handled, and processed adequately in order to maintain the fertility of the spermatozoa. Breeders, farm managers, and veterinarians often perform a cursory analysis of semen that will be used for fresh or cooled AI, but depending on the intended use, semen must be handled differently. This chapter will describe the handling procedures of stallion semen that is going to be used within a few hours and up to 48 hours after collection.

There are many ways and reasons for semen evaluation. A lengthy discussion of a complete semen evaluation can be found in Chapter 6, but a very simple semen evaluation should always be done when semen is going to be processed. However, the most important factor is the proper handling of the raw semen in order to avoid artifacts or iatrogenic damage to the sperm that could affect the results and the calculations performed for the estimation of a breeding dose. Sperm concentration and sperm motility are perhaps the two key factors that must be evaluated accurately in order to properly prepare breeding doses.

HANDLING OF RAW SEMEN

Semen is the combination of sperm cells and the fluids in which they are suspended. The fluid portion is known as seminal plasma, and since seminal plasma has a very low buffering capacity and there is a rapid accumulation of by-products because of high metabolic activity of the sperm, raw semen has to be processed very quickly to avoid damage that might affect the integrity of the sperm and the evaluation results.

Evaluation of the raw semen every time a stallion is collected is a critical part of processing semen for AI. Stallion managers and veterinarians must realize that it is critical to evaluate the sperm during each step of the process. Failure to do so could result in poor semen quality without knowing where or why the process failed.

Immediately after collection, raw semen must be maintained at body temperature (35°–38°C), and so does the equipment that will come in contact with it. Therefore, it is necessary and highly recommended for laboratories that process semen to have a 37°C incubator available. Sudden temperature changes will cause temperature shock, causing irreversible and detrimental changes to sperm. *Thermal shock* is a sudden temperature reduction of more than 8°–10°C to sperm cells and can cause *cold shock*. This irreversible damage to sperm is evidenced microscopically by a typical forward or backward tight circular motility pattern of the spermatozoa. Cold shock also affects the

longevity as well as the fertilizing potential of the sperm. The reduction in fertilizing potential, as well as the abnormal motility observed, is a consequence of the reduction in the fluidity of the lipid component of the plasma membrane.[1] The rigidity of the structure of the membrane caused by this sudden change makes the sperm less able to accommodate to volume changes when exposed to different osmotic pressures. The reasons for cold shock include cold incubators, cold receptacles for semen collection, cold slides and cover slips, or cold ambient temperatures without proper protection of the semen.

Although it does not happen as often as cold shock, exposure of sperm to temperatures over 10°C above body temperature for short periods will also cause irreversible changes to sperm. *Heat shock* is often evidence under the microscope by a change in the motility pattern from a linear and progressive motion to a small circular tight pattern. Longevity of sperm motility is also significantly reduced. Heat shock is most often induced by either exposure of semen to high temperatures in the artificial vagina liner, by accidentally having incubators or slide warmers too hot, or by prolonging the thawing time of frozen semen longer than what is recommend when temperatures are above 37°C. Another type of shock is the *osmotic shock,* which can be induced by exposing the sperm to hyperosmotic (>400 mOsm) or hypo-osmotic (< 250 mOsm) environments. This type of shock can be induced when extenders are improperly made or have too little or too much water, respectively. Hypo-osmotic shock can be shown by the typical swelling of the plasma membrane, resulting in a characteristic coiling of the sperm tail. Hyperosmotic shock can be induced by the leaking of inappropriate artificial vagina lubricants into the semen receptacle, resulting in a significant reduction in the longevity of motility of the spermatozoa.[2] Hypo-osmotic shock can be evidenced by a typical coiling of the tail either as hair pins or a complete wrap around the sperm head as the plasma membrane swells, drawing water to the inside of the cell.

SPERM CONCENTRATION

Although the ultimate goal when counting sperm is to determine the total number of sperm cells in an ejaculate in billions (10^9), this number cannot be calculated unless the volume is accurately measured and the number of sperm per milliliter in millions is calculated. Counting of sperm cells can be done in several ways.

Manually Counting with the Use of a Hemocytometer

In order to count with a Neubauer hemocytometer, the individual performing the procedure should dilute the sample at a known ratio. This can be done by diluting the sample with buffered formalin or water. To make a 1:100 dilution, 0.1 ml of semen is added to 9.9 ml of diluent. Another system that can be used is the *Unopette system* (B&D), where 50 or 100 μl of semen are loaded in a capillary and added to a predetermined amount of fluid. The final dilution using this system is 1:200 or 1:100, respectively. Once that dilution ratio is determined, the hemocytometer chamber is loaded without overflowing. After a few minutes, before the chamber starts to dry and when the sperm have settled, the total number of sperm in the red or white blood cell cross-hatched area should be counted. To calculate the number of sperm per milliliter, the following formula is used:

$$\text{Sperm/ml (millions)} = \text{Number counted} \times \text{dilution ratio} \times 10,000$$

Ten thousand is the conversion factor from 0.01 cubic ml (volume of the chamber) to 1.0 cubic centimeter (ml). Calculation of the total number of sperm is done by multiplying sperm concentration per ml by the total volume of the ejaculate.

$$\text{Total no. of sperm } (10^9) = \text{Sperm / ml (millions)} \times \text{volume (ml)}$$

Automated Counters

Although spectrophotometers or densimeters are easy to use compared with the hemocytometer, individuals using these counters need to have good knowledge of its use and basis for measuring. If it is not used correctly, both hemocytometers and densimeters can be a source of profound error. Because of the ease of use, many breeding farms and laboratories have adopted the use of automatic sperm counters. All automated sperm counters work under the same principle. The addition of an aliquot of semen to the transparent fluid will cause a certain degree of turbidity. The higher the turbidity, the higher the sperm concentration. Although counting in this way is fast, the equipment is more expensive than a hemocytometer. In addition, any particles that increase the turbidity of the fluid such as red or white blood cells, urine, epithelial cells, dirt, or extender will raise the sperm concentration, giving inaccurate readings. Furthermore, extremely high or low concentrations per milliliter of semen in the raw ejaculate are not accurately determined by these counters. It is important that all laboratories that collect semen be equipped with some counting device. To avoid or reduce the error factor, proper dilution and clean samples should be used for counting.

When using automated semen counters, the use of extenders prior to counting should be avoided since all extenders will increase the turbidity of the diluent. When determining the concentration with automated sperm counters, counts must be made on raw semen.

A recent study by Texas workers using the hemocytometer as the gold standard concluded that all types of concentration calculating devices that are based on semen turbidity are very accurate over a small range of sperm concentrations (150–300 million/ml). However, sperm concentrations lower than that were overestimated while higher concentrations were underestimated.[3] Recently, a new sperm counter known as the Nucleo-Counter SP-100 (Allerod, Denmark) uses fluorochromes to stain sperm and therefore appears to be able to differentiate sperm from other particles. Since it detects sperm nuclei and is not based on turbidity, the NucleoCounter SP-100 can be used to count sperm in the presence of extenders.[4]

SPERM MOTILITY

The total number of sperm cells moving (total motility), the number of sperm cells moving in a forward motion (progressive motility), and the relative sperm velocity (0–4) should be determined. Unless motility is estimated, proper semen dilution for AI purposes cannot be performed.

Contrary to counting, accuracy of motility determination is enhanced when a proper semen extender is added to it prior to evaluation. In order to determine the percentage of motile cells, a warm slide and cover slip should be used. A small drop (5–10 μl) of semen should be placed on a clean warm slide and a cover slip placed on top. It is important that only a single layer of cells be visualized under a 10×, 20×, or 40× objective. In addition, several fields free of debris and air bubbles should be observed, since air bubbles and dirt will affect motility estimations. In addition, the evaluation should be performed on several fields while avoiding the edges of the cover slip. Although evaluation of the percentage of motile sperm cells is a subjective test, experienced individuals can provide accurate estimates that reflect the quality of the ejaculate. Inexperienced individuals should at least try to determine if more than half (>50%) or less than half (<50%) of the sperm cells are moving forward. Every laboratory processing semen should have a good microscope for motility evaluation. Some microscopes are adapted to a monitor for ease of use.

Computer-Assisted Semen Analysis

In order to increase the objectivity of motility readings, there are several computerized motility analyzers.[5] This equipment, although very costly, will provide information such as velocity of sperm, amplitude of lateral head displacement, and other parameters that would be very difficult to assess with a regular microscopic evaluation. Since the computer analyzes particles the size of a sperm head, when semen is extended and evaluated with the motility analyzer, one has to ascertain that particular matter in the extender does not interfere with the motility estimates. Although computer-assisted semen analysis (CASA) systems are commonplace in most human and andrology laboratories, its use in veterinary medicine has been restricted to a few laboratories because of the cost of the equipment. However, semen samples can be videotaped and sent to referral laboratories where the analysis can be performed. A more detailed discussion is found in Chapter 6.

Morphological Evaluation

In order to have a better idea of the quality of the semen and probably of the potential fertility of a semen sample, the character of the cells that make up that ejaculate should be evaluated. Although it is recognized that the percent of motile cells in an ejaculate should parallel the number of morphologically normal sperm, the two numbers are not exactly the same. That is because not all motile cells have normal morphology and not all morphologically normal cells are motile.

Numerous studies have tried to explain different levels of fertility by correlating the number of normal or abnormal sperm present in an ejaculate. Jasko et al.[6] reported that the number of abnormal heads, midpieces, and proximal droplets accounts for 60% of the variation in stallion fertility.

In order to perform accurate morphological evaluations, it is important to ensure that no iatrogenic defects are inflicted on the sperm. These would include heat or cold shock causing reflected midpieces or hypo-osmotic shock causing coiled tails.

Morphological evaluation of sperm cells can be performed by evaluating at least 100 cells on a stained smear with the oil immersion objective (100×). Routine stains used for this purpose include: eosin nigrosin, aniline blue, or India ink.[7] However, if the sperm have been diluted with an extender, it is necessary to dilute the sample in 10% buffered formal saline or glutaraldehyde to fix the sperm. Evaluation will be done on a wet sample with the oil immersion objective and a phase contrast microscope. The morphological categories that should be recorded include the number of normal sperm, abnormal heads or nuclei, abnormal acrosomes, abnormal necks, tailless heads, proximal droplets, distal droplets, abnormal midpieces, abnormal tails, and round spermatids (cells).

Fig. 14-1 shows some of the most common morphological features observed in stallion spermatozoa. Sperm cells that have more than one defect should be recorded and the frequency of them noted on at least 100 cells. It is important to realize that the morphological evaluation should record the frequency of defects in at least 100 cells and not the number of abnormal cells out of 100. It is not clear how an individual sperm abnormality affects the fertility of a stallion. It can be assumed that stallions with a higher number of sperm abnormalities will have lower fertility compared with one with higher numbers of morphologically normal sperm. However, the different levels of fertility reduction are not well established. Sperm abnormalities are the result of testicular or epididymal insult.[8,9] A slight increase in bull's testicular temperature (3.1°C) for 48 hours causes a significant increase in sperm defects that are evidenced as early as 8 days after. This is followed by a peak in abnormalities around 18 days. Furthermore, after 39 days the animals in this study still had not regained their pre-treatment morphology.[9] Interestingly, in this study sperm motility was only slightly and transiently affected. The transient effect of increased testicular temperature had no effect on sperm output. The authors suggest that the type of defect depends on the stage of the spermatogenic cycle where the cell was at the time. In other words, when sperm with increased cytoplasmic droplets were at the epididymal level, tailless heads were in the process of spermiation, nuclear vacuoles were germ cells in early stages showing a lack of DNA condensation, and head changes would be inflicted to spermatids that were elongating. Stallions are exercised and competed during the hot summer months, which could have a significant impact on sperm morphology, particularly on stallions with both duties (performance and breeding).

High testicular temperatures can also be self induced by stallions that carry their testicles high in the inguinal area during

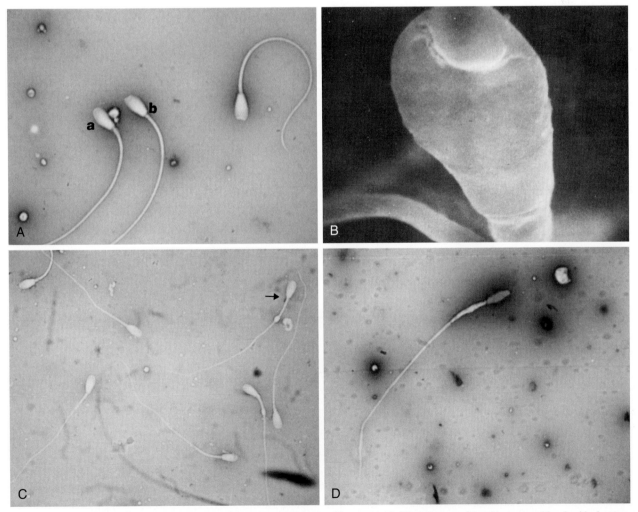

Figure 14-1. Common morphological characteristics found during evaluation of stallion sperm. **A,** Normal sperm *(a)* and a sperm with a knobbed acrosome *(b).* **B,** Scanning electron micrograph of sperm in **A. C,** Sperm with distal cytoplasmic droplet *(arrow).* **D,** Sperm with abnormally thickened midpiece and abnormal head.

Continued

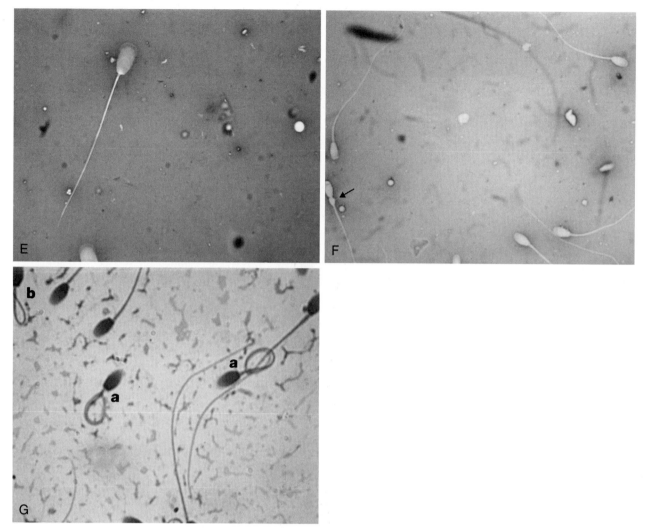

Figure 14-1.— (cont'd) E, Swollen acrosome. **F,** Proximal droplet *(arrow)*. **G,** Coiled tail caused by hypoosmotic stress *(a)*; hairpin tail bend *(b)*.

periods of stress, pain, or competition. The morphology of the sperm cells can be affected not only by high scrotal temperatures, but also by prolonged stress during training of competition, exogenous hormones such as progesterone or anabolic steroids, and sexual rest.[9-11] The individual stallion's susceptibility to factors that affect sperm morphology remains to be investigated.

MICROBIOLOGY OF SEMEN

Individuals evaluating semen should be aware that the ejaculate is very often contaminated with microorganisms.[12] The challenge is to determine whether these microorganisms are pathogenic and therefore likely to reduce the fertility of a stallion and the efficiency of the breeding program. Bacterial and viral microorganisms are the most common pathogens and of most concern. Chapter 10 provides an excellent discussion on this topic.

TECHNIQUES FOR ARTIFICIAL INSEMINATION

AI is the technique whereby an adequate number of live normal sperm are deposited into the clean uterus at the optimal time. Although this procedure can seem quite simple, the adequate

coordination of events will result in optimum pregnancy rates. In horses, there are three methods of AI.

Fresh Semen

Fresh semen is used when the stallion is collected at the farm and the semen is used either immediately in its raw state or diluted.[13]

Fresh Cooled Semen

After collection, semen is diluted with an extender and slowly cooled to 5°–8°C and transported to be used within 12–36 hours afterward.

Frozen Semen

Frozen semen is collected and processed in the appropriate way and then stored in liquid nitrogen to be used several days, months, or years after collection. Depending on the final intended use of the semen, several factors have to be considered to adequately retain the fertilizing potential of spermatozoa (see Chapter 15).

COLLECTION OF SEMEN FOR ARTIFICIAL INSEMINATION

Semen collection has been addressed elsewhere in this book. All methods described in Chapter 3 are adequate to process semen for AI. Perhaps the most important aspect of collecting and processing semen for AI is the quality of the raw ejaculate. The quality of the raw ejaculate is determined principally by the individual stallion. Factors such as age, exogenous hormones, and debilitating or pyrexic periods can affect the quality of the semen. In a healthy stallion, the period of sexual rest is probably the most important aspect of determining quality of semen. To maximize the quality of raw ejaculate, it is very important to have the stallion sexually active. The capacity of stallions to store viable sperm in the external duct system (ampullae or tail of the epididymis) is perhaps dependent on the stallion himself, but as much as 60% of the total daily sperm production can be stored in the epididymal tail.[14] Therefore, the frequency of collection should be tailored to the individual stallion depending on his capacity to store viable sperm. Semen collection from some stallions once a week is sufficient to maintain good semen quality, whereas others will need daily collections to maintain semen quality. For the average stallion, one ejaculate every 2–3 days can maintain normal semen quality.

Although there is a great variation between stallions in their ability to store viable sperm, sexually rested males in general will produce semen with an abnormally high concentration, regular to poor motility and longevity, and high numbers of morphologically abnormal spermatozoa. Although these ejaculates often contain enough sperm to impregnate mares, it is not recommended to use them for transported semen or freezing programs until the stallion has been collected several times. Fig. 14-2 exemplifies an extreme case of a stallion that needed seven collections to stabilize its extragonadal sperm reserves. It has been reported that an average of four collections is enough to stabilize extragonadal sperm numbers.[15]

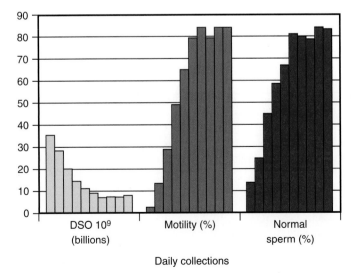

Figure 14-2. Total daily sperm output in billions (DSO × 10⁹), sperm motility (%), and percent morphological normal sperm of a sexually rested stallion through 10 daily collections.

EVALUATING SEMEN FOR ARTIFICIAL INSEMINATION

A detailed discussion of semen evaluation is described in Chapter 6. Veterinarians or farm managers who are not familiar with a particular stallion should perform a more detailed evaluation of the semen. This evaluation should include the following:

- Sperm concentration per milliliter
- Total number of sperm
- Total and progressive motility
- Longevity of motility either at room temperature or at 5°–8°C for 6, 12, 24, and 48 hours
- Morphological evaluation to determine the total number of normal sperm

For stallions that are being collected routinely for which the management knows the stallion's semen quality, concentration and progressive motility are perhaps the most important parameters that should be evaluated routinely. However, the extent of the evaluation depends on the final intended use of the semen and the way it will be processed. For instance, if semen is intended to be used in frozen insemination programs, a more comprehensive evaluation should be conducted. This would include post-thaw motility as well as longevity, morphology, special stains, filtration, and bacteriological evaluation. Unfortunately, as stated in Chapter 6, most of the semen evaluation assays either have low correlations with fertility or have not had their relationship investigated. This is particularly noticeable when evaluating frozen semen.

PROCESSING AND COOLING OF FRESH SEMEN

The way semen should be processed depends on its final intended use. Semen used fresh at the farm or transported chilled or frozen should be processed in different ways to properly preserve its fertility potential. Semen used fresh shortly after collection should be diluted with an appropriate extender (Table 14-1). If semen is to be used within 6 hours after collection, addition of the warm extender at a ratio of 1:1 or 1:2 and maintained at room temperature (20°C) would be sufficient to maintain motility and fertilizing potential. On the other hand, semen that is going to be maintained in its liquid state and used at the farm or transported to inseminate 12–48 hours after collection should be diluted at higher rates. In general, dilution ratios of 1:3–1:10 (semen:extender) are done depending on the total volume and total sperm count. Semen intended for transport should be diluted so that the final sperm concentration per milliliter is 25–50 million/ml.[14] In addition, this semen should be slowly cooled (0.3°C/min) down to 5°–8°C, so that the metabolic activity of the sperm is reduced. However, in stallions producing ejaculates of high volume of semen and low sperm concentrations per milliliter, the amount of extender added is often not sufficient to neutralize the detrimental effects of seminal plasma on spermatozoa. In these cases the raw ejaculate should be centrifuged so that a soft sperm pellet is formed and reconstituted in the appropriate amount of extender, leaving about 5% seminal plasma.[16,17]

Although AI can be performed with raw semen immediately after collection, it is highly recommended that an extender be used. Addition of the extender helps prevent cold shock, preserves longevity of sperm, neutralizes the detrimental effects of seminal plasma, and reduces the amount of bacterial contamination when an appropriate antibiotic is added.

Table 14-1 | **Commonly Used Extenders for Diluting and Transporting Fresh, Chilled Semen**

KENNY EXTENDER	CREAM GEL EXTENDER	SKIM MILK GEL	GLYCINE EGG YOLK	INRA—96
Nonefat dried milk 2.4 g Glucose 4.9 g Distilled water to equal 100 mL	Knox gelatin 1.3 g 10 mL of heated distilled water Half and half cream 90 mL	Knox gelatin 1.3 g Skim milk 100 mL Heat for 10 min at 97° F	#1 Glucose 12 g Fructose 12 g Water 600 mL #2 Na citrate 20 g Glycine 9.4 g water 1000 mL Mix# 1and #2. Supplement with 20% egg yolk. Centrifuge for clarification.	Glucose 12.2 g Lactose 45.4 g Phosphocaseinate 27 g Hanks salts 7.27 g Distilled water to equal 1L

Table 14-2 | **Dilution Rates According to the Number of Progressively Motile Sperm/mL in Raw Semen from Stallions**

MOTILE SPERM (MILLION/ML) IN RAW EJACULATE	DILUTION RATIO (SEMEN:EXTENDER)	NUMBER OF SPERM IN FINAL DOSE (MILLION/ML)	VOLUME IN ML FOR 500 MILLION AI DOSE
100–150	1:3	25–37.5	20–13.3
150–200	1:4	30–40	16.6–12.5
200–250	1:5	33.3–41.6	15.1–12.1
250–300	1:6	35.7–42.8	14–11.7
300–350	1:7	37.5–43.7	13.3–11.5
350–400	1:8	38.9–44.4	12.9–11.3
400–450	1:9	40–45	12.5–11.1
450–500	1:10	40.9–45.5	12.3–11

AI, Artificial insemination.

Factors Affecting Preservation

Methods of semen preservation should be done according to the projected time between collection and insemination. Several factors will determine the longevity and the retention of fertility potential of preserved semen, including quality of the raw ejaculate, dilution rate,[18] rate of cooling and storage temperature,[19] storage time and container,[20] and type of extender.[21]

Quality of the Ejaculate

Several parameters must be taken into account when semen is going to be used for AI: the volume, number of sperm per milliliter, total number of sperm, total number of progressively motile sperm, and total number of morphologically normal sperm. In order to maximize the number of morphologically normal and motile sperm, stallions should be collected on a regular basis. Sexually active stallions have better semen quality than inactive stallions.[15] As explained previously, the number of times a stallion should be collected to increase the semen quality depends on the individual stallion. Sperm from the first ejaculate of the year or the first few ejaculates collected after periods of prolonged sexual rest in general have a high number of morphological abnormalities, higher concentrations, and lower motility. In addition, these ejaculates have a shorter longevity and therefore should not be used for long-term preservation. However, these ejaculates can be used for insemination within 15 minutes after collection, preferably using the entire ejaculate, provided that there is at least 25%–30% progressively motile sperm. A stallion's whole ejaculate, which has <50% morphologically

normal and progressively motile sperm, are not good for long semen preservation programs such as transported cooled or frozen semen programs. Owners of mares as well as veterinarians breeding to stallions with semen of such characteristics should be advised about the stallion management of the semen quality so that unrealistic expectations are not created.

DILUTION RATES

Longevity of sperm is related to the sperm concentration per milliliter and the rate at which it is diluted. Therefore, semen that is highly concentrated should be diluted at a higher ratio than ejaculates of lower sperm concentrations. Dilution ratios have to be calculated according to the total volume of the ejaculate and sperm concentration. In general, sperm concentration per milliliter is negatively related to ejaculate volume. Ejaculates that have higher volumes and have lower sperm per milliliter are more difficult to find the appropriate dilution rate. The ideal concentration for diluted semen is 25–50 million sperm/ml.[22,23] The key is to add enough extender to reduce the detrimental effects of seminal plasma as well as to dilute the metabolic products released from the active sperm. Table 14-2 gives a general guideline for dilution of ejaculates of different concentrations. Ejaculates with <100 million sperm/ml and a high volume (>150 ml) should be centrifuged. Centrifugation at 300–500 × g for 10–15 minutes will recover sufficient sperm. The seminal plasma is removed, leaving 5%–10 % of the initial volume to resuspend the sperm.[24] At this point the dilution with extender is performed according to Table 14-2.

Insemination Dose and Volume

For several years it has been accepted that the minimum dose required to maximize fertility in horses is 500 million progressively motile sperm.[25] Although this might be true for some stallions, it could be more for others and far less for a number of stallions. It has been demonstrated in the bull that the number of sperm in the insemination dose needed to reach the maximum fertility is a male-dependent phenomenon.[26] The maximum fertility that a male can reach also varies. The insemination dose for horses is perhaps more sensitive to the individual stallion, the quality of the spermatozoa, and the site of deposition than to the volume of the inseminate. It is suggested that volumes over 100 ml are too large, particularly in young and maiden mares, resulting in a fairly large reflux of semen into the vagina. However, Bedford and Hinricks[27] inseminated pony mares with 135 ml and found no reduction in fertility. On the other hand, mares inseminated with frozen, thawed semen are sometimes bred with volumes ranging between 0.5 and 5 ml with acceptable pregnancy rates. Therefore, volume of the inseminate does not seem to be an important factor affecting fertility.

Rate of Cooling and Storage Temperature

The final storage temperature at which semen should be kept depends on the storage time for which the semen will be maintained. In general, raw semen should always be maintained at 35°–38°C. However, raw semen storage time should not exceed 15–20 minutes. When semen is expected to last more than 15 minutes, it should be diluted with an appropriate extender. Semen that is intended for use within 6 hours after collection can be diluted at 1:1 or 1:2 (semen to extender) and placed in a dark location at room temperature (18°–20°C). The cooling rate for semen on a counter top should not exceed 1.5°–2°C/min. When the ejaculate is expected to last more than 6 hours, semen should be placed in a passive cooling device such as an Equitainer. The cooling rate achieved with this system is around 0.3°C/min.[28] The important feature of the cooling device is its ability to maintain a controlled cooling curve and a temperature of 5°–8°C for up to 48 hours.

The importance of cooling resides in the fact that the sperm's metabolism is significantly reduced, and sperm will save energy and diminish the amount of metabolic products released into the fluid in which they are suspended.

There are several positive cooling devices in the market besides the Equitainer. Some of those are the boxes known as Equine Express, Bio-Flite, and Expecta-A-Foal. These containers are basically Styrofoam boxes of different sizes and shapes; however, they all have frozen packs placed above, below, or at the side of the cup, syringes, or tubes containing the extended semen. Although these systems provide a good system for passive cooling, their ability to maintain a constant low temperature is poor, and therefore the temperature will start to rise again at or before 24 hours. This becomes more critical when there is a great deal of variation in the ambient temperatures at which the containers are exposed. In an experiment done by Texas[20] and Finland[21] researchers reported that the cooling rate and ability to maintain the temperature was evaluated under different conditions. They concluded that the Equitainer system, including the disposable version, maintained progressive motility and semen temperature longer than any of the other containers evaluated. It is suggested that these Styrofoam box containers be used only

for shipments when semen is going to be used <36 hours after collection and not to expose the boxes to extreme outside temperatures. The advantage of the disposable containers is the cost and the lack of need to return them to the stallion farm.

Type of Extenders

There are several extenders that have been used for preservation of liquid or frozen semen. Extenders for cooled transported semen are based mostly on a mixture of non-fat dried milk and glucose with an antibiotic.[29] However, several other extenders have been used for the same purpose. It is important to add antibiotics to the extenders. The final solution should contain 100–150 mg/ml of Gentamicin, Amikacin with K Penicillin, Ticarcillin, or Timentin.[30,31]

Over the years, a variety of extenders have been proposed for cooling, storage, and transport of stallion semen.[21,32] Fractionation techniques for milk have allowed preparation of purified milk fractions in order to test them on stallion sperm survival. French researchers identified native phosphocaseinate (NPPC) as having a protective effect on sperm.[33] A new extender, INRA96, based on modified Hanks' salts supplemented with NPPC, was developed for use with cooled/stored semen. Experiments comparing INRA96 with other milk-based extenders showed that semen diluted in INRA96 extender and stored at 15°C can be an alternative to semen diluted in milk-based extenders and stored at 4°C. Furthermore, INRA96 extender can be as efficient at 15°C as at 4°C for preserving sperm motility and fertility and could be an alternative for some stallions.[34]

EVALUATION OF COOLED SHIPPED SEMEN

Although semen evaluation techniques are discussed in detail elsewhere in this book, a few considerations should be taken into account when evaluating shipped semen at the receiving end. Individuals evaluating cooled transported semen should be aware that the evaluation is generally limited. The parameters that can be evaluated accurately are motility, morphology, and sperm concentration.

Motility

The percentage of motile sperm is highly influenced by the temperature and the thickness of the drop evaluated. It has been shown that there can be as high as 25% reductions in progressive motility when sperm are evaluated at 22°C compared with 37°C.[5,35] Temperatures over 37°C were also detrimental to motility estimates.

A common question is whether an individual evaluating shipped semen should warm it before evaluation. When a single drop is placed on a slide at 37°C, there is no need to warm the entire shipment. In addition, there is no need to warm the semen prior to insemination. Very often the initial motility pattern is not progressive and might have several sperm moving in small circles, but within a few minutes the character of the motility changes to a more progressive pattern.

Morphology

It is recommended that extended semen be morphologically evaluated under a wet mount with phase contrast microscopy. Although morphological evaluations are not routinely performed by the receiver, they should be performed, particularly when the shipments from a particular stallion are not resulting in pregnancies or are of poor quality. Several of the stains that are used for raw semen will not work properly when sperm have been in contact with some types of extenders, particularly those containing egg yolk. If a practitioner were to stain sperm with different acrosome dyes, a rigorous washing procedure would have to be done on the cells in order to have an accurate evaluation. Egg yolk particles in extenders interfere with the fluorescent stains that are used for membrane evaluations; besides, they are not practical for use at the farm. Perhaps the easiest and most accurate way to evaluate the morphology of a semen shipment is by placing one to two drops of semen in buffered formal saline and the evaluation done on a wet mount with the oil immersion objective (100×) with phase contrast microscopy. Alternatively, use of conventional stains such as eosin-nigrosin can be used provided that the sperm are fixed first in buffered formal saline and then stained from this solution.

Sperm Concentration

Sperm concentrations of extended semen can only be evaluated manually with the use of the hemacytometer since the extender will interfere with turbidity-based sperm counters. An alternative to the hemacytometer is the use of computer-assisted semen analyzers or the NucleoCounter SP-100.[4] These instruments work on a different principle (particle size or uptake of fluorochromes) rather than turbidity of the sample. Therefore, accurate readings can be obtained provided that the analyzer has been set correctly and that the sperm suspension does not have large egg yolk particles of similar size to the sperm head.

The total number of motile sperm in the shipment is estimated by multiplying the volume received by the sperm concentration per milliliter by the estimated motility of the sample. In the author's opinion shipments that have >30% motility with adequate sperm numbers of good morphology should achieve pregnancy rates of over 50% per cycle when the mares are bred within 24–36 hours prior to ovulation. In a review of mares bred with cooled shipped semen, Metcalf[36] showed that good quality semen received at her practice results in higher pregnancies per cycle and lower cycles per pregnancy compared with poor semen. Good quality semen had >50% morphologically normal sperm and >50% progressive motility. Individuals shipping cooled semen are encouraged to send an information sheet accompanying the shipment. In addition to showing respect for the breeder, it is a good way of informing receivers of what they should expect and perhaps finding reasons for unexplained deterioration of the semen during transport. Fig. 14-3 shows the form that accompanies the shipments sent at the author's practice. Individuals involved in the insemination of mares with cooled shipped semen should always evaluate the semen prior to or immediately after inseminating the mare.

SEMEN DEPOSITION

The site of semen deposition by the stallion in the mare is believed to be the anterior cervix, but with forceful ejaculatory jets, most of the spermatozoa end up in the uterine body. During routine AI, semen is deposited in the uterine body. Prior to insemination, the mare's tail is bandaged and tied away from contact with the vulva and perineum. The vulva is scrubbed clean and rinsed thoroughly with water. The vulva and perineal area should then be dried. The inseminator dons a sterile sleeve

VETERINARY REPRODUCTIVE SERVICES

J.C.Samper DVM, MSc, PhD Diplomate A.C.T.
2943 216TH St., Langley, BC V2Z2E6 Canada
Telephone: (604) 530-0223 Fax (604) 530-0299

SHIPPED SEMEN INFORMATION

STALLION NAME: _____ BREED:____ OWNER:_____

DATE:_____ TIME OF COLLECTION:_____

RAW SEMEN: VOLUME:_____ML CONCENTRATION/ML:_____X10⁶

DILUTION RATE: _____ EXTENDER TYPE: _____

MOTILITY: _____% VOLUME /DOSE: _____ML TOTAL DOSES: _____

TOTAL NUMBER OF MOTILE SPERM/ DOSE: _____

THE SHIPPING CONTAINER DOES NOT STORE SEMEN WELL FOR LONG PERIODS OF TIME. SPERM WILL LIVE FOR 4-5 DAYS IN THE MARE'S REPRODUCTIVE TRACT. THEREFORE WE RECOMMEND TO INSEMINATE THE MARE WITH THE ENTIRE DOSE AS SOON AS POSSIBLE.

PLEASE EVALUATE THE SEMEN JUST PRIOR OR JUST AFTER INSEMINATION. IF THE SEMEN DOES NOT LOOK VIABLE PLEASE CONTACT US IMMEDIATELY AT THE ABOVE NUMBERS TO ORDER A REPLACEMENT SHIPMENT. THANK YOU FOR YOUR BUSINESS.

Figure 14-3. Form currently in use at the author's practice to accompany shipments of transported semen.

and grasps a sterile insemination pipette between thumb and palm to ensure that the tip is protected in a sterile environment (Fig. 14-4). Non-spermicidal sterile lubricant is applied sparingly to the sleeve covering the forefinger. Prepared semen should be contained in a non-spermicidal syringe and protected in the non-sterile hand from adverse environmental conditions such as direct UV light or extreme cold or heat. The procedure is performed by inserting the sleeved hand, continuing to protect the tip of the insemination pipette, proceeding through the lips of the mare's vulva and into the vaginal vault, and inserting one to two fingers through the cervical os. The finger(s) then acts as a guide for advancement of the insemination pipette through the cervix, which is advanced approximately 1 cm. into the mare's uterus. Extreme care must be taken to avoid damaging the endometrium while advancing the pipette. Once the pipette is satisfactorily in place, the plunger of the syringe is depressed slowly and semen is deposited into the uterus.

With the increasing popularity of rectally guided deep horn insemination,[37,38] it is now possible that doses of semen from stallions that have poor quality of motility or concentration can be centrifuged upon arrival to the mare's location. Semen is loaded in 2-5 × 0.5 ml straws and inseminated as described in Chapter 15.

THE MARE AS A STORAGE PLACE

It has become common practice in cool shipped semen programs to send two insemination doses in the container with instructions of inseminating one dose upon arrival and the second 12–24 hours later. Several experiments have shown that

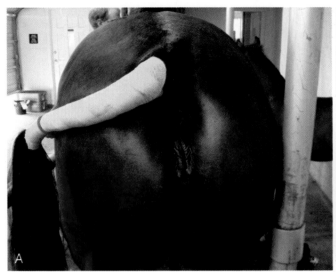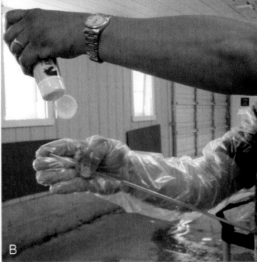

Figure 14-4. A, Perineal area of a mare washed and ready to be inseminated. **B,** Gloved hand with non-spermicidal lube protecting the catheter tip for a uterine body insemination.

spermatozoa reach and attach to the oviductal epithelium of the mare within 2–4 hours after insemination. Furthermore, the attached sperm will live for more than 72 hours in that environment.[39] On the other hand, it is known that most stallion's sperm will lose motility and perhaps fertilizing ability with prolonged times in the transport container. It is the author's opinion that transporting systems are just for that purpose, and that the storage and retention of fertilizing ability of the sperm is best maintained in the mare's oviduct. Therefore, all semen shipped should be inseminated upon arrival.

A considerable amount of controversy exists regarding the number of insemination doses and the number of times that the mare should be inseminated.[40,41] In the author's opinion, there is no clear answer and it would depend on the quality of the stallion's semen and the reproductive history of the mare. If the semen is of good quality and the mare is a young fertile mare, she could be inseminated once or twice at 12- or 24-hour intervals. However, if the semen has poor quality, it would be important to breed the mare as close to ovulation with the entire dose. On the other hand, if the semen is of good quality but the mare is a problem mare with a tendency to accumulate uterine fluid, she should be bred only once within 24–48 hours prior to ovulation. The problem mare bred with poor quality semen should be avoided since she will be a source of aggravation for the mare owner, the stallion owner, and the veterinarian.[42] However, if there is no option, these mares should be bred as close as possible to ovulation with all the semen that is available.

REFERENCES

1. Watson PF, Plummer IM, Allen WE: Quantitative assessment of membrane damaged in cold shocked spermatozoa of stallions. *J Reprod Fertil Suppl* 35:651, 1987.
2. Samper JC, Garcia A, Burnett K: The effect of different lubricants on longevity of motility and velocity of stallion spermatozoa. *Theriogenology* 69:436, 2007.
3. Rigby SL, Varner DD, Thompson JA, et al: Measurement of sperm concentration in stallion ejaculates using photometric or direct enumeration techniques. *Proc Am Assoc Eq Pract* 47:236–238, 2001.
4. Comerford KL, Love CC, Brinsko SP, et al: Validation of a commercially available fluorescence-based instrument to evaluate stallion spermatozoal concentration. *Anim Reprod Sci* 107:316–317, 2008.
5. Amann RP: Computerized evaluation of stallion spermatozoa. Proc 36th Annu AAEP Conv. Dallas, TX: 1988, p 453.
6. Jasko DI, Lein DH, Foote RH: Determination of the relationship between sperm morphologic classifications and fertility in stallions: 66 cases (1987-1988). *J Am Vet Med Assoc* 197:389,1990.
7. Dott HM, Foster GC: A technique for studying the morphology of mammalian spermatozoa which is eosinophilic in a differential "livedead" stain. *J Reprod Fertil* 29:443, 1972.
8. Aman RP: Physiology and endocrinology. In McKinnon AO, Voss JM, eds: *Equine Reproduction*. Philadelphia: Lea & Febiger, 1993, p 658.
9. Squires EL, Todter GE, Brendston WE, et al: Effect of anabolic steroids on reproductive function of young stallions. *J Anim Sci* 54:576, 1982.
10. Love CC, Kenney RM: Scrotal heat stress induces altered sperm chromatin structure associated with a decrease in protamine disulfide bonding in the stallion. *Biol Reprod* 60(3):615-620, 1999.
11. Vogler CI, Bame IH, DeIarnette IM, et al: Effects of elevated temperature on morphology characteristics of ejaculated spermatozoa in the bovine. *Theriogenology* 40:1207, 1993.
12. Samper JC, Tibary A: Disease transmission in horses. *Theriogenology* 66:551–559, 2006.
13. Pickett BW: Collection and evaluation of stallion semen for artificial insemination. In McKinnon AO, Voss IM, eds: *Equine Reproduction*. Philadelphia: Lea & Febiger, 1993, p 705.
14. Amann RP, Thompson DL, Squires EL, et al: Effects of age and frequency of ejaculation on sperm production and extragonadal sperm reserves in stallions. *J Reprod Fertil Suppl* 27:1, 1979.
15. Thompson JA, Love CC, Stich KL, et al: A Bayesian approach to prediction of stallion daily sperm output. *Theriogenology* 62(9):1607-1617, 2004.
16. Jasko DI, Moran DM, Farlin ME, et al: Effect of seminal plasma dilution and removal on spermatozoal motion characteristics of cooled stallion semen. *Theriogenology* 35:1059, 1991.
17. Rigby SL, Brinsko SP, Cochran M, et al: Advances in cooled semen technologies: seminal plasma and semen extender. *Anim Reprod Sci* 68(3-4):171-180, 2001.
18. Brinsko SP: Insemination doses: how low can we go? *Theriogenology* 66(3):543-550, 2006.
19. Katila T, Combes GB, Varner DD, Blanchard TL: Comparison of three containers used for the transport of cooled stallion semen. *Theriogenology* 48(7):1085-1092, 1997.
20. Brinsko SP, Rowan KR, Varner DD, Blanchard TL: Effects of transport container and ambient storage temperature on motion characteristics of equine spermatozoa. *Theriogenology* 53(8):1641-1655, 2000.
21. Aurich C, Seeber P: Müller-Schlösser F: Comparison of different extenders with defined protein composition for storage of stallion spermatozoa at 5 degrees C. *Reprod Domest Anim* 42(4):445-448, 2007.
22. Batellier F, Vidament M, Fauquant J, et al: Advances in cooled semen technology. *Anim Reprod Sci* 68(3-4):181-190, 2001.

23. Pickett BW, Burwash LD, Voss JL, Back DG: Effect of seminal extenders on equine fertility. *J Anim Sci* 40(6):1136-1143, 1975.

24. Love CC, Brinsko SP, Rigby SL, et al: Relationship of seminal plasma level and extender type to sperm motility and DNA integrity. *Theriogenology* 63(6):1584-1591, 2005.

25. Voss JL, Pickett BW, Squires EL: Stallion spermatozoal morphology and motility and their relationships to fertility. *J Am Vet Med Assoc* 178(3):287-289, 1994.

26. den Daas N: Prediction of bovine male fertility. Doctoral thesis, University of Utrecht, The Netherlands. 1997.

27. Bedford S, Hinricks K: Effect of insemination volume on pregnancy rates of pony mares. *Theriogenology* 32:515, 1994.

28. Hamilton DH, Osol R, Osol G, et al: A field study on the fertility of transported equine semen. *Theriogenology* 22:291, 1984.

29. Kenney RM, Bergman RY, Cooper WL: Minimal contamination techniques for breeding mares: Technique and preliminary findings. Proc 22nd Annu AAEP Conv. Lexington, KY: 1975, p 327.

30. Aurich C, Spergser J: Influence of bacteria and gentamicin on cooled-stored stallion spermatozoa. *Theriogenology* 67(5):912-918, 2007.

31. Varner DD, Blanchard TL, Thompson JT: Proceedings of the Second International Symposium on Stallion Semen Preservation. Amersfoort, The Netherlands: 1996.

32. Padilla AW, Foote RH: Extender and centrifugation effects on the motility patterns of slow-cooled stallion spermatozoa. *J Anim Sci* 69(8):3308-3313, 1991.

33. Leboeuf B, Guillouet P, Batellier F, et al: Effect of native phosphocaseinate on the in vitro preservation of fresh semen. *Theriogenology* 60(5):867-877, 2003.

34. Batellier F, Duchamp G, Vidament M, et al: Delayed insemination is successful with a new extender for storing fresh equine semen at 15 degrees C under aerobic conditions. *Theriogenology* 50(2):229-236, 1998.

35. Amann RP, Graham JK: Spermatozoal function. In McKinnon AO, Voss JM, eds: *Equine Reproduction*. Philadelphia: Lea & Febiger, 1993, p 715.

36. Metcalf ES: Pregnancy rates with cooled equine semen received in private practice. Proc 22nd Annu AAEP Conv. 44:16-18, 1998.

37. Lyle SK, Ferrer MS: Low-dose insemination: Why, when and how. *Theriogenology* 64(3):572-579, 2005.

38. Morris L: Advanced insemination techniques in mares. *Vet Clin North Am Eq Pract* 22(3):693-703, 2006.

39. Ellington IE, Ball BA, Blue BI, et al: Capacitation like changes and prolonged viability in vitro of equine spermatozoa cultured with oviduct epithelial cells. *Am J. Vet Res* 1993;54:1505.

40. Shore MD, Macpherson ML, Combes GB, et al: Fertility comparison between breeding at 24 hours or at 24 and 48 hours after collection with cooled equine semen. *Theriogenology* 50(5):693-698, 1998.

41. Squires EL, Brubaker JK, McCue PM, Pickett BW: Effect of sperm number and frequency of insemination on fertility of mares inseminated with cooled semen. *Theriogenology* 49(4):743-749, 1998.

42. Sieme H, Bonk A, Hamann H, et al: Effects of different artificial insemination techniques and sperm doses on fertility of normal mares and mares with abnormal reproductive history. *Theriogenology* 62(5):915-928, 2004.

ARTIFICIAL INSEMINATION WITH FROZEN SEMEN

ROBERTO SANCHEZ, ISABEL GOMEZ, AND JUAN C. SAMPER

In the last decade significant accomplishments have been achieved in the processing, freezing, and insemination of frozen equine semen. Although the techniques are far from optimal, there is wider acceptance of the technique by horse owners and veterinarians with more and more mares being bred with frozen semen worldwide. The advantages of using frozen semen are well established and include: (1) lower cost of transportation of a tank, (2) continuous availability of semen, (3) better timing of insemination, (4) decrease in the risk of transmitting venereal diseases, and (5) increase of the genetic pool. However, there are some disadvantages, including: (1) lower pregnancy rates from some stallions and lack of reassurance from the stallion owner to mare owners regarding quality of the product, (2) increased cost to the mare owner, (3) increased labor, (4) risk of disease transmission, and (5) lack of standard protocols for breeding mares with frozen thawed semen.

Pregnancy rates of mares bred with frozen semen are, on average, around 50%.[1,2] However, it is becoming more obvious that the quality of the frozen semen that is commercialized is improving and pregnancy rates are steadily increasing with the majority of stallions that are offered in the open market. This is perhaps due to the improvement in the freezing techniques and the freezing extenders used. In addition, it is almost standard that frozen stallion semen is now exclusively packed in 0.5-ml straws. Although it is evident that the average semen quality and the fertility are improving, one has to look at averages with a certain degree of caution since these numbers can sometimes be misleading. It is well accepted that although an average pregnancy rate per cycle with frozen semen is around 40% when properly used,[3] there is significant variation in the results, and it is not uncommon to have per cycle pregnancy rates ranging between 0% to over 70%.[4] In addition to this variation, there is a lack of standardization in the information that is available regarding time of an insemination and semen handling procedures.[5,6] Individuals involved in the insemination should know the factors that affect the fertility of frozen semen, so that they can convey realistic expectations to the stallion and mare owners. These factors are (1) the stallion and its semen quality, (2) the fertility of the mare, and (3) the reproductive management and the handling of the semen.

STALLION FACTORS

Thousands of foals are born every year using frozen, thawed semen. Although the technology is still far from optimal, it has gained, and is still gaining, wider acceptance in the industry. An increasing number of stallion and mare owners are taking advantage of the benefits of using frozen semen. Perhaps one of the most important reasons why frozen equine semen is still far from optimal is because there is wide variability in the ability of semen from individual animals to tolerate the freezing and thawing process. It is thought that only 25% of stallions will achieve pregnancy rates compared with those of stallions used for fresh semen or natural cover when inseminated into healthy mares at the proper time.[6] Although the other 75% of the stallions will produce suboptimal pregnancy rates on a per cycle basis, end-of-season pregnancy rates for some of these stallions can reach more than 80%.[7] The drawback is that the number of breeding cycles needed to achieve acceptable pregnancy rates is often too high, making this technique too expensive for the mare owner. Table 15-1 shows the variability in pregnancy rates obtained with frozen semen from different stallions when bred at the uterine body.

It is still uncertain why there is so much variation in the ability of semen to tolerate the freezing and thawing process. Among other reasons, constituents of the seminal plasma or molecules of the sperm itself may be responsible. But stallion owners must also realize that the selection criteria for stallions rarely, if ever, involve semen quality or fertility. Therefore, breeding to stallions that have poor semen could affect the semen quality of the offspring. It is well accepted that there are sire lines known for poor semen quality as well as others known for good quality.[8] There are also sire lines known for good frozen semen quality.

Previous work has shown that this inherent stallion variability is one of the most important factors in determining the pregnancy rates with frozen, thawed semen.[3] Because sperm from individual males responds differently to the freezing and thawing process, several investigators and laboratories have tried numerous systems to try to improve the survival of equine sperm after thawing.[9]

It is still well accepted that one of the most important factors affecting the quality of frozen stallion semen is the quality of the raw ejaculate.[10] The technique for semen collection, processing, and extender type is perhaps just one of the factors. However, if the quality of the raw ejaculate is an important factor in determining the post-thaw quality, it seems that sperm should not be collected for freezing while the stallion is sexually rested. Collection of at least two to four ejaculates before the first freezing should be done to maximize the quality of the raw semen. This procedure should be done even when the semen apparently looks to be of good quality under the microscope.

Recent experimental data have indicated that stallions with apparent suboptimal semen quality for cooling and freezing can be moderately improved by increasing the levels of omega fatty acids in their diet.[11] In addition it is very important that the stallion be in a stress-free environment with the ability to be exercised.

Table 15-1 | Variation in First Cycle and Seasonal Pregnancy Rates of Stallions Used with Frozen Semen and Deposited in the Uterine Body*

STALLION	NO. OF MARES	PACKAGE (ML)	MOTILITY (%)	FIRST CYCLE PREGNANCY (%)	SEASONAL PREGNANCY (%)	CYCLES PER PREGNANCY
A	37	2.5	38	51	81	2.3
B	33	2.5	40	66	83	1.8
C	32	0.5(8)	45	64	80	1.7
D	22	2.5	50	78	94	1.5
E	19	0.5 (8)	43	40	67	2.8
F	17	0.5 (6)	60	54	77	1.6
G	16	2.5	55	42	67	2.8
H	15	5.0	35	30	60	3.0
I	14	2.5	35	50	90	2.8
J	13	4.0	30	44	78	3.1
L	12	0.5 (8)	65	66	100	1.3
M	12	5.0	35	14	71	3.5
N	10	0.5 (12)	25	17	83	4.1
O	9	0.5 (1)	60	33.3	66.6	3.0
P	9	0.5 (8)	50	80	80	1.0
Q	9	0.5 (4)	55	0	20	5.0
R	8	5.0	30	20	75	3.0
S	7	4.0	35	66	66	1.0
T	7	2.5	25	100	100	1.3
U	6	0.5 (1)	50	0	50	4.0
V	6	5.0	30	50	100	1.5
W	6	2.5	30	50	50	4.0
X	5	0.5 (1)	45	0	0	0
Y	5	2.5	35	100	100	1.0
Z	2	0.5 (6)	45	50	50	2.0
N = 25	N = 338		AV = 43	AV = 46	AV = 70.2	AV = 2.4

Note that stallion N, although with a low first cycle pregnancy rate, can end up with an acceptable rate after several cycles, whereas stallion X was unable to achieve any pregnancies at all.

AV, average.

SEMEN PROCESSING

The protocol for processing semen for cryopreservation (freezing) involves the following:

1. The collection and evaluation of gel-free semen
2. The dilution 1:1 of the ejaculate with a centrifugation extender
3. The removal of the cushion and supernatant, leaving a soft sperm pellet
4. The addition of a freezing extender that contains proteins and cryoprotectant(s) necessary to protect the sperm during freezing
5. The final packaging cooling equilibration and controlled freezing
6. Thawing and evaluation of the semen

Once the stallion's extragonadal reserves are stabilized and a detailed evaluation has been previously performed, the evaluation of the raw semen immediately prior to cryopreservation includes the estimation of motility and the calculation of the total number of sperm in the ejaculate. Previously centrifugation extender consisted of mostly a glucose-EDTA solution.[12] Currently it is almost standard practice that the raw semen is quickly diluted at a ratio of 1:1 with any of the milk-based extenders described in Chapter 14.

The centrifugation process has been significantly improved in recent years. The addition of a high-viscosity carbohydrate cushion to the bottom of the centrifugation tube prevents the sperm pellet from compacting against the bottom of the tube (Fig. 15-1). The quality of the sperm pellet is also a critical aspect of the process of semen processing for cryopreservation. The advantage of using the sperm cushion includes a higher recovery of sperm due to higher gravitational centrifugation force ($800–1000\times$ g) compared with the centrifugation force of $300–500\times$ g) for semen without a cushion.[13] Commercial cushion preparations are available from MiniTube or IMV.

Although it has been argued that differences in the composition of the extender will improve the quality of frozen-thawed semen from certain stallions, experimental data have not supported this concept. Stallions considered to be "good freezers" based on post-thaw motility and/or pregnancy rates were not affected by extender type, whereas semen from stallions whose semen did not freeze well could not be improved by simply changing the extender.[14] However, it must be noted that most of the experiments done with changing the extender composition have used 3%–5% glycerol as the cryoprotectant. Recent evidence has shown that a combination of glycerol with

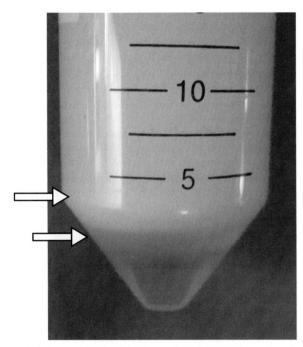

Figure 15-1. Semen centrifuged in Kenney Extender at 1000× g using a bottom cushion preventing the sperm from compacting at the bottom of the tube. Note the band of sperm between the arrows above the clear cushion area.

methylformamide has significantly improved post-thaw motion characteristics as well as pregnancy rates of frozen thawed semen.[15] Preliminary results[16] have also indicated that the use of DMSO as a cryoprotectant and L-ergothioneine as supplement and antioxidant or glutamine to the extender has the potential of improving motion characteristics of sperm after thawing.[17] The amount of freezing extender added to the pooled sperm pellet should be no less than two thirds of the total volume and the practitioner must be careful of not overextending the semen before packaging.

As mentioned previously, semen-handling procedures such as time and force of centrifugation, type of package, and freezing rate have the potential to have a greater impact on the quality of the semen and its potential fertility than changing one single component of the extender.

Semen for freezing has been placed in a variety of packages including 5.0-, 4.0-, 2.5-, 0.5-, and 0.25-ml straws, aluminum tubes, glass ampoules, glass cryovials, and polyethylene bags.[18] The current standard package is the 0-5-ml straw with 500-800 million total motile sperm loaded in one or up to eight straws per insemination dose prior to freezing.

The freezing process starts by an initial cooling of the semen at 0.5°C/min until 6°C. Once that temperature has been reached, a 30- to 60-minute equilibration time is done. Freezing rates for 0.5-ml straws vary between stallions and range from −15°C to −40°C/min until −130°C, at which time the straws are plunged into the liquid nitrogen. Semen can also be frozen successfully by placing the loaded straws on a rack horizontally 2.5–4 cm above the liquid nitrogen. A recent report has also shown that straws can be frozen in plastic goblets containing 5 × 0.5 straws, avoiding further manipulation of individual straws.[19]

It has been shown experimentally that the raw semen from stallions that are considered "good freezers" have lower volumes, higher sperm concentrations, and higher sperm motility compared with semen from those classified as "poor freezers."[20]

In contrast to these results, Brinsko et al.[21] reported a lack of correlation between raw semen parameters and those of cooled stored or frozen semen. Selection criteria of these stallions could explain some of the conflicting results found by these two groups.

The standard procedure has been to collect the stallion and freeze semen at a location where the equipment and technology are centralized or to have a mobile unit that will go to the stallion location. One report indicates that it is possible to ship the stallion's entire ejaculate overnight to a central location in order to be frozen with the appropriate technique. Although not ideal, it could solve the problems of stallions that are located in remote areas.[22]

Freezing of semen from stallions that have suddenly died can be performed by shipping the testicles and epididymides in a cool pack to a central location. Freezing of epididymal semen with extenders containing a combination of glycerol and formamide as cryoprotectant seems to optimize the results.[23,24]

Post-Thaw Evaluation

Post-thaw evaluation of frozen semen is a difficult and controversial topic. Evaluation is generally based on sperm motility, longevity of motility, and morphology. It is thought that frozen, thawed semen having longer longevity tends to produce better pregnancy rates. It is becoming a routine procedure to evaluate the longevity of thawed semen at 37°C, 20°C, or 5°C. Motility, besides being a fairly subjective measure of quality, is a poor predictor of fertility.[14] Hence, it is important for veterinarians using frozen semen routinely to evaluate the morphology of the sperm. It is not uncommon to have stallion sperm with fairly good motility and poor morphology, which could account for some sperm with poor fertility despite good motility after thawing. Bioassays such as zona binding or oviductal epithelial binding may prove to be better indicators of sperm viability and potential for fertilization.[25,26]

Although there are no standards, minimum criteria required for semen to be used commercially seem to be 30%–35% progressively motile with >600 million total sperm per insemination dose. With a small group of mares, Squires et al.[27] recommend that a dose of 250 million progressively motile sperm optimizes fertility when semen was inseminated in the uterine body. Furthermore, Colorado investigators recently reported that stallion semen frozen in 0.5-ml straws that had 320 million progressively motile sperm after thawing resulted in higher pregnancy rates.[28] There is still no consensus on the minimum number of progressively motile sperm per dose needed to maximize fertility; this perhaps is a stallion-dependent factor, as has been reported for the bull. Semen frozen in The Netherlands needs to meet a minimum number of 300 million progressively motile and morphologically normal sperm in order to be sold commercially. However, the site of deposition of the semen could influence the pregnancy rates dramatically. A detailed discussion can be found later in this chapter.

For each of the cryopreservation steps previously mentioned, there are a number of alternatives and variations that are used.[29] This has resulted in a great number of variations in the techniques and in the results of the quality of frozen-thawed semen.

For a good percentage of the stallions, the process of cryopreserving semen results in some degree of reduction in their fertility. This is due to the effect of freezing and thawing on some of the characteristics that sperm must retain to be able to achieve fertilization. Spermatozoa that have been frozen have an impaired ability to reach the oviduct or site of fertilization. Fewer sperm reach the site of fertilization, or perhaps sperm take a longer time to reach it.[30] Sperm attach to the oviductal epithelium through a complex interaction of the carbohydrates present on the plasma membrane.[31] It is not clear whether sperm that have been frozen and thawed have a reduction in their oviductal binding capacity as a result of sperm-extender-carbohydrate interactions or because there are changes in the carbohydrate composition around the membranes as a result of the physical stress of freezing and thawing. Whatever causes this change, it results in a decrease in the capacity of the sperm to attach to the fallopian tube, where they need to capacitate or acquire their capacity to penetrate the egg.[32] Furthermore, sperm cells that are frozen and thawed have changes in their level of calcium, which is also an important factor during the time that sperm cells need to prepare for fertilization. The high levels of intracellular calcium in frozen, thawed sperm compared with that of fresh sperm is perhaps one of the reasons why inseminations with frozen semen have to be performed closer to ovulation.[33,34] All of these changes that happen during the freezing and thawing process of the sperm affect the ability of the mare to form a sperm reservoir, which would normally happen when mares are bred by natural cover or with a fresh semen.[35] These are some of the reasons why it is important that frozen, thawed semen be inseminated within a few hours of ovulation (<12 hours) to maximize fertility. However, this involves more labor for both veterinarians and mare owners.

MARE FACTORS

Mare Fertility Status and Management

The average cycle pregnancy rate for mares inseminated with frozen semen is between 30% and 60%. However, it is not uncommon to have pregnancy results ranging between <10% per cycle or for the season to >70% per cycle (see Table 15-1). Some of the factors that affect the pregnancy rates of frozen semen have been analyzed in the past.[14] Data generated from this analysis of more than 200 mares bred with approximately 400 doses of semen indicated that, on the average, 1.5 doses of semen were used per cycle in all mares and it took an average of 1.7 cycles to produce pregnancy.[36] Mares were examined daily during the first days of their heat period and then at least twice daily when close to ovulation. Every attempt was made to breed the mares within 12 hours before ovulation. Mares that did not ovulate after the first insemination were rebred with a second dose as soon as ovulation was detected if semen was available.

Besides the wide range of inherent fertility rates of the stallions, mare status was the major factor determining the pregnancy rates with frozen semen.[20] Mares were allocated into one of four groups: (1) young maiden mares (<7 years old), (2) older maiden mares (>8 years of age), (3) barren mares, and (4) mares with foal at foot. The average per cycle pregnancy rates were 67.3%, 34%, 50.7%, and 50.9%, respectively. However, mares that had undergone treatment for uterine infections during the cycle before the insemination had an overall first cycle pregnancy rate of 43% compared with an average of 50.5%.[37] Mares that are going to be bred with frozen semen should be carefully and routinely examined at short intervals and bred only once, as late as possible before ovulation. To determine the ideal breeding time, routine ultrasound examinations should be performed to determine uterine and follicular echotexture. Furthermore, in order to time the insemination more accurately and to minimize

the number of breeding doses, the use of ovulatory-inducing agents such as deslorelin or 2500 IU of human chorionic gonadotropin (hCG) is highly recommended. Inseminations with frozen semen that is in short supply or that is very expensive are performed almost exclusively not more than 4 hours after ovulation to avoid inseminations when anovulatory follicles develop.

When young healthy mares with good reproductive histories are to be inseminated, and if there are enough doses available, a reasonable fertility rate can be expected by breeding mares at fixed times. For this, mares that are in good estrus with marked uterine edema and a dominant follicle >35 mm, 2500 IU IV of hCG are given. Mares are bred at 24 and 40 hours after hCG administration.[37] However, this system is far from practical when semen supply is limited or when mares have dubious fertility histories or tend to accumulate uterine fluid.

In addition to depositing the semen at the appropriate time, an examination after ovulation is a crucial component of the insemination process. This examination helps the veterinarian determine possible fluid accumulation in the uterus or severe inflammatory reactions after insemination. This is particularly important in the old maiden group and in those mares susceptible to uterine infections.[38]

Insemination Techniques

As with cooled shipped artificial insemination (AI), the standard site for semen deposition has been the body of the uterus. The increasing popularity in the use of frozen semen and the need to find techniques to maximize the fertility of semen samples with low numbers or semen of low availability has provided considerable incentive to find alternatives to the standard site of semen deposition. In 1998, two reports[39,40] suggested that insemination or deposition of relatively low numbers of spermatozoa at the uterotubal papilla could result in pregnancy in mares. Although pregnancy rates were low (22%–30%) after insemination less than 4 million motile sperm, these studies demonstrated the possibility of significantly reducing the sperm numbers to achieve pregnancies in the horse. These initial studies were performed using a flexible endoscope to deliver the semen, and since then several studies have been performed using various sperm numbers and using rectally guided or hysteroscopic techniques. Table 15-2, adapted from work done by Morris et al.,[41] indicates that although pregnancies can be established with as low as 1000 sperm delivered by hysteroscopic insemination in a 200-μl volume, it is necessary to have at least 1 million sperm or more to be able to achieve

Table 15-2 | **Effect of Sperm Numbers Deposited by Hysteroscopic Insemination on Fertility of Mares**

SPERM NUMBER (MILLION)	PREGNANCY RATE (%)	NO. OF MARES
0.001	10	10
0.1	22	11
0.5	29	14
1	64	25
5	75	8
10	60	10

Modified from Morris LH, Hunter RH, Allen WR: Hysteroscopic insemination of small numbers of spermatozoa at the uterotubal junction of preovulatory mares. *J Reprod Fertil* 118:95-100, 2000.

acceptable pregnancy rates (>50%) under laboratory conditions. This study clearly shows that the number of sperm needed to establish pregnancies is far less than the 500 million originally suggested.

Today there are three common techniques to inseminate mares with frozen semen: (1) body insemination, (2) rectally guided deep horn insemination, and (3) hysteroscopic or endoscopic deep horn insemination. All of these three require different equipment and skills with different advantages and disadvantages.

All inseminations with frozen semen require proper facilities with running water to be able to wash the mares; an ultrasound machine; and basic AI equipment including latex gloves, non-spermicidal lubricant, pipettes, syringes, a warming plate, slides, cover slips, small pipettes, microscope, an incubator, a warm water bath or access to warm water, a thermometer, scissors, and liquid nitrogen storage.

Uterine Body Insemination

The insemination in the uterine body is the most common technique and is performed as described in Chapter 14. Briefly, a clean glove is put over the technician's hand and a sterile pipette is advanced vaginally past the cervix. Volumes of 0.5–5 ml are inseminated using air or a small amount of extender to flush the pipette. Failure to do this will result in a significant amount of sperm left in the pipette, particularly with the smaller volumes. It is not recommended to dilute the semen in an extender in order to increase the inseminate volume. The major disadvantages of this technique are the need for higher volume and sperm numbers, increasing the inflammatory reaction of the mare and causing a delay in uterine sperm transport; however, the technique is easy and very inexpensive.[42]

Rectally Guided Deep Horn Insemination (DHI)

The rectally guided technique starts by washing the perineum thoroughly and under light sedation. A 65-cm flexible pipette is passed through the cervix (Fig. 15-2). The inseminator's hand is then placed in the previously emptied rectum. The pipette is moved by rectal manipulation toward the tip of the horn ipsilateral to the ovary that has the recent ovulation. Once the pipette

is placed in the desired location, the first straw of semen is inserted into the pipette with the cotton plug toward the outside of the pipette. A steel plunger is used to push the straw to the tip of the horn (Fig. 15-3). With the pressure of the plunger, the open end of the straw will lodge into the pipette's tip nipple (Fig. 15-4), avoiding any backflush of semen into the lumen of the pipette. If multiple straws are used for one insemination, the MiniTube system provides an easy and effective way of delivering the semen and removing empty straws from the pipette without having to replace the pipette. The rectally guided deep horn insemination (DHI) technique has several advantages. It is inexpensive, and only two people are needed. With experience it can be performed very rapidly. The major disadvantage is that

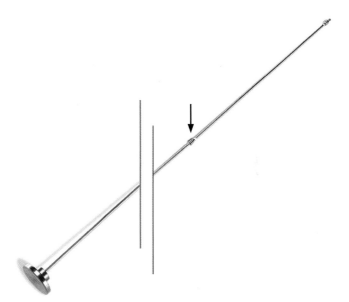

Figure 15-3. Flexible stainless steal Stylette for use with the pipette shown in Fig. 15-2. The inverted cone *(arrow)* is located at approximately 10 cm from the tip so that it can pull back an empty straw. (Courtesy of Minitube, Verona, Wisc.)

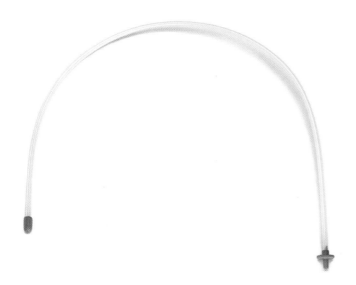

Figure 15-2. Flexible pipette is used for the rectally guided deep horn insemination technique. (Courtesy of Minitube, Verona, Wisc.)

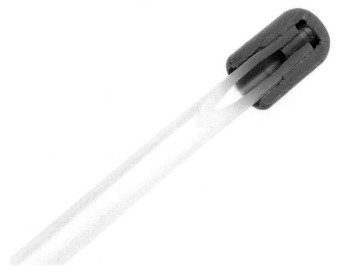

Figure 15-4. Sagittal view of the tip of the flexible pipette shown in Fig. 15-2. The inside of the tip has a 4-mm nipple-like protrusion that lodges the tip of the 0.5-ml straw when it is pushed by the Stylette, avoiding any backflush of semen into the lumen of the pipette. (Courtesy of Minitube, Verona, Wisc.)

carelessness might cause trauma to the uterus or the rectum during the manipulation. In addition, it can be difficult to manipulate the large uterus of a post-partum mare to deposit the small volume of semen in the appropriate location.

Hysteroscopic (Endoscopic) Insemination (EDHI)

As with any vaginal procedure, the perineal area is washed and disinfected. The mare is sedated with the use of butorphanol tartrate (5 mg IV) coupled with either xylazine (150 mg IV) or detomidine (4 mg IV). As with DHI, evacuation is essential. A prewarmed 1.2- or 1.6-m flexible videoscope or endoscope previously cold sterilized with glutaraldehyde and rinsed with abundant lactated Ringer's solution is inserted into the uterine body of the mare. The endoscope operator removes the hand from the vagina and places it in the rectum and, as described for DHI, the endoscope is moved toward the tip of the horn by rectal manipulation toward the horn ipsilateral to the ovary that has or had the preovulatory follicle. Once the endoscope is in the proximal third of the desired horn, the uterine horn is distended with air in order to observe the tip where the oviductal papilla is identified. When the papilla is easily observed and the endoscope is close to it, the delivery system, which has been placed previously in the endoscope biopsy channel and loaded with the semen at the distal third of the tube, is advanced so that it touches the papilla. The semen is then slowly delivered onto the oviductal papilla (Fig. 15-5). Volumes of >1 ml delivered endoscopically usually tend to run down the horn after delivery, particularly if the uterine lumen is tightly distended with air. Once the semen is delivered, the endoscope is removed. With experience, the entire procedure should not take more than 5 minutes. Fig. 15-5 shows the areas of the uterus where semen can be deposited.

The use of endoscopic AI should be limited to frozen semen, sexed sperm, or very valuable sperm in very low volumes (0.5 ml). Although it would appear that endoscopic insemination

should result in better pregnancy rates, it is difficult to justify considering the additional expense in personnel and equipment needed to conduct the procedure. Table 15-3 shows a comparison of the two techniques under field conditions reported by the authors. In this study mares were bred with frozen semen using a maximum of 100 million total sperm in 500–1500 µl. Results indicate that although there is a slight and consistent advantage of the endoscopic technique, veterinarians must weigh the advantages and disadvantages as well as semen availability before deciding what technique should be used. However, if the number of sperm is in a volume of 250 µl or less, we strongly advocate the use of the endoscopic technique. Fig. 15-6 depicts the oviductal papilla and the endoscopic delivery tube approaching the papilla to deliver the semen.

Previous reports have indicated that as the number of sperm inseminated in the uterine body decreases, so does the expected fertility rate. Maximum fertility was achieved when insemination doses deposited in the uterine body contained over 600 million total sperm.[36,37] However, recent research as well as clinical experience is starting to show that in stallions with very good semen quality, sperm numbers can be significantly reduced in the insemination dose without compromising fertility rates in commercial settings if semen is deposited closer to the oviduct. However, sperm numbers to achieve maximal fertility for a particular animal appear to be dependent on the individual. Therefore, some stallions achieve their maximal level of fertility with 50 million sperm whereas others might need 10 times that number to achieve the same level of fertility. Regardless of the insemination method used, the stallion remains the biggest variable accounting for fertility in frozen semen breeding programs. Table 15-4 shows the variation amongst stallions used in a commercial breeding program.

The question that still remains to be answered is if fertility rates can be further increased or changed significantly by changing the site of semen deposition. Experience by the authors would indicate that fertility will not be improved if the stallion already has a good fertility rate. However, fertility of some stallions with poor fertility can be slightly improved by doubling or tripling the number of sperm from 100 to 200 or 300, whereas others will remain severely subfertile. Further increases in fertility were not detectable when inseminating higher numbers of sperm. It appears that only some stallions can be helped when using the deep horn insemination techniques (Fig. 15-7).

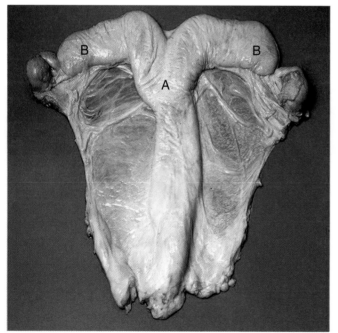

Figure 15-5. Uterus of the mare showing the place of semen deposition. *A,* Body of the uterus; *B,* tip of the horn close to the oviductal papilla.

Table 15-3 | **Deep Horn Insemination Pregnancy Rates During Three Breeding Seasons with Frozen Semen Deposited by Rectally Guiding a Flexible Pipette (DHI) or with the Use of an Endoscope (EDHI)***

	DHI		EDHI	
YEAR	NO. AI	PREGNANCY (%)	NO. AI	PREGNANCY (%)
2005	107	42	490	47
2006	408	41	555	45
2007	759	44	225	42
Total	1274	43	1270	45

*A slight consistent but not significant pregnancy rate is detected with the endoscopic deep horn insemination.

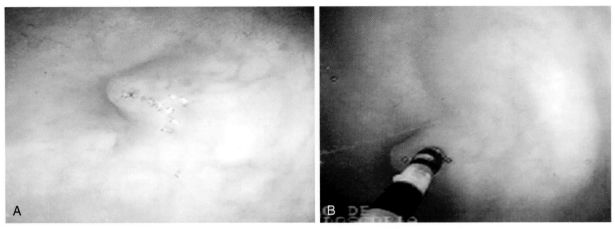

Figure 15-6. A, Endoscopic view of the oviductal papilla. **B,** Endoscopic catheter approaching the papilla to deliver a small volume of semen.

Table 15-4 | **Stallion Effect on Pregnancy Rates Expressed As Embryo Recovery with Frozen Semen Using Low-Dose Inseminations**

STALLION	NO. AI	PREGNANCY (%)
A	135	42
B	61	61
C	32	81
D	23	22
E	22	50
F	20	45
G	18	61
H	15	33
I	14	29
J	10	60
K	10	10

We have used the rectally guided DHI technique to deposit cooled shipped sperm that appears to be of poor quality or is very diluted on arrival. The sperm are centrifuged at $1000\times$ g for 15 minutes using a sperm centrifugation cushion. Once the supernatant is discarded, 2 ml of concentrated sperm are aspirated into one to four 0.5-ml straws and inseminated as described previously. Clinical impressions support an increase in fertility from these stallions.

Pregnancy Rates with Endoscopically Deposited Semen or by Rectally Guided Insemination

The perception that some mares accumulate excessive amounts of fluid because of an allergic reaction has been recently addressed by Dutch, Finnish, and American investigators. Their data indicated that fluid accumulation in the uterus after insemination is a normal process, is not an allergic reaction, and is not dependent on the type of extender or any of its components (such as egg yolk or glycerol). Small amounts of uterine fluid can be detected on most mares shortly after breeding and is a transient uterine inflammatory and normal process in all mares. Seminal plasma appears to be a modulator and delays the physiological uterine reaction to semen.[43] Since the processing of semen for thawing involves the removal of the seminal plasma, this perhaps exacerbates this transient inflammatory response from the mare. Small to moderate amounts of fluid are drained through the cervix within a few hours of breeding in the normal mare.[44] Excess fluid accumulation is perhaps the result of poor cervical relaxation coupled with poor lymphatic drainage in the old maiden mare, or poor uterine contractility in mares susceptible to uterine infections.[45] Mares that are in these categories should be routinely checked and a uterine lavage performed, and therapy with oxytocin, carbetocin, and/or cloprostenol should be implemented to drain this excess amount of fluid, particularly when bred with frozen semen. Recently, steroidal anti-inflammatory drugs such as prednisolone or dexamethasone have been used to modulate the inflammatory response of the uterus of mares. Mares with hyperedema or those that have an increased grade of endometrial edema after insemination or ovulation are good candidates to treat with these products.[46]

In summary, veterinarians involved in AI with frozen semen are often presented with frozen semen accompanied by an array of different instructions with respect to type of package, thawing, and timing of examination. The lack of consensus among laboratories processing semen invariably places the industry in a precarious position and makes the technique lose credibility among some of the users. Individuals purchasing frozen semen should inquire regarding the previous fertility of the stallion with frozen semen. The fact that some stallions have very good conception rates with natural breeding or shipped semen does not guarantee their fertility with frozen semen. Mare owners are also encouraged to ask their veterinarian to evaluate the semen immediately after thawing to determine parameters such as motility, morphology, sperm concentration, number of doses used, and type of package. In the long run, this type of information from large numbers of inseminations will be the only way to standardize some of the basic parameters needed to increase pregnancy rates. Although it is very evident that there has been a tremendous increase in the quality of the frozen semen that is commercialized now compared with 10 years ago, the creation of realistic expectations regarding breeding mares with frozen semen, together with higher pregnancy rates per cycle, will be the best proponents for the use of cryopreserved semen in the equine industry.

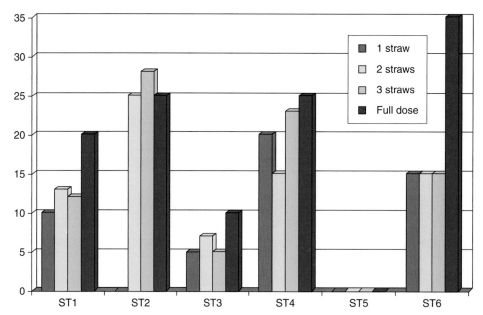

Figure 15-7. Effect of number of straws on the level of fertility achieved by frozen semen in stallions with poor reproductive performance. Note that stallion #5 was unable to achieve pregnancies while other stallions had marked improvement.

REFERENCES

1. Nishikawa Y, Shinomiya S: Results of conception tests of frozen horse semen during the past ten years. Proc Intl Congress Animal Reproduction and Artificial Insemination. 4:1034, 1976.
2. Muller Z: Practicalities of insemination of mares with deep frozen semen. J Reprod Fertil Suppl 35:121, 1987.
3. Samper JC, Hellander IC, Crabo BG: Relation between fertility of fresh and frozen stallion semen and its quality measured as sperm motility and with glass wool/sephadex filters. *J Reprod Fertil Suppl* 44:107-114, 1991.
4. Samper JC: Are there industry standards for the production and utilization of frozen equine semen? Proc Society Theriogenology. Montreal: 1997.
5. Samper JC, Morris CA: Current methodology for stallion semen cryopreservation: an international survey. *Theriogenology* 49:895, 1998.
6. Amann RP, Pickett BW: Principles of cryopreservation of stallion spermatozoa. *Eq Vet Sci* 7:145, 1987.
7. Samper JC: Stallion semen cryopreservation: Male factors affecting pregnancy rates. Proc Society for Theriogenology. San Antonio, TX: 1995, pp 160–165.
8. Weber AF, Buoen L, Hurtgen JP: Cytogenetic and hereditary sources of infertility in stallions. Proc Stallion Reproduction Symposium, Society for Theriogenology. Baltimore: 1998, p 45.
9. Samper JC: Current techniques for artificial insemination. In Youngquist RM, ed: *Current Therapy in Large Animal Theriogenology.* Philadelphia: WB Saunders, 1997, p 36.
10. Sieme H, Harrison RA, Petrunkina AM: Cryobiological determinants of frozen semen quality, with special reference to stallion. *Anim Reprod Sci* 107(3-4):276-292, 2008.
11. Brinsko SP, Varner DD, Love CC, et al: Effect of feeding a DHA-enriched nutraceutical on the quality of fresh, cooled and frozen stallion semen. *Theriogenology* 63(5):1519-1527, 2005.
12. Martin JC, Klug E, Günzel AR: Centrifugation of stallion semen and its storage in large volume straws. *J Reprod Fertil Suppl* 27:47-51, 1979.
13. Waite JA, Love CC, Brinsko SP, et al: Factors impacting equine sperm recovery rate and quality following cushioned centrifugation. *Theriogenology* 70:704-714, 2008.
14. Dell'Aqua JA, Papa FO, Alvarenga FC, et al: Effects of warming rate on sperm parameters and of insemination and dose on the fertility of equine frozen semen. *Anim Reprod Sci* 68:344-346, 2001.
15. Samper JC, Garcia A: Post-thaw characteristics and fertility of stallion semen frozen in extenders with different cryoprotectant. *Anim Reprod Sci* 107:348-349, 2008.
16. Metcalf ES, Dideon BA, Blehr R, et al: Effects of DMSO and L-ergothioneine on post-thaw semen parameters in stallions: preliminary results. *Anim Reprod Sci* 107:332-333, 2008.
17. Khlifaoui M, Battut I, Bruyas JF, et al: Effects of glutamine on post-thaw motility of stallion spermatozoa: an approach of the mechanism of action at spermatozoa level. *Theriogenology* 63(1):138-149, 2005.
18. Samper JC: Artificial insemination. In Samper JC, ed: *Equine Breeding Management and Artificial Insemination.* Philadelphia: WB Saunders, 2000.
19. Love CC, White RD, Varner DD: Prepackaging of equine semen in goblets prior to cryopreservation. *Anim Reprod Sci* 89(1-4):248-250, 2005.
20. Samper JC, Hearn P, Ganheim A, et al: Pregnancy rates and effect of extender and motility and acrosome status of frozen-thawed stallion spermatozoa. Proc 40th Annual AAEP Convention. Vancouver: 1994, pp 41-43.
21. Brinsko SP, Van Wagner GS, Graham IK, Squires EL: Motility morphology and triple stain analysis of fresh, cooled and frozen stallion spermatozoa. Proc 7th Int Symp Equine Reproduction. Pretoria, South Africa: 1998.
22. Crockett EC, Graham JK, Bruemmer JE, Squires EL: Effect of cooling of equine spermatozoa before freezing on post-thaw motility: preliminary results. *Theriogenology* 55(3):793-803, 2001.
23. Neild D, Miragaya M, Chaves G, et al: Cryopreservation of cauda epididymis spermatozoa from slaughterhouse testicles 24 hours after ground transportation. *Anim Reprod Sci* 94:250-252, 2006.
24. Papa FO, Melo CM, Fioratti EG, et al: Freezing of stallion epididymal sperm. *Anim Reprod Sci* 107(3-4):293-301, 2008.
25. Fazeli AR, Steenweg W, Bevers MM, et al: Relation between stallion sperm binding to homologous hemizonae and fertility. *Theriogenology* 44:751, 1995.
26. Samper JC, Ellington IE, Burnett K: Use of sperm and oviduct co-culture as a test for stallion field fertility. Proc 42nd Annu AAEP Convention. Lexington, KY: 1996, p 3.
27. Squires EL, Pickett BW: Pregnancy rates with cryopreserved semen. In *Proceedings of Symposium on Techniques for Handling and Utilization of Transported Cool and Frozen Semen.* Ft Collins, CO: 1995, p 106.
28. Leipold SD, Graham IK, Squires EL, et al: Effect of spermatozoal concentration and number on fertility of frozen equine semen. *Theriogenology* 49:1537, 1998.
29. Pickett BW, Amann RP: Cryopreservation of semen. In McKinnon AO, Voss JM, eds: *Equine Reproduction.* Philadelphia: Lea & Febiger, 1993, p 769.
30. Bader H: An investigation of sperm migration into the oviducts of the mare. *J Reprod Fertil Suppl* 32:59, 1982.
31. Lefebvre R, DeMott RP, Suarez SS, Samper JC: Specific inhibition of equine sperm binding to oviductal epithelium. *Biol Reprod Mono Ser* 11995:689–696, 1998.

32. Dobrinski I, Thomas PGA, Ball BA: Cryopreservation reduces the ability of equine sperm to attach to oviductal epithelial cells and zona pellucida. *J Androl* 16:536, 1995.

33. Leopold S, Samper JC, Curtis E, Buhr MM: Effect of cryopreservation and oviductal cell conditioned media on calcium flux in equine spermatozoa. Proc 7th Int Symp Equine Reproduction. Pretoria, South Africa: 1998.

34. Dobrinski I, Smith TT, Suarez SS, et al: Membrane contact with oviductal epithelium modulates the intracellular calcium concentration of equine spermatozoa in vitro. *Biol Reprod* 56:861-869, 1997.

35. Woods I, Bergfelt DR, Ginther OJ: Effects of time of insemination relative to ovulation on pregnancy rate and embryonic loss in mares. *Eq Vet J* 22:410, 1990.

36. Samper JC: Why are pregnancy rates lower with frozen semen? Proc Stallion Reproduction Symposium, Society for Theriogenology. Baltimore: 1998, p 71.

37. Metcalf ES: The efficient use of equine cryopreserved semen. *Theriogenology* 68(3):423-428, 2007.

38. Pycock JF: Breeding management of the problem mare. In Samper JC, ed: *Equine Breeding Management and Artificial Insemination.* Philadelphia: WB Saunders, 2000.

39. Vazquez JJ, Medina VM, Liu IKM, et al: Nonsurgical uterotubal insemination in the mare. Proc Annu Conv Am Assoc Equine Pract 44:68-69, 1998.

40. Manning ST, Bowman PA, Fraser LM, et al: Development of hysteroscopic insemination of the uterine tube in the mare. Proc Annu Conv Am Assoc Equine Pract 44:70-71, 1998.

41. Morris LH, Hunter RH, Allen WR: Hysteroscopic insemination of small numbers of spermatozoa at the uterotubal junction of preovulatory mares. *J Reprod Fertil* 118:95-100, 2000.

42. Morris L: Advanced insemination techniques in mares. *Vet Clin North Am Eq Pract* 22(3):693-703, 2006.

43. Katila T: Onset and duration of uterine inflammatory response of mares after insemination with fresh semen. *Biol Reprod Mono Ser* 1:515, 1995.

44. LeBlanc MM, Neuworth L, Jones L, et al: Differences in uterine position of reproductively normal mares and those with delayed uterine clearance detected by scintigraphy. *Theriogenology* 50:49, 1998.

45. Dell'Aqua JA Jr, Papa FO, Lopes MD, et al: Modulation of acute uterine inflammatory response after artificial insemination with equine frozen semen. *Anim Reprod Sci* 94:321, 2006.

46. Samper JC: How to interpret endometrial edema in mares. *Proc Am Assoc Eq Pract* 53:571–572, 2007.

EQUINE EMBRYO TRANSFER

FERNANDO L. RIERA

An increasing amount of work has been done in the area of embryo transfer (ET) since it was first reported in 1972 by Oguri and Tsutsumi.[1] Despite the efforts of many clinicians and laboratories working in the equine field, progress has been slow compared with that accomplished in bovine, ovine, and swine. Perhaps the major reason why equine ET has lagged behind is the lack of interest by most breed associations in registering foals born by ET. More recently some associations have become more flexible and accept ET as an alternative to regular breeding. Although there are products in the market that can be used to induce multiple ovulations, the results obtained with such products have been inconsistent and not yet very practical, which still renders ET inefficient in the horse.[2] Since the development of blood typing and DNA parentage verification, parentage errors or frauds can be easily avoided. Even so, many breed registries either do not accept registration of offspring produced by ET or have restrictions on the number of registerable ET foals produced from one mare during a breeding season.

At our clinic, ETs are performed primarily from polo pony mares. In addition, Warmblood, Quarter Horse, Arabian, and Peruvian Paso mares are commonly used as embryo donors. The Argentinian Polo Pony Breeders Association (AACCPP) has no restrictions on the number of foals that can be registered every season. Since the first ET in polo ponies was performed in 1989,[3] there has been a significant number of foals produced using this technology. During the 2007-2008 ET season, approximately 4000 pregnancies were produced by ET in Argentina. It is common for a donor mare to produce four to five pregnancies in the remainder of a breeding season after the polo season. At Doña Pilar, up to 13 foals have been produced from the same mare during one breeding season.

This chapter describes the practical aspects related to a large-scale commercial ET program in Argentina. In addition, some of the factors that have been determined to influence the success of the program are discussed. Fig. 16-1 shows the distribution from 10,256 uterine lavages for embryo collection performed on 2174 donor mares over the last 11 years. These mares were bred by artificial insemination to one or more of 160 stallions. This graph is a reference for the discussion of several factors affecting the overall success of ET.

For optimal results, it is necessary to keep donors, recipients, and stallions at the same facility. Working with a large number of donors requires an efficient system for teasing and examination of mares. On an average day during the peak of the breeding season at Doña Pilar, it is common to examine over 300 mares by palpation via rectum and ultrasonography. In addition, approximately 30–50 donors are artificially inseminated with semen collected from 10–20 stallions. Approximately 12–20 flushings are performed per day, which requires good organization and a skillful team, as well as proper facilities.

Embryos at our center are recovered non-surgically by means of a uterine lavage performed 6–8 days after donor ovulation. Embryos are transferred non-surgically into synchronized intact mares or non-cycling mares supplemented with exogenous progesterone. To maximize the number of pregnancies achieved per season, most embryo donor mares are injected with a luteolytic dose of prostaglandin-$F_{2\alpha}$ ($PGF_{2\alpha}$) after each uterine lavage. Pregnancy diagnosis is performed on recipient mares 7–14 days after ET and then confirmed at 45–60 days and again immediately before sending to the embryo owner.

APPLICATIONS OF EMBRYO TRANSFER IN THE EQUINE INDUSTRY

Young Mares

Frequently, a 2-year-old mare that becomes pregnant fails to carry a foal to term. Immaturity, stress, abortion, or embryonic loss have been implicated.[4] Two-year-old mares, particularly late in the spring, are good embryo donors, provided that they are of a similar body size compared with mature mares.[5]

Old Subfertile Mares

Old mares with uterine conditions such as periglandular fibrosis, endometrosis,[6] or endometritis[7] can become pregnant, but early embryonic death (EED) or abortion may occur. In such cases, transfer of the embryo to a healthy uterus increases the chances of obtaining offspring from that mare.[8,9] At Dona Pilar, many old subfertile mares consistently produce several foals every year.[10]

Old retired donor mares 18 to 25 years old are a minor group within the embryo donors. Most of these mares have histories of infertility or are too old to carry a foal to term. Despite their uterine condition, some of them still have normal cycles and produce embryos that can be transferred to normal recipients.

Mares in Competition

ET allows pregnancies in mares without interfering with their athletic careers. By obtaining embryos from competition mares, the time interval to the next generation can be shortened for a mare, which otherwise would not be able to deliver offspring until later in her life. Through ET, mares can produce several foals each breeding season, even though they are competing.[4,11]

Some studies have indicated that exercising can be detrimental to embryo recovery rates and can increase the incidence

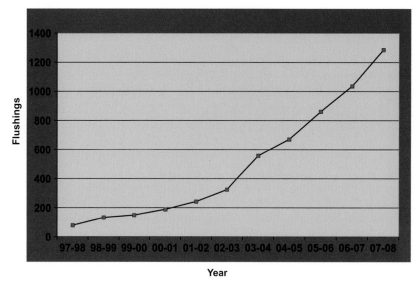

Figure 16-1. Number of embryo transfer recover attempts (flushings) at the Embryo Transfer Center Doña Pilar between 1997 and 2008.

of morphologic abnormalities, which can be related to thermal stress.[11] We believe that this depends on the conditions of the exercising. Embryo recovery rate and embryo morphology rate was not affected in competing Warmbloods in Germany[12] or in performance polo ponies in England.[13]

Progeny Testing

It is common to have a mare bred to different stallions during a single season, thus producing several foals that are trained simultaneously. ET becomes a valuable tool to identify the good polo sires as well as the dams.

PROCESS INVOLVED IN AN EMBRYO TRANSFER PROGRAM

Selection and Management of Embryo Donors

There are several reasons why mares are enrolled in an ET program. Because ET is an expensive technique, its application is usually restricted to those mares of superior quality with characteristics that are thought to be highly heritable. Most mares brought to our center are polo ponies (Thoroughbred or Thoroughbred-crosses) ranging in age from 5 to 18 years and weighing 400–500 kg. Many of these mares are still at the peak of their athletic careers. They are enrolled in the program for 3–4 months after the polo tournaments and during this time undergo intensive reproductive management to produce as many pregnancies as possible.

Breeding Soundness Evaluation

Before admission to the center, every mare should have been tested for equine infectious anemia. Once the mare arrives, a general physical examination is performed. All mares are dewormed, and vaccinations, including that for strangles, are updated. Records and fertility history, including previous ET records, are carefully reviewed. This review provides useful information regarding general and reproductive management. Previous records can show the mare's temperament, teasing behavior, susceptibility to endometritis, and characteristics of the

estrous cycle (e.g., length, time from prostaglandin administration to ovulation, and incidence of double ovulations). Most of these findings are repeated from year to year.

Each donor mare should provide the following information upon arrival: number of pregnancies to achieve, sires to be used on each cycle, and type of housing and feeding to which the mare is accustomed. The mares are carefully identified with tags, and samples are submitted for DNA typing.

Every mare undergoes a breeding soundness evaluation after arrival at the ET center. This examination includes visual inspection of the external genitalia and evaluation of the internal genitalia by transrectal palpation and ultrasonography. Cervical evaluation is done by direct digital palpation to assess its integrity and to detect abnormalities such as tears or adhesions.

In some cases, a uterine cytological evaluation, culture of an endometrial swab, and histological evaluation of an endometrial biopsy sample are performed. Because it is common for polo pony mares to have had a Caslick's operation to prevent air aspiration into the vagina while in competition, many times it is necessary to open the mare's vulva enough to allow for the evaluation procedures to be conducted. On some old mares with defective perineal conformation, surgical correction should be performed.

If a fertility problem is detected, appropriate therapy is instituted. The most common therapy performed at our clinic is a uterine lavage, using large volumes of prewarmed sterile saline[14] on mares with clinical signs of endometritis. Several lavages are performed until the effluent is clear; then 20 IU of oxytocin is given intravenously to induce uterine contractions. The treatment is repeated several times until signs of endometritis have disappeared. Intrauterine infusion of antibiotics, which are selected based on culture and sensitivity, is sometimes performed.[15] In some cases, response to therapy is evaluated by an endometrial biopsy and graded according to Kenney's grading system.[6]

Ideally, one or preferably two estrous cycles of each embryo donor are evaluated before starting the program. This allows for evaluation of teasing behavior, ovarian follicular dynamics, and palpable and ultrasonographic changes in the uterus and ovaries throughout the cycle. This becomes of great relevance if no previous records of the mare are available. Donor mares must be cycling normally before being started in the program. Because of time constraints, most mares are started in the program immediately after arrival and normal cyclicity cannot be evaluated. Owners who plan to have a mare in an ET program are warned regarding the effects of anabolic steroids on the mare's fertility and are discouraged from giving potential embryo donors hormones during training and competition.

Management of Embryo Donors

At Doña Pilar, embryo donors are housed in groups of 10 to 25 to optimize management and decrease stress and chances of injuries. Once a mare is introduced and adapted to a social group, it will stay with that group for the rest of the season. Donor groups are assigned to one of two different examination facilities directed by two different veterinarians in each team. An average of 150 donor mares will be examined, inseminated, and flushed in each team.

Selection and Management of Recipients

One of the most critical aspects that determines the success of an ET program is the selection, management, and quality of the recipient mares. Good recipient mares should meet all of the following requirements: (1) good health and body condition, (2) easy to handle and halter broken, (3) body size similar to that of the embryo donor, (4) 4–10 years of age, (5) sound breeding condition and a uterine biopsy grade 1 or IIA according to Kenney,[6] (6) good estrus displayed when teased, and (7) regular cycling.

We prefer mares that have foaled normally at least once and that have shown good ability to nurse the foal. Although primiparous mares can be used, it is important to advise the owner of the embryo that the mare may need more attention at the time of foaling and that foals can be of smaller size at birth. Mean placental parameters and foal birthweights were shown to be lower in primiparous mares when compared with mares on the second or subsequent parities. The primiparous mares showed a significant reduction in the areas of microcotyledons compared with mares in their second or subsequent parities.[16]

Our recipient herd consists of crossbred mares weighing between 400 and 600 kg. Health requirements for recipient mares are the same as those for donor mares. In addition, all recipient mares are freeze branded. Careful records include identification information, age, markings, vaccination status, deworming status, and reproductive history, if available.

Careful attention is given to the size of the recipients. Polish workers have shown the effect of the size of the recipient on the size of the offspring.[17] In this study, embryos obtained from Polish pony mares (380–400 kg) and transferred into large recipients (560–780 kg) developed into foals that were larger and heavier than their siblings born to the genetic mothers. Embryo transfer into larger mares also resulted in foals that grew faster during the nursing period.

Lagneaux and Palmer[18] in 1989 suggested that the uterus of a pony mare responds differently from that of a large mare to the cervical stimulation induced during non-surgical ET performed on day 7 after ovulation. The investigators demonstrated that prostaglandin release resulting from mechanical stimulation or endometritis induces luteolysis more frequently in pony mares than in large Selle-Francaise mares. Nine embryos transferred transcervically to pony mares resulted in no pregnancies, whereas nine embryos transferred to Selle-Francaise mares yielded four pregnancies.[18]

The breeding soundness examination for the recipient mare is similar to that performed on the donor mare. Special emphasis is given to the size and tone of the uterus and cervix. We prefer to use recipient mares with documented, well-known reproductive histories.

Recipient mares are kept in mixed pastures of grass and alfalfa. Pregnant and transferred recipients receive the best pastures, especially from the day of ET up to 40 days of gestation. Non-pregnant mares are kept in groups of approximately 50 to 100. These groups are examined periodically depending upon the synchronization requirements to determine follicular activity and day of ovulation.

One of the most critical aspects that affect pregnancy rates in a large-scale ET program is related to recipient management. Stress should be avoided as much as possible. It is very common for recipient mares added to the program on the last trimester of the breeding season not to become pregnant and go into anestrus earlier than the rest of the group. Many times these mares will be infected with strangles, which is a common disease in Argentina. The ability to overcome this problem is one of the major challenges in a large commercial program.

During the breeding season of 2008, we introduced a managerial change with respect to strangles in the recipient herd. New recipient mares went into a quarantine and were vaccinated twice 15 days apart against strangles. With this system we have been able to avoid strangles infections and pregnancy rates have been higher than in previous years.

Synchrony between Donor and Recipient Mares

One of the most time-consuming activities in an ET center is related to the examination of donors and recipients to determine ovulation dates and degree of synchrony between them. This examination is routinely performed by transrectal palpation[19] and ultrasonography[20] of the ovarian structures. Serum progesterone levels are also used for this purpose.[21,22]

Donor mares in estrus should be examined daily once a dominant follicle has been detected. This is essential for deciding the timing for either natural mating or artificial breeding and for determining the day of ovulation (day 0).

Several authors have shown that pregnancy rates are similar when transferring the embryos to recipient mares that have ovulated 24 hours before (−24) and up to 72 hours after (+72) donor ovulation.[23-30] However, a retrospective analysis of 544 embryos transferred non-surgically to mares that ovulated within −24, 0, +24, and +48 hours of the donor indicated that pregnancy rates were similar for 0, +24, and +48 hours (58.4%, 62.3%, and 62.3%, respectively) but were lower (50%) for the mares that ovulated 24 hours before the donor. When a smaller number of embryos were transferred to recipients ovulating 72 hours after the donor, pregnancy rates were further enhanced (83.8%). Based on these data, we prefer recipients to ovulate on the same day or after the donor. Furthermore, because it appears that pregnancy rates are not affected by day of ovulation, as long as recipients ovulate after the donor, we examine recipients every other day or every 2 days, based on recipient demand.

The method used for synchronization depends on the number of donors and recipients involved in the program. If there is a large number of recipients, synchronization may be performed by administration of a luteolytic dose of $PGF_{2\alpha}$ or an analogue given to one or two recipients 1 or 2 days after administration to the donor. In large programs recipient availability can sometimes be a limitation. The optimal ratio should not be lower than 1.2 recipients per donor. Ovulation usually occurs 6–8 days after treatment if prostaglandin is given between days 6 and 9 of the cycle. However, response to treatment and time to ovulation can depend on the follicular status of the ovaries at the time of treatment. Mares with large follicles when given prostaglandin tend to show heat and ovulate sooner than do mares with small follicles. Ovulation occurs in approximately two thirds of mares given prostaglandin that have a large pre-ovulatory size follicle; in approximately one third, the follicle regresses and a second one grows.[31] This phenomenon occurs, perhaps, because there is a certain degree of atresia in some of those large follicles at the time of treatment. The use of ovulatory inducing agents such as human chorionic gonadotropin (hCG) is common in ET programs. Injection of 1500 IU of hCG intravenously when there is a 35-mm follicle induces ovulation 36–48 hours after injection.[32,33] Other ovulatory inducing agents such as deslorelin or Ovuplant are also commonly used in ET programs to tighten the synchrony between donors and recipients. These agents are also used when donor mares have more than one dominant follicle to promote multiple and synchronous ovulations. In our experience, hCG has been useful to synchronize ovulations but not to promote double ovulations.

Meclofenamic acid is a non-steroidal anti-inflammatory drug that has been used successfully to increase the window of synchrony between donors and recipients. It was first used in goats and dromedary camels. Administration of 1 gm daily of meclofenamic acid to recipient mares that had ovulated up to 4 days before the donors showed that acceptable pregnancy rates can be achieved.[34]

Progesterone Supplementation

The use of ovariectomized mares as embryo recipients was first reported by Hinrichs.[35] To use ovariectomized recipients, mares are injected daily with 300 mg of progesterone starting 2 days after donor ovulation. This treatment is continued for 100–110 days if the mare is pregnant. Long-acting progesterone preparations are commercially available that can be administered every 6–7 days.[36] Alternatively, the synthetic progestin altrenogest has been used successfully to prepare ovariectomized mares as embryo recipients.[37-42] Mares are started on altrenogest orally at a dosage of 0.044 mg/kg of body weight daily from the day of donor ovulation up to day 35 of pregnancy. After this stage, the dose can be lowered to 0.022 mg/kg up to 100–110 days. After 100 days of gestation, both progesterone- and altrenogest-treated mares produce fetal placental progestins that maintain the pregnancy. Endocrine profiles for the remainder of gestation, parturition, and lactation have been reported to be normal.[43] The main advantage of using ovariectomized mares is to reduce the number of recipients per donor. In addition there is a significant reduction of labor expenses because there is no need for ovarian control of the recipients. At our clinic, because inexpensive mares are available, we routinely use intact mares.

The use of intact anestrous mares supplemented with progesterone to mimic a regular cycle has been a useful alternative when recipients stop cycling at the end of breeding season. As previously mentioned, it is common that new mares added to the program at the end of the season enter anestrus. In these cases we administer 2 days of estradiol benzoate (2 mg/day) and then 300 mg of progesterone daily for 4–5 days before using the mare as a recipient. On the day that anovulatory mares receive an embryo, they are treated with progesterone in oil, 300 mg IM, plus biorelease progesterone, 1.8 gm IM. The biorelease progesterone treatment is repeated on a weekly basis thereafter, until day 110 of gestation.

In a study conducted at our clinic (Fig. 16-2), a total of 469 transfers were performed between February 15 and April 30, 2008, comparing pregnancy rates achieved in normal cycling mares vs. intact non-cycling mares supplemented with progesterone.[44] The results comparing both groups were analyzed in 15-day periods. Overall, pregnancy rates in anovulatory, progesterone-treated recipients were significantly lower than those for ovulatory recipients (164/192 [56.1%] vs. 197/277 [71.1%]).

This finding was probably related to the season in which this study was conducted (early fall); mares that become anovulatory early in the fall are typically those with lower body scores or condition. Later in the anovulatory season, many mares, regardless of body score, will be transitional or anestrus and the

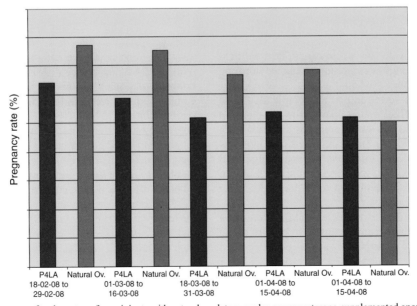

Figure 16-2. Pregnancy rates of embryo transfer recipients with natural ovulatory cycles or progesterone-supplemented anovulatory mares *(P4LA)*.

pregnancy rates obtained in either group are similar. However, the use of noncycling progesterone-treated mares is still a viable alternative to extend the ET season by 1 or 2 months.

Artificial Insemination in Embryo Transfer Programs

In our program, mares are artificially inseminated with fresh, extended semen collected at the center. Only in rare occasions is semen collected at other farms and transported to our center. Mares that are inseminated and ovulate within 24–48 hours after breeding are not rebred if the semen is of good quality and sperm longevity is adequate. Mares that are susceptible to endometritis are inseminated using minimal contamination breeding procedures.[45] Ovulations are routinely induced with hCG (1600 IU IV) and artificial insemination performed on the same day or the day after. If ovulation is detected in a mare that has not been inseminated, she is bred immediately as long as she displays good estrous behavior to the teaser and the cervix is still open. Embryo recovery rate in mares inseminated within 12 hours of ovulation resulted in a reduction of recovered embryos (63% vs. 83%). There was no significant difference in the proportion of grade 1 embryos between the groups (76/85 [89%] pre-ovulation vs. 13/19 [68%] post-ovulation). There was no difference in recipient pregnancy rate at days 14–21 (73% pre-ovulation vs 68% post-ovulation).[46]

Susceptible mares may show signs of endometritis such as heavy uterine edema, fluid accumulation, or vaginal discharge 24 hours after insemination. In such cases, mares undergo a uterine lavage with 2–4 L of sterile saline at body temperature. This procedure can be repeated daily for up to 3 days after ovulation, followed by injection of 20 IU of oxytocin. In some cases, this therapy appears to be beneficial at cleaning the uterine environment to allow for a clear uterine lavage 6–8 days after detection of ovulation. Corticosteroids (0.1 mg/kg of prednisolone acetate) have been used in donor mares with history of intense inflammatory uterine response after AI.[47]

Uterine Lavage (Flushing) for Embryo Recovery

The equine embryo stimulates oviductal movement and embryo transport through the production of prostaglandin-E_2 (PGE_2).[48,49] The embryo enters the uterus from 5 days 10 hours to 5 days 22 hours after ovulation.[48-50] The possible reasons for this variability could be the variable delay between ovulation and fertilization (depending on individual oocytes), embryonic factors related to timing of PGE_2 secretion, sex of the embryo, or other individual factors. Because of this variability in the oviductal transport period, uterine lavage or flush for embryo recovery is performed between days 6 and 8 after ovulation. Most authors agree that recovery rate is lower when performed at day 6.[24,25] It has been postulated that this can be due to one or more of the following reasons: (1) failure of the embryo to descend into the uterus by day 6, (2) failure of the technician to recover the embryo from the uterus because of a higher gravity weight of the embryo, (3) failure of the technician to find the embryo because of its smaller size, and (4) loss of the embryo at some point during the process.

We prefer to attempt embryo recovery on day 8 after ovulation. At this stage, embryos are large enough to be easily found, so chances of missing or losing the embryo are decreased. In addition to their smaller size, day 6 embryos have higher specific gravity, which might also account for the lower embryo recovery on this day.

Flushing Technique

The uterine lavage, or uterine flush, is a simple procedure performed with the mare restrained in stocks. Before the flushing, the mare's rectum is evacuated of feces, and the size and tone of the uterus and cervix are evaluated. In addition, follicular status of the ovaries is established to determine whether the mare will receive prostaglandin immediately after the uterine flush. When the mare has a follicle >35 mm, prostaglandin treatment is delayed to prevent premature ovulation. We prefer to delay $PGF_{2\alpha}$ administration for at least 48 hours. This allows the uterus to recover from the uterine flushing and increases the chances of a normal subsequent heat before re-insemination.

Depending on the mare's temperament, a wide band is placed over the loin and in front of the chest to prevent unruly mares from jumping forward or kicking during the procedure. If necessary, the mare is twitched during the procedure. Tranquilization is usually not necessary, but some mares may require a light sedation with 50–100 mg of xylazine intravenously. Acepromazine maleate can also be used for this purpose, but we prefer not to use it because it induces relaxation of the uterus, making it more difficult to recover the fluid in some instances.

Once the mare has been examined, her tail is wrapped and hung in a vertical position (Fig. 16-3). The perineal area is carefully washed with soap, rinsed with tap water, and dried with a clean paper towel. A small piece of wet cotton is used to clean the vestibule. Uterine lavage is currently performed with lactated Ringer's solution with addition of 0.5% fetal calf serum.[51] Use of fetal calf serum prevents the embryo from sticking to the tubing and filter. Use of fetal calf serum is controversial, and some authors report no differences in recovery rates with or without serum.

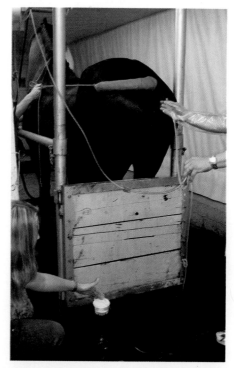

Figure 16-3. The mare is placed in stocks with the tail wrapped and hung in a vertical position. The technician, who is wearing a sterile sleeve, holds the sterile catheter while examining the integrity of the air cuff. The system is completed by a large-volume filter and a plastic container with flushing medium, both connected to the catheter by means of Silastic tubing and a V-junction. The flushing medium is recovered in a graduated recipient to measure the volume recovered.

The technician, wearing a sterile sleeve with a small amount of lubricating jelly in the dorsal part of the hand, introduces the arm in the vagina to identify the external os of the cervix. With the index finger, the technician dilates the external os to a size large enough to pass the tip of a 24-gauge Foley catheter into the body of the uterus. The air cuff is inflated with 30–50 ml of air, and the catheter is pulled back gently, forming a tight seal at the internal cervical os (Fig. 16-4). A total of 2–3 L of flushing media is infused by gravity flow in aliquots of 500–1000 ml, depending on the size of the uterus.

The flushing catheter is connected with a Y junction to the delivery tubing on one end and to a large-volume filter on the other end. The system should be completely purged with flushing medium to eliminate all air before the procedure is started. This prevents the formation of foam and bubbles. Several brands of catheters can be used. Integrity of the air cuff should be checked before the catheters are introduced in the mare (Fig. 16-4).

The fluid is passed through the filter connected in line with the catheter by means of the Y junction and Silastic tubing. The amount of fluid recovered is measured in a graduated recipient and should be more than 95% of the volume infused in the uterus.

In some cases, especially in old mares with a large pendulous uterus, fluid recovery can be difficult. In such cases, the use of 20 IU of oxytocin intravenously during the flushing procedure can aid in the recovery of the flushing medium. The use of ultrasonography to locate pockets of fluid can be helpful during the subsequent manipulation of the catheter toward these areas. Gentle massage of the uterus is performed to ensure that the medium has reached the entire uterus. This also produces a slight turbulence to get the embryo in suspension, thereby increasing the chances of recovery. If excessive manipulation is performed, fluid recovered can be slightly tinged with blood. Although we have not detected this to be a problem in terms of recovery, nor has it been associated with lower pregnancy rates after transfer, we will carefully wash the embryo several times before transfer in these cases.

Handling and Evaluation of the Embryo

After the uterine flush is completed, the filter is drained so that approximately 20 ml of fluid are left in the filter. This content is swirled gently to prevent the embryo from sticking to the filter walls, and then it is poured into a sterile Petri dish (Fig. 16-5). The filter is then rinsed with flushing medium to ensure that the embryo is not lost in the filter. Many of the expanded blastocysts recovered at day 7 and almost all embryos recovered at day 8 can be found with the naked eye or with a small magnifying glass if the effluent is clean. Consequently, the embryo can be easily found and transferred within a short period (approximately 10 minutes). If we fail to find the embryo with the naked eye, we search with a dissecting microscope first at a lower magnification and then with a higher magnification to grade the embryo quality. Embryo searching is facilitated when bubbles or foam are not present in the Petri dish. Once the embryo is found, it is rinsed at least three or four times and then transferred to a small Falcon dish containing holding media (VIGRO, AB Technology, Pullman, WA) by means of a 10- to 20-ml Unopette adapted to a 1-ml syringe. Large embryos will be handled with a 0.25-ml sterile straw since they are too large to be loaded in a Unopette.

Embryos can be kept a room temperature in holding media for 2 or 3 hours before transfer. If transfer is delayed more than this, we usually cool them to 18°C.

Embryo Transfer

Surgical Technique

Embryos can be transferred into the uterus of a recipient mare by either surgical or non-surgical technique. Although no controlled studies have been done comparing results obtained with surgical and non-surgical techniques, it is suggested that higher pregnancy rates are achieved by transferring embryos surgically.[52] However, surgical methods are time-consuming, are more expensive,

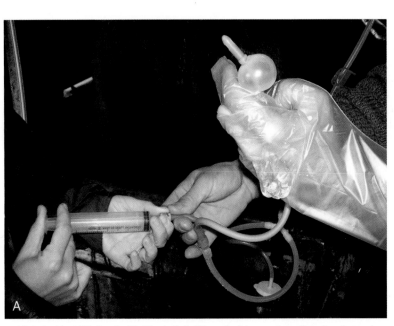
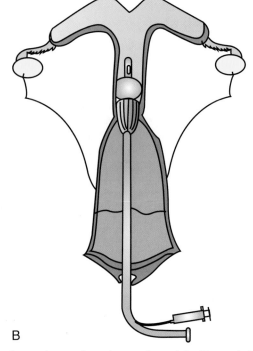

Figure 16-4. A, Air cuff inflated with 30 ml of air. We prefer 24-gauge latex French catheters because they are inexpensive and very soft, so minimal trauma is done to the uterus during flushing. **B,** Correct placement of the flushing catheter, forming a tight seal at the internal cervical os after the cuff has been inflated.

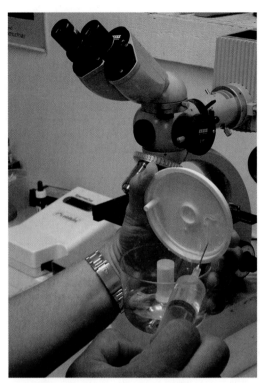

Figure 16-5. The filter content is poured off in a sterile cross-hatched Petri dish, and the filter and lid are rinsed with flushing medium to reduce the risk of the embryo's sticking to them.

require surgical facilities, are more labor intensive, and demand post-surgical care of the recipient. Although it may be convenient in some occasions, it is not practical in a large commercial program when it may be necessary to transfer more than 10–20 embryos per day and labor is limited. Nowadays there are probably very few places where ET is performed surgically.

Initial transfers at Colorado State University were done under general anesthesia through a midline incision. The horn of the uterus ipsilateral to the side of ovulation was retracted through the incision and the uterine wall perforated with a cutting edge needle in a low vascular area. The embryo was loaded in a fire-polished pipette and transferred with a small volume of sterile transfer medium.

A more practical alternative to the midline incision is a flank laparotomy under local anesthesia with the mare standing mildly sedated. The paralumbar fossa is scrubbed for surgery. A vertical incision large enough to permit retraction of the horn of the uterus is performed between the last rib and tuber coxae. Muscle layers are bluntly separated and the peritoneum is perforated. This technique is simpler and fast if it is performed by an experienced surgeon. Muscle layers and skin are then closed.

Because of the mobility of the equine embryo during the first 15–16 days of pregnancy, there is no need to transfer the embryo to the horn ipsilateral to the side of ovulation; however, it has been suggested that there is a beneficial effect of progesterone if the embryos are transferred to the horn ipsilateral to the ovary having the corpus luteum.[53]

Non-Surgical Technique

The non-surgical technique is faster and less costly than the surgical technique.[54] At our center, we have attempted two different transfer techniques, called technique A and technique B.

Preparation for Transfer

To achieve good pregnancy rates it is essential to follow these steps:
1. Select the recipient to be used among the ones available: The records of the recipients available should be carefully reviewed. It is important to note if the mare has received an embryo on the same season and did not get pregnant, or if the mare was pregnant and suffered EED. It is important to note if there were any signs of uterine abnormality during the cycle such as presence of fluid or any evidence of endometritis. The recipients are evaluated before transfer and notes are taken about tone of the uterus and cervix and the presence of a corpus luteum.
2. Prepare the recipient carefully; the mare is restrained in stocks and prepared as for any other intrauterine procedure. It is essential that the recipient mare be properly restrained at the time of transfer. Xylazine hydrochloride (Rompun, Bayer Animal Health), which is an alfa-2 adrenergic receptor agonist that causes an increase in the uterine tone, is routinely given at our clinic before transfer. We use 50–100 mg IV. In rare cases we may use detomidine (Dormosedan, Pfizer) at a dose of 1 mg IV given before transfer.[55] We do not use acepromazine maleate before the transfer, although some do because of its effects of relaxation of the uterus and cervix.

Technique A. The first technique was described by Douglas et al.[9] and modified by Sertich.[54] The embryo is aseptically aspirated between two columns of air and two columns of transfer medium into a 55-mm sterile insemination pipette attached to a 10-ml sterile syringe. The pipette is guided through the cervix alongside a gloved index finger, and the embryo is deposited within the body of the uterus. The pipette can be guarded with a plastic sheath. We sometimes use this technique when transferring day 8 or 9 embryos that are too large to be transferred with a regular transfer gun.

Technique B. The second technique was described by Pashen.[27] The embryo is aseptically aspirated into a 0.5-ml straw in the following manner: 0.2 ml medium + 0.05 ml air + 0.10 ml medium with the embryo + 0.05 ml air + 0.1 ml medium. This volume is not enough to fill the straw, so the air is expelled with the plunger after the straw is fitted in the transfer gun (Fig. 16-6). An assistant separates the mare's vulvar lips and the operator penetrates the vagina with a sterile gloved hand. The external os of the cervix is located with the index finger. Care should be taken not to dilate the cervix in this procedure, which in our experience will lower pregnancy rates. The index finger should be used just to find the external os but not to dilate it. A sanitary protector is used to pass through the vagina and halfway into the cervix. The anterior end of the transfer gun is introduced gently halfway into the cervix where the sanitary sleeve is punctured by the gun. The operator removes his or her hand from the mare's vagina and introduces it into the rectum. Manipulation of the body and right horn of the uterus through the rectal wall is performed to position the transfer gun at the tip of the right horn. It is essential to avoid scratching the endometrium, which would induce prostaglandin release and could cause pregnancy failure. The embryo is transferred by gentle pressure to the transfer gun plunger (Fig. 16-7). Many ET centers perform Caslick's suturing after each non-surgical transfer. We usually do not do so unless perineal conformation of the recipient is poor.

Pregnancy rates reported using techniques A and B are similar. No evidence has shown an advantage of one over the other.

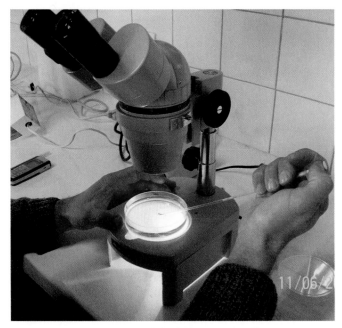

Figure 16-6. Embryo is loaded in a 0.5-ml sterile straw.

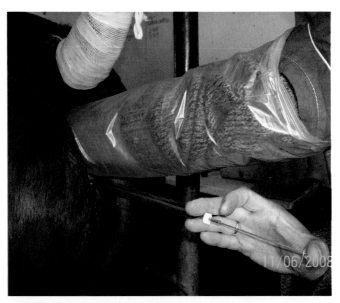

Figure 16-7. After the embryo is aspirated into a 0.5-ml straw, it is placed into a disposable sterile transfer gun. The embryo is transferred to the tip of a uterine horn by gentle pressure on the transfer gun plunger.

Technician experience is critical to achieve good pregnancy rates with non-surgical transfer. Colorado workers have reported significant differences in pregnancy rates after transfer by different technicians. In our program, we classify each transfer according to quality. We have seen an effect of transfer on pregnancy rate, particularly between transfers classified as very good or good and poor (Table 16-1).

Embryos are classified as grade 1 to 5 depending on morphologic characteristics.[56] At our program we classified embryos from grade 1 to 3 only. Pregnancy rates obtained with grade 2 and 3 embryos are lower than with grade 1 (Table 16-2). The incidence of embryos with morphologic abnormalities is low in the mare. At our laboratory, poor quality embryos are rare, perhaps

Table 16-1 | Effect of Transfer Quality on Pregnancy Rates and Early Embryonic Death (EED)

QUALITY	EMBRYOS TRANSFERRED	PREGNANCY AT 14 DAYS (%)	PREGNANCY AT 90 DAYS
Very good	6115	3871 (63%)	3382 (12% EED)
Good	405	273 (67%)	246 (10% EED)
Poor	62	25 (40%)	22 (12% EED)

Table 16-2 | Effect of Embryo Quality on Pregnancy Rates

QUALITY	EMBRYOS TRANSFERRED	PREGNANCY AT 14 DAYS (%)	PREGNANCY AT 90 DAYS
Grade 1	5967	3823 (64%)	3361 (12% EED)
Grade 2	514	302 (58%)	248 (17% EED)
Grade 3	86	29 (33%)	25 (15% EED)

EED, Early embryonic death

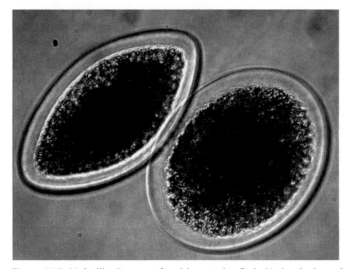

Figure 16-8. Unfertilized oocytes found in a uterine flush. Notice the loss of spherical shape.

because most of the mares are young, fertile individuals. Occasionally we can find unfertilized oocytes of different morphology in the uterine flush (Fig. 16-8). However, it has been shown that mare age has a definite impact on embryo quality, with older mares having a higher incidence of embryonic defects, particularly extruded blastomeres (Figs. 16-9 and 16-10).

A method for non-surgical transfer that involves the use of a vaginal forceps to grasp the external os of the cervix has been recently reported. This method is advantageous because a great deal of skill is not necessary in order to achieve a good pregnancy rate. The mare is restrained in stocks and a vaginoscope is used so the operator can visualize the external os. Then the embryo is loaded in a regular AI pipette protected by a sanitary guard. The operator will then pass the pipette into the uterus and deposit the embryo in the body of the uterus. In our opinion this is a good option for those technicians that lack the expertise to transfer embryos. It is not practical in large programs because it requires a large number of forceps and vaginoscopes. In addition, it is crucial to be able to work in a very clean area not exposed to dust of wind blow to avoid contamination of the vagina.

Several studies have shown that manipulation of the cervix during non-surgical transfer can induce prostaglandin and oxytocin release, decrease of progesterone levels, and shorten

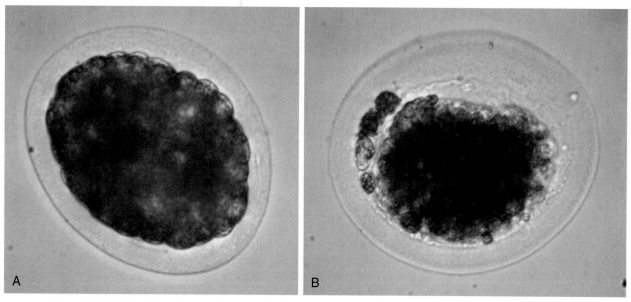

Figure 16-9. A, A grade 1 equine morula recovered at 6.5 days after ovulation. **B,** A grade 2 morula with extruded blastomeres.

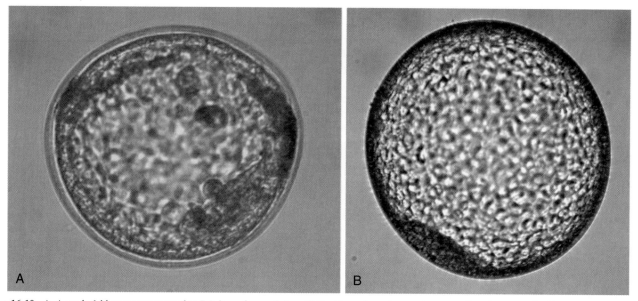

Figure 16-10. A, A grade 1 blastocyst recovered at 7.5 days after ovulation. Notice the embryonic capsule surrounding the zona pellucida. **B,** An expanded grade 1 blastocyst recovered 8 days after ovulation.

the cycle. Therefore, it is a common practice in many centers to administer a prostaglandin synthesis inhibitor prior to the transfer. Flunixin meglumine has been used in many centers. At the author's center, every recipient receives long-acting progesterone (1.8 gm) at the time of transfer.

SYSTEMATIC APPROACH FOR EVALUATING AN EMBRYO TRANSFER PROGRAM

The final success or failure of an ET program depends on a multitude of small details that have to be carefully synchronized and performed. Once the program is in progress and most aspects are under control, it is not difficult to detect details that will lower the general results. When lower pregnancy rates are detected, however, oftentimes there is not a single factor involved. Because the ET season is usually short, by the time a problem is recognized and its cause is identified, the season might be over.

When a problem is detected, it is imperative to implement a systematic investigation to resolve the issue in a timely manner. The following discussion is my view on how to investigate causes of lower pregnancy rates and the factors involved.

Many of the factors that affect efficiency in an ET program are well described, but there are many others that are not yet known. These factors could be classified in the following groups:

1. Organization and logistics: In a large-scale program, it is essential that every item needed for the program to be operated is available at the right time.
2. General management of donors, recipients and stallions: This is related to the animal's well-being. It is very important to avoid stress, which is the major cause of pregnancy failure in large ET programs. It includes proper feeding and water supply as well as protection from heat stress. It is quite common that pregnancy rates will drop during the summer, which is at least partially due to the effect of heat stress.

3. Recipient availability: This is a very important factor that will affect pregnancy rates. The best recipients usually get pregnant early in the season. This is another cause of low pregnancy rates at the end of the season. Oftentimes new recipients added to the program in the middle of the season will have a lower pregnancy rate, so every effort is made to have all the recipients at the facility at the beginning of the ET season.
4. Fertility of mares and stallions
5. Technician skill

SOME FACTORS THAT CAN AFFECT EMBRYO RECOVERY RATE

Normal recovery rates calculated on the basis of simple ovulation cycles is approximately 70% (65%–75%). If this figure is below this value, the cause should be analyzed.

Some factors affecting embryo recovery rate are as follows:
1. Factors related to general management, feeding, sanitary conditions
2. Factors related to reproductive management of donors
3. Factors related to the flushing technique

Technical factors, such as flushing technique, must also be considered when investigating a low embryo recovery rate. It is important to ensure that the uterus does not overflow and fluid is lost through the cervix into the vagina. In such a case, the mare may show signs of discomfort because there is high intrauterine pressure resulting from an excessive amount of flushing media introduced into the uterus by gravity flow. On the other hand, in a pluriparous mare that has a large uterus or that has been recently foaled, the fluid does not reach both uterine horns. We prefer to evaluate the uterus by rectal palpation and ultrasonography when flushing this category of mares.

Overinflation of the air cuff makes fluid recovery difficult. For most donor mares, 30–35 ml of air is enough to properly seal the cervix and prevent fluid reflux into the vagina. If recycled catheters are used, the air cuff should be checked before being used because ethylene oxide can damage it. If the air cuff breaks during the uterine lavage, the flushing medium leaks into the vagina and often the embryo is lost. If uterine lavage does not progress, the catheter should be gently pushed forward by pressure on the caudal part of the cuff. In some mares with a large uterus, the fluid may not be reached by the tip of the catheter if it is located in the body of the uterus, so we attempt to complete the lavage by reaching each horn with the tip of the catheter. Ultrasonography can be used to find pockets of fluid or to better evaluate whether the fluid has reached the entire uterus.

Factors Related to Timing of Flushing

Detection of ovulation within a 48-hour period is important to plan the uterine lavage to recover transferable embryos. If the uterine lavage is scheduled too early, lower recovery rates may be expected. In contrast, flushing too late results in collection of large, fragile, non-transferable embryos or of embryos with lower viability after transfer.

Post-ovulation Breeding

If the mare was inseminated after ovulation, it is better to perform the uterine lavage on day 8 or even 9. We have observed that embryos recovered from post-ovulation breeding are smaller and retarded in their development. We have had the same observation in mares inseminated with frozen semen.

Multiple Ovulations

In cases of multiple ovulations, the uterine lavage is scheduled so embryos are between 6.5 and 8.5 days old. If ovulations have occurred more than 48 hours apart, it is necessary to perform two uterine lavages. In most cases, the second lavage is cloudy because of the uterine reaction induced by the previous lavage. In our experience, the second embryo is recovered in only a few cases.

Although multiple ovulations increase the embryo recovery per cycle, it does not double the one achieved in single ovulation cycles.[57] In a retrospective analysis of 1300 double ovulation cycles classified as ipsilateral or contralateral double ovulation, the embryo recovery rate per follicle ovulated was less in unilateral than bilateral ovulating mares (752/1398 [54%] vs. 790/1202 [66%], respectively; $P<.001$). Concomitantly, the proportion of flushings yielding two embryos was less in the unilateral group (247/699 [35%]) than in the bilateral group (290/601 [48%]; $P<.001$). Both unilateral and bilateral ovulation types yielded more flushes with two embryos or no embryos, and fewer flushings with single embryos, than would be expected if the recovery rate for that ovulation was consistent for each follicle ovulated ($P<.001$).

The lesser embryo recovery in unilaterally ovulating mares indicates that some mechanism at the level of the ovary or oviduct may interfere with ovulation or oocyte pick-up in multiple-ovulating mares and may explain the reduction in embryo recovery per follicle ovulated in superovulated mares.

Increased prevalence of flushes with two or no embryos in double-ovulating mares suggests that either both or no oocytes are fertilized rather than each individual oocyte being a separate event doubling the chances of conception.

Old Mares

Old mares may experience a delay before an embryo descends into the uterus. We documented a case of a donor mare that had not yielded embryos for 4 years. When the mare's uterine lavage could not be performed on the scheduled day 7 because of a severe colic of the mare, it was performed on day 9 and an expanded blastocyst compatible with development seen by day 7 was recovered and transferred. The recipient mare was examined by ultrasonography on day 14 after donor ovulation, and although the mare had good tone in the uterus, an embryonic vesicle could not be identified. The recipient mare was re-examined on day 17 and a small vesicle was detected. If these mares with embryos that have a severe delay in growth and development can be identified, embryo recovery should be attempted on days 9 or 10 because at day 7 the embryo has not yet descended in the uterus.

Factors Related to Donors' Fertility

Besides the flushing technique, factors such as the fertility of embryo donors and stallions can affect pregnancy rates and therefore embryo recovery. Individual stallion or mare problems are simpler to detect because not all the population is affected. Donors with a low recovery rate should be evaluated carefully with a complete breeding soundness evaluation. Recovery rates should be analyzed according to the different categories of donor mares. Young fertile mares, bred to normal stallions, yield embryo recovery rates that should be close to 75%–80%. There is a significant reduction in embryo recovery rates in aged mares as well as in those with history of infertility. Uteri of mares susceptible to endometritis or with delayed uterine clearance may provide a hostile environment for embryo survival. Regardless of uterine environment, some old mares with a normal uterus produce a higher incidence of embryos with age-associated defects, which occur before the day the embryo enters the uterus. Carnevale et al.[58] in 1993 demonstrated that embryos from old mares had significantly more morphologic abnormalities and fewer embryonic cells at day 3 of gestation. On day 11, there were significantly fewer pregnancies in older mares, and smaller embryonic vesicles were present in embryos recovered from old mares than from young ones.

It is a donor owner's concern whether the procedures involved in an ET program could affect future fertility of the mare. Most donor mares at our center are flushed on successive cycles during the entire breeding season with no obvious consequences on future fertility. Some of them are flushed up to 10 times per season. We have not seen any detrimental effect on embryo recovery rate or on pregnancy rate after transfer in these mares on consecutive cycles. This may be because most of the mares are fairly young donors. It is possible to have problems in old, subfertile mares that are susceptible to endometritis. Susceptible mares may show signs of endometritis the day after insemination. In such cases, we perform uterine lavage as described previously.

Normal Donors

A normal donor could be defined as the mare that assumedly is mated with a fertile stallion under good management conditions of insemination, and uterine flushing will render at least 70% embryo recovery in single ovulation cycles with a 65%–80% pregnancy rate at 14 days after transfer into a normal recipient mare by an experienced technician. The pregnancy loss should be <12%, and the interovulatory interval using prostaglandins should average 17 days.

Categories of Difficult Donors

MARES THAT DO NOT CYCLE NORMALLY. Mares coming out of training commonly will show the effect of stress, anabolic steroid administration, or different hormones that are commonly used to prevent ovulation and/or signs of heat. Some mares will take longer than others to wear off the effect of these drugs. Some mares will consistently develop anovulatory follicles on subsequent cycles. There are several known causes of anovulatory follicles and probably many others that are still unknown.[59,60] Pastures with a high proportion of clover particularly after the rainfalls could cause anestrus or delayed ovulation because of the effect of phytoestrogens.

MARES THAT CYCLE NORMALLY BUT RENDER A LOW EMBRYO RECOVERY RATE. The most common mares in this group are those with reproductive problems associated with the uterus (e.g., endometritis, pyometra). Causes related to the cervix or oviducts are uncommon.[60-62]

MARES WITH A NORMAL RECOVERY BUT WITH A LOW PREGNANCY RATE. We have identified donor mares that produce embryos at a normal rate but show a very low pregnancy rate after transfer. We believe that the effect of stress on embryo donors can produce not only low embryo recovery rates, but also low embryo viability after transfer.

Strategic Management of the Donors

Since uterine lavages for embryo recovery can be scheduled either on day 7 or 8 after ovulation on most donor mares, and since AI can be performed up to 48 hours before expected ovulation on

stallions with normal sperm longevity, we can use this flexibility in order to decrease the number of examinations on each donor. This is particularly useful in large commercial programs when there is not enough time to examine the mares every day. It is also very helpful for those practitioners who are performing embryo transfer in the field and cannot examine the mare everyday. A dose of 1600 IU IV of human chorionic gonadotropin (HCG) is given to the mare in the morning when findings indicate that the mare is ready for induction of ovulation. The mare is artificially inseminated the same afternoon or the next day depending upon semen availability. Examination is performed 48 hours after HCG administration to confirm that ovulation has occurred. The flushing is scheduled 7.5–8 days after detected ovulation. When comparing the embryo recovery of mares examined every day or every other day, 1079 embryo recovery attempts from mares examined every day until yielded 679 embryos (63%) whereas 181 flushes from mares examined 48 hours after HCG administration yielded 127 embryos (70%). A possible explanation for this result is that the donor mares evaluated everyday included all the problem breeders.

Stallion Factors

To recover embryos at a normal rate, it is necessary that fertile mares be bred with semen from fertile stallions with normal sperm longevity within 48 hours before detection of ovulation. When artificial insemination is used, semen should be adequately collected and processed so sperm viability is optimized.

In addition to the inherent fertility of the mare, embryo recovery and pregnancy rates after transfer can be significantly affected by the stallion, depending on his intrinsic fertility and his management (Fig. 16-11). It is important to evaluate recovery rates for the different stallions. In a retrospective analysis of 34 stallions of different breeds and of 1274 cycles, the embryo recovery rate between days 6 and 8 after donor ovulation ranged between 26.3% and 100%, and the pregnancy rate after transfer ranged between 20% and 100%. The EED rate between 14 and 60 days ranged between 0% and 50%. In some cases, embryo recovery and pregnancy rates can be enhanced with appropriate stallion management.

Although we discourage our clients from using stallions with fertility problems, there are still some stallions that have been involved in our program. The most common stallion problems seen in our clinic are as follows.

Stallions with Decreased Sperm Longevity

Depending on the composition of the stallion's seminal plasma, sperm concentration, and probably other unknown factors, in some stallions sperm do not live very long. Removal of the seminal plasma by low-speed centrifugation to produce a soft pellet and resuspension with Kenney extender seems to enhance sperm longevity in some of these stallions. When using sperm of stallions with these characteristics, every effort is made to breed the donor mares within 6 hours of ovulation.

Oligospermic Stallions

Stallions with low sperm numbers most commonly resulting from age-related testicular degeneration or genetics are frequently used in ET programs. In these cases, we attempt to synchronize donor cycles in such a way that the stallion has several days of rest between collections. Mares are bred with complete ejaculates without the gel fraction in an effort to maximize the sperm numbers deposited in the uterus.

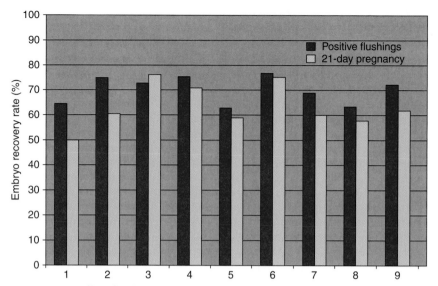

Figure 16-11. Effect of stallion on embryo recovery and pregnancy rates at 21 days after transfer.

Urospermic Stallions

A few stallions consistently urinate during semen collection. Urination usually occurs toward the end of ejaculation. In these cases, the sperm-rich fraction can be collected before urination by means of an open-ended artificial vagina. In most cases, embryo recovery and pregnancy rates achieved with semen obtained by this method have not been different from the ones of normal stallions.[63]

Even among stallions of good fertility, there are still differences in embryo recovery rates, pregnancy rates at 14–20 days, and EED rates. It appears that even in stallions with good fertility, pregnancy rates always lag behind embryo recovery rates. This finding highlights the effect of EED, which occurs at different rates with different stallions. At least part of the difference between embryo recovery and pregnancy rate may be the tailing off of the ongoing EED process.

Management of Artificial Insemination

If fertility of donor mares and stallions has been evaluated and cannot be incriminated as a cause of low embryo recovery rate, management factors should be carefully investigated. Most mares at our center are mated by AI. It is important to minimize contamination during the AI procedure. Artificial vaginas should be perfectly washed and rinsed and sterilized by immersion in isopropyl alcohol. All the materials used should be sterile and non-toxic to sperm. If semen extender is added to semen, every sample should be evaluated to rule out the possibility of spermicidal factors on each of its components. In rare occasions mares are artificially inseminated with frozen semen at our center. In general, these breedings result in a lower embryo recovery rate even if the semen quality of the stallions used is not optimal and of proven fertility.

Seasonality

The pregnancy rate achieved after transfer and the incidence of embryonic death and pregnancy loss will vary significantly along the breeding season. At our program, the highest efficiency is achieved during October and November and then decreases slightly from December to March. It is lowest at the end of the season in April and May. Some of the factors involved are heat stress, recipient quality and availability, and nutritional factors.

FACTORS THAT CAN AFFECT PREGNANCY RATES AFTER TRANSFER

If embryos are recovered at a normal rate but pregnancy rates achieved at 14–21 days are low, several factors should be investigated.

1. Embryo quality: Because the incidence of abnormal embryos is low compared with that in other domestic species where superovulation treatments are used, the effect of morphologic abnormalities on the general results should not be significant.

2. Embryo age: Embryos collected on day 8 or later may be too large to be loaded in a 0.5-ml straw. In some instances, they can fit in the straw but may be larger in diameter than the opening of the transfer gun, which means that the embryo will be destroyed at time of the transfer attempt. In such cases, embryos should be transferred either surgically or by means of an AI pipette. Large embryos may be less resistant to temperature stress and osmolarity changes than smaller embryos. Pregnancy rates appear to be higher if large day 8 or 9 embryos are transferred surgically.[52,64] If pregnancy rates achieved with day 9 embryos were similar to day 7 or 8, this would be very valuable for scheduling flushings in large commercial programs or even in those cases when ET is performed "on farm."

3. Materials and media: All materials and tubing should be sterile and free of residues toxic to embryos. Although many materials are disposable, equipment that is to be reused is washed with deionized water and sterilized. Tubing, catheters, and filters are sterilized with ethylene oxide for 24 hours. We allows 7–10 days for ventilation because ethylene oxide is toxic to embryos and spermatozoa. The embryo should not be exposed to direct sunlight. Although temperature of the media is not critical, we prefer working with media between 24°C and 30°C.

4. Transfer technique: There is a significant effect of technician skill on pregnancy rates achieved by non-surgical ET. An experienced technician could achieve a 75% pregnancy

rate if every factor affecting pregnancy rate is under control. This is not a difficult figure to achieve during a limited period, but in a large-scale ET program, it is difficult to maintain optimal conditions during the entire ET season, so overall pregnancy rates at the end of the season are usually close to 60%–70%.

5. Recipient factors and nutrition of recipients: In our laboratory, the most important factors that affect pregnancy rates after transfer are recipient availability, recipient management, and nutrition. Recipient mares should be gaining weight during the ET season. Recipient mares that receive an embryo are immediately switched to a different pasture and higher quality grain. Pregnancy rates can be dramatically affected in recipient mares that are losing weight, even when they are in good body condition. Nutrition level also affects EED rates, which can be high if the mares are losing weight.

6. Repeated transfers in the same recipient: If performed properly, while using sterile materials and a clean technique, non-surgical transfer is not a harmful procedure and does not affect immediate fertility if the mare did not become pregnant after the transfer. Recipient mares that received an embryo are examined by ultrasonography 14–20 days after donor ovulation. At this stage, transrectal ultrasonography is 98% accurate for pregnancy diagnosis. If the mare is not pregnant and there are no signs of endometritis, she is reused when needed again. Pregnancy rates after transfer among recipient mares that received one, two, or three embryos in the same season were not significantly different.

7. Seasonality. Pregnancy rates are usually higher during the spring, probably because the best recipients are used early in the season and because nutrition is generally better in spring than in summer. Also, the heat stress of the summer can affect pregnancy rates. The efficiency will drop significantly during the last third of the breeding season.

ECONOMICS OF A LARGE-SCALE EMBRYO TRANSFER CENTER

The efficiency of the ET program should be measured with a parameter such as embryo recovery attempts or flushings per pregnancy. This concept is essential in a commercial ET program. At Doña Pilar our clients will be charged on a per pregnancy basis

so that any decrease in our efficiency will dramatically affect the economical result of the program.

Most of the expenses involved in an ET program are independent of the results achieved. In other words, fixed costs incurred are the same whether the recipients become pregnant or not. Then the efficiency of a commercial program, indicated as number of flushings required to produce a pregnancy (flushings per pregnancies), becomes crucial to determine the final economic viability of the program. As an example, during 2006 our expenses were classified as: salaries, 34%; feeding of horses, 22%; laboratory and veterinary supplies, 21%; taxes, 10%; maintenance, administration, and horse transportation, 13%. The pregnancy rate achieved on this season had very little or no impact on these expenses. Fig. 16-12 is an example of how the efficiency will affect the economic outcome of the season. If the efficiency is four flushings per pregnancy, there will be no profit. However, if we decrease the number of flushings per pregnancy from four to two, the increase in economic profitability increases from 0% to 25%.

Another consideration in large commercial programs is that it becomes necessary to invest large amounts of money on recipient mares every year. Our program owns approximately 2000 recipients. Since the number of pregnancies is increasing every year, this means that it is mandatory not only to replace old recipients, but also to add new mares in the program. In the 2006 season we invested 17% of our total expenses on recipient mares. Facilities also need to be constantly improved. During 2006 we invested 9% of our expenses on improving our facilities.

FUTURE CONSIDERATIONS

If ET programs are successful, the technique will be widely accepted and will be, perhaps, the most practical alternative to regular breeding in fertile mares that need to develop a sport career and probably the most feasible option for producing offspring of mares with severe fertility problems. Once breed registries accept offspring produced by ET and the general efficiency of the procedure is increased, it is not difficult to foresee this technique being performed in a similar way to that in cattle. Most of the cost of ET in the horse resides in the labor and time spent following the mare's cycles to ensure proper synchronization of donor and recipients. To reduce costs and use the technique on a wider scale, it becomes imperative to solve the following problems:

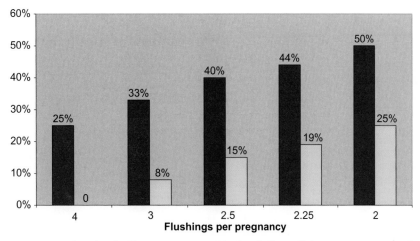

Figure 16-12. Efficiency of an ET program evaluated as flushings per pregnancy. Blue bars indicate efficiency per pregnancy. Yellow bars reflect the profit margin.

1. Diagnosis of the day of ovulation by a practical, reliable, and inexpensive method. This would eliminate the need of daily examinations during heat. The veterinarian would attend the farm only on the day of the uterine lavage to recover the embryo.

2. The use of progesterone-supplemented recipients could become very useful in ET programs. Intact anestrous mares supplemented with progesterone would be very useful in commercial ET programs. For this to be practical, however, it is essential to develop a method of progesterone supplementation that does not depend on daily or weekly administration either orally or systemically. Implants of slow-rate progesterone release could be a great aid for this purpose. Such products are being investigated.

3. Development of a practical, reliable, inexpensive, and harmless system to induce multiple ovulations in the mare would increase the efficiency of the procedure, having an immediate effect on the final cost of each ET pregnancy. Although many studies have succeeded in inducing multiple ovulations, the embryo recovery rate per ovulation still remains low. Some studies indicate that there may be a mechanism at the level of the ovary or the oviduct that interferes with normal pick-up or transport of the ova.

4. Development of techniques to recover and freeze morulae that produce high pregnancy rates would involve ET centers in national and international transport of frozen embryos as is common with transported cooled embryos in the United States and Europe. In addition, development of hormonal regimens that reliably induce cyclicity of mares during the winter would increase the availability of donor mares in ET programs. Finally, ET centers will perhaps become equine fertility clinics where more sophisticated techniques such as oocyte transfer, *in vitro* fertilization, gamete intrafallopian transfer, and intracytoplasmic sperm injection procedures are conducted for valuable mares with idiopathic or tubal infertility.

REFERENCES

1. Oguri N, Tsutsumi Y: Non-surgical recovery of equine eggs and an attempt to non-surgical embryo transfer in the horse. *J Reprod Fertil* 31:187-195, 1972.
2. Carmo MT, Losinno L, Aguilar JJ, et al: Oocyte transport to the oviduct of superovulated mares. *Anim Reprod Sci* 94:337-339, 2006.
3. Pashen RL, Lascombes FA, Darrow MD: The application of embryo transfer to polo ponies in Argentina. Embryo Transfer 3. *Eq Vet J Suppl* 15:119-121, 1993.
4. Mitchell D, Allen WR: Observations on reproductive performance in the yearling mare. *J Reprod Fertil Suppl* 23:531, 1975.
5. Savage NC, Woodcock LA, de Gannes G: Use of two year old mares as embryo donors in a commercial embryo transfer programme. *Eq Vet J* 8(Suppl):68-70, 1989.
6. Kenney RM: Cyclic and pathologic changes of the mare endometrium as detected by biopsy, with a note on early embryonic death. *J Am Vet Med Assoc* 172:241-262, 1978.
7. Hughes JP, Loy RG: Investigations on the effect of intrauterine inoculation of *Streptococcus zooepidemicus* in the mare. Proc AAEP Conv., 1969.
8. Ball BA: Embryonic loss in mares: Incidence, possible causes and diagnostic considerations. *Vet Clin North Am Eq Pract* 4:263-290, 1988.
9. Douglas RH, Burns PJ, Hershman L: Physiological and commercial parameters for producing progeny from subfertile mares by embryo transfer. Equine Embryo Transfer. *Eq Vet J* 3 (Suppl):111-114, 1985.
10. Riera FL, MacDonough J: Commercial embryo transfer in polo ponies in Argentina. Embryo Transfer 3. *Eq Vet J* 15(Suppl):116-118, 1993.
11. Mortensen C, Choi YH, Hinrichs K, et al: Effects of exercise on embryo recovery rates and embryo quality in the horse. *Anim Reprod Sci* 94: 395-397, 2006.
12. Sanchez R: Personal communication.
13. Riera.FL, Roldan JE, Campos M, Tomlinson EC: Equine Embryo Transfer in performing polo ponies in England.
14. Brinsko SP, Varner DD, Blanchard TL, Meyers SA: The effect of post-breeding uterine lavage on pregnancy rates in mares. *Theriogenology* 33:785, 1990.
15. Love CC, Strzemienski PI, Kenney RM: Endometrial concentrations of ampicillin in mares after intrauterine infusion of the drug. *Am J Vet Res* 51:256, 1990.
16. Wilsher S, Allen WR: The influence of maternal size, age and parity on placental and fetal development in the horse. *Theriogenology* 58: 833-835, 2002.
17. Tischner M: Embryo recovery from Polish pony mares and preliminary observations on foal size after transfer to large mares. *Eq Vet J* 3(Suppl):100-103, 1985.
18. Lagneaux D, Palmer E: Are pony and larger mares similar as recipients for non-surgical transfer of day 7 embryos? *Eq Vet J* 8(Suppl):64-67, 1989.
19. Greenhoff GR, Kenney RM: Evaluation of reproductive status of non-pregnant mares. *J Am Vet Med Assoc* 167:449, 1975.
20. Ginther OJ: *Ultrasonic Imaging and Reproductive Events in the Mare.* Cross Plains, WI: Equiservices, 1986.
21. Boyle MS, Sanderson MW, Skidmore I, Allen WR: Use of serial progesterone measurements to assess cycle length, time of ovulation and timing of uterine flushes in order to recover equine morulae. *Eq Vet J* 18(Supp):1013, 1989.
22. Lofstead RM: Control of the estrous cycle. *Vet Clin North Am* 4:177-195, 1988.
23. Douglas RH: Some aspects of equine embryo transfer. *J Reprod Fertil* 32(Suppl):405-408, 1982.
24. Imel KI, Squires EL, Elsden RP, Shideler RK: Collection and transfer of equine embryos. *J Am Vet Med Assoc* 179:987-991, 1981.
25. Squires EL, Garcia RH, Ginther OJ: Factors affecting success of equine embryo transfer. *Eq Vet J* 3(Suppl):20-22, 1985.
26. Squires EL, Ilmel KK, Iuliano MF, Shideler RK: Factors affecting efficiency in an equine embryo transfer program. *J Reprod Fertil* 32(Suppl):409-414, 1982.
27. Pashen RL: Embryo transfer in the horse. Proceedings of the Society for Theriogenology, Sacramento, CA: 1985.
28. Pashen RL: Current developments in embryo transfer. Equine Embryo Transfer. *Eq Vet J* 3(Suppl):25-27, 1985.
29. Vogelsang SG, Bondioli KR, Massey JM: Commercial application of equine embryo transfer. Equine Embryo Transfer. *Eq Vet J* 3(Suppl): 89-91, 1985.
30. Squires EL, Voss JL, Shideler RK: Equine embryo transfer up-date. Proc AAEP Convention, Dallas, TX: 1984, pp 357-363.
31. Loy RG, Buell IR, Stevenson W, Hamm D: Sources of variation in response intervals after prostaglandin treatment in mares with functional corpora lutea. *J Reprod Fertil* 27(Suppl):229-235, 1979.
32. Hughes IP: The effect of human chorionic gonadotrophin on ovulation, length of estrous and fertility in the mare. *Comel Vet* 56:41-50, 1966.
33. Gastal EL, Silva LA, Gastal MO, Evans MJ: Effect of different doses of HCG on diameter of the preovulatory follicle and interval to ovulation in mares. *Anim Reprod Sci* 94:186-190, 2006.
34. Wilsher S, Kolling M, Allen WR: Meclofenamic acid extends donor-recipient asynchrony in equine embryo transfer. *Eq Vet J* 38(5):428-432, 2006.
35. Hinrichs K; Use of ovariectomized mares as embryo transfer recipients. Proc Soc Theriogenology. Rochester, NY: 1986.
36. Alvarenga M: Long-acting progesterone. Personal communication.
37. McKinnon AO, Squires EL, Carnevale EM, Hermenet MI: Ovariectomized steroid-treated mares as embryo transfer recipients and as a model to study the role of progestins in pregnancy. *Theriogenology* 29:1055-1063, 1988.
38. Hinrichs K, Riera FL, Klunder L: Establishment of pregnancy after embryo transfer in mares with gonadal dysgenesis. *J In Vitro Fertil Embryo Trans* 6:155, 1989.
39. Shideler RK, Squires EL, Voss IL, et al: Progesterone therapy of ovariectomized pregnant mares. *J Reprod Fertil* 32(Suppl):459-464, 1982.
40. Hinrichs K, Sertich PL, Kenney RM: Use of altrenogest to prepare ovariectomized mares as embryo transfer recipients. *Theriogenology* 26:455-460, 1986.
41. Pashen RL, Downie C, McCue P: An attempt to use progesterone treated XO mares as embryo recipients. *Eq Vet J* 8(Suppl):95-97, 1989.
42. Squires EL, Seidel GE, McKinnon AO: Transfer of cryopreserved equine embryos to progestin treated ovariectomized mares. *Eq Vet J* 8(Suppl):98, 1989.

43. Sertich PL, Hinrichs K, Schiereck DE, Kenney RM: Periparturient events in ovariectomized embryo transfer recipient mares. *Theriogenology* 30:401, 1988.

44. Riera FL, Roldan JE, Hinrichs K: Pregnancy rate after embryo transfer in ovulating vs progesterone-treated-anestrous recipient mares in a commercial embryo transfer programme. 7th Equine Embryo Transfer Symp. Magdalene College, Cambridge: July 9-11, 2008.

45. Kenney RM, Bergman RV, Cooper WL, Morse GW: Minimal contamination techniques for breeding mares: Technique and preliminary findings. Proc AAEP Convention. Boston, MA: 1975.

46. Riera FL, Roldan JE, Hinrichs K: Effect of insemination timing on embryo recovery rate, pregnancy rate after transfer and pregnancy loss rate in a commercial embryo transfer programme. Proc 5th Int Symp Equine Embryo Transfer. Saari, Finland.

47. Dell'Aqua JA Jr, Papa FO, Lopes MD, et al: Modulation of acute uterine inflammatory response after artificial insemination with equine frozen semen. Anim Reprod Sci 94:270-273, 2006.

48. Weber IA, Freeman DA, Vanderwall DK, Woods GL: Prostaglandin E2 secretion by oviductal transport-stage equine embryos. *Biol Reprod* 45:540-543, 1991.

49. Boyle MS, Sanderson MW, Skidmore J, Allen WR: Use of serial progesterone measurements to assess cycle length, time of ovulation and timing of uterine flushes in order to recover equine morulae. *Eq Vet J* 8(Suppl): 10-13, 1989.

50. Battut I, Grandchamp des Raux A, Nicaise JL, et al: When do equine embryos enter uterine cavity? An attempt to answer. Equine Embryo Transfer. Proc 5th Int Symp Equine Embryo Transfer. Saari, Finland.

51. Alvarenga MA, Landim FC, Meira C: Modifications in the technique used to recover equine embryos. Embryo Transfer 3. *Eq Vet J* 15 (Suppl):111-112, 1993.

52. Iuliano MF: The effect of age of the equine embryo and method of transfer on pregnancy rate. MS Thesis. Colorado State University, Fort Collins, CO: 1983.

53. McKinnon AO, Squires EL: Equine embryo transfer. *Vet Clin North Am Eq Pract* 4:305-333, 1988.

54. Sertich PL: Transcervical embryo transfer in performance mares. *J Am Vet Med Assoc* 195:940-944, 1989.

55. Gibbs HM, Troedsson MH: Effect of acepromazine, detomidine and xylacine on myometrial activity in the mare. *Biol Repro Mono* 1:489-493, 1995.

56. McKinnon AO, Squires EL: Morphological assessment of the equine embryo. *J Am Vet Med Assoc* 192:401-406, 1988.

57. Riera FL, Roldan JE, Hinrichs K: Patterns of embryo recovery in mares with unilateral and bilateral double ovulations. *Anim Reprod Sci* 94:398, 2006.

58. Carnevale EM, Griffin PG, Ginther OJ: Age associated subfertility before entry of embryos into the uterus in mares. *Eq Vet J* 15(Suppl): 31-34, 1993.

59. McCue PM, Vanderwall DK, Squires EL: Embryo recovery in mares with echogenic preovulatory follicles. Proc 5th Int Symp Equine Embryo Transfer. Saari, Finland.

60. Aurich JE, Hoppen HO, Trampler R, et-al: Effects of mycotoxins on reproductive function in mares. Animal reproduction recovery rates in mares with echogenic pre-ovulatory follicles. Proc 5th Int Symp Equine Embryo Transfer. Saari, Finland.

61. Kenney RM: A review of the pathology of the equine oviduct. *Eq Vet J Suppl* 15: 1993.

62. Allen WR, Wilsher S, Morris L, et al: Re-establishment of oviductal patency and fertility in infertile mares. *Anim Reprod Sci* 94:242-243, 2006.

63. Love CC: personal communication, 1998.

64. Jasko DJ: Comparison of pregnancy rates following non-surgical transfer of day 8 equine embryos using various transfer devices. *Theriogenology* 58:713-715, 2002.

COOLING AND CRYOPRESERVATION OF EQUINE EMBRYOS

ELAINE M. CARNEVALE

Equine embryos can be stored for short periods at reduced temperatures or stored for long periods after cryopreservation. Embryos are often stored at reduced temperatures (approximately 5°C) during transport intervals of <24 hours. In contrast, after cryopreservation, embryos can be maintained for very long periods. Reasons for embryo cryopreservation include genetic preservation, long transport intervals, and storage for transfer at a later date. Embryos of various sizes can be stored at reduced temperatures; however, the success of cryopreservation with large embryos (>300 μm) is limited. In this chapter, factors affecting embryo preservation are reviewed and procedures are described.

REDUCED TEMPERATURE STORAGE OF EMBRYOS

Development of Methods to Cool Embryos

The potential to store equine embryos was first demonstrated in 1982, when Yamamoto[1] cooled equine embryos to 0° or 20°C for minutes to hours and produced foals from embryos stored at either temperature. The research used as a basis for commercial transport of embryos was reported in 1987.[2] In the study, embryos were stored in a tissue culture medium (Ham's F-10 with 10% fetal calf serum) that was gassed with 5% CO_2, 5% O_2, and 90% N_2 or buffered with HEPES. The gassed medium was determined to be preferential to medium with HEPES for storage of embryos for 24 hours. At 14 days, pregnancy rates were similar for control embryos, which were transferred immediately after collection, and embryos stored in the gassed medium; however, by 35 days, pregnancy rates were significantly higher for control than stored embryos (80% and 55%, respectively). The researchers concluded that storage procedures were acceptable for embryo transport. This system was modified to provide a commercial shipping regimen, and pregnancy rates at 12, 35, and 50 days were not different for embryos that were cooled and shipped versus transferred directly into recipients at the location of embryo collection.[3] However, pregnancy losses tended to be higher when embryos were transported for more versus less than 12 hours.[3]

Because methods for the short-term storage of equine embryos were developed primarily to allow embryo transport between collection and transfer facilities, embryos had to remain viable for at least 12 hours in the storage system. Storage at reduced temperatures retarded embryo metabolism and growth. During an interval of 12 hours, embryos increased in diameter 1.5%, 9.3%, and 37% at 5°, 24°, or 37°C, respectively.[4] After storage for 24 hours at 5°C, the mean embryo diameter increased by only 35 μm over 24 hours, for embryos with a mean diameter of 490 ± 43 μm at the onset of storage; the embryos did not advance in developmental stage.[2] The success of storage at reduced temperatures does not appear to be strictly dependent on embryo size,[5] although researchers have suggested that smaller embryos may be more susceptible to deleterious effects of cooling.[2,4,6,7]

Packaging of Embryos

Different methods have been used to package embryos for storage or transport. However, in most systems, the embryo is immediately identified, washed, and packaged in a holding medium within a secure container. The packaging system needs to maintain an appropriate temperature for the duration of storage. Packaging systems for transporting cooled semen have been used for embryo transport. These systems vary in their ability to maintain temperatures over time and to protect against heat and cold. Therefore, prior to use, the packaging system should be investigated. One of the most commonly used systems is the Equitainer (Hamilton Research, Inc., South Hamilton, MA). In a previous study,[2] the medium within an Equitainer initially decreased in temperature 0.3°C/min to 10°C at 5 hours; the temperature was maintained at 5°–10°C between 5 and 24 hours.

The medium for embryo storage must maintain a constant pH and sustain embryo viability. A protein source and antibiotic are usually added or supplied with the medium. Published data are available for Ham's F-10 medium, gassed (5% CO_2, 5% O_2, and 90% N_2) or with HEPES.[2] Other media, containing zwitterionic buffers to maintain pH, are currently available; these media were initially designed for washing and holding embryos prior to transfer. Similar pregnancy rates were reported for embryos stored in gassed Ham's F-10 medium (Sigma Chemical, St Louis, MO) and an embryo-holding medium (EmCare Holding Solution, ICP, Auckland, NZ).[6,8] The two media were compared *in vitro* to another medium (ViGro Holding Plus, Bioniche, Athens, GA)[6,9]; although the percentage of dead cells per embryo increased with storage time, no differences were observed among media.[9] These media are currently being used in clinical programs to transport embryos.

When collecting equine embryos for cooling and transport, media and materials needed for the procedure should be organized before collecting the embryo (Fig. 17-1, *A*). Ideally, the interval of time that the embryo is kept in a holding medium before being cooled should be limited. Although holding media are designed to accommodate the embryo, any artificial environment has the potential to cause deleterious effects. When embryos are cooled, the reduced temperature lowers embryo metabolism and

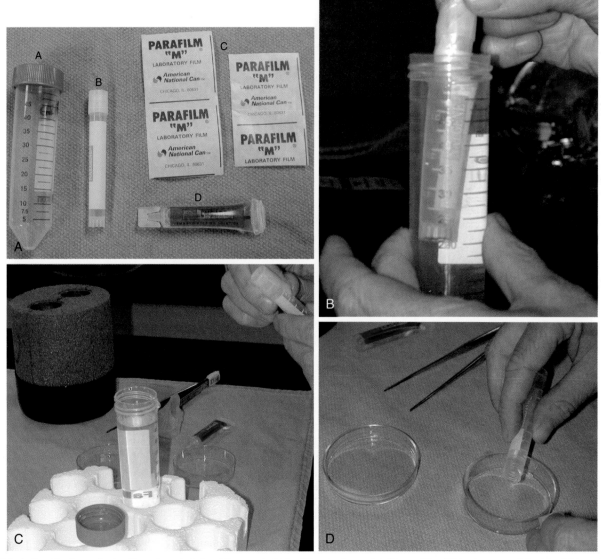

Figure 17-1. A, Supplies for packaging the embryo include a 50-ml conical tube *(A)*, a 5-ml cryovial *(B)*, parafilm *(C)* to place around the tubes' lids, and embryo-holding medium *(D)*. **B,** The embryo is packaged within the small tube. The large tube is filled with embryo flush medium, and the small tube is being placed within the large tube. **C,** To unpack the embryo, the small tube is removed with a pair of forceps, and the parafilm is unwrapped from around the cap. **D,** The holding medium and embryo are gently poured from the small vial into a tissue culture plate.

helps to protect the embryo from a suboptimal environment. Therefore, the embryos should be collected, washed, and packaged for cooling in the shortest possible interval.

For packaging embryos, an Equitainer or other appropriate packaging can be used. The container is typically held at room temperature before packing. Coolant cans or packs should be prepared as instructed.

Upon collection, the embryo is washed through three to six drops of medium to remove debris. The medium should be at a consistent temperature (room to body temperature) for washing, holding, and packaging the embryo; major temperature fluctuations should be avoided. A cryovial or snap-cap tube, usually containing 4–6 ml of medium, can be used to hold the embryo during transport. Prior to loading the embryo, medium is used to fill the vial or tube about three-quarters full with medium. The embryo is pulled into a pipette or 0.25-ml straw for transfer into the tube. If a straw is used to transfer the embryo, the end

of the straw containing the cotton plug can be attached to a ureteral catheter connector (Cook Urological, Spencer, IN) and a 1-ml syringe. The open end of the straw should not be handled to minimize bacterial contamination of the transport medium. The embryo is pulled into the straw, being careful to avoid getting fluid into the cotton end of the plug, which will seal the straw. To transfer the embryo, the end of the straw is inserted into the holding medium within the tube. The author likes to do this while holding the tube of medium against a light source (overhead or microscope light) and placing the straw 1–2 cm into the medium. In this way, the embryo can be seen as it exits the straw. The embryo should not be released near air bubbles, and air bubbles should not be pushed from the straw during the transfer, since the embryo can adhere to air bubbles and float to the top of the tube. After being placed into the medium, the embryo should begin to sink toward the bottom of the tube. The tube can then be completely filled with medium. Properly filling the tube is important. Air in the tube can allow agitation of media and formation of air bubbles during transport; however, if the tube is too full, the medium can overflow as the cap is closed. After being secured on the tube or vial, a strip of parafilm is placed around the cap. A 50-ml, conical tube is used as a second container. The 50-ml tube is filled with embryo-collection medium at the same temperature as the holding medium. The vial containing the embryo is then placed within the 50-ml tube, and the lid is placed upon the larger tube (Fig. 17-1, *B*). The 50-ml tube helps to protect the smaller tube and would contain the embryo if the smaller tube breaks or loses its cap. The large tube also provides additional temperature and shock insulation for the embryo. Parafilm is placed around the cap of the large tube. Although the embryo should not be exposed to the medium in the large tube, the medium should not be contaminated. Therefore, the tubes should be handled minimally and kept as clean as possible. Identification information for the embryo should be printed clearly on the large tube. Paperwork should be included, containing contact information and a description of the embryo (stage and quality). This will allow personnel at the receiving facility to determine if the embryo has changed in quality during transport. Also, if the clinician is not certain if the structure is an embryo vs. debris or an unfertilized oocyte, this should be noted. After packaging of the embryo, the large tube can then be placed directly into a tube holder if one is present within the cooling container. If not, ballast bags or insulation material can be placed around the tube before packaging within the container. Embryos have been shipped as cargo on airplanes or on overnight carriers. The receiving facility should be contacted since they may have specific packaging and shipping instructions, and they will need tracking information for the package on the day of shipment. Insuring the package during transport should be discussed with the owner of the donor mare, in case of failure or delay in delivery.

Removal of the Embryo

To unpack the embryo, the smaller tube is grasped with a pair of forceps and removed from the 50-ml tube (see Fig. 17-1, *C*). The large tube and its contents are kept intact until the embryo is identified. If the embryo is not found within the smaller vial, the medium within the large tube can be searched. To remove the embryo, the outside of the small tube is wiped dry, and the parafilm is removed. The vial is gently tilted back and forth so the embryo will float from the bottom of the tube. Care is taken to avoid the formation of bubbles that can make finding the embryo more difficult. The contents of the small tube are gently poured into a tissue culture dish (see Fig. 17-1, *D*). If the embryo is not immediately imaged as the medium is poured into the culture dish, the tube and its cap are immediately filled with medium; if the embryo is not found in the culture dish, the tube and cap can be rinsed and the media searched. Upon identification, the embryo is washed in clean medium and placed within a holding medium for immediate transfer. Because embryos do not significantly advance in developmental stage, recipients should be synchronized for the day of embryo collection or within an approximate window of 5–7 days from ovulation of the recipient.

Alternative Methods

An alternate method for embryo storage has been described.[7] Donor mares' uteri were flushed with 1500 ml of collection solution (EmCare). The flush was collected in three 500-ml bottles and allowed to sit for 10 minutes. Approximately 80% of the supernatant was removed, and the remaining media were pooled in a 500-ml bottle. Fresh flush medium at 30°–35°C was added to fill the bottle, and the bottle was placed in a refrigerator (5°C). The bottles were refrigerated for 6 or 24 hours before the embryo was recovered and evaluated. The percentage of dead cells was lower for embryos stored in 500-ml bottles for 6 hours than after packaging in an Equitainer for 24 hours, as described previously. However, embryos stored in 500-ml bottles for 24 hours had significantly more dead cells than the other groups. Storage of embryos in 500-ml bottles would not be feasible for long-distance transportation of embryos using commercial carriers. However, under field conditions, the procedures could be useful, especially if mares are flushed in a location distant to a stereoscope and recipients. The embryos in the study by Moussa and associates[7] were evaluated only on cellular characteristics, and pregnancy rates were not obtained.

CRYOPRESERVATION OF EMBRYOS

The first foal was produced from a cryopreserved embryo more than 25 years ago.[1] Since then, methods to cryopreserve equine embryos have been investigated and refined[10,11]; however, clinical use of embryo cryopreservation has been limited. Changes in breed registration rules and new procedures have helped to renew the interest of the equine industry in embryo cryopreservation.

Embryo Diameter and Stage

Size and stage of development are important factors in the success of embryo cryopreservation. Equine embryos entered mares' uteri at approximately 5.5 days after ovulation, with morula the earliest stage of development within the uterus.[12] After entering the uterus, embryos grew rapidly, almost doubling in diameter each day. Mean diameters for embryos collected on different days after the detection of ovulation were 208 μm at 6 days, 406 μm at 7 days, and 1132 μm at 8 days; however, mares were examined once daily for ovulation, and embryo flushes were done at different times of the day. Therefore, the range of embryo diameters were wide (132–756 μm on day 6, 136–1460 μm on day 7, and 120–3980 μm on day 8).[13] The optimal time to collect small embryos is limited to approximately 1 day, because the embryo does not enter the uterus until approximately 5.5 days, and it grows rapidly after entering in the uterus. By 7 days, many equine embryos are too large for cryopreservation.

For many routine breeding procedures, mares' ovaries are examined using transrectal palpation or ultrasound once daily; therefore, the actual time of ovulation could be ±24 hours. Different strategies have been used to collect small embryos for cryopreservation. Mares can be examined for the detection of ovulation at 6- to 12-hour intervals. When ovulation is detected, the optimal time of embryo collection can be determined; however, this method is very time consuming. Recently, embryos were collected based on the anticipated time of ovulation after administration of human chorionic gonadotropin (hCG, 2000 IU, IV).[14] The hCG was administered to young, light-horse mares when the following criteria were observed: (1) follicle ≥35 mm, (2) relaxed uterine and cervical tone, and (3) endometrial edema. Ovulation was anticipated at approximately 36 hours after the administration of hCG. Therefore, embryos were collected 8 days after hCG or 6.5 days after the anticipated time of

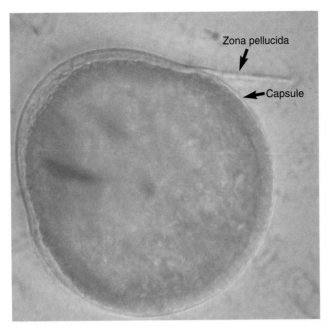

Figure 17-2. Equine blastocyst surrounded by the capsule. The zona pellucida has thinned and broken.

ovulation. The embryo collection rate per ovulation was high (78%), and all of the collected embryos were small (140–250 μm in diameter). Although embryo development appears to be relatively consistent for younger mares bred with fresh or cooled semen, development may be delayed in older mares or after insemination with frozen semen. In these cases, additional palpations may be necessary to properly time embryo collection.

Embryos of different diameters have been cryopreserved.[10,11] Although conventional cryopreservation or vitrification has been successful with smaller embryos, cryopreservation of larger embryos is more difficult.[10,11,14-16] Researchers have speculated that unique aspects of the equine embryo are responsible for the failure of larger embryos to cryopreserve. The equine blastocyst grows rapidly with a large, hypotonic blastocoele. It is surrounded by a mucin glycoprotein layer called the *capsule* (Fig. 17-2). The formation of the capsule occurs at the approximate stage when embryo cryopreservation fails, and although the capsule can be penetrated by large molecules, it has been postulated to reduce access of cryoprotectants to the embryo. However, the growing equine embryo also has a unique tolerance to hypertonic environments, and changes in the yolk sac wall could result in an altered embryonic response to cryoprotectants.[17] For most studies, embryos were considered small when <300 μm in diameter and at the morula to early blastocyst stage of development. Ideal embryos for cryopreservation have been defined as ≤250 μm. Embryos were defined as large for cryopreservation at >300 μm; these embryos are usually blastocysts.

Methods of Cryopreservation

Two basic methods have been used to cryopreserve equine embryos: conventional, slow-cooling and vitrification. Both methods have been successful for the cryopreservation of small embryos, but neither technique has proved reliably successful with embryos >300 μm.

Before cryopreservation, embryos are exposed to cryoprotectants.[10] Cryoprotectants are classified as intracellular or extracellular. Intracellular cryoprotectants have low molecular weight and can permeate cells; these include ethylene glycol, glycerol, and dimethyl sulfoxide (DMSO). Extracellular cryoprotectants, including sucrose and serum albumin, have relatively high molecular weights and do not penetrate embryonic cells. Combinations of cryoprotectants are used to minimize the potential deleterious effects of a high concentration of a single cryoprotectant. Cryoprotectants are often added and removed in steps to prevent sudden osmotic changes within cells. Osmotic changes are more apt to damage cells during removal than addition of cryoprotectants. Much higher concentrations of cryoprotectants are used for vitrification than conventional freezing, since embryos are packaged in straws and exposed to liquid nitrogen during vitrification prior to equilibration with cryoprotectants.

Conventional Freezing

During conventional freezing, the embryo is exposed to cryoprotectants and slowly cooled. As the temperature is reduced, ice crystals begin to form in the extracellular medium. The formation of ice crystals causes the cryoprotectant solution to become more hypertonic, and additional water is drawn from the embryo. The desired result is the movement of water from the embryo and into the extracellular solution, where ice crystals begin to form. The typical cooling rate is approximately 0.5°C.[10] The rate of cooling is designed to minimize the detrimental effects of large ice crystal formation and of exposure to hyperosmotic solutions. To prevent cooling below the freezing point (supercooling), ice crystal formation is usually induced (seeding) at approximately −6°C. Seeding is often accomplished by dipping forceps into liquid nitrogen and then touching the straw with the frozen forceps.

Embryos can be damaged during thawing. Rapid thawing can result in an influx of water into blastomeres and osmotic swelling. To minimize damage, embryos are often placed into solutions with decreasing concentrations of cryoprotectants and/or into solutions with high concentrations of extracellular cryoprotectants. The desired result is a gradual hydration of the embryo.

METHODS AND SUCCESS OF CONVENTIONAL CRYOPROTECTION. Equine embryos have been frozen with variable success.[10,11] Different methods and cryoprotectants were used to freeze embryos, although freezing in straws with glycerol as the primary cryoprotectants was most common. One relatively simple and successful method was reported by Slade and associates in 1985.[16] In the study, glycerol was used as a cryoprotectant in a base medium of modified Dulbecco's phosphate-buffered saline with 5% fetal calf serum. Embryos were exposed to glycerol in two steps (5% v/v for 10 minutes and 10% v/v for 30 minutes) and packaged in 0.5-ml straws. The straws were cooled (4°C/minute) to −6°C, seeded, and held for 15 minutes. The temperature of the straw was slowly reduced to −30°C at 0.3°C/minute and to −33°C at 0.1°C/minute before plunging in liquid nitrogen. Thawing was accomplished by immersing the straw in a water bath at 37°C. Embryos were then moved through solutions of decreasing glycerol concentrations (10%, 8.3%, 6.7%, 5.0%, 3.3%, and 1.6% glycerol, 10 minutes per solution) to dilute the cryoprotectant, before the embryo was placed in base medium. The method described by Slade and associates[16] was simplified by Maclellan and associates.[15] Although cooling rates were similar, embryos were exposed to glycerol in two steps (5% for 10 minutes and 10% for 20 minutes). Embryos were frozen in 0.25-ml straws and thawed by exposing the straw to air for 10 seconds before placing the straw in a water bath at 37°C for 30 seconds. Cryoprotectant was removed by placing the embryo in 8%, 6%, 4%, 2%, and 1% glycerol, before moving it to the base medium (SOF/HEPES + 0.6% BSA). These methods achieved pregnancy rates of approximately 55% with small embryos.

For conventional freezing, an automated cell freezer is often used, and the freezing and thawing procedures can be time consuming. Therefore, use of conventional freezing is often impractical under farm conditions.

Vitrification

Vitrification is the conversion of a liquid into glass. During vitrification, viscosity of a solution is increased until a solid state is achieved. High concentrations of cryoprotectants (6 to 7 molar [M]) are used to obtain this effect. The embryo is not allowed to reach equilibrium with the cryoprotectants in the final vitrification solution. Therefore, precise timing of cryoprotectant exposure is essential to prevent deleterious solution effects. The slow-cooling rates used with conventional freezing are not necessary. Procedures for vitrification are rapid and require less-specialized equipment than conventional freezing.

VITRIFICATION PROCEDURES. Pregnancies were first produced from vitrified and warmed embryos in 1994, when equine embryos were vitrified in 40% ethylene glycol, 18% Ficoll (a macromolecule), and 0.3 M sucrose.[18] More recently, a vitrification procedure that had been used for ovine and water buffalo embryos was modified for use with equine embryos. The initial work in this area was reported in 2004,[19] with embryos exposed to serial dilutions of cryoprotectants after warming. Subsequently, the procedure was modified for dilution of cryoprotectants in the straw, and embryos were transferred directly from straws into recipients' uteri.[14,20]

This vitrification process requires sequential exposure of embryos to three vitrification solutions. The first vitrification solution (VS1) contains 1.4 M glycerol; VS2 contains 1.4 M glycerol and 3.6 M ethylene glycol; and VS3 contains 3.4 M glycerol and 4.6 M ethylene glycol. The base medium for vitrification solutions is a modified phosphate-buffered saline without calcium and magnesium and supplemented with 0.3 mM sodium pyruvate, 3.3 mM glucose, and 20% fetal calf serum (PBS).[19] Methods to prepare vitrification solutions have been published.[20] and similar media are commercially available (Bioniche Animal Health, Athens, GA).

Vitrification procedures are performed at room temperature (22° to 24°C). Media can be placed in four-well dishes or organized in droplets within a tissue culture dish (Fig. 17-3, *A*). However, the system needs to allow movement of the embryo between solutions at precise intervals and with small volumes of medium. The embryo is placed into VS1 for 5 minutes, and then into VS2 for 5 minutes. Protracted exposure to the high concentrations of cryoprotectants in VS3 can be deleterious; therefore, the embryo should be in VS3 for <1 minute before being placed in liquid nitrogen vapor.

The embryo in VS3 will be loaded into a 0.25-ml, non-irradiated, polyvinyl chloride straw. Dilution solution (DS, 0.5 M galactose) is also loaded in the straw. The DS is important in moderating the movement of water into the embryo during warming. The volumes of solutions within the straw are important. Precise volumes can be pipetted into a tissue culture dish (see Fig. 17-3, *A*), or they can be pulled up based on length of the column in the straw.

Because the embryo should be exposed to VS3 for <1 minute, the straw should be labeled before loading. The straw is loaded with 90 μl of DS; 5 μl of air; 30 μl of VS3 with the embryo; 5 μl of air; 90 μl of DS (Figs. 17-3, *B* and *C*). The DS is pulled into the cotton plug of the straw to seal the end. The open end of the straw can be heat sealed or plugged. Straw adaptors can

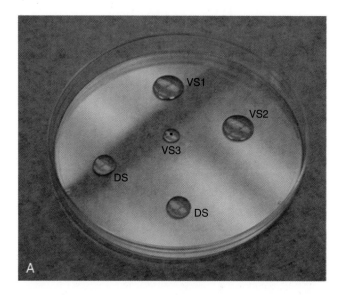

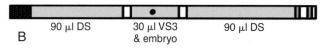

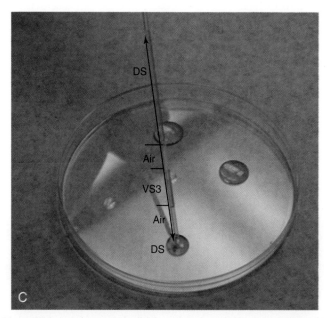

Figure 17-3. **A,** A tissue culture dish is used to place vitrification solutions (VS) and dilution solution (DS) before beginning vitrification procedures. Approximately 200-μl drops of VS1 and VS2 are placed on the plate, with a 30-μl drop of VS3 *(center)* and two 90-μl drops of DS. The VS3 and DS will be used to load the straw. The embryo is placed in VS1 for 5 minutes, in VS2 for 5 minutes, and in VS3 for <1 minute. **B,** The straw is loaded with 90 μl of DS, approximately 5 μl of air, 30 μl of VS3 with the embryo, approximately 5 μl of air, and 90 μl of DS. The DS is pulled into the cotton plug to seal the cotton end of the straw, and the open end is heat sealed or plugged. **C,** Once packaged, the straw contains two columns of DS and a column of VS3. The columns are separated by air.

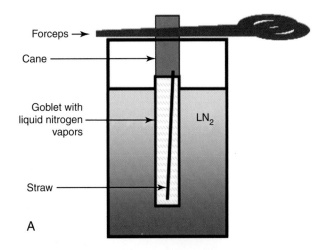

Forceps →

Cane

Goblet with
liquid nitrogen
vapors

LN_2

Straw

A

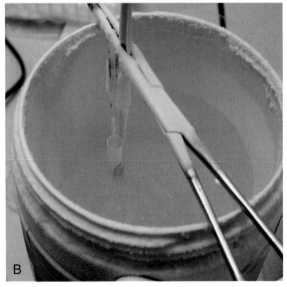

B

Figure 17-4. A, An insulated container is filled with liquid nitrogen. A plastic goblet is placed on a cane. The cane is held by forceps, and the goblet is surrounded by liquid nitrogen, but only vapors are within the goblet. The straw is placed within the goblet for 1 minute and exposed to vapors. The forceps are then removed, and the goblet is plunged into the liquid nitrogen. **B,** A cane and goblet are being held by forceps in liquid nitrogen. The 0.25-ml straw is attached to a 0.5-ml straw by an adapter. The larger straw has been labeled.

be used that plug the 0.25-ml straw and fit into a 0.5-ml straw. The larger straw can be flattened and labeled to aid in identification. The adaptors and straw should be tested to ensure a firm fit before their use. Within 1 minute of embryo exposure to VS3, the straw is placed into liquid nitrogen vapor. This can be done by suspending a plastic goblet (10 × 20 mm) within a container of liquid nitrogen (Fig. 17-4). The goblet should be filled with vapors, but not with liquid nitrogen. The straw is held in the vapors for 1 minute and then plunged into the liquid nitrogen. A second goblet can be inverted and placed on the cane over the first goblet and straw; this will help to keep the straw in the goblet during storage. The cane containing the embryo can then be placed into a tank of liquid nitrogen for storage.

The embryo is warmed by removing the straw from liquid nitrogen. The straw is held in room air for 10 seconds, before being placed into a cold water bath (20°–22°C) for 10 seconds. The straw is wiped of excess water and flicked to mix the VS3

and DS. The straw can be placed on a stereoscope to locate the embryo. If the embryo is near the sealed ends of the straw, the straw can be tilted to move the embryo toward the center of the straw. The straw should be placed flat on a room-temperature surface until placement into an embryo transfer gun. The embryo should be transferred into a recipient's uterus at 6–8 minutes after warming. For transfer, the straw adaptor can be removed or the straw can be cut if it was heat sealed. The straw is loaded into a transfer rod ("Deep Chamber" for full-length straws and "Shallow Chamber" for cut straws; Agtech, Manhattan, KS or IMV, Maple Grove, MN), and the embryo can be transferred using standard procedures. In our laboratory, we have preferentially used recipients at 5 days after ovulation, although recipients from 4 to 6 days after ovulation should be acceptable.

VITRIFICATION OF COOLED EMBRYOS. The effects of cooling equine embryos at approximately 5°C before vitrification were studied[21] to determine if embryos could be shipped to a facility for cryopreservation. Embryos were collected and vitrified directly using methods previously described[14,20] or held at 5°–8°C for 12–19 hours before vitrification using the same technique. For cold storage, embryos were packaged as previously described in this chapter using an embryo-holding medium (ViGro). Early pregnancy rates were not different for embryos that were or were not cooled before vitrification (15/20, 75% and 13/20, 65%, respectively).

CONCLUSIONS

Equine embryos can be successfully preserved for transport or long-term storage. Storage at low temperatures has been used to transport embryos, although the time of storage is limited to <24 hours. Cryopreservation of equine embryos has been successful for small embryos, but difficult for embryos >300 μm. Embryos can be cryopreserved by conventional, slow-cooling methods or by vitrification. Vitrification with direct transfer provides a rapid procedure that requires limited equipment and time.

REFERENCES

1. Yamamoto Y, Oguri N, Tsutsumi Y, et al: Experiments in the freezing and storage of equine embryos, *J Reprod Fertil* 32(Suppl):399-403, 1982.
2. Carnevale EM, Squires EL, McKinnon AO: Comparison of Ham's F10 with CO₂ or HEPES buffer for storage of equine embryos at 5°C for 24 H. *J Anim Sci* 65:1775-1781, 1987.
3. Carney NJ, Squires EL, Cook VM, et al: Comparison of pregnancy rates from transfer of fresh versus cooled, transported equine embryos. *Theriogenology* 36:23-32, 1991.
4. Clark KE, Squires EL, McKinnon AO, et al: Viability of stored equine embryos. *J Anim Sci* 65:534-542, 1987.
5. Fleury JJ, Fleury PDC, Landim-Alvarenga FC: Effect of embryo diameter and storage period on pregnancy rates obtained with equine embryos stored in Ham's F-10 with HEPES buffer at a temperature of 15-18°C — preliminary results. *Theriogenology* 58:749-750, 2002.
6. Moussa M, Duchamp G, Mahla R, et al: In vitro and in vivo comparisons of Ham's F-10, EmCare holding solution and ViGro holding plus for the cooled equine embryos. *Theriogenology* 59:1615-1625, 2003.
7. Moussa M, Duchamp G, Daels PF, et al: Effect of embryo age on the viability of equine embryos after cooled storage using two transport systems. *J Equine Vet Sci* 26:529-534, 2006.
8. McCue PM, Scoggin CF, Meira C, et al: Pregnancy rates for equine embryos cooled for 24 h in Ham's F-10 versus EmCare™ embryo holding solution. Proc Annu Conf Soc Theriogenology:2000, p 147.

9. Moussa M, Tremoleda JL, Duchamp G, et al: Evaluation of viability and apoptosis in horse embryos stored under different conditions at 5°C. *Theriogenology* 61:921-932, 2004.
10. Seidel GE: Cryopreservation of equine embryos. *Vet Clin North Am Equine Pract* 12:85-99, 1996.
11. Squires EL, Carnevale EM, McCue PM, et al: Embryo technologies in the horse. *Theriogenology* 59:151-170, 2003.
12. Freeman DA, Weber JA, Geary RT, et al: Time of embryo transport through the mare oviduct. *Theriogenology* 36:823-830, 1991.
13. Squires EL, Cook VM, Voss JL: Collection and Transfer of Equine Embryos, Animal Reproduction Laboratory Bulletin No. 1. Fort Collins, CO:, 1985.
14. Eldridge-Panuska WD, Caracciolo di Brienza V, Seidel GE, Jr. et al: Establishment of pregnancies after serial dilution or direct transfer by vitrified equine embryos. *Theriogenology* 63:1308-1319, 2005.
15. Maclellan LJ, Carnevale EM, Coutinho da Silva MA, et al: Cryopreservation of small and large equine embryos pretreated with cytochalasin-B and/or trypsin. *Theriogenology* 58:717-720, 2002.
16. Slade NP, Takeda T, Squires EL, et al: A new procedure for the cryopreservation of equine embryos. *Theriogenology* 24:45-57, 1985.
17. Crews LJ, Waelchli RO, Huang CX, et al: Electrolyte distribution and yolk sac morphology in frozen hydrated equine conceptuses during the second week of pregnancy. *Reprod Fertil Dev* 19:804-814, 2007.
18. Hochi S, Fujimoto T, Braun J, et al: Pregnancies following transfer of equine embryos cryopreserved by vitrification. *Theriogenology* 42:483-488, 1994.
19. Caracciolo di Brienza V, Squires EL, Zicarelli L, et al: Establishment of pregnancies after vitrification of equine embryos. *Reprod Fertil Dev* 16:165, 2004.
20. Carnevale EM, Eldridge-Panuska WD, Caracciolo di Brienza V: How to collect and vitrify equine embryos fro direct transfer. Proc 50th Ann Conv Am Assoc Equine Pract 2004, pp 402-405.
21. Hudson J, McCue PM, Carnevale EM, et al: The effects of cooling and vitrification of embryos from mares treated with equine follicle-stimulating hormone on pregnancy rates after nonsurgical transfer. *J Equine Vet Sci* 26:51-54, 2006.

New Assisted Reproductive Techniques Applied for the Horse Industry

MARCO A. ALVARENGA AND FERNANDA DA CRUZ LANDIM-ALVARENGA

The development of assisted reproductive technologies (ARTs) in the horse dates back to the late nineteenth century with the establishment of the first equine pregnancies obtained by artificial insemination.[1] Since then, ARTs have helped to produce offspring from valuable mares that cannot produce embryos and are considered infertile. Besides artificial insemination, which is discussed in detail elsewhere, embryo transfer has been the most common ART in mares. However, there are a number of mares that cannot produce embryos because of various pathological conditions of the reproductive tract. Therefore, other embryo production techniques using both *in vivo* and *in vitro* procedures have been developed. These techniques include (1) oocyte transfer (OT), (2) intracytoplasmic sperm injection (ICSI), (3) *in vitro* fertilization (IVF), and (4) nuclear transfer or cloning. All of these techniques are intended to increase the chances of producing offspring from severely subfertile mares or stallions. ARTs involve the endocrine stimulation of the gonads and the *in vitro* and *in vivo* manipulation of gametes. In addition, it is not uncommon to use surgical procedures to accomplish some of these techniques.[2]

The development of techniques such as ultrasound-guided aspiration of follicles,[3-6] which allows recovery of *in vivo* matured oocyte from live mares, has led to some clinical interest in the standardization of IVF, which includes the culture of mature oocytes with capacitated sperm. However, this procedure has not resulted in an efficient method to produce equine offspring. The main reasons for the limited progress of IVF in the horse include the scarce availability of abattoir ovaries, poor *in vivo* recovery of immature oocytes, the difficulty in developing efficient systems for oocyte maturation *in vitro,* and problems in defining and achieving sperm capacitation *in vitro*. The lack of basic scientific information on both of these fields has made IVF an expensive and inefficient technique in the horse.

To date, only two foals have been produced after IVF of oocytes matured *in vivo*.[7] Because of the inefficiency of IVF, researchers and clinicians have opted for different approaches in order to fertilize equine oocytes both *in vivo* and *in vitro*. As mentioned previously, these techniques include OT, gamete intrafallopian transfer (GIFT), and ICSI. In addition, several recent reports describe successful cloned horses, some of which are performing the procedure commercially.[8] Of the *in vitro* ARTs, OT has been the most repeatable and affordable in horses. However, recent improvements in the efficiency with the use of ICSI have also increased the interest for the use of these techniques by horse breeders.

This chapter focuses on recent progress in OT, ICSI, and nuclear transfer or cloning, and it highlights the procedure of ovum pick up (OPU) that is key in the development and implementation of the previously mentioned techniques.

OOCYTE COLLECTION AND *IN VITRO* MATURATION

The first successful maturation of equine oocytes in vitro was achieved by Fulka and Okolski,[9] which coincided with the time when research on the technology of in vitro maturation of ruminant oocytes was at its peak. This was in great part enhanced by the unlimited availability of abattoir-collected bovine oocytes and the lack of restrictions to conduct research with such material.[2] In contrast, in the case of the horse, availability of abattoir ovaries is scarce and in vivo oocyte recovery rate; with the use of ultrasound-guided follicular aspiration is far from providing enough viable oocytes.

In the equine, the anatomy of oocyte attachment to the follicular wall interferes with the efficiency of oocyte recovery both *in vivo* and *in vitro*. In the mare, the follicle has a thecal pad beneath the cumulus cell attachment. These processes are the extension of the granulosa cells into the thecal layer. The position of the pad, the granulosa cell processes that extend into it, and the acid polysaccharide component of the pad seem to act as an anchor for the cumulus attachment.[10] In addition, the equine ovary has a much smaller number of antral follicles compared with other species, with the average number of visible follicles in the horse's ovaries being six per ovary.[2,11,12] Several investigators have reported the number of harvested cumulus oocyte complexes (COCs) using different techniques. Okolski et al.[13] and Hinricks and DiGiorgio[12] reported an average of 1.5 and 2.7 COC per ovary, respectively, when aspirating the follicles. Zhang et al.[14] reported a COC recovery of 3.1 COC per ovary when the follicular wall is scraped. Choi et al.[15] obtained 4.14 oocytes per ovary when the ovaries were sliced and washed.

In vivo or *in vitro* follicular aspiration results in an average recovery of 1.5 oocytes per ovary in horses compared with an average of 10 oocytes per ovary in the cow. However, harvest of *in vitro* recovered cumulus intact oocytes or COCs is greatly increased (50% to 80% of aspirated follicles) if follicles are opened and the granulosa layer is scraped from the follicle using a curette[12,16] (Fig. 18-1). Unfortunately, this process significantly increases the time and number of personnel required to collect oocytes from a given number of slaughterhouse ovaries. The difficulties in obtaining large numbers of oocytes represent a major limitation for research on technologies such as IVF, ICSI, embryo culture, and cloning.

Palmer et al.[17] were the first to describe a standing *in vivo* aspiration technique for horses, where the operator held the ovary via rectum and guided a needle through the flank toward the preovulatory follicle. The recovery rate reported in this pioneering work was 63%. The same year, McKinnon et al.[18] reported a recovery rate of 71.4% when using a trocar cannula and a larger needle (9.8 mm) to aspirate preovulatory follicles via the flank. A similar procedure was described by Hinrichs and DiGiorgio[12] with recovery rates of 73%. To aid in the fixation of the ovary for the flank technique, a colpotomy incision was made in the cranial vagina, enabling the operator to introduce his hand into the peritoneal cavity and to fix the ovary directly against the abdominal wall.[11]

The first group of researchers to describe the ultrasound-guided transvaginal aspiration (TVA) approach to harvest oocytes in the standing mare was Brück et al.[3] Based on a similar approach used in humans and cattle IVF programs, a finger-shaped transducer connected to an ultrasound and equipped with a needle guide that showed the puncture line on the screen was used to aspirate preovulatory follicles (Fig. 18-2). A single lumen needle attached to a 50-ml syringe was used to flush the follicular cavity up to three times with Dulbecco's PBS. One oocyte was recovered out of four follicles.

Cook et al.[5] performed a study comparing single- and double-lumen needles. The 12-gauge double-lumen resulted in the highest recovery rate (84%) of preovulatory follicles compared with the single lumen needle (52%). The double-lumen needle allowed the fluid to drip continuously into the follicle while suction was being applied.

The aspiration of immature follicles increases the number of follicles punctured. Cook et al.[19] aspirated oocytes on days 7 to 9 of diestrus when an average of four follicles measuring 10 to 25 mm was detected. A total of 135 diestrus follicles were aspirated and 25 oocytes (18.5%) were recovered,[20] indicating that follicle size significantly influenced the COC recovery. More oocytes were collected from small follicles measuring 5 to 15 mm (52%) than from subordinate follicles measuring 20 to 27 mm (22%). The scraping technique of the follicular wall is easier to perform when the follicle diameter is smaller.[21,22] Although there are abundant data in the literature concerning

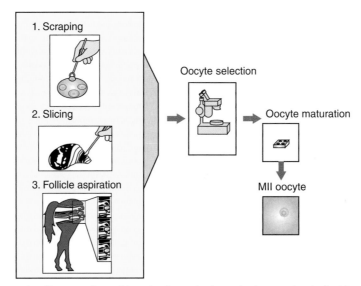

Figure 18-1. Oocyte collection and maturation. Oocytes to be used in assisted reproductive technology can be obtained by transvaginal follicular aspiration in live mares. Higher oocyte numbers can be recovered by scraping the follicular cavity or slicing the ovaries obtained from mares at an abattoir.

Pre-ovulatory follicle aspiration from donor

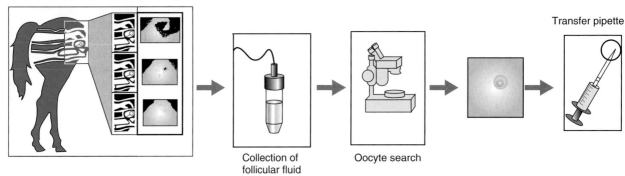

Figure 18-2. Donor management for oocyte transfer. A transrectal ultrasound probe, equipped with a needle guide, indicates the puncture line on the screen and is often used to aspirate the donor and recipient mare follicles. Each follicle is flushed at least three times. The fluid is then examined under a stereomicroscope to identify cumulus oocyte complexes.

the aspiration of immature oocytes, very little is known about the developmental potential of such oocytes for producing horse embryos. Furthermore, comparisons and data interpretation are difficult because of the great variation in procedures between laboratories. For example, Squires[22] reported a range between 8% and 31% embryo development, while Bezard et al.[21] reported between 22% and 52% and Galli et al.[2] reported between 26.7% and 71.1%.

One significant factor is whether oocytes are collected from immature or preovulatory follicles. The loss of junctions between cumulus cells and cells from the follicular wall, during the LH surge before ovulation, results in a much higher oocyte recovery from preovulatory follicles compared with non-preovulatory follicles (78% vs. 43%).

The pregnant mare has also been considered a source of oocytes. Meintjes et al.[23] Ginther,[24] and Ginther and Bergfelt[25] have described the occurrence of follicular waves during early pregnancy in mares. Follicular activity is variable among early pregnant mares, ranging from periodically to sporadically occurring major waves (largest follicle ≥35 mm) in some mares to only minor waves (largest follicle ≤35 mm) in others. Oocyte recovery rates from pregnant mares seem to be higher compared with cycling mares. Goudet et al.[26] reported 54% oocyte recovery rates in pregnant mares vs. 47% in cyclic mares. Meintjes et al.[23] reported 75.8% oocyte recovery for pregnant mares vs. 42.9% for pre-ovulatory follicles used as control. In a first study by Meintjes et al.,[23] eleven aspirations were performed per mares between days 22 and 66 of gestation with a maximum of seven oocytes recovered per aspiration session. In a second study, the same authors[27] extended the aspirations until day 150 of gestation. The mean number of aspirations per mare was around 7.6 and the average number of oocytes obtained was 18.9 per mare. They concluded that an average of 2.5 oocytes could be collected every 7 to 10 days from pregnant mares. It was estimated that 19 oocytes could be retrieved from a mare between days 21 and 150 of gestation compared with 12 collected during 130 days in cycling mares without any hormonal treatment. In another study, Cochran et al.[28] reported an average of 13 follicles per procedure, and an oocyte recovery rate of 66% for 20 aspirations performed between days 14 and 70 of pregnancy.

Oocyte Maturation

After the oocytes are collected and selected on the basis of cumulus morphology, they are transferred to a maturation medium and allowed to mature *in vitro* for 24 to 36 hours. Oocyte maturation consists of nuclear and cytoplasmic modifications that prepare the oocyte for fertilization. *In vivo,* maturation is a process coinciding with follicular development, changing hormone levels, and meiotic progression. Nuclear maturation is referred to as the finalization of the meiotic process with the reduction of DNA content in the oocyte. Resumption of meiosis is marked by extrusion of the first polar body and formation of a metaphase II plate. In most species, the resumption of meiosis is mediated by LH-receptor interaction in the cumulus cell membrane, mediating the increase of the MPF in the ooplasm.[29,30]

A detailed description of meiotic changes was reported by Grondahl et al.,[31] who used transmission electron microscopy to visualize the process. According to the stage of nuclear maturation observed using light microscopy, oocytes are classified as follows:
- GV (germinal vesicle)—when a spherical oocyte nucleus is located centrally or peripherally in the ooplasm

- GVBD (germinal vesicle breakdown)—when the oocyte nucleus presents an irregular envelope surrounding disperse condensed chromatin
- M-I (metaphase I)—characterized by the presence of metaphase chromosomes at the periphery of the ooplasm
- M-II (metaphase II)—presence of metaphase chromosomes in the ooplasm's periphery and presence of an extruded polar body in the peri-vitelline space

The occurrence of meiotic maturation is accompanied, and probably regulated, by changes in the phosphorylation patterns of various cellular proteins. One such protein is the MPF reported by Masui and Makert,[32] which is known to be a universal cell cycle regulator of both mitosis and meiosis.[33] Active MPF induces chromosome condensation, nuclear envelope breakdown, and cytoplasmic reorganization with entry into M-phase of either mitotic or meiotic cell cycle.[34-36] During oocyte meiotic maturation of mammalian species, MPF activity is very low in the germinal vesicle stage and peaks at metaphase I and II stages (mouse: Hashimoto and Kishimoto,[37] Choi et al.[38]; rabbit: Naito and Toyoda[39]; goat: Jelinkova et al.[40]; pig: Dedieu et al.[41]; bovine: Wu et al.[42]) (Fig. 18-3). Other kinases are also involved in the regulation of meiotic events, such as mitogen-activated protein kinase (MAPK).[103]

Cytoplasmic maturation is characterized by several changes in the shape and localization of the organelles. Grøndahl et al.[31] described a breakdown of the intermediate junctions between the cumulus cell projections and the oolemma with an enlargement of the peri-vitelinic space. In addition, they described the formation and arrangement of a large number of cortical granules immediately beneath the cytoplasmic membrane and the structural change of the mitochondria to a round shape. The migration of the cortical granules is believed to be an important step in cytoplasmic maturation[43] and can be used to assess general oocyte maturity.[23,44] The redistribution of the cortical granules provides the ovum the capacity to initiate the block of polyspermy and to induce sperm nuclear decondensation.[43]

Factors that may affect cytoplasmic maturation include presence of cumulus cells, addition of gonadotropins to the

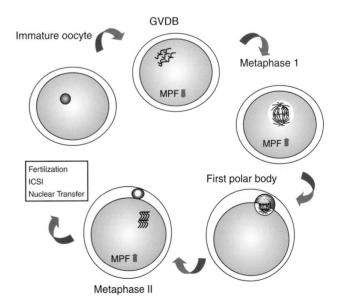

Figure 18-3. Oocyte maturation. During oocyte meiotic maturation, the maturation promoting factor (MPF) activity is low at the germinal vesicle stage and peaks at metaphase I and II stages.

maturation media, and time of culture. The structure of the oocyte and its associated granulosa cells is collectively called the cumulus oocyte complex (COC). The presence of granulosa cells during *in vitro* maturation has proven to be beneficial in humans,[45] rabbits, and cows.[46] The inner layer of the COC is called the corona radiata and is connected with the oocyte membrane, permitting the transfer of molecules from the outer granulosa cells to the oocyte.[47] The association between germinal cells and somatic granulosa cells regulates the level of synthesis of specific proteins and the pattern of protein phosphorylation in growing oocytes, thus directly regulating their metabolism.

The *in vitro* maturation of equine oocytes reviewed by Galli et al.[2] ranges from 20% to 85%, and comparisons between *in vitro* maturation procedures in horses are difficult because each study has a different protocol.

An interesting aspect, peculiar to the horse oocyte, is that oocytes with expanded cumulus mature have normal developmental competence. In other species such as ruminants and pigs, the presence of expanded cumulus is linked to the collection of oocytes from atretic follicles, and these oocytes are generally discarded immediately because of their extremely low developmental capacity.[48] Hinrichs et al.,[49-51] in a series of studies demonstrated that oocytes with expanded cumulus were more capable of complete maturation than oocytes with compact cumulus.

Another aspect is that the maturation rate will be directly linked with the quality of the ovaries used and especially with the time between slaughter and collection of the oocytes. Better maturation rates are obtained when oocytes are transferred directly into the maturation media after aspiration. Delaying this process will result in reduced maturation rates.[52] In our laboratory, ovaries must be transported 500 km and the total time between slaughter and beginning of maturation is about 8 to 9 hours. It is important to mention that it is not always clear from the literature how the maturation rate of equine oocytes is calculated and whether degenerated oocytes are taken into account. In our laboratory, degenerating oocytes identified after *in vitro* maturation are taken into account to establish our maturational rates.

The majority of studies in equine oocyte IVM use TCM-199 as a culture medium with the addition of serum, follicular fluid, or hormones (LH, FSH, and estradiol 17β).[50,53-56] However, the source and levels of LH and FSH have not been optimized. LH of ovine,[53] bovine,[53,57,58] equine origin,[20,23] and equine pituitary extract (EPE)[59] have been used, but none of these has increased the efficiency of conventional equine IVF.

OOCYTE TRANSFER IN MARES

The OT procedure involves several steps where the recipient reproductive tract will provide a healthy environment for sperm survival and transport, oocyte fertilization, and embryo development. The first successful OT in the horse was performed in 1988 by McKinnon et al.,[60] and 10 years later the first commercial program was established at Colorado State University.[61] Since then, more than 200 pregnancies from very valuable mares have been obtained.[62]

Results from this program have demonstrated that pregnancies can be obtained consistently from older, subfertile mares using OT. In spite of a low efficiency (30% to 40% pregnancy per transferred oocyte), at least one pregnancy from 80% of the mares has been achieved in the last 11 years.[62] For mares

<15 years, higher pregnancy rates (60% to 70%) per OT are reported.[63] OT is usually performed in valuable mares from which embryos cannot be collected because of poor oocyte viability, high incidence of ovulatory failure in mares of advanced age (>18 years), oviductal pathology, and advanced uterine or cervical pathology. Most OT candidates are older mares whose expected embryo recovery rate is around 30%. Carnevale et al.[62] reported that in mares with histories of repeated ovulatory dysfunction, if aspirations are done before the luteinization and/or echogenic debris on follicular fluid is observed, the retrieved oocyte quality is better, thus increasing the chances of pregnancy.

OOCYTE TRANSFER TECHNIQUE

Preparation of the Donor

Difficulties in the retrieval of oocytes from immature follicles, as well as *in vivo* and *in vitro* maturation techniques, have forced investigators and clinicians to collect oocytes from pre-ovulatory follicles. Ovulation of donor mares is induced with a combination of hCG (1500 to 2000 UI IV) and deslorelin acetate (1 mg IM) when a pre-ovulatory follicle is observed. The combination of these two drugs appears to induce a better follicle response and better oocyte quality in old mares.[61] However, it is important to remember that response to ovulation-inducing drugs is more variable in old mares, and sometimes the oocyte aspiration must be performed before the expected ovulation time. This is particularly evident in mares with a history of ovulatory problems.

Oocyte Collection and Culture

Several approaches have been used for follicular aspiration in the live mare. These include flank laparotomy, transcutaneous flank puncture, or TVA. The method of choice for oocyte retrieval is TVA using a linear or a sector ultrasound (see Fig. 18-1). TVA has the advantage of being a non-surgical procedure, allowing repeated aspiration attempts on consecutive cycles. Donor mares are sedated with a combination of butorphanol (0.01 mg/kg) and xylazine (0.33 mg/kg). In addition, 0.04 mg/kg of propantheline bromide can also be used to promote rectum relaxation. During the TVA, the ultrasound transducer is placed in a plastic casing containing a needle guide and is inserted into the vagina. The ovary is positioned over the ultrasound transducer by rectal manipulation, and the follicle from which the oocyte will be collected is visualized. A double-lumen needle is advanced and punctures the follicular wall. The fluid is aspirated by gentle suction (150 mmHg) and the follicular cavity is rinsed with 50 to 100 ml of Dulbecco's phosphate buffer saline supplemented with 10 IU/ml of heparin. After the aspiration process is finished, the recovered fluid is transferred to a Petri dish and searched for the COC. Although the presence of the large cumulus cell mass makes the COC easy to visualize in the blood-tinged fluid, the large mass makes it more difficult to manipulate the oocyte.

The interval between ovulation induction and OT must be between 36 and 44 hours. Most oocytes collected at 24 hours after hCG injection are in metaphase I and require a supplementary culture time to complete maturation.[62] After collection and classification, recovered oocytes are transferred to tissue culture medium TCM-199 supplemented with 10% fetal calf serum and 0.2 mM of pyruvate, and then incubated at 38.5° to 39°C in an atmosphere containing 5% to 6% CO_2 in air for 12 to 18 hours before transfer. Most oocytes are expected to recover at 36 hours after hCG administration are in metaphase II and can be transferred

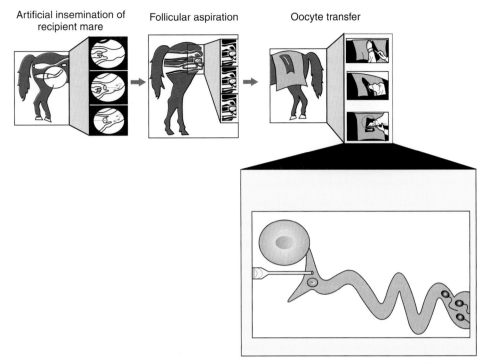

Figure 18-4. Oocyte transfer. Oocytes are transferred by standing flank laparotomy into the oviduct of an inseminated recipient mare. The ovary and oviduct are exposed through the incision, and the oocyte, previously loaded into a fire-polished glass pipette, is introduced approximately 2 to 3 cm into the oviduct from the infundibulum. The ovary is then returned into the abdominal cavity, and the muscle layers and skin are sutured.

immediately into a recipient's oviduct. In 2002 Carnevale et al.[64] reported similar oocyte collection rates and embryo development rates for oocytes collected at 24 or 36 hours after hCG administration and transferred directly. Furthermore, no differences were detected when oocytes were aspirated 24 hours after hCG injection and immediately transferred or incubated *in vitro* during the next 12 to 16 hours.[64] These results eliminate the necessity of an expensive CO_2 incubator, making the procedure more practical and possible to be performed under clinical conditions.

Preparation of Recipient Mares

During OT, sperm transport, capacitation, fertilization, and embryo development occur within the recipient's reproductive tract; therefore, it is very important that a selection of good quality recipient mares be used in an OT program. Young mares (3 to 10 years) are selected after a complete clinical and reproductive examination. During the reproductive examination, it is important to evaluate the length of the broad ligaments to determine if the ovaries can be easily exposed during OT. Oocyte recipients can be cyclic or non-cyclic mares. Use of cyclic mares as oocyte recipients involves estrous cycle synchronization of donor and recipient mares and the removal of the recipient's oocytes to be sure that the pregnancy will result from fertilization of the donor oocyte. Recipient mares receive 2000 IU of hCG at the same time as the donors, and the recipient's oocyte is collected approximately 24 hours after hCG administration. Only recipient mares from which an oocyte is collected are used as oocyte recipients. Use of non-cyclic recipients eliminates the need to synchronize donors and recipients and eliminates the need to retrieve the pre-ovulatory oocytes from the recipients before transfers. Non-cyclic recipients receive 3 mg of estradiol benzoate daily for approximately 2 to 5 days before transfer. Following

the estradiol treatment 200 mg per day of injectable progesterone in oil or 0.044 mg/kg of oral progestagen (Altrenogest), supplementation is required until OT. Regardless of whether the mares are cycling or not, progesterone supplementation must be continued for pregnancy maintenance until day 110 to 120. Although a corpus luteum forms after aspiration of the preovulatory follicle,[65] progesterone secretion can be delayed or reduced in cyclic mares. In non-cyclic mares, the absence of corpus luteum obviously requires progesterone supplementation.

Oocytes are transferred into the oviduct of the recipient mares preferably by standing flank laparotomy. After sedation and local anesthesia, an incision is made between the last rib and the tuber coxae. Prior to OT the ovary and oviduct are exposed through the incision. The oocyte is loaded into a fire-polished glass pipette with a low volume of medium (<0.1 ml). The pipette is introduced approximately 3 cm into the infundibular end of the oviduct and the oocyte is gently deposited (Fig. 18-4). The ovary is returned into the abdominal cavity, and the muscle layers and skin are sutured separately. Recipients are routinely treated with parenteral non-steroidal anti-inflammatory drugs and broad spectrum antibiotic for 5 to 7 days after surgery.

Insemination of Recipients

Before transferring the oocyte to the recipient, mare sperm must be present in the oviduct for fertilization. Therefore, recipients should be inseminated with at least 500 million progressively motile fresh or cooled sperm before OT. It is important to encourage owners to use semen from highly fertile stallions.

Oocyte recipients can be inseminated only once, at approximately 12 hours before transfer. In a study conducted by Carnevale et al.[64] oocyte recipients were inseminated 12 hours before and 2 hours after OT with cooled semen from different stallions; they observed that 94% of the embryos resulted from the first insemination. However if poor-quality semen is used, it is recommended to re-inseminate the mare 2 hours after the transfer. There is a tendency for uterine fluid accumulation when the second insemination is performed,[62] probably due to uterine relaxation associated with the surgical sedatives. It was also reported that pregnancy rates are significantly reduced when recipient mares are only inseminated once 2 hours after OT.[64] Recipient mares that accumulate uterine fluid should be treated with oxytocin (20 IU) and uterine lavage every 12 hours until no fluid is detected in the uterus.

GAMETE INTRAFALLOPIAN TRANSFER (GIFT)

The main difference between OT and GIFT is that the latter involves the transfer of oocytes together with a low number of sperm (2 to 5×10^5) into the oviduct. Because GIFT requires a lower number of sperm, the technique is useful for producing pregnancies from stallions in which sperm numbers are low (subfertile stallions), from frozen semen, and from sexed sorted sperm. The first successful GIFT in horses was performed in 1998 at Colorado State University (reported by Carnevale et al.[66]).

During GIFT, sperm are deposited in the infundibular or ampullary region of the oviduct, bypassing the uterus and the uterotubal junction. Percoll gradient centrifugation has been the method of choice to select the best sperm population for GIFT.[61,66-68] Sperm are centrifuged through a discontinuous (90/45%) Percoll gradient, and 100,000 to 200,000 sperm cells are transferred into the oviduct together with the oocyte using a fire-polished glass pipette. Embryo development rates of GIFT using fresh (raw) semen ranged from 20% to 80%, demonstrating that GIFT can be an alternative to OT when sperm numbers are low.

Disappointing results using GIFT with cooled or frozen semen have been reported by Coutinho da Silva et al.[67] When oocytes were transferred to recipient mares inseminated in the uterus, embryo development rate was 83% (19/23) compared with 25% (4/16) using the GIFT technique. Embryo development rates were even lower when frozen semen was used for GIFT 8% (1/12). It is speculated that the low fertilization and embryo development rates obtained with the use of cooled and frozen semen in GIFT could be related to impaired fertilization after intraoviductal inseminations. Further studies are needed in this area in order to make GIFT a commercially viable technique for horses.

IN VITRO FERTILIZATION AND ICSI

The fertilization process of the horse *in vivo* has been elegantly described,[69-72] and blastocyst formation and establishment of pregnancy have been achieved following transfer of IVM oocytes to oviducts of mated recipient mares.[73,74]

On the other hand, reports on conventional IVF of *in vitro* or *in vivo* matured equine oocytes are few, and the data are difficult to interpret because of variations in techniques used by different laboratories. Parameters for assessing fertilization include: the presence of swollen sperm heads in association with sperm tail or mid piece,[14] the presence of two pronuclei,[75] or cleavage. However, in the mare the success of producing embryos using IVF procedures remains extremely low.

The first cleavage after IVF of *in vivo* matured oocytes has been reported by Bezard et al.[71] The fertilization rate was low, with 26% of oocytes fertilized and only 18% cleaved. However,

two successful pregnancies were obtained after 14 surgical transfers of these fertilized oocytes.[7]

The reason(s) for poor IVF and subsequent development rates of equine oocytes remains unclear. Sperm cell capacitation,[76] oocyte maturation,[77] and changes in the zona pellucida[59,78,79] have all been offered as possible reasons for the poor IVF rates. The most encouraging method for capacitation induction and acrosome reaction of equine sperm cells is the use of calcium ionophore A23187, reaching 17% to 33% fertilization rates.[14,31,75] The use of caffeine or heparin for sperm capacitation did not improve the fertilization rate ($<17\%$[14,31,80]). The question of whether stallion spermatozoa are exceptional in their requirements for these agents remains to be answered.

In order to increase the IVF rates in the horse, fertilization techniques such as partial zona dissection (PZD) or partial zona removal (PZR), sub-zonal sperm injection (SUZI), zona drilling (ZD), and ICSI have been used.

Choi et al.[81] used PZR and PZD in an attempt to fertilize equine oocytes *in vitro*. For PZD, a slit in the zona pellucida of the oocyte is made; for PZR, a piece of the zona pellucida is removed, facilitating access of the spermatozoa to the oocyte membrane. Sperm penetration rates evaluated by staining were 52% for PZR and 12% for PZD oocytes. Although polyspermy was evident in some of these oocytes with a large slit in the zona pellucida, monospermic penetration rates were found to be between 57% and 58%.

For ZD, a small hole is made in the zona pellucida with a drop of acidic Tyrode's solution, facilitating the mobile sperm cells to overcome the zona barrier. Li et al.[82] obtained 33% to 79% of cleavage after ZD of *in vitro* matured oocytes obtained from pregnant mares. The best results were achieved after sperm exposure to 1.0 μM concentration of Ca++ ionophore A23187. In this experiment, 45.5% of the oocytes that cleaved developed to the morula and blastocyst stages.

At the end of the twentieth century, ICSI had been introduced in human IVF with great success (PALERMO et al., 1992). For ICSI, a direct injection with a fine pipette of one spermatozoon, after crushing its tail, is performed into the cytoplasm of a mature oocyte, exhibiting the first polar body in the peri-vitelinic space. Whereas other methods depend on the presence of a functional capacitated and acrosome-reacted spermatozoon for fusion with the membrane of the oocyte, ICSI does not seem to require capacitation or acrosome reaction; the only prerequisites are that the injected spermatozoon is motile. Sperm injection circumvents the problem of having sperm bind to the oocyte, penetrate the oocyte, and initiate fertilization. With ICSI, spermatozoa are injected directly into the oocyte, initiating fertilization.

ICSI requires a mature oocyte in metaphase II. Spermatozoa used for ICSI are usually frozen-thawed, but fresh or cooled sperm can also be used. Choi et al.[84] found that there is no significant difference in embryo development when using cooled or frozen-thawed sperm. Sperm is selected through a discontinuous Percoll gradient, and under micromanipulation one sperm cell is picked up in a micropipette (Fig. 18-5) and transferred into the cytoplasm of the oocyte. ICSI is a way to simulate *in vitro* fertilization by injecting a single spermatozoon into a mature oocyte (Fig. 18-6). It seems to be important that the sperm membrane be ruptured before transfer, ensuring that it is immotile and that sperm cytosolic factors important in oocyte activation are released.[52]

Studies on ICSI procedures in mammals started in 1976 when Uehara and Yanagamachi[85] first reported that human sperm cells develop into male pronuclei when injected into the cytoplasm

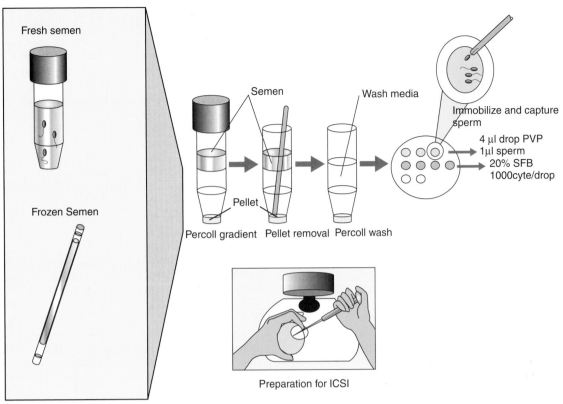

Figure 18-5. Sperm selection for intracytoplasmic sperm injection. Fresh or frozen-thawed sperm is selected through centrifugation in a discontinuous Percoll gradient. Viable sperm is transferred to a drop of solution containing PVP to slow down tail movement. A single sperm is then immobilized and inserted into a fine glass pipette for ICSI.

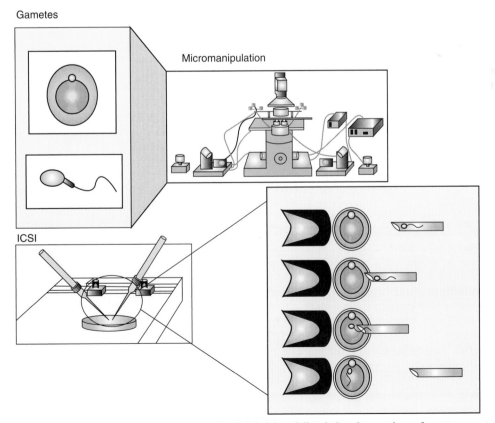

Figure 18-6. Intracytoplasmic sperm injection. The selected sperm (see Fig. 18-5) is injected directly into the cytoplasm of a mature oocyte in metaphase II (MII). Oocyte maturity is evidenced by the presence of an extruded first polar body.

of hamster eggs. Twenty years after Yanagamachi's report, the first foal was born from ICSI at Colorado State University.[58] In this pioneering work, the authors injected four *in vitro*–matured oocytes with sperm and transferred them to the oviducts of recipient mares. Although several other researchers have successfully produced foals from ICSI,[2,28,86,87] subsequent studies showed that this success rate was difficult to repeat. Initially, laboratories working with ICSI in the horse had difficulty in achieving good rates of embryo development after sperm injection. However, in 2002, use of the Piezo drill for ICSI was reported to increase cleavage rates from 69% to 89%.[55,86] The Piezo drill is a device that causes minute vibrations in the injection pipette; these not only facilitate penetration of the zona pellucida, but also ensure breakage of the sperm and oocyte plasma membranes.

One of the main advantages on the use of ICSI, over IFV, or OT is the possibility of using semen with very low fertility rates and poor quality since only one sperm is needed. Fresh,[88,89] cooled,[28,90] and frozen-thawed[54,77,78,91] semen have all been used for ICSI procedures in the horse. According to Choi et al.,[84] the difference in using different sperm sources appears to be related to the necessity of oocyte activation treatment after ICSI. Researchers working with fresh semen achieved minimal pronuclei formation without chemical activation of the oocyte after ICSI.[88,89,92] On the other hand, chemical activation for pronuclei formation when using cooled semen has been controversial. Li et al.[90] reported the necessity for sperm activation, whereas Cochran et al.[28] did not see the need for oocyte activation. When frozen-thawed semen was used, pronuclei formation was obtained without activation[54,78,86,91] at rates of approximately 50%. Because spermatozoa injected into the oocyte by ICSI are still surrounded by their plasma membrane, it is possible that the process of freezing, which may result in changes on the sperm membrane, has a beneficial effect on the diffusion of sperm factors into the cytoplasm of the oocyte, leading to activation. When fresh sperm with an intact membrane is used, chemical activation seems to be more important.[84]

A study from Lazzari et al.[93] compared the developmental capacity of *in vitro* matured oocytes fertilized by ICSI with frozen-thawed stallion semen of different motility and/or fertility. No difference in either cleavage or advanced embryo development rates among oocytes injected with spermatozoa from stallions of good, poor, and no fertility was observed, as long as a motile spermatozoon was selected for ICSI. In contrast, when a nonmotile sperm from samples having very poor motility after thawing and low fertility was used, significantly lower cleavage rates were observed and no embryos were capable of developing to the compact morula or blastocyst stage. However, in an experiment performed and reported by Choi et al.,[94] a blastocyst was formed after the injection of an *in vitro*–matured oocyte with an immotile sperm obtained from a frozen-thawed sample.

Before the injection of the spermatozoa into the oocyte, semen is either centrifuged through a Percoll gradient or obtained by swim-up procedures in order to select a viable sperm. The sperm suspension is then diluted in a Tyrode's medium with 10% (w/v) polyvinylpyrrolidone to slow down flagellar beating and allow capturing of the sperm cell. The injection pipette used for ICSI in horses has to be between 7 and 8 μm in outside diameter while a 120 to 140–μm outside diameter pipette is used to hold the oocyte (see Figs. 18-5 and 18-6). The entire procedure is done with a micromanipulator under oil in an inverted microscope. The selected sperm is immobilized by applying a few pulses with the Piezo drill to the tail immediately before injection. It is important that injected oocytes be held at room temperature for at least

20 minutes to allow the healing of the oocyte punctured plasma membrane. After this time the oocytes can be placed in culture or directly transfer to a recipient's mare oviduct.

Initially, the ICSI procedure presented limited clinical use because of the lack of standardization in the technique. Because of the absence of a standard protocol for culturing fertilized equine oocytes to the blastocyst stage, it was necessary to transfer the zygotes directly to the oviduct of a recipient mare immediately after injection. Choi et al.[95] obtained a blastocyst recovery rate of 36% after collection of ICSI-injected IVM oocytes transferred immediately after injection, showing that ICSI can result in efficient embryo production if embryos are cultured in an optimal environment. However, the direct transfer of an ICSI embryo to the oviduct of a recipient mare seems to have very little benefit over performing OT. Although some advantages can be noticed, especially concerning the use of poor-quality semen or semen with low numbers of spermatozoa, the ICSI procedure has a very high cost in equipment and technical personnel. Moreover, the inefficiencies associated with the ICSI procedure, including the time needed for micromanipulation, the risk of lyses of the oocyte during the injection procedure, and the reduced rate of embryo cleavage, render ICSI a less efficient method than oocyte transfer when one oocyte and semen of normal fertility is used.[8]

For the ICSI procedure to become a commercially available technique, the development of a suitable embryo culture system is necessary. In cattle, typically 25% to 35% of fertilized oocytes develop to blastocysts *in vitro*. In contrast, most of the work with *in vitro* culture of equine embryos has been disappointing, with blastocyst rates remaining between 4% and 16%. The development of successful IVM and ICSI technologies has resulted in increased pressure to design suitable culture systems for early embryos. Culture media that has been reported to sustain preimplantation embryo development of ICSI fertilized horse oocytes includes defined media such as G1.2,[87] DMEM-F12 and CZB,[84] and modified SOF.[55]

Recently, the culture of ICSI-produced equine embryos in DMEM-F12 medium, in a mixed-gas environment, was able to support >35% blastocyst development,[51,94] which is similar to the rates reported from *in vivo* culture. The range of blastocyst formation, using this system, is 27% to 44% with pregnancy rates of 50%.[94] This exciting result opens the possibility of offering the technique commercially in some laboratories around the world. It is important to realize, however, that when comparing cell numbers between *in vivo*– and *in vitro*–produced embryos,[96]—day 7 of development—the *in vitro*–produced embryos had significantly fewer cell numbers, resembling a day 5 rather than a day 7 embryo. This difference must be taken into account when embryos are transferred to synchronized recipients.

The clinical use of ICSI in horses is mainly for the production of foals from stallions that have very few sperm or perhaps stallions that have died and a limited quantity of frozen semen is still available. Another promising application is to obtain embryos from mares, after their untimely deaths, by recovering the mare's oocytes. In this case, multiple immature oocytes are recovered from the follicles present in the ovaries and are matured *in vitro*. Use of ICSI under these circumstances has a major advantage over OT because of the increased number of oocytes that can be available for fertilization. After the oocytes have been collected and matured *in vitro*, those in metaphase II are fertilized by ICSI and placed into embryo culture. Blastocysts are identified after 7 to 8 days of *in vitro* culture, and each blastocyst may be transferred separately to a recipient mare by transcervical transfer.

The consistency of obtaining ICSI-produced embryos in the horse has led to the establishment of commercial clinical programs in America (CSU) and Italy (Select Breeder Services). In addition to the production of live offspring, sperm injection is a powerful tool that can be use to evaluate *in vitro* oocyte maturation systems, study fertilization, and the production of *in vitro*–produced embryos for subsequent studies.

CLONING

Cloning is the production of genetically identical individuals by non-sexual means.[97] The first results on mammalian cloning were obtained by Willesden,[98] when cloned sheep were borne after the split of 8 to 16 cell embryos. In the late 1990s Wilmut et al.[99] surprised the world by producing the first clone obtained from an adult cell. Since then, the production of clones by nuclear transfer has been a success in many mammalian species, including the horse.

The cloning process using somatic or body cells is a powerful instrument for the multiplication of animals with a unique genotype, or for the preservation of endangered species, representing one of the most extraordinary achievements on developmental biology research.[99] However, the efficiency of the technique is still low because of the complexity of the process involving a combination of biological and technical factors, not all fully understood.[2] In addition, nuclear transferred or cloned embryos, fetus, or offspring have had several developmental problems with high rates of miscarriage and perinatal deaths.[99-101] However, it is not clear if the developmental failure on embryo development is linked with the reprogramming of the somatic nuclei or is intrinsic to the cloning process itself.[102]

The nuclear transfer or cloning technique involves obtaining of somatic (body) cells from the genetic donor, as well as *in vivo–* or *in vitro*–matured oocytes of any female of the same species to be used as recipient cytoplasm. By delicate micromanipulation the oocyte's chromatin (nucleus) is removed, creating an oocyte with no genetic component (also known as a cytoplast) (Fig. 18-7).

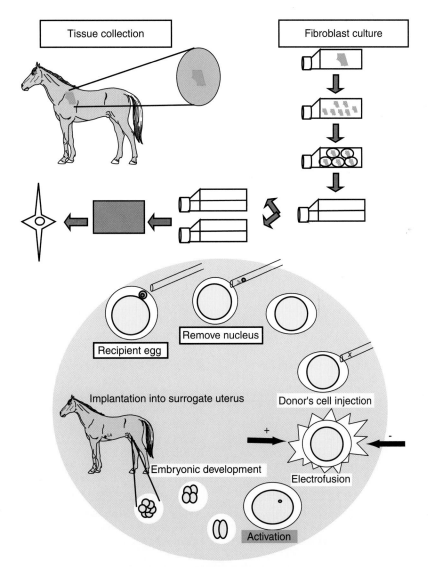

Figure 18-7. Cloning by nuclear transfer. Nuclear transfer involves obtaining somatic cells from a genetic donor, as well as several matured oocytes from any female of the same species. By micromanipulation the oocyte's chromatin (nucleus) is removed, and the enucleated oocytes are used as recipient cytoplasms. A whole somatic donor cell is inserted into the perivitelinic space of the recipient ooplasma. The fusion of the two cells is induced by electric pulses, and chemical activation is performed to induce embryo development.

The production of cytoplasts requires the removal of the nuclear material from an already mature oocyte. This procedure is essential for the maintenance of the normal number of chromosomes of a given species. In horses, the visualization of the metaphase plate containing the chromosomes may be difficult because of the high amount of lipids present in the oocyte cytoplasm. Moreover, the metaphase plate is not always located next to the released polar body. These features make the enucleation of the oocyte in absence of a specific DNA stain very difficult. The main stain used to mark DNA in nuclear transfer procedures is the Hoechst 33342, which allows the visualization of the chromosomes under UV light during enucleation.

The selected somatic cells from the donor animal, grown *in vitro* from a tissue sample (e.g., a skin cell), are combined with the cytoplast either by fusing the two cells by electric pulsation or by breaking the donor cell's membrane and injecting the cell directly into the cytoplasm of the oocyte. The recombined oocyte now contains the nucleus (all genetic information) of the genetic donor and needs to be artificially activated to start embryo development.

In the mature MII oocyte prior to fertilization, there is an arrest in meiosis mainly due to the high levels of MPF and MAPK (see Fig. 18-3). During normal fertilization the sperm activates the egg. After fertilization these levels drop in response to the elevation of intracellular calcium.[103] The blockage of the MPF and the MAPK allows the occurrence of the initial events that result in embryo development. In nuclear transfer the activation of the reconstructed embryo is essential for the success of cloning and is performed by using a combination of several chemicals that interfere with the cellular cycle. Most protocols for oocyte activation in horses use a combination of drugs that increase the intracellular calcium, such as ionomycin, and reduce the activity of the MPF and MAPK, such as 6-dimethylaminopurine (6-DMAP) and/or cycloheximide.[104-106] Galli et al.[2] found that either of the two used alone, after ionomycin exposure, was not providing satisfactory results. However, by using a combination of the two, the activation rate was around 90%. Hinrichs et al.[107] have used a combination of injection of sperm extract and culture in 6-DMAP to produce embryos that result in successful foaling of cloned offspring. Once the cleavage starts, the embryo is then transferred to a recipient mare.[8]

The first equids born from somatic cell nuclear transfer were three mules whose genetic donor was a 45-day-old fetus. *In vivo*–matured oocytes were used as cytoplast and the embryos were transferred directly to the oviduct of the recipient mares.[108] This same group reported establishment of seven pregnancies from transfer of 62 oocytes subjected to adult somatic cell nuclear transfer, but all pregnancies were lost before 80 days of gestation. Galli et al.[2] also reported the birth of a cloned horse from an adult somatic cell transferred to an *in vitro*–matured oocyte. The embryo was then cultured to the blastocyst stage before transcervical transfer to the uterus of the recipient mare. One of the most exciting aspects of the birth of this cloned horse is that the recipient mare of that delivery of the clone was also the somatic cell donor. In that report, 841 recombined oocytes were cultured, and 22 blastocysts developed (3%). Seventeen blastocysts were transferred, and four pregnancies resulted (24% pregnancy rate after transfer). Of the four pregnancies, two were lost around 30 days, one was lost at 6 months of gestation, and one was carried to term for a normal birth. Recently, another group reported the birth of a cloned horse at Texas A&M.[52] In this study, 423 recombined oocytes resulted in 6 blastocysts (1.4%) and one pregnancy (17% pregnancy rate), which produced a viable foal.

One major limitation of equine cloning is the low availability of cytoplasts suitable for nuclear transfer. Since a critical factor determining the success of the technique is the quality of the oocyte, the availability of younger healthy mares with good-quality MII oocytes that can undergo proper cytoplasmic maturation is important.

The increasing efficiency of equine cloning makes it potentially clinically applicable at this time. However, although animals from different species have been cloned, the fate of these cloned individuals is still uncertain. Until now, the low efficiency of the method is a consequence of the technical problems that affect the embryos during their development.[109] The main abnormalities found are dysfunction of the mitotic fibers,[110] chromosomal abnormality,[111] and low number of cells in the inner cell mass. Although a great number of reconstructed embryos are capable of beginning cleavage and develop until the blastocyst stage, the pregnancy rate is much lower and the embryonic death is much higher than the ones observed in normal pregnancy. Although Hinrichs et al.[51,52] have found a pregnancy rate of 50% after transfer of *in vitro*–produced embryos, half of these are lost in early gestation. In other species the main problems with cloned offspring are respiratory dysfunction, immunological deficiency, cardiac and vascular abnormalities, renal failures, and hepatic congestion and fibrosis.[101,112-114] However, in horses, all animals that have been born do not seem to have these abnormalities; a larger number of animals still need to be evaluated critically.

Besides the many clinical options, the possibility of cloning opens up many new areas for study and raises many ethical questions. One very important aspect that should be understood is that a cloned foal will not be an exact copy of the original horse. Based on spontaneous twins and the few split-embryo identical twins produced, it is known that the intra-uterine environment affects not only the size of the foal at birth, but also the adult size and phenotype, especially concerning the distribution of the white hair areas. Because of that, the cloned animal frequently does not have the exact same coat as the donor animal.

Another important aspect is that although the reconstructed embryo will have the nuclear DNA of the genetic donor, the mitochondrial DNA will be from the recipient oocyte. A very small proportion of the donor cell mitochondria will also be present but proportionately in much lower numbers. The impact of the source of mitochondria or a mixture of mitochondria on the traits of the progeny is currently unknown.[8] In a cloned female horse, all their oocytes will have a heterogeneous mitochondria population, and it will be passed down to her offspring. However, in the case of a male clone, since the mitochondria present in the sperm do not contribute to the mitochondria of the embryo after fertilization, the cloned colt could be considered to produce the same progeny that its genetic donor would have produced.[8]

The development of the cloned foal will also be influenced by epigenetic effects. Although the genetic makeup of the clone will be exactly the same as the donor, within the genome certain genes may be "turned off" while the transcription of others is enhanced. The differences in which genes will be active are due to the reprogramming of the clone nuclei. The state of activity of the DNA during fetal life may affect the phenotype of the animal at birth and after birth. However, what is important is that the offspring of the cloned embryos will carry the exact same genetics as the original donor.[8]

Even though there is significant variation in the efficacy of the nuclear transfer technique in equids, the cloned equid foals reported so far have all been healthy at birth and have developed normally after birth. Because of this accomplishment, at least two companies offer commercial cloning for horses, with more than 15 commercially produced clones born up to 2008. Clinically, cloning can be used to prolong the use of genetically exceptional individuals with acquired infertility, such as males that have been castrated and/or animals that die before being able to reproduce. However, it is important to point out that nuclear transfer will never become a common clinical procedure, but can be used to solve exceptional problems. Registry limitations on cloned animals or registry restrictions of the offspring produced from cloned stallions or mares will determine the extent in which the technique will be used.

REFERENCES

1. Heape W. On the artificial insemination of mares, *Veterinarian* 71:202-212, 1989.
2. Galli C, Olleoni S, Duchi R, et al: Developmental competence of equine oocytes and embryos obtained by in vitro procedures ranking from in vitro maturation and ICSI to embryo culture, cryopreservation and somatic cell nuclear transfer. *Anim Rep Sci* 98:39-55, 2007.
3. Brück I, Raun K, Synnestvedt B, Greve T: Follicle aspiration in the mare using a transvaginal ultrasound-guided technique. *Equine Vet J* 24:58-59, 1992.
4. Bracher V, Parlevliet J, Fazeli AR, et al: Repeated transvaginal ultrasound-guided follicle aspiration in the mare. *Eq Vet J Suppl* 15:75-78, 1993.
5. Cook NL, Squires EL, Ray BS, Jasko DJ: Transvaginal ultrasound-guided follicular aspiration of equine oocytes. *Equine Vet J Suppl* 15:71-74, 1993.
6. Dippert KD, Ray BS, Squires EL: Maximizing ultrasound guided retrieval of equine oocytes (abstract). *Theriogenology* 41:190, 1994.
7. Palmer E, Bezard J, Magistrini M, Duchamp G: In vitro fertilization in the horse: a retrospective study. *J Reprod Fertil Suppl* 44:375-384, 1991.
8. Hinrichs K: Update on equine ICSI and cloning. *Theriogenology* 64:535-541, 2005.
9. Fulka J, Okolski A: Culture of horse oocytes in vitro. *J Reprod Fertil* 61:213-215, 1981.
10. Hawley LR, Enders AC, Hinrichs K: Comparison of equine and bovine oocyte-cumulus morphology within the ovarian follicle. *Biol Reprod Mono* 1:243-252, 1995.
11. Hinrichs K, DiGiorgio LM: Embryonic development after intra-follicular transfer of horse oocytes. *J Reprod Fertil Suppl* 44:369-374, 1991.
12. Hinrichs K, Schmidt AL, Friedman PP, et al: In vitro maturation of horse oocytes: characterization of chromatin configuration using fluorescence microscopy. *Biol Reprod* 48:363-370, 1993.
13. Okolski A, Babusik P, Tischner M, Lietz W: Evaluation of mare oocyte collection methods and stallion sperm penetration of zona-free hamster ova. *J Reprod Fertil Suppl* 34:191-196, 1987.
14. Zhang JJ, Muzs LZ, Boyle MS: In vitro fertilization of horse follicular oocytes matured in vitro. *Mol Reprod Dev* 26:361-365, 1990.
15. Choi YH, Hochi S, Braun J, Oguri N: In vitro maturation of equine oocytes collected by aspiration and additional slicing of ovaries. *Theriogenology* 40:959-966, 1993.
16. Del Campo MR, Donoso X, Parrish JJ, Ginther OJ: Selection of follicles, preculture oocyte evaluation, and duration of culture for in vitro maturation of equine oocytes. *Theriogenology* 43:1141-1153, 1995.
17. Palmer E, Duchamp G, Bezárd J, et al: Non-surgical recovery of follicular fluid and oocytes of mares. *J Reprod Fertil Suppl* 35:689-690, 1987.
18. McKinnon AO, Wheeler MB, Carnevale EM, Squires EL: Oocyte transfer in the mare: preliminary observations. *Eq Vet Sci* 6:306-309, 1987.
19. Cook NL, Squires EL, Ray BS et al: Transvaginal ultrasonically guided follicular aspiration of equine oocytes: preliminary results. *J Eq Vet Sci* 12:104-107, 1992.
20. Bezard J, Mekarska A, Goudet G, et al: Meiotic stage of the preovulatory equine oocytes at collection and competence of immature oocytes for in vitro maturation: effect of interval from induction of ovulation to follicle puncture. *Theriogenology* 47(1):386, 1997, Abstr.
21. Kanitz W, Becker F, Alm H, Torner H: Ultrasound-guided follicular aspiration in mares. *Biol Reprod Mono* 1:225-231, 1995.
22. Squires EL: Maturation and fertilization of equine oocytes. *Vet Clin North Am* 12:31-45, 1996.
23. Meintjes M, Bellow MS, Paul JB, et al: Transvaginal ultrasound-guided oocyte retrieval from cyclic and pregnant horse and pony mares for in vitro fertilization. *Biol Reprod Mono* 1:281-292, 1995.
24. Ginther OJ: *Reproductive Biology of the Mare*, ed 2. Cross Plains, WI: Equiservices: CHP8, 1992.
25. Ginther OJ, Bergfelt DR: Associations between concentrations and major and minor follicular waves in pregnant mares. *Theriogenology* 38:807-821, 1992.
26. Goudet G, Leclerq L, Bezárd J, et al: Chorionic gonadotropin secretion is associated with an inhibition of follicular growth and an improvement on oocyte competence for in vitro maturation in the mare. *Biol Reprod* 58:760-768, 1998.
27. Meintjes M, Graff KJ, Paccamonti D, et al: Effects of follicular aspiration and flushing, and the genotype of the fetus on the circulating progesterone levels during pregnancy in the mare. *Eq Vet J Suppl* 25:25-32, 1997.
28. Cochran R, Meintjes M, Reggio B, et al: Live foals produced from sperm injected oocytes derived from pregnant mares. *J Eq Vet Sci* 18:736-740, 1998.
29. Lee M, Nurse P: Cell cycle control genes in fission yeast and mammalian cells. *Trends Genet* 10:287-290, 1988.
30. Cran DG, Moor RM: Programming the oocyte for fertilization. In BD Bavister, J Cummins, ERS Roldan, eds: *Fertilization in Mammals*. Serono Symposia, Norwell, USA: 1990, pp 241-251.
31. Grøndahl C, Host T, Brück I, et al: In vitro production of equine embryos. *Biol Reprod Mono* 1:299-307, 1995.
32. Masui Y, Markert CL: Cytoplasmic control of nuclear behavior during meiotic maturation of frog oocytes. *J Exp Zool* 177:129-146, 1971.
33. Nurse P: Universal control mechanism regulating onset of M-phase. *Nature* 344:503-508, 1990.
34. Murray AW: The cell cycle as a cd2 cycle. *Nature* 342:14-15, 1989.
35. Murray AW, Kirschner MW: Dominos and clocks: the union of two views of the cell cycle. *Science* 246:614-621, 1989.
36. Motlík A, Kubelka M: Cell cycle aspects of growth and maturation of mammalian oocytes. *Mol Reprod Dev* 27:366-375, 1990.
37. Hashimoto N, Kishimoto T: Regulation of meiotic metaphase by a cytoplasmic maturation-promoting factor during mouse oocyte maturation. *Dev Biol* 126:242-252, 1988.
38. Choi T, Aoki F, Mori M: Activation of P34 cdc2 protein kinase activity in meiotic and mitotic cell cycle in mouse oocytes and embryos. *Development* 113:789-795, 1991.
39. Naito K, Toyoda Y: Fluctuation of histone H1 kinase activity during meiotic maturation in porcine oocytes. *J Reprod Fertil* 93:467-473, 1991.
40. Jelinkova L, Kubelba M, Motlik J, Guerrier P: Chromatin condensation and histone H1 kinase activity during growth and maturation of rabbit oocytes. *Mol Reprod Dev* 37:210-215, 1994.
41. Dedieu T, Gall L, Crozet N: Mitogen-activated protein kinase activity during goat oocyte maturation and the acquisition of meiotic competence. *Mol Reprod Dev* 45:351-358, 1996.
42. Wu B, Ignotz G, Currie WB, Yang X: Dynamics of maturation-promoting factor and its constituent proteins during in vitro maturation of bovine oocytes. *Biol Reprod* 56:253-259, 1997.
43. Cran DG: Cortical granules distribution during oocyte maturation and fertilization. *J Reprod Fertil Suppl* 38:49-62, 1989.
44. Long CR, Damiani P, Pinto-Correia C, et al: Morphology and subsequent development in culture of bovine oocytes matured in vitro under various conditions of fertilization. *J Reprod Fertil* 102:361-369, 1994.
45. Kennedy JF, Donahue RP Human oocytes: maturation in chemically defined media. *Science* 164:1292-1293, 1969.
46. Robertson JE, Baker RD: Role of female sex steroids as possible regulators of oocyte maturation. Second Annual Meeting of the Society for the Study of Reproduction (Abstract). University of California, Davis, CA: 1969, p 57.
47. Okolski A, Bezard J, Magistrini M: Maturation of oocytes from normal and atretic equine ovarian follicles as affected by steroid concentrations. *J Reprod Fertil* 44:385, 1991.
48. de Loos F, van Vliet C, van Maurik P, Kruip TA: Morphology of immature bovine oocytes. *Gamete Res* 24:197-204, 1989.
49. Hinrichs K, Williams KA: Relationships among oocyte-cumulus morphology, follicular atresia, initial chromatin configuration, and oocyte meiotic competence in the horse. *Biol Reprod* 57:377-384, 1997.

50. Hinrichs K, Schmidt AL: Meiotic competence in horse oocytes: interactions among chromatin configuration, follicle size, cumulus morphology, and season. *Biol Reprod* 62:1402-1408, 2000.

51. Hinrichs K, Choi YH, Love LB, Varner DD: Transfer of in vitro produced equine embryos, Proc Sixth Inter Equine Embryo Transfer Symp: 2005, pp 38-39.

52. Hinrichs K, Choi YH, Love LB, et al: Chromatin configuration within the germinal vesicle of horse oocytes: changes post-mortem and relationship to meiotic and developmental competence. *Biol Reprod* 72:1142-1150, 2005.

53. Willis P, Caudle AB, Fayrer-Hosken RA: Equine oocyte *in vitro* maturation: influences of sera, time, and hormones. *Mol Reprod Dev* 30:360-368, 1991.

54. Dell'Aquila ME, Cho YS, Minoia P, et al: Intracytoplasmic sperm injection (ICSI) versus conventional IVF on abattoir-derived and *in vitro* matured equine oocytes. *Theriogenology* 47:1139-1156, 1997.

55. Galli C, Crotti G, Turini P, et al: Frozen-thawed embryos produced by ovum pickup of immature oocytes and ICSI are capable to establish pregnancies in the horse. *Theriogenology* 58:705-708, 2002.

56. Lagutina I, Lazzari G, Duchi R, et al: Somatic cell nuclear transfer in horses: effect of oocyte morphology, embryo reconstruction method and donor cell type. *Reproduction* 130:559-567, 2005.

57. Shabpareh V, Squires EL, Seidel GE Jr, Jasko DJ: Methods for collecting and maturing equine oocytes *in vitro*. *Theriogenology* 40:1161-1175, 1993.

58. Squires EL, Wilson JM, Kato H, Blaszcyk A: A pregnancy after intracytoplasmic sperm injection into equine oocytes matured *in vitro* (abstract). *Theriogenology* 45(1):306, 1996.

59. Landim-Alvarenga FC, Choi YH: *In vitro* maturation of equine oocytes without hormones (Abstract). *Theriogenology* 51:383, 1999.

60. McKinnon AO, Carnevale EM, Squires EL, et al Heterogenous and xenogenous fertilization of in vivo matured equine oocytes. *J Equine Vet Sci* 8:143-147, 1988.

61. Carnevale EM, Maclellan LJ, Coutinho da Silva MA, et al: Comparison of culture and insemination techniques for equine oocyte transfer. *Theriogenology* 54:981-987, 2000.

62. Carnevale EM, Coutinho da Silva MA, Panzani D, et al: Factors affecting the success of oocyte transfer in a clinical program for subfertile mares. *Theriogenology* 64:519-527, 2005.

63. Carnevale EM, Ginther OJ: Use of a linear ultrasonic transducer for the transvaginal aspiration and transfer of oocytes in the mare. *J Eq Vet Sci* 13(6):331-333, 1993.

64. Carnevale EM, Coutinho da Silva MA, Maclellan LJ, et al: Effects of culture media and time of insemination on oocyte transfer. *Theriogenology* 58:759-762, 2002.

65. Hinrichs K: The relationship of follicle atresia to follicle size, oocyte recovery rate on aspiration, and oocyte morphology in the mare. *Theriogenology* 36:157-168, 1991.

66. Carnevale EM, Alvarenga MA, Squires EL, Choi YH: Use of non-cycling mares as recipients for oocyte transfer and GIFT. Proc Ann Conf Soc Theriogenology: 1999, p 44.

67. Coutinho da Silva MA, Carnevale EM, Maclellan LJ, et al: Oocyte transfer in mares with intrauterine or intraoviductal insemination using fresh, cooled, and frozen stallion semen. *Theriogenology* 61:705-713, 2004.

68. Coutinho da Silva MA, Carnevale EM, Maclellan LJ, et al: Effect of time of oocyte collection and site of insemination on oocyte transfer in mares. *J Anim Sci* 80:1275-1279, 2002.

69. Betteridge KJ, Eaglesome MD, Mitchell D, et al: Development of horse embryos up to twenty-two days after ovulation: observations on fresh specimens. *J Anat* 135:191-209, 1982.

70. Enders AC, Liu IK, Bowers J, et al: The ovulated ovum of the horse: Cytology of nonfertilized ova to pronuclear stage ova. *Biol Reprod* 37:453-466, 1987.

71. Bezard J, Magistrini M, Duchamp G, Palmer E: Chronology of equine fertilization and embryonic development in vivo and in vitro. *Eq Vet J Suppl* 8:105-110, 1989.

72. Grøndahl C, Grøndahl NC, Greve T, Hyttel P: *In vivo* fertilization and initial embryogenesis in the mare. *Eq Vet J Suppl* 15:79-83, 1993.

73. Zhang JJ, Boyle MS, Allen WR, Galli C: Recent studies on in vivo fertilization of *in vitro* matured horse oocytes. *Eq Vet J Suppl* 8:101-104, 1989.

74. Fernandes CB, Peres KR, Alvarenga MA, Landim-Alvarenga FC: The use of transmission electron microscopy and oocyte transfer to evaluate In vitro maturation of equine oocytes in different culture conditions. *J Eq Vet Sci* 26(4):159-167, 2006.

75. Del Campo MR, Donoso MX, Parrish JJ, Ginther OJ: *In vitro* fertilization of *in vitro* matured equine oocytes. *Eq Vet Sci* 10:18-22, 1990.

76. Alm H, Torner H, Blottner S, et al: Effect of sperm cryopreservation and treatment with calcium ionophore or heparin on *in vitro* fertilization of horse oocytes. *Theriogenology* 56:817-829, 2001.

77. Li X, Morris LH, Allen WR: Influence of co-culture during maturation on the developmental potential of equine oocytes fertilized by intracytoplasmic sperm injection (ICSI), *Reproduction* 121:925-932, 2001.

78. Dell'Aquila ME, De Felici M, Massari S, et al: Effects of fetuin on zona pellucida hardening and fertilizability of equine oocytes matured in vitro. *Biol Reprod* 61:533-540, 1999.

79. Hinrichs K, Love CC, Brinsko SP, et al: *In vitro* fertilization of *in vitro*-matured equine oocytes: effect of maturation medium, duration of maturation, and sperm calcium ionophore treatment, and comparison with rates of fertilization *in vivo* after oviductal transfer. *Biol Reprod* 67:256-262, 2002.

80. Dell'Aquila ME, Fusco S, Lacalandra GM, Mariato F: *In vitro* maturation and fertilization of equine oocytes recovered during the breeding season. *Theriogenology* 45:547-560, 1996.

81. Choi YH, Okada Y, Hochi S, et al: *In vitro* fertilization rate of horse oocytes with partially removed zona. *Theriogenology* 42:795-802, 1994.

82. Li LY, Meintjes M, Graff KJ, et al: *In vitro* fertilization and development of *in vitro* matured oocytes aspirated from pregnant mares. *Biol Reprod Mono* 1:309-317, 1995.

83. Palermo G, Joris H, Devroey P, Van Steirteghem AC: Pregnancies after intracytoplasmic injection of single spermatozoon into an oocyte. *Lancet* 340:17-18, 1992.

84. Choi YH, Love CC, Love LB, et al: Developmental competence *in vivo* and *in vitro* of *in vitro*-matured equine oocytes fertilized by intracytoplasmic sperm injection with fresh or frozen-thawed spermatozoa. *Reproduction* 123:455-465, 2002.

85. Uehara T, Yanagamachi R: Microsurgical injection of spermatozoa into hamster eggs with subsequent transformation of sperm nuclei into male pronuclei. *Biol Reprod* 15:467-470, 1976.

86. McKinnon AO, Lacham-Kaplam O, Trounson AO: Pregnancies produced from fertile and infertile stallions by intracytoplasmic sperm injection (ICSI) of single frozen/thawed spermatozoa into *in vivo* matured mare oocytes. Seventh International Symposium on Equine Reproduction, Pretoria (South Africa):1998, 137.

87. Choi YH, Love CC, Chung YG, et al: Production of nuclear transfer horse embryos by Pies-Driven injection of somatic cell nuclei and activation with stallion sperm cytosolic extract. *Biol Reprod* 67:561-567, 2002.

88. Kato H, Seidel GE Jr, Squires EL, Wilson JM: Treatment of equine oocytes with A23187 after intracytoplasmic sperm injection. *Eq Vet J Suppl* 25:51-53, 1997.

89. Schmid RL, Kato H, Herickhoff LA, et al: Effects on follicular fluid of progesterone on in vitro maturation of equine oocytes before intracytoplasmic sperm injection with non-sorted and sex-sorted spermatozoa. *J Reprod Fertil Suppl* 56:519-525, 2000.

90. Li X, Morris LHA, Allen WR: Effects of different activation treatments on fertilization of horse oocytes by intracytoplasmic sperm injection. *J Reprod Fertil* 119:253-260, 2000.

91. Grøndahl C, Hansen TH, Hossaini A, et al: Intracytoplasmic sperm injection of in vitro-matured equine oocytes. *Biol Reprod* 57:1495-1501, 1997.

92. Guignot F, Ottogalli M, Yvon JM, Magistrini M: Preliminary observations in in vitro development of equine embryo after ICSI. *Reprod Nutri Dev* 38:653-663, 1998.

93. Lazzari G, Crotti G, Turini P, et al: Equine embryos at the compacted morula and blastocyst stage can be obtained by intracytoplasmic sperm injection (ICSI) of in vitro matured oocytes with frozen-thawed spermatozoa from semen of different fertilities. *Theriogenology* 58:709-712, 2002.

94. Choi YH, Love CC, Varner DD, Hinrichs K: Equine blastocyst development after intracytoplasmic injection of sperm subjected to two freeze-thaw cycles. *Theriogenology* 6:808-819, 2006.

95. Choi YH, Rosa LM, Love CC, et al: Blastocyst formation rates in vivo and in vitro of in vitro-matured equine oocytes fertilized by intracytoplasmic sperm injection. *Biol Reprod* 70:1038-1231, 2004.

96. Tremoleda JL, Stout TA, Lagutina I, et al: Effects of in vitro production on horse embryo morphology, cytoskeletal characteristics, and blastocyst capsule formation. *Biol Reprod* 69:1895-1906, 2003.

97. Seidel GE: Cloning mammals by microsurgery to embryos. Proc Second Symp Advanced Topics Animal Reproduction:1983, pp 141-158.

98. Willadsen SM: Nuclear transplantation in sheep embryos. *Nature* 320:63-65, 1986.

99. Wilmut I, Schnieke AE, McWhir J, et al: Viable offspring derived from fetal and adult mammalian cells. *Nature* 385:810-813, 1987.

100. Heyman Y, Chacatte-Palmer P, Lebourhis D, et al: Frequency and occurrence of late-gestation losses from cattle cloned embryos. *Biol Reprod* 66:6-13, 2002.
101. Hill JR, Rousse AJ, Cibelli JB, et al: Clinical and pathological features of cloned transgenic calves and fetuses (13 case studies). *Theriogenology* 51:1451-1465, 1999.
102. Han YM, Kang YK, Koo DB, Lee KK: Nuclear reprogramming of cloned embryos produced in vitro. *Theriogenology* 59:33-44, 2003.
103. Nurse PA: A long twentieth century of the cell cycle and beyond. *Cell* 100:71-78, 2000.
104. Galli C, Duchi R, Moor RM: Mammalian leukocytes contain all the genetic information necessary for the development of a new individual. *Cloning* 1:161-170, 1999.
105. Wells DN, Misica PM, Tervit HR: Production of cloned calves following nuclear transfer with cultured adult mural granulosa cells. *Biol Reprod* 60:996-1005, 1999.
106. Wells DN, Misica PM, Tervit HR, Vivanco WH: Adult somatic cell nuclear transfer is used to preserve the last surviving cow of the Enderby Island cattle breed. *Reprod Fertil Dev* 10:369-378, 1998.
107. Hinrichs K, Choi YH, Varner DD, Hartman DL: Efficient production of cloned horse pregnancies using roscovitine-treated donor cells. *Anim Reprod Sci* 94:309-310, 2006.
108. Vanderwall DK, Woods GL, Aston KI, et al: Cloned horse pregnancies produced using adult cumulus cells (Abstract). *Reprod Fertil Dev* 16:160, 2004.
109. Bordignon V, Keyston R, Lazaris A: Transgene expression of green fluorescent protein and germ line transmission in cloned calves derived from in vitro-transfected somatic cells. *Biol Reprod* 68:2013-2023, 2003.
110. Simerly C, Dominko T, Navara C, et al: Molecular correlates of primate nuclear transfer failures. *Science* 300:297, 2003.
111. Booth PJ, Viuff D, Tan S, et al: Numerical chromosome errors in day 7 somatic nuclear transfer bovine blastocysts. *Biol Reprod* 68:922-928, 2003.
112. Chavatte-Palmer P, Heyman Y, Richard C: Clinical, hormonal and hematologic characteristics of bovine claves derived from nuclei form somatic cells. *Biol Reprod* 66:1596-1603, 2002.
113. Renard JP, Chastant S, Chesné P, et al: Lymphoid hypoplasia and somatic cloning. *Lancet* 353:1489-1491, 1999.
114. Cibelli JB, Campbell KH, Seidel GE: The health profile of cloned animals. *Nat Biotechnol* 20:13-14, 2002.

THE EARLY PREGNANCY

Chapter 19

Tom A.E. Stout

Early pregnancy in the mare is a fascinating period that encompasses numerous profound developmental changes and events, many of which are unique to the horse. Moreover, a number of the unusual aspects of early equine pregnancy are of clinical relevance because they significantly affect our ability to monitor, or intervene to influence the success of, a breeding program. For example, aspects of early embryonic development and embryo-maternal interaction dramatically influence the way, exact timing of how, and success with which embryo recovery and transfer can be performed, whereas disturbances in normal development may trigger or increase the likelihood of early pregnancy loss (EPL). In addition, the fact that the early conceptus expands very rapidly while maintaining a spherical shape is diagnostically useful because it enables us to accurately detect the presence or absence of a conceptus before the expected onset of the subsequent cyclical estrus; this greatly improves our ability to monitor and maintain the efficiency of a breeding program. The ability to accurately detect pregnancy during the early intra-uterine period has also been critical in the development of techniques to successfully manage twin pregnancy and for detecting abnormal conceptus development, pregnancy loss, or threatened pregnancy loss. This chapter discusses the essentials of early embryonic development and conceptus-maternal signaling up to around day 40 of gestation, when formation of the definitive chorioallantoic placenta begins in earnest; this is also the period in which the vast majority of equine EPL occurs. Where possible, developmental processes are discussed with respect to their significance to the success or otherwise of natural or assisted equine-breeding programs.

INTRA-OVIDUCTAL EMBRYO DEVELOPMENT

At ovulation, the oocyte is released into the relatively small oviductal fimbria and descends to the ampullary region where, if capacitated sperm are present, fertilization will take place.[1,2] Once fertilized, the newly formed "zygote" embarks on a series of regular cell divisions, such that it reaches the two-cell stage within 24 hours, four to six cells within 48 hours, and by 72 hours contains eight to ten cells.[3] Between days 4 and 5, a "morula" is formed, and the as yet undifferentiated cells "compact" into a homogenous ball until late on day 5 or early on day 6 when the embryo starts to develop into a "blastocyst" (i.e., to form a central cavity while the constituent cells differentiate visibly into either inner cell mass [ICM] or trophectoderm). At around the same time, day 6–7 after ovulation, the embryo finally enters the uterus,[4,5] generally at the late morula or early blastocyst stage of development,[6] containing around 600 cells[7] and still surrounded by its original protective coat, the zona pellucida.[4,6] As a result of the recent increase in commercial embryo transfer (ET), it has become apparent that embryonic development up to the blastocyst/uterine entry stage can be retarded by as much as 1–2 days by factors such as advancing maternal age, use of frozen-thawed semen, and insemination early in the breeding season,[8] or by in vitro embryo production[9,10]; this needs to be taken into account when attempting to recover embryos for immediate transfer or cryopreservation, and when selecting a suitably synchronized recipient for ET.

Selective Oviductal Transport

In the horse, only developing embryos are transported into the uterus; unfertilized oocytes (UFOs) instead lodge in the ampulla of the oviduct where they slowly degenerate.[11,12] Although UFOs will occasionally enter the uterus along with an embryo from the same or a subsequent cycle,[13] independent transport of a UFO to the uterus is very uncommon. For this reason, if only a UFO is identified during an embryo flush, it is advisable to recheck the lavage equipment and/or repeat the flush in the expectation that the oocyte accompanied an embryo into the uterus.[8]

In an elegant series of experiments by Weber et al.,[14-17] the oviduct's ability to differentiate between fertilized embryos and UFOs was shown to be based not on any subtle fertilization-induced difference in shape or zona pellucida composition, but rather on embryonic secretion of prostaglandin E_2 (PGE$_2$). In short, Weber et al.[14,15] demonstrated that equine embryos not only secrete PGE$_2$ from around day 4–5 after ovulation, but that continuous local (intra-oviductal) administration of PGE$_2$ is sufficient to induce premature uterine entry of embryos.[15] Weber et al.[17] summarized their findings by proposing that a developing embryo lodges at the ampullary-isthmic junction as a result of tonic contraction of the isthmic circular smooth muscle until PGE$_2$ secretion by the compact morula is sufficient to relax the isthmic "sphincter" and allow the embryo to pass rapidly into the uterus. Robinson et al.[18] made use of these discoveries to develop a technique for hastening oviductal passage so that embryos could be collected reliably by uterine lavage at a stage of development when they were, for example, still suitable for cryopreservation; laparoscopic application of PGE$_2$ gel to the oviduct on day 4 after ovulation allowed embryos to be recovered from the uterine lumen 24 hours later. This technique has not, however, been adopted in clinical practice, largely because laparoscopic administration requires the mare to be starved, requires her flank to be surgically prepared, and involves entry into the abdominal cavity; all of these reduce its appeal to the owners of valuable mares.[19]

223

Early Pregnancy Factor

Although selective oviductal transport is an important example of early embryo-maternal interaction, it does not result in any immediate, measurable changes in maternal physiology that could serve as the basis of an early pregnancy test. On the other hand, as in other species, there have been reports of an "early pregnancy factor" (EPF) that can be detected in the serum of pregnant mares from as early as day 2 after ovulation using the Rosette Inhibition Test (RIT).[20] Although the precise identity and function(s) of the equine EPF are not known,[21] it is clear that a reliable and practical EPF assay would improve our ability to examine the scale and timing of embryonic death, investigate unexplained infertility, and improve the efficiency of ET programs in particular, and breeding programs in general. Whereas the RIT is too laborious and expensive to be of use in practice, an "early conception factor" test that aims to detect the EPF protein in blood serum has been marketed for mares inseminated 3–30 days previously (Horse ECF cassette test, Concepto Diagnostics, Knoxville, TN). Unfortunately, early field trials indicated a high incidence of false positives in known non-pregnant mares, and a general low ability to discriminate between pregnancy and non-pregnancy.[22] for these reasons, the ECF test is not currently recommended for determining pregnancy status in mares.

Embryonic Death During the Oviductal Period

Early pregnancy loss is a common and economically important problem in brood mares. However, pregnancy loss during the oviductal period appears to be primarily a cause of reduced breeding success in aged mares, and much less common in young, fertile mares.[23] Indeed, while fertilization rates in experimental settings are similarly high in both aged and young mares (approaching 90%[23]), embryo recovery rates at days 4 and 7 after ovulation are significantly lower in older mares,[23-25]

suggesting significant early losses in the latter group. Furthermore, the embryos recovered from older mares are significantly less likely to result in an ongoing pregnancy after transfer to a fertile recipient. There are, of course, two major possible contributors to embryonic loss during the oviductal period, namely an inadequate oviductal environment, or intrinsic abnormalities of the embryo arising from a defective oocyte or a defective sperm. Since equine embryos spend an unusually long part of their early development within the oviduct, it is probable that an inadequate oviductal microenvironment— for example, due to salpingitis (which is more common in aged mares[26]) or impaired oviduct secretory activity—would adversely affect embryonic survival. On the other hand, both oviductal pathology and insufficiency are difficult to diagnose or treat and, furthermore, oocyte-transfer (OT) experiments suggest that embryonic abnormality arising from age-related poor oocyte quality is by far the most significant contributor to intra-oviductal embryonic death.[27] The significance of embryonic abnormalities to EPL will be discussed further in the section relating to EPL during the early intra-uterine period.

EARLY INTRAUTERINE DEVELOPMENT: THE PRE-FIXATION PERIOD

Very soon after its arrival in the uterus, the equine early blastocyst begins to form an acellular glycoprotein "tertiary embryo coat," the so-called "blastocyst capsule."[28] The capsule first becomes visible as patches of iridescent material between the trophectoderm and the zona pellucida of the late morula/early blastocyst; these patches soon coalesce to form a confluent layer by about day 7 after ovulation, when blastocyst formation is complete (Fig. 19-1).[29] The blastocyst then embarks on a period of rapid expansion during which it sheds its zona pellucida to emerge fully enveloped by a complete capsule; at this stage (i.e., day 7 after ovulation) the embryo has a diameter of approximately 250 μm[6]

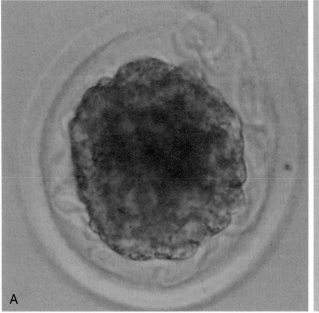 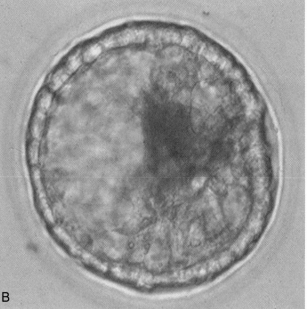

Figure 19-1. Equine embryos at around the time of blastulation. **A,** The zona pellucida around this early blastocyst has been incised so that the disorganized fibrils of capsule during formation can be appreciated. **B,** An early blastocyst around which the newly formed capsule can be seen as a complete layer of iridescent material between the trophectoderm and zona pellucida.

and contains a few thousand cells.[7,9] During the following week, the conceptus remains spherical and continues to expand rapidly, reaching 3–5 mm in diameter (and in excess of 45,000 cells) on day 10 after ovulation and 15–20 mm by day 14. Expansion is predominantly a result of yolk sac fluid accumulation[6] and is accompanied by a corresponding increase in the size and dry weight of the capsule, which remains as a protective envelope around the conceptus.[6,30] During the same period, the blastocyst cavity becomes lined with primitive endoderm to form a true "yolk sac" and the small ICM expands and develops to form the bi-layered embryonic disc (trophectoderm and yolk-sac endoderm). Between days 10 and 12, the embryonic disc becomes macroscopically visible and at around day 12 the primitive streak, the precursor of the embryo proper, becomes microscopically visible (Fig. 19-2); subsequently, cells migrate through the primitive streak and differentiate to create mesoderm in a process known as gastrulation, which heralds the formation of a recognizable multi-cellular embryo.[31,32]

One of the defining characteristics of pre-fixation horse conceptus development is the presence of the blastocyst capsule. Although the exact functions of the capsule are not known, its tough, elastic nature almost certainly allows it to provide mechanical protection (Fig. 19-3) to the delicate conceptus during the day 10–16 period when it is propelled around the uterine lumen by myometrial contractions.[33] The proposed anti-adhesive properties of the capsular glycoproteins presumably further facilitate conceptus migration.[30] Although not proven, the capsule has also been proposed to provide protection against microorganisms and the maternal immune system,[34] and to act as an interface for storing or transferring molecules involved in conceptus-maternal communication (e.g., insulin-like growth factor binding protein 3 [IGF-BP3][35]) or transfer of nutrients (e.g., uterocalin/P19).[36,37]

The blastocyst capsule also appears to be instrumental in maintaining the characteristic spherical form of the early equine conceptus,[38] a feature that differs markedly to the rapid elongation seen in the other large domestic species at an equivalent stage of development (pigs and ruminants[39]). As discussed later, the maintenance of the spherical shape, together with an unusually prolonged period of intrauterine mobility, are linked to the manner in which the equine conceptus achieves "maternal recognition of pregnancy." In addition, expansion of the conceptus as a sphere confers the considerable practical advantage of enabling ultrasonographic detection from as early as day 9–10 after ovulation.[40] In practice, because detection of a 2-3–mm vesicle on day 10 after ovulation has a sensitivity of no more than 70%, routine scanning for pregnancy is generally delayed until at least day 12 after ovulation and is most commonly performed on days 14–16 when the conceptus is visible as an approximately 2-cm fluid-filled vesicle with characteristic hyperechogenic artefacts known as "specular echoes" at the dorsal and ventral poles (Fig. 19-4).[41,42] Indeed, day 16 after ovulation is late enough to definitively diagnose non-pregnancy and identify most asynchronous twins (e.g., even if a second ovulation took place 3–4 days after the first), while retaining plenty of time to plan mating at the subsequent spontaneous estrus, should that be necessary. Prior to the widespread use of ultrasonography, early pregnancy diagnosis was generally performed by strategic teasing or transrectal manual palpation of uterine and cervical tone, where the latter typically increases beyond those of normal diestrus from around day 16 after ovulation.[43] And although manual pregnancy diagnosis alone is insufficient to either detect multiple pregnancy or EPL or to reliably differentiate between early pregnancy and prolonged diestrus, "palpation" is still an important part of determining whether a pregnancy is progressing normally.

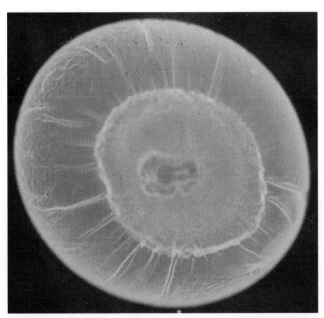

Figure 19-2. Day 15 equine conceptus showing a roughly circular embryonic disc at the center of which the early embryo is macroscopically distinguishable. Whereas the bulk of the conceptus membrane is bilaminar, comprising endoderm and ectoderm, the embryonic disc is trilaminar and also contains the mesoderm in which vascularization begins and the embryo proper forms.

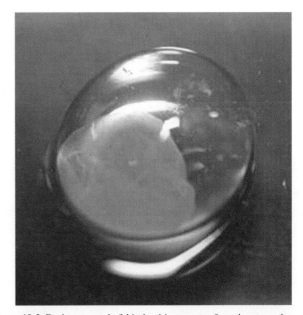

Figure 19-3. During removal of this day 14 conceptus from the uterus through a large bore flushing catheter, the delicate conceptus membrane ruptured while the tough, elastic capsule remained intact. It is thought that the physically resilient capsule provides vital mechanical protection for the delicate conceptus during the mobile phase when it is propelled around the uterine lumen by myometrial contractions.

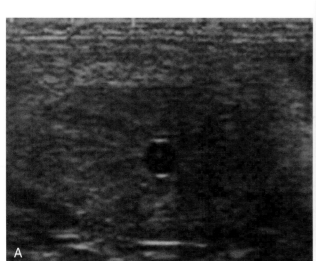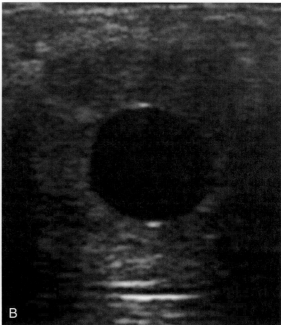

Figure 19-4. Ultrasonographic images of day 11 **(A)** and 15 **(B)** equine conceptuses. The former at approximately 5 mm in diameter is recorded soon after the conceptus would first be visible ultrasonographically, whereas the latter at approximately 2 cm in diameter is taken at a more typical time for pregnancy diagnosis. Both show the dorsal and ventral "specular echoes" characteristic of the spherical conceptus.

Conceptus Migration

In the period following its arrival in the uterus, the equine conceptus does not form a stable attachment to the endometrium but instead remains mobile and migrates continuously throughout the uterine body and horns,[40,44] propelled by myometrial contractions induced by prostaglandins produced either directly or indirectly (by stimulating local production in the endometrium) by the conceptus.[33] The mobile phase eventually comes to an end when the combination of increasing conceptus size and the pregnancy-related increase in uterine tone cause the conceptus to lodge at the base of one of the uterine horns on day 16 or 17 after ovulation.[45] Changes in capsule composition also appear to play a role in fixation, since fixation is accompanied by structural changes in the capsule (loss of sialic acid residues) consistent with a loss of anti-adhesive properties.[46] The physiological function of conceptus migration in the mare appears to be two-fold: (1) to allow the conceptus to interact with, and send biochemical signals to, sufficient endometrial area to prevent luteolysis (i.e., to effect maternal recognition of pregnancy), and (2) to improve the ability of the growing conceptus to harvest nutrients from the uterine milk or "histotrophe," in the period before the formation of a stable placental attachment (Fig. 19-5).[38,47]

Maternal Recognition of Pregnancy

Short[48] coined the term *maternal recognition of pregnancy (MRP)* to describe the process by which a female mammal determines that a conceptus is present in her uterus and makes the appropriate physiological changes to ensure that an adequate environment is established for the growth and development of that conceptus. Since the primary determinant of an "adequate environment" is the continued supply of progesterone, MRP is now more commonly taken to refer specifically to the

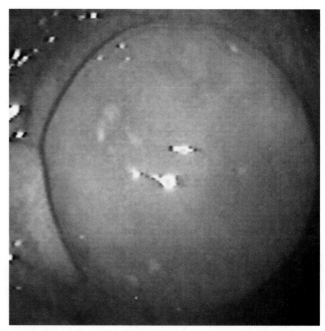

Figure 19-5. Day 15 conceptus imaged within the uterine lumen using a video-endoscope. The white areas on the surface of the translucent capsule are thought to be proteinaceous secretions of the type that the conceptus must harvest by migration during the period before fixation.

conceptus-initiated events that result in the prolonged lifespan and secretory activity of the primary corpus luteum (CL). In the horse, MRP appears to depend on an absolute suppression of the endometrium's ability to release the luteolytic hormone prostaglandin $F_{2\alpha}$ ($PGF_{2\alpha}$) in response to oxytocin[49,50] secreted by either the hypothalamus-anterior pituitary unit[51] or the endometrium itself.[52-54] Since the oxytocin responsiveness that underpins cyclical luteolysis develops at around day 10 after ovulation,[49,55] it is assumed that conceptus signaling to achieve MRP also begins at around this time. At the other extreme, pregnancy removal experiments[56] suggest that signaling to complete MRP is not complete until at least day 14 after ovulation, and it is generally thought that MRP consists of a complex continuum of conceptus-maternal signaling events that together ensure prolonged CL survival.[57]

MRP in the mare is known to depend critically on conceptus migration, where the latter ensures that the anti-luteolytic signal is distributed (repeatedly) to all parts of the uterus, thereby allowing it to suppress $PGF_{2\alpha}$ release from sufficient endometrium to avert luteolysis. Indeed, when McDowell et al.[58] surgically restricted horse conceptuses to a single uterine horn, $PGF_{2\alpha}$ release was not inhibited sufficiently to block luteolysis and the pregnancies failed. In practice, it is thought that large single intraluminal uterine cysts or local accumulations of cysts may present sufficient impediment to conceptus migration to endanger MRP, particularly if they are located at the base of a uterine horn; this is one of the reasons for recommending the removal of large intraluminal endometrial cysts when they are detected during a pre-breeding examination (Fig. 19-6).[59]

Given its critical importance in pregnancy maintenance and potential use for diagnosing pregnancy and detecting incipient pregnancy loss, it is surprising that the equine conceptus MRP signal has still not been identified. Molecules proven to function as MRP signals in the other large domestic species, such as interferon-τ in the ruminants and estrogens in the pig (for review, see Spencer et al.[60]), are either not secreted by equine conceptuses (interferon-τ: 57) or are secreted but do not reliably extend CL lifespan (estrogens[33]). Studies to investigate the size of the conceptus product that inhibits $PGF_{2\alpha}$ secretion by equine endometrium incubated *in vitro* concluded that the equine MRP signal must have a molecular weight of 1-6 Kda[61] or 3-10 Kda[62]; however, further characterization has proven elusive. On the other hand, MRP stage equine conceptuses have been shown to secrete a variety of hormones, including PGE_2 and $PGF_{2\alpha}$,[63] IGF-1,[64] and estrogens[65,66] that, although they may not be directly involved in inhibiting endometrial $PGF_{2\alpha}$ secretion, almost certainly play significant roles in processes essential to pregnancy maintenance, such as conceptus migration,[33] increased uterine vascularity,[67] and qualitative and quantitative alterations in the composition of the uterine secretions that make up histotrophe.[68]

Early Management of Twin Pregnancy in the Mare

The conceptus mobile phase has proven to be of particular clinical use with respect to the management of twin or multiple pregnancy. Before the introduction of ultrasonography for the early detection of pregnancy in the 1980s,[69,70] twin pregnancy was one of the most common causes of abortion in the mare.[71] Ultrasonography made the early detection of multiple conceptus vesicles possible, and it soon became clear that diagnosis of twins before conceptus fixation on day 16-17 after ovulation was beneficial because, even if the conceptuses were adjacent at the time of examination, they could be gently massaged apart or allowed to separate spontaneously (e.g., by returning the mare to a stable and reexamining her 30–60 minutes later) and thereby allow crushing of one of the vesicles between the fingers and the palm of the hand or between the ultrasound probe and pelvic brim, while leaving the second vesicle intact (Fig. 19-7, A-C). In experienced hands, success rates for the manual reduction of a twin to a singleton pregnancy between days 14 and 16 after ovulation are high (>90%[72-74]), whereas spontaneous reduction to a singleton during the mobile phase is rare and only likely if one of the conceptuses is abnormal.[75] After day 17, separation or preferential crushing of one of two unilaterally fixed vesicles without accidentally disrupting both becomes increasingly difficult (Fig. 19-7, D), and the success rate drops accordingly.[76]

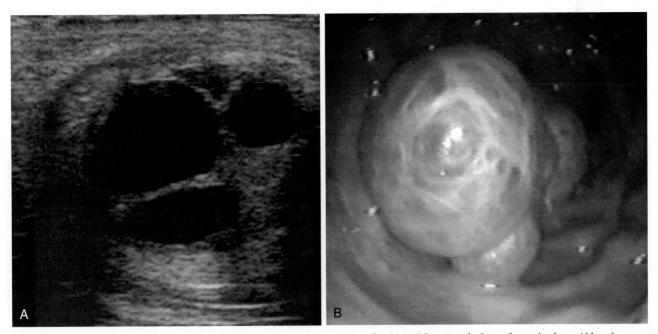

Figure 19-6. Ultrasonographic (**A**) and videoendoscopic (**B**) images of an accumulation of endometrial cysts at the base of a uterine horn. Although conceptuses have been documented to squeeze their way past cysts, large or numerous cysts may present sufficient impediment to conceptus migration to interfere with normal conceptus-maternal signaling and thereby prevent maternal recognition of pregnancy.

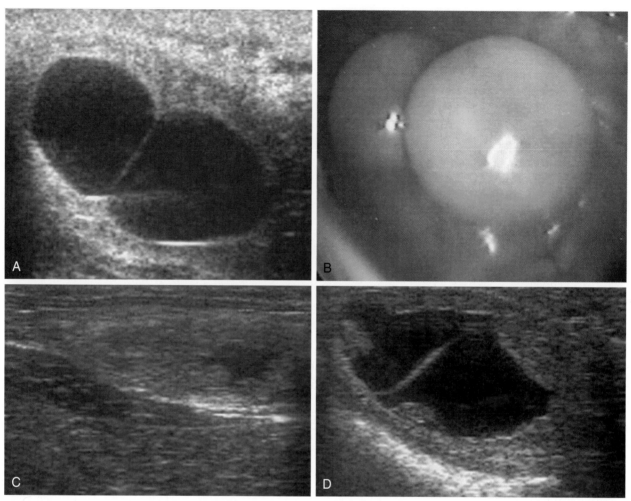

Figure 19-7. Ultrasonographic (**A**) and videoendoscopic (**B**) images of pre-fixation equine twins. At this stage, the conceptuses can still be massaged away from each other to enable transrectal crushing of one of the vesicles. **C,** Immediately after crushing, the fluid from the disrupted vesicle assumes the shape of the uterine lumen before dispersing throughout the uterus. **D,** Day 22 unilateral twins; once the vesicles lose their spherical shape and assume a single outer contour, separation and selective crushing of one vesicle becomes extremely difficult.

EARLY INTRAUTERINE DEVELOPMENT: THE POST-FIXATION PERIOD

Following fixation, conceptus expansion slows and the vesicle finally loses its perfectly spherical shape, becoming first "guitar-pick"–shaped and then irregular in cross-section.[45] It is probably no coincidence that this change in form is associated with cessation in growth and then attenuation of the blastocyst capsule, which eventually disappears completely at around day 23 of gestation.[34] Although the rate of increase in conceptus diameter during days 16–35 may be modest when compared with early expansion, the increase in complexity is anything but. In particular, the mesoderm that first appeared at around day 12 continues to expand and differentiate within the so-called "trilaminar omphalopleure" and gives rise to the first primitive blood vessels—the vitelline artery and sinus terminalis—to aid the transport and distribution of nutrients, respiratory gases, and waste products. The embryo proper also undergoes a period of rapid development that includes organogenesis and is exemplified by the formation of a primitive heart and blood vessels (Fig. 19-8) and the development of the allantois as a small sac-like diverticulum protruding from the hindgut. By day 23, the extraembryonic mesoderm covers most of the conceptus, leaving only

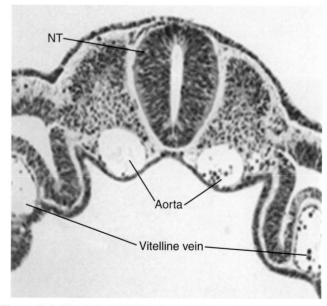

Figure 19-8. Histological (H&E stained) section through a day 18 equine embryo showing the development of the neural tube *(NT)* and, within the mesodermal tissue, the major vessels (aorta and vitelline veins) that already contain primitive blood cells.

a small area of "bilaminar omphalopleure" at the abembryonic pole; furthermore, all the major internal organs are discernible in the embryo, the limb buds are beginning to develop, and the allantois has greatly enlarged.[77] Two days later the vascularized allantois fuses with the outermost chorion to form the chorioallantois, the future fetal component of the true placenta. At the point where the enlarging allantois meets the by-now regressing yolk sac, a discrete annulate band of chorion develops that is not underlain by vascularized mesoderm; the specialized trophoblast cells within this band proliferate rapidly during days 25–35 of gestation and accumulate in simple folds in the distinctive pale band known as the "chorionic girdle."[78,79] During this same period, the chorioallantois enlarges progressively and the yolk sac shrinks such that, by day 35, the allantois accounts for about 75% of the cross-section of the roughly spherical conceptus.

The Endometrial Cup Reaction and Formation of the True Placenta

The endometrial cup reaction and onset of placentation were comprehensively reviewed by Allen.[47] At around day 36, the entire chorionic girdle detaches from the conceptus and adheres to the overlying endometrium, enabling its cells to actively invade the maternal tissue and initiate the process of endometrial cup development.[79] During invasion, the girdle cells push through or between the luminal and glandular epithelial cells, penetrate the underlying basement membrane and migrate into the endometrial stroma where they abruptly stop moving, enlarge, and become tightly packed together to form the temporary endocrine organs known as the "endometrial cups."[79,80] The endometrial cup cells secrete the peptide hormone, equine chorionic gonadotrophin (eCG), into nearby lymph sinuses from which it passes into the systemic circulation and stimulates, as a result of its predominantly LH-like biological activity, continued progesterone secretion by the primary CL and the ovulation, or luteinization without ovulation, of any large follicles developing on the ovaries as a result of the continued waves of pituitary FSH secretion.[81] This leads to a series of rise(s) in the circulating progesterone concentrations in the dam, which ensure that ovarian progesterone secretion remains elevated until the chorioallantoic placenta is sufficiently well developed to assume the role of providing the progestagens necessary to maintain pregnancy, which occurs somewhere between days 70 and 100 of gestation.[82] The endometrium cups persist until days 100–120 of gestation, when, in most mares, they are sloughed as a result of an increasingly intense, maternal, cell-mediated immune response to what are, in essence, immunologically foreign cells.[83]

Although the endometrial cups are themselves not ultrasonographically visible, their effects usually are; the "secondary" or "accessory" corpora lutea that form as a result of eCG can be seen as multiple CL-like or anovulatory hemorrhagic follicle-like structures on the ovaries (Fig. 19-9). Because it is necessarily associated with pregnancy, elevated blood eCG concentrations between days 45 and 120 of pregnancy have been described as a test to confirm pregnancy.[84] However, although eCG analysis is still occasionally used as an indicator of pregnancy in miniature breeds[85] or horses that, for other reasons, cannot be examined *per rectum*, it should be noted that the size and duration of eCG secretion varies considerably between mares (e.g., is considerably lower in the case of donkey or mule pregnancies[86]), and that pregnancies can develop normally in the absence of endometrial cups, eCG, and secondary CLs.[87] In addition, pregnancy

loss after the formation of the endometrial cups is not accompanied by loss of the cups (Fig. 19-10).[84,88] The cups persist until the normal 100–120 days and, in some cases, much longer.[89] Of course, persistence of the endometrial cups after pregnancy loss can lead to a false-positive pregnancy diagnosis when an eCG assay is used and can also make attempts to rebreed mares that suffer from pregnancy loss after day 35 frustrating since many of the developing follicles luteinize instead of ovulating normally.

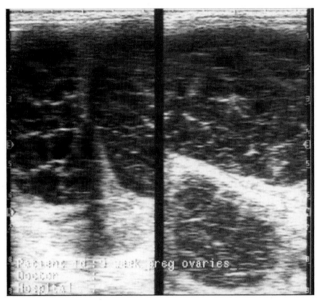

Figure 19-9. Ultrasonographic image of the ovaries of a mare at day 50 of pregnancy. Both ovaries contain multiple large (>6 cm) hemorrhagic follicle-like accessory corpora lutea formed as a result of the LH-like activity of the equine chorionic gonadotrophin secreted by the endometrial cups.

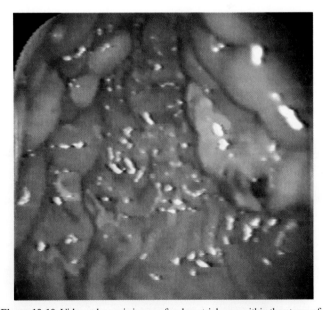

Figure 19-10. Videoendoscopic image of endometrial cups within the uterus of a mare that lost her pregnancy at day 38 of gestation. Following such a pregnancy loss, the cups would be expected to persist for at least another 2–3 months, and the eCG that they secrete would interfere with ovulation so that it would be difficult to establish a new pregnancy.

Soon after the start of the endometrial cup reaction, between days 40 and 45, the chorioallantoic membrane finally begins to interdigitate with the endometrium to form the true placenta (for reviews see Allen[38] and Allen and Stewart[47]); over the next 40 days, the interdigitations become increasingly complex to form the classical microcotyledons of the non-invasive, epithe-liochorial placenta.[90]

Ultrasonographic Monitoring of Post-Fixation Conceptus Development

The developmental changes that occur between approximately days 16 and 20 are essentially invisible to the clinician. However, from around day 20, the more obvious developmental changes can be visualized ultrasonographically, which is useful for monitoring conceptus development. Between days 19 and 22, the developing embryo proper becomes ultrasonographically visible as a tiny projection,[91] usually at the ventral/anti-mesometrial pole of the vesicle; soon after, the embryonic heartbeat also becomes detectable. Since there is a degree of variation between mares and pregnancies regarding when exactly the embryonic heartbeat can be detected, it is common to perform a second pregnancy check—to confirm embryonic viability—at around days 25–28 of gestation (Fig. 19-11). Although it is not yet common practice, embryonic blood flow and therefore viability can be detected earlier and more reliably using color or power-flow ultrasonography (Fig. 19-12). From around day 24 of gestation, characteristic changes within the conceptus membranes can also be used to verify the stage of embryo development and confirm that a pregnancy is developing normally. In particular, the developing allantois becomes ultrasonographically visible at around this time, and its subsequent expansion coupled with the previously mentioned yolk sac regression leads to an apparent dorsal migration of the embryo, suspended at the interface of the two sacs. By day 28, the allantois accounts for approximately 50% of total conceptus volume, and by day 32 this has increased to 75%.[42] On days 37–38, the embryo reaches the dorsal pole of the conceptus vesicle, the yolk sac becomes incorporated into the umbilical cord, and, over a further 7–8 days, the cord elongates so that the *fetus*—note that the nomenclature changes because it now has primitive stages of all its major organs—descends back down to the floor of the chorioallantoic vesicle (Fig. 19-13).[42]

Twin Pregnancy During the Post-Fixation Period

For reasons outlined previously, resolution of twin or multiple pregnancies by transrectal crushing of supernumerary vesicles is preferably performed during the pre-fixation period. However, in some instances a twin may be missed at an initial pregnancy scan or a mare may be presented for a first pregnancy examination after conceptus fixation. Although a monozygotic, monochorionic twin (i.e., identical twins derived from the same yolk sac) will also not be apparent until formation of the embryos and their allantoic sacs,[92] monozygotic twins appear to be rare in the mare, and the vast majority of twins probably result from multiple ovulations.

In the case of post-fixation twins, the synchrony of conceptus development and the distribution of the conceptuses within the uterus after fixation (i.e., unilateral or bilateral) will affect the likelihood of early spontaneous reduction, the success of any attempts to preferentially disrupt one vesicle, and, therefore, the desired time at which and technique with which twin reduction should be considered. In this respect, around 70% of twin vesicles appear to fix unilaterally (i.e., at the base of the same uterine horn[93]) with the tendency to unilateral fixation even more pronounced when the vesicles differ in size. Unilateral fixation is advantageous in that it leads to a very high incidence of spontaneous reduction to a singleton pregnancy before day 40 of gestation (approximately 85%[94]), leaving the remaining conceptus to develop normally. Even for unilaterally fixed conceptuses, however, the likelihood of spontaneous reduction is influenced by relative conceptus size; in a survey of 68 twin pregnancies,[94] spontaneous reduction to a singleton occurred in 100% of mares in which a clear difference in conceptus size was evident, and mostly occurred very soon after fixation (i.e., by day 20 after ovulation). By contrast, spontaneous reduction before day 40

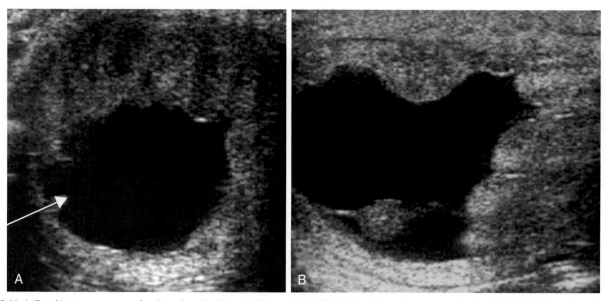

Figure 19-11. A, Day 21 pregnancy soon after the embryo has become ultrasonographically visible at the anti-mesometrial pole. **B,** By day 27, the embryonic heartbeat should be easily visualized and the embryo seen suspended between the expanding allantois (ventrally) and the regressing yolk sac (dorsally).

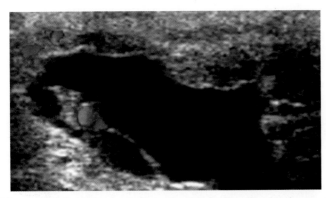

Figure 19-12. Day 26 conceptus imaged with color-flow Doppler ultrasonography demonstrating blood flow within the embryo proper. Color-flow Doppler ultrasonography allows detection of fetal blood flow even when the heartbeat is difficult to visualize with standard B-mode ultrasound.

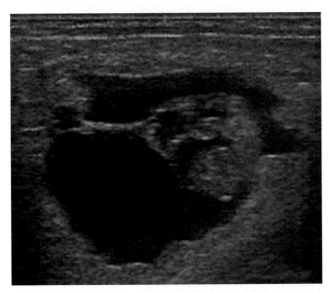

Figure 19-13. Day 42 fetus with distinguishable head and limbs suspended in the allantoic cavity, at the end of an umbilical cord that has the yolk sac remnant at its base.

occurred in "only" 73% of unilateral twin pregnancies in which the conceptuses were equally developed.[94] Two similar but conflicting "deprivation" hypotheses have been proposed to explain why spontaneous reduction of unilateral twins is very common, but not 100%. Ginther[95] and Allen[47] both proposed that the orientation of the bilaminar (trophectoderm and endoderm) and trilaminar (trophectoderm, endoderm, and vasculature-containing mesoderm) portions of the conceptuses in relation to each other is critical; however, whereas Ginther suggested that adequate contact between the vascularized trilaminar membrane and the endometrium is vital for post-fixation conceptus-maternal nutrient exchange, Allen proposed that the "highly absorptive" bilaminar omphalopleure must contact the endometrium to ensure adequate nutrient uptake. In practical terms, we can conclude that in the case of unilateral twins, the viability of one twin is frequently compromised because, following final vesicle orientation—note that after fixation, a vesicle normally orientates with the embryo ventrally/anti-mesometrially—a large proportion of its absorptive surface is in contact with its co-twin rather than the endometrium, thereby predisposing to

pregnancy loss by nutritional failure. When one twin is smaller (asynchronous or poorly developed), a greater proportion of its absorptive surface is likely to rest against its co-twin such that embryonic death is almost certain and more rapid.

In the 30% of twin pregnancies that fix bilaterally (i.e., one at the base of each uterine horn), spontaneous reduction before day 40 of gestation is rare, for the simple reason that the conceptuses have not yet contacted each other and do not, therefore, impinge on each other's ability to uptake nutrients.[96] Soon after day 42, and coincident with the time of true placenta formation, the conceptuses finally make contact and, if left to develop undisturbed, the most common outcome (10/15 cases monitored by Ginther and Griffin[96]) is loss of both fetuses either soon after contact is made or, more disturbingly for an owner, at 8–11 months of gestation.

Management of Post-Fixation Twins

Management of twins discovered after fixation was reviewed by MacPherson and Reimer.[97] In essence, the "best" approach depends on a combination of the exact time of diagnosis and the relative size and distribution of the vesicles. For practical purposes, in the period between fixation and true placenta formation (day 45), the approach to managing twin pregnancy can be divided into three categories:

1. Bilateral twins—Because spontaneous reduction will not occur until after day 40 and is most likely to involve loss of both pregnancies, intervention should be carried out as soon as possible after diagnosis. This is emphasized by reports that transrectal manual crushing of one vesicle by an experienced clinician before day 30 of gestation offers a good chance of an ongoing singleton,[71,75,98] whereas crushing later in gestation usually results in the loss of both pregnancies (e.g., 20% live single foals after manual crushing at days 35–45).[99] An alternative to manual crushing is transvaginal ultrasound-guided reduction; however, existing reports of this procedure for bilateral twins are few, are based on low numbers, and suggest only moderate success (<31% live foals[97]). In the author's clinic during 2000–2005, transvaginal-guided aspiration of one of bilateral twins at days 20–72 of gestation in 34 mares resulted in only 12 live singleton foals (35%); in contrast to earlier suggestions, however, the success rate was not worse if transvaginal aspiration was performed after day 35 of gestation. It therefore appears that transvaginal aspiration is probably preferable to manual crushing after approximately day 30 of gestation.

2. Unequally sized unilateral twins—A conservative approach involving regular monitoring until one conceptus either disappears or shows signs of compromise is advised, because spontaneous reduction before endometrial cup formation is very likely. Intervention should only be considered if, early in the breeding season, a pregnancy is approaching day 35 and there are still no clear signs of impending death of one conceptus. In the author's clinic, color-flow Doppler ultrasonography to assess embryonic blood flow is proving useful for the more sensitive detection of embryonic compromise (Fig. 19-14).

3. Equally sized/developed unilateral twins (Fig. 19-15)—This is the most difficult group with regard to the decision as to how and when to intervene. Although there are reports of a high success of manual crushing between days 17 and 20 if the vesicles are still distinctly spherical and can be separated

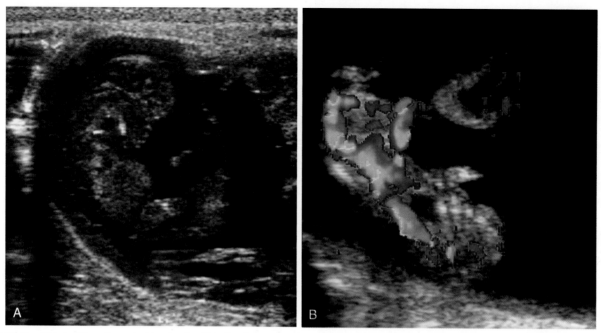

Figure 19-14. Day 50 twin fetuses imaged with color-flow Doppler ultrasonography showing definitively that one is dead (**A**) and the other alive (**B**).

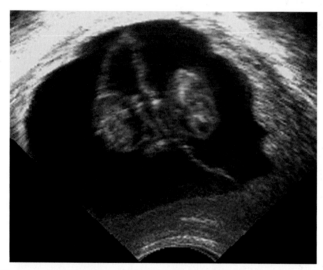

Figure 19-15. Unilateral equally sized twins imaged with a transvaginal probe and positioned such that, with the help a biopsy guideline, a needle can be introduced into one vesicle without disrupting the other.

(>90%[75,98]), manually disrupting one conceptus when the two vesicles present a single outer contour is difficult, likely to result in the loss of both conceptuses and not, therefore, recommended. Similarly, manual reduction of equally sized unilateral twins between days 20 and 29 is discouraged[75] because the high risk of damaging both conceptuses is outweighed by the 70% chance of spontaneous reduction to a singleton. In this respect, while Mari et al.[100] reported an impressive 70% single live foal following transvaginal ultrasound-guided reduction of 20 unilateral twins during days 16–25 after gestation, the success rate is no better than would be expected for spontaneous reduction during this period; it is therefore still questionable whether early transvaginal aspiration is beneficial in the case of unilateral twins. The current approach in the author's clinic is to monitor development of unilateral twins up to approximately day 30 of gestation and, if there is still no sign of a difference in size or viability between the two conceptuses, to intervene. Early in the breeding season in a fertile mare, the preferred intervention is termination of both pregnancies by systemic administration of a $PGF_{2\alpha}$ analogue supplemented, if the mare is close to day 35, by removing the conceptuses from the uterus by manual crushing and uterine lavage or transcervical videoendoscopic puncture and aspiration; removing the membranes removes any risk of endometrial cup formation and subsequent disturbance of cyclicity. The rationale for starting anew is that, in our experience, a surprisingly high percentage of mares in which transvaginal aspiration appears to be successful (one surviving pregnancy 7–10 days after intervention) go on to lose the remaining pregnancy 1–2 months later, at which point it is too late to consider rebreeding. On the other hand, when a twin is presented late in the breeding season or when a subfertile mare or subfertile stallion is involved, and starting anew is therefore not an option, transvaginal ultrasound-guided reduction is attempted at around day 30. During 2000–2005, live foals were born to 10 of 32 mares (31%) in which transvaginal reduction of a unilateral twin was performed between days 25 and 35 of gestation.

PREGNANCY LOSS DURING THE EMBRYONIC PERIOD

Recent surveys have confirmed that pregnancy loss remains a significant cause of financial loss and frustration to horse breeders; approximately 15%-20% of all pregnancies detected at day 15 after ovulation fail to develop to term.[74,101,102] Moreover, the majority of these pregnancy losses (approximately 63%[103]) occur in the period before day 40 after ovulation when, as described previously, critical developmental processes such as the maternal recognition of pregnancy, development of the primitive streak to an embryo and then a fetus, dissolution of the blastocyst capsule, the endometrial cup reaction, and initiation of true placental formation must all occur. Moreover, for the majority of this early intra-uterine period, the conceptus is entirely dependent on progesterone produced by the primary CL for its continued survival.[103]

Although many potential causes of EPL have been suggested (for review, see Ball[104]), surprisingly little is known about how common or significant each of the potential problems is or, therefore, what should be done to reduce the likelihood of, or prevent, EPL. This is largely because EPL is most commonly diagnosed retrospectively (i.e., the conceptus has already disappeared) when it is no longer possible to determine the initiating cause. Nevertheless, recent reproductive surveys, incorporating more frequent ultrasonographic monitoring of pregnancy, and planned studies have increased our understanding of some of the likely causes of EPL. The latter are commonly divided into embryonic abnormalities, inadequacy of the maternal environment and "external" factors but, as will be clear in the following discussion, there is considerable overlap between these categories.[104]

Embryonic Factors Resulting in EPL

In the section relating to embryonic death during the oviductal period, it was concluded that embryonic abnormalities were an important contributor to EPL, without elaborating on what these embryonic abnormalities might involve and how they might arise. During the intrauterine period, it is similarly clear that abnormalities of the embryo *per se* play an important role in EPL, not least because EPL often occurs in the absence of any obvious external trigger or change in maternal physiology (e.g., loss of the primary CL) and may even be associated with ultrasonographically detectable abnormalities of the conceptus such as abnormally slow expansion or failure to develop an embryo with a heartbeat (i.e., an anembryonic vesicle) (Fig. 19-16).[105] In species other than the horse, it has long been clear that the

most common underlying cause of embryonic abnormality, and indeed of pregnancy loss in general, is chromosomal aberration.[106-107] Chromosomal aberrations can basically arise in two different ways; namely, as the result of a pre-existing parental abnormality transmitted to the gamete or, more commonly, as a result of a spontaneous aberration arising either during gametogenesis, at fertilization, or during early embryonic development.[106] Although it has long been assumed that chromosomal abnormalities were a major contributor to EPL in the mare, it was not until the development of more sophisticated techniques for detecting abnormalities of chromosome number (e.g., fluorescent in situ hybridization) that Rambags et al.[7] were able to prove that chromosomally abnormal cells are a common finding, even in normal-looking equine embryos (Fig. 19-17); moreover, the proportion of abnormal cells is occasionally high enough to make embryonic survival extremely unlikely. Although it is not

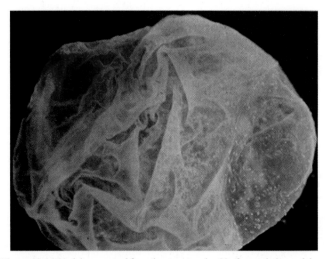

Figure 19-16. Vesicle recovered from the uterus on day 33 after ovulation and demonstrating failure to develop any of an embryo, a normal pattern of vascularization, or a discernible division between bilaminar and trilaminar areas of membrane.

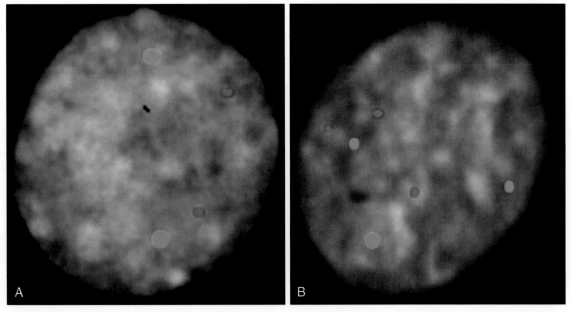

Figure 19-17. Photomicrographs of the cell nuclei of day 7 equine blastocysts stained with fluorescent probes labeling two red and two green chromosomes. The nuclei shown are from an apparently normal diploid cell (**A**) and from a cell that is either triploid or double trisomic (**B**) (three copies of each chromosome). A high proportion of chromosomally abnormal cells in the inner cell mass/embryonic disc would be expected to lead to embryonic death.

clear how and why such abnormalities arise in equine embryos, in women the primary cause is failure of normal chromosome dysjunction during either fertilization or early cell division, as a result of a maternal age-related reduction in oocyte quality.[107] In the mare, it is similarly clear that rising maternal age beyond approximately 14 years is accompanied by a marked increase in the incidence of EPL.[74,101,104] Moreover, since this effect persists when the oocyte[27] or very early embryo[23,25] is transferred to the oviduct or uterus of a young healthy mare, it is clear that a significant part of the effect is related to oocyte quality *per se,* rather than deterioration of the oviductal and/or uterine environment, and it has been suggested that diminished mitochondrial number or function may play a role in reduced embryo quality.[108] A more accelerated form of oocyte degeneration leading to embryonic abnormality presumably explains the increased rate of EPL noted in mares mated or inseminated more than 12 hours after ovulation.[109]

Although poor oocyte quality may be the most important source of embryonic abnormalities, there is also clear evidence of a stallion contribution to EPL[104] that could, at least in part, be due to chromosomal or DNA abnormalities carried by the sperm. In two recent surveys in the United Kingdom, approximately 20% of Thoroughbred breeding stallions were associated with significantly higher EPL rates than all other stallions (13%–33% versus 0%–12%,[101] $26 \pm 5\%$ vs. $7 \pm 6\%$[74]). The origin of stallion-related EPL was not examined further in these surveys, and although managerial factors, venereal diseases, and mare–stallion genetic incompatibility (e.g., caused by recessive embryonic lethal genes) cannot be ruled out, there are also indications that genetic abnormalities of the stallion or sperm DNA instability could play a role. In this respect, Kenney et al.[110] demonstrated that some subfertile stallions are indeed karyotypically abnormal; however, stallions with a normal karyotype were also associated with elevated rates of EPL. Similarly, while Love and Kenney[111] used the sperm chromatin structure assay to demonstrate an association between increased sperm DNA instability and poor fertility in stallions, there is as yet no clear evidence for the link between sperm DNA instability and pregnancy loss that has been reported for people.[112]

Although there are, thus, indications that both oocyte and sperm factors may contribute to EPL, failure of embryonic development is also thought to occasionally result from interventions that preferentially damage cells of the ICM,[105] such as embryo freezing.[113] In this respect, it is probable that the apparently increased rates of EPL following the production of embryos *in vitro* by intracytoplasmic sperm injection or cloning by nuclear transfer[10] result either from poor development of the ICM or from an increased incidence of chromosomal abnormalities.[7] Studies to examine the causes of embryonic death in horse pregnancies showing clear signs of abnormal development have, however, not yet been performed.

Inadequacies of the Maternal Environment and EPL

Inadequacy of the maternal environment is a broad concept encompassing diverse factors such as insufficiency of the maternal progesterone supply on which pregnancy maintenance depends (reviewed by Allen[103]), inadequate provision of essential nutrients from an aged or damaged endometrium, and infection/inflammation as a result of either unresolved post-breeding endometritis or subsequently acquired endometritis. EPL caused by endometritis is predominantly a problem of aged mares that are either less able to adequately resolve the physiological inflammatory response to mating (e.g., because of deficiencies in uterine contractility, lymphatic drainage, cervical and/or vulval conformation[114]) or are more prone to ascending infection because of inadequate vulval, vestibular-vaginal, and/or cervical barrier function. EPL caused by endometritis is sometimes ultrasonographically evident as a visible accumulation of uterine fluid despite the presence of a conceptus (Fig. 19-18); subsequent conceptus death may result either by direct infection or via luteolysis caused by $PGF_{2\alpha}$ release from an irritated endometrium.[115] In theory, post-breeding endometritis would be expected to affect the embryo immediately after its entry into the uterus; however, a more slowly developing infection has been proposed (e.g., by Villahoz et al.[116]) to explain the increased incidence of EPL noted, in some surveys, in mares bred at the first post-partum estrus (e.g., Morris and Allen,[74] Allen et al.,[101] and Merkt and Gunzel[117]).

Given that progesterone is an absolute requirement for pregnancy maintenance, it is tempting to assume that inadequate progesterone—caused by failure to maintain the primary CL, for example—would be a common cause of EPL. Although contested, this assumption is supported by the findings that in

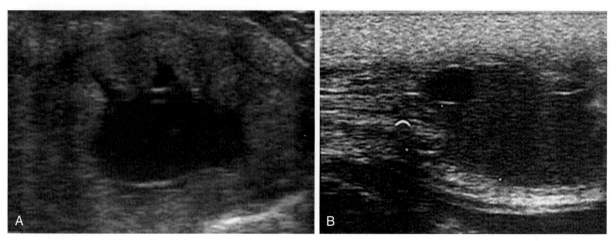

Figure 19-18. Ultrasound images of pregnancies accompanied by free intrauterine fluid. **A,** Normally developed day 16 pregnancy surrounded by a small amount of free fluid that probably represents an early endometritis. **B,** A small for date (<1 cm) day 15 vesicle floating in a large accumulation of flocculent fluid that is definitely the result of endometritis.

10 of 13[118] and 5 of 11[119] mares that lost a pregnancy before day 20 of gestation, EPL was associated with a fall in maternal circulating progesterone concentrations at the expected time of cyclical luteolysis. Newcombe[119] did note, however, that most of the failed pregnancies were "small for dates" and therefore already showed signs of possible abnormality. Although Irvine et al.[120] conversely recorded a fall in maternal progesterone in only 1 of 17 instances of EPL, it may be significant that initial pregnancy diagnosis in this study was not performed until day 17 or 18 after ovulation, when EPL caused by failure of MRP may already have been complete. Since specific cases of EPL associated with failed MRP have also been documented,[105,121] and there are numerous anecdotal cases of day 16–18 pregnant mares showing clear signs of a return to estrus (i.e., atonic uterus and cervix, endometrial edema; Fig. 19-19), it is clear that EPL caused by failure of MRP does occur; it is less clear how often this problem is partially due to irresolvable conceptus abnormalities.

Beyond the MRP period, although mechanisms for luteal failure have been proposed, their significance to EPL is not clear. Certainly, luteolysis can be induced by $PGF_{2\alpha}$ release from organs other than the uterus, such as in the case of systemic disease (e.g., severe gastro-intestinal disease) accompanied by pyrexia and/or endotoxemia.[122] In addition, since it is clear that MRP depends on a potent suppression of the endometrial $PGF_{2\alpha}$ release capacity during days 10–16 of pregnancy, the possible consequences of the waning of this suppression during days 18–35 are intriguing.[63] In short, it appears that the day 18–35 horse pregnancy is vulnerable to luteolysis, which could theoretically be triggered by any manipulation or hormone release capable of stimulating uterine $PGF_{2\alpha}$ secretion; there are a surprising number of the latter. During the day 18–35 period, both the uterine manipulation necessary to reduce a twin pregnancy[73] and oxytocin administration[50,123] have been reported to provoke $PGF_{2\alpha}$ release, whereas administration of both estrogens[124] and hCG[125,126] have been shown to induce partial or complete luteolysis. Interestingly, hCG administration also led to pregnancy loss in most instances if the mare was first treated before, but not after, day 38 of gestation.[125] As noted previously, however, there is little current evidence that complete luteolysis and a return to estrus is a common cause of EPL during the day 18–35 period; it is therefore possible that a second as yet uncharacterized MRP pathway exists to protect the CL during this period. It is also possible that EPL caused by progesterone deficiency does not always require complete luteolysis; in this respect, both Ball[104] and Allen[103] have suggested that there may be an individual mare threshold for progesterone below which pregnancy may be endangered, presumably as a result of compromised ability of the uterus to secrete the proteins a developing conceptus requires.[68]

Although an effect of maternal circulating progesterone concentrations on the ability of the endometrium to provide the conceptus with adequate nutritional support is speculative, it is clear that the age-related drop in endometrial quality that begins at an average of 13 years[127] can markedly affect the supply of nutrients to the conceptus. The detrimental effects of chronic endometrial damage and fibrosis beyond day 40 of gestation are well established,[128] but it is also quite possible that severe endometrial inadequacy could cause earlier pregnancy loss. In this respect, Newcombe[91] proposed that fixation of a conceptus next to an endometrial cyst (Fig. 19-20) could predispose to EPL by nutritional inadequacy in a modification of Ginther's[95] "deprivation hypothesis" for the spontaneous reduction of twins; in short, if too much of the absorptive surface was apposed to the cyst, pregnancy might fail because of inadequate nutrient uptake.

External Factors Contributing to EPL

There are numerous anecdotal reports that stress predisposes to EPL in the mare. Factors proposed to act as stressors include pain and/or systemic disease, weaning,[129] transport,[130] changes

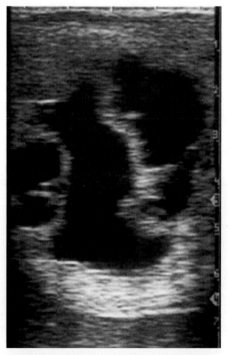

Figure 19-20. A day 20 pregnancy nestled between multiple large endometrial cysts. A conceptus positioned in this fashion may be at risk of early embryonic death because of inability to derive sufficient nutrition or form an adequate placenta over the unproductive cystic endometrium.

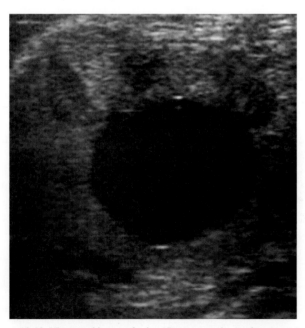

Figure 19-19. Ultrasound image of a day 17 pregnancy in an edematous uterus. This image suggests failure of maternal recognition of pregnancy and return to estrus despite the presence of a normally sized conceptus.

in group structure, poor nutrition,[131] and extremes of temperature. In the case of at least social disturbances, weaning, transport, and poor nutrition, the predisposition to pregnancy loss is thought to occur primarily via a reduction in plasma progesterone concentrations stimulated by circulating corticosteroid elevations.[129] Although the exact role of stress and/or corticosteroids in EPL is not clear, it is certainly prudent to minimize avoidable stress (e.g., weaning, mixing, long-distance transport) during early pregnancy, at least until the endometrial cups have formed to provide luteal protection. In the case of extremes of temperature, anecdotal experiences from ET programs suggest that prolonged heat can lead to reduced day 7–8 embryo quality likely to increase the risk of EPL.

Management of Pregnancy Loss

It is often not clear whether or how best to avert EPL in mares showing ultrasonographic indications of impending pregnancy loss. However, when a mare shows clear signs of returning to estrus despite the presence of an apparently normal conceptus in her uterus,[91] has a history of repeated EPL associated with a return to estrus, is systemically sick, or has recently undergone severe stress that might adversely affect circulating progesterone concentrations, the most logical approach is to treat the mare with a suitable progestagen (e.g., altrenogest[132]) from as soon as CL failure is suspected or, in cases of repeated EPL, from before the onset of MRP. In fact, it appears that normal conceptuses can survive at least 2 days in the absence of maternal progesterone, since progesterone supplementation[133] or ovulation[134] 4 and 3 days, respectively, after the induction of luteolysis with a $PGF_{2\alpha}$ analogue have been reported to rescue pregnancy. Once initiated, progestagen supplementation should be continued until adequate maternal progesterone production can be confirmed by measuring endogenous progestagen concentrations, detecting secondary ovulations or waiting until at least day 100 of gestation, when placental progestagens should be sufficient to maintain pregnancy. When stopping progesterone administration, it is sensible to stop gradually since there are indications that exogenous progestagen administration suppresses endogenous production in both mid-gestation[87] and early pregnancy (unpublished observations).

As previously discussed, however, luteal failure may result in some cases because of abnormal conceptus development (e.g., the "small for dates" vesicle[91]) and in these cases progesterone therapy may not prevent EPL. Although progesterone supplementation therefore has a clear place in protecting pregnancies clearly threatened by maternal progesterone deficiency (i.e., the mare is in estrus or is systemically ill), the large-scale use of exogenous progesterone therapy is questionable, if only because it will do no more than delay or mask EPL caused by embryonic abnormalities[91] and exacerbate uterine infection in those caused by endometritis. Moreover, since EPL after the MRP period most commonly occurs despite continued luteal activity,[120] there is a need to better define the causes of pregnancy loss and determine how often progesterone supplementation is really necessary and helpful, and how often it is actually contraindicated or should be substituted by more frequent monitoring of conceptus development; frequent monitoring is definitely preferable in cases of (suspected) abnormalities of conceptus growth or development.[91,105]

Another treatment proposed to reduce the incidence of EPL is a single systemic administration of the GnRH analogue, buserelin, during days 8–12 after ovulation.[135] However, while subsequent studies have confirmed a positive effect of GnRH administration on day 12 pregnancy rates,[136,137] they do not support a reduction in subsequent pregnancy losses. Moreover, it is not clear how GnRH administration might protect pregnancy in mares since, despite inducing an immediate release of LH,[137] it neither increases circulating progesterone levels[137] nor inhibits the ability of the endometrium to secrete $PGF_{2\alpha}$,[122] the proposed mechanisms of the pregnancy protective effect in cattle.[138] Nevertheless, if administration of GnRH on days 8–12 after ovulation really does improve pregnancy rates 2–4 days later by approximately 10%, the mechanism of action must involve some form of EPL prevention that demands further investigation.

Finally, it is clear that there are instances of threatened pregnancy loss where attempts to preserve the conceptus in the uterus are either futile or contraindicated. For example, when a previously normal conceptus fails to develop a heart beat during days 25–30 after ovulation, it is sensible to terminate that pregnancy as soon as the clinician is confident of the diagnosis "anembryonic," to avoid losing time in a short breeding season.[91,105] Similarly, when signs of uterine or conceptus infection (e.g., intrauterine free-fluid or echogenic conceptus fluids) are noted before day 35 of pregnancy and early in the breeding season, it is pragmatic to terminate the pregnancy and resolve the endometritis rather than trying to rescue the pregnancy using systemic antibiotics and progestagen therapy; the latter is mostly unsuccessful, and there is always a chance that the damaged conceptus may survive in the short term but die later, thereby condemning the mare to a barren year.

CONCLUSIONS

During the first 40 days of pregnancy, the equine conceptus develops from a single cell "zygote" to a multi-organ fetus with recognizable body parts. Many critical developmental events take place during this period that are unusual to the equids and affect both the success of pregnancy establishment and maintenance and our ability to assist or monitor conceptus development. Indeed, the advent of ultrasonography to monitor conceptus development has enabled successful resolution of twin pregnancy and improved our understanding of the timing of EPL. Nevertheless, there is still much that we do not understand about how the early equine pregnancy develops; how often this is compromised by maternal, paternal, or embryonic abnormalities arising before, at, or soon after fertilization; how vulnerable pregnancy really is to luteolysis during the period when it is totally dependent on the primary CL; how the conceptus derives its nutrition before the formation of a definitive placenta; and how we can better predict or prevent EPL. In short, while management and monitoring of breeding and early pregnancy have improved greatly during the last 30 years, there is still considerable room for further improvement.

REFERENCES

1. Boyle MS, Cran DG, Allen WR, et al: Distribution of spermatozoa in the mare's oviduct. *J Reprod Fertil Suppl* 35:79-86, 1987.
2. Hunter RH: The fallopian tubes in domestic mammals: how vital is their physiological activity? *Reprod Nutr Dev* 45:281-290, 2005.
3. Bezard J, Magistrini M, Duchamp G, et al: Chronology of equine fertilization and early embryonic development in vivo and in vitro. *Equine Vet J Suppl* 8:105-110, 1989.
4. Freeman DA, Weber JA, Geary RT, et al: Time of embryo transport through the mare's oviduct. *Theriogenology* 36:823-830, 1991.

5. Battut I, Colchen S, Fieni F, et al: Success rates when attempting to nonsurgically collect equine embryos at 144, 156 or 168 hours after ovulation. *Equine Vet J Suppl* 25:60-62, 1997.

6. Betteridge KJ, Eaglesome MD, Mitchell D, et al: Development of horse embryos up to twenty two days after ovulation: observations on fresh specimens. *J Anat* 135:191-209, 1982.

7. Rambags BPB, Krijtenburg PJ, Drie HF, et al: Numerical chromosomal abnormalities in equine embryos produced in vivo and in vitro. *Mol Reprod Dev* 72:77-87, 2005.

8. Stout TAE: Equine embryo transfer: review of developing potential. *Equine Vet J* 38:467-478, 2006.

9. Tremoleda JL, Stout TA, Lagutina I, et al: Effects of in vitro production on horse embryo morphology, cytoskeletal characteristics, and blastocyst capsule formation. *Biol Reprod* 69:1895-1906, 2003.

10. Galli C, Colleoni S, Duchi R, et al: Developmental competence of equine oocytes and embryos obtained by in vitro procedures ranging from in vitro maturation and ICSI to embryo culture, cryopreservation and somatic cell nuclear transfer. *Anim Reprod Sci* 98:39-55, 2007.

11. van Niekerk CH, Gerneke WH: Persistence and parthenogenetic cleavage of tubal ova in the mare. *Onderstepoort J Vet Res* 31:195-232, 1966.

12. Flood PF, Betteridge KJ, Irvine DS: Oestrogens and androgens in blastocoelic fluid and cultures of cells from equine conceptuses of 10-22 days gestation. *J Reprod Fert Suppl* 27:413-420, 1979.

13. Freeman DA, Woods GL, Vanderwall DK, et al: Embryo-initiated oviductal transport in mares. *J Reprod Fert* 75:535-538, 1992.

14. Weber JA, Freeman DA, Vanderwall DK, et al: Prostaglandin E_2 secretion by oviductal transport-stage equine embryos. *Biol Reprod* 45:540-543, 1991.

15. Weber JA, Freeman DA, Vanderwall DK, et al: Prostaglandin E_2 hastens oviductal transport of equine embryos. *Biol Reprod* 45:544-546, 1991.

16. Weber JA, Woods GL, Freeman DA, et al: Prostaglandin E_2 secretion by day 6 to day 9 equine embryos. *Prostaglandins* 43:55-59, 1992.

17. Weber JA, Woods GL, Lichtenwalner AB: Relaxatory effect of prostaglandin E_2 on circular smooth muscle isolated from the equine oviductal isthmus. *Biol Reprod Monog Ser* 1:125-130, 1995.

18. Robinson SJ, Neal H, Allen WR: Modulation of oviductal transport in mares by local application of prostaglandin E_2. *J Reprod Fertil Suppl* 56:587-592, 2000.

19. Allen WR: The development and application of the modern reproductive technologies to horse breeding. *Reprod Domest Anim* 40:310-329, 2005.

20. Takagi M, Nishimura K, Oguri N, et al: Measurement of early pregnancy factor activity for monitoring the viability of the equine embryo. *Theriogenology* 50:255-262, 1998.

21. Ohnuma K, Ito K, Takahashi J, et al: Partial purification of mare early pregnancy factor. *Am J Reprod Immunol* 51:95-101, 2004.

22. Horteloup MP, Threlfall WR, Funk JA: The early conception factor (ECF™) lateral flow assay for non-pregnancy determination in the mare. *Theriogenology* 64:1061-1071, 2005.

23. Ball BA, Little TV, Hillman RB, et al: Pregnancy rates of days 2 and 14 and estimated embryonic loss rates prior to day 14 in normal and subfertile mares. *Theriogenology* 26:611-619, 1986.

24. Ball BA, Little TV, Weber JA, et al: Viability of day-4 embryos from young, normal mares and aged subfertile mares after transfer to normal recipient mares. *J Reprod Fert* 85:187-194, 1989.

25. Vogelsang SG, Vogelsang MM: Influence of donor parity and age on the success of commercial equine embryo transfer. *Equine Vet J Suppl* 8:71-72, 1989.

26. Henry M, Vandeplassche M: Pathology of the oviduct in mares. *Vlaams Diergeneeskundig Tijdschrift* 50:301-325, 1981.

27. Carnevale EM, Ginther OJ: Defective oocytes as a cause of subfertility in old mares. *Biol Reprod Mono* 1:209-214, 1995.

28. Flood PF, Betteridge KJ, Diocee MS: Transmission electron microscopy of horse embryos three to 16 days after ovulation. *J Reprod Fertil Suppl* 32:319-327, 1982.

29. Stout TAE, Meadows SM, Allen WR: Stage-specific formation of the equine blastocyst capsule is instrumental to hatching and to embryonic survival in vivo. *Anim Reprod Sci* 87:269-281, 2005.

30. Oriol JG, Sharom FJ, Betteridge KJ: Developmentally regulated changes in the glycoproteins of the equine embryonic capsule. *J Reprod Fertil* 99:653-664, 1993.

31. Enders AC, Schlafke S, Lantz KC, et al: Endoderm cells of the equine yolk sac from day 7 until formation of the definitive yolk sac placenta. *Equine Vet J Suppl* 15:3-9, 1993.

32. Betteridge KJ: Comparative aspects of equine embryonic development. *Anim Reprod Sci* 60-61:691-702, 2000.

33. Stout TAE, Allen WR: Role of prostaglandins in intrauterine migration of the equine conceptus. *Reproduction* 121:771-775, 2001.

34. Betteridge KJ: The structure and function of the equine capsule in relation to embryo manipulation and transfer. *Equine Vet J Suppl* 8:92-100, 1989.

35. Herrler A, Pell JM, Allen WR, et al: Horse conceptuses secrete insulin-like growth factor-binding protein 3. *Biol Reprod* 62:1804-1811, 2000.

36. Crossett B, Suire S, Herrler A, et al: Transfer of a uterine lipocalin from the endometrium of the mare to the developing equine conceptus. *Biol Reprod* 59:483-490, 1998.

37. Suire S, Stewart F, Beachamp J, et al: Uterocalin, a lipocalin provisioning the preattachment equine conceptus: fatty acid and retinol binding properties, and structural characterization. *Biochem J* 356:369-376, 2001.

38. Allen WR, Stewart F: Equine placentation. *Reprod Fertil Dev* 13:623-634, 2001.

39. Amoroso EC: Placentation. In Parkes AS, ed: *Marshall's Physiology of Reproduction*, ed, 3, vol. 2 London: Longmans Green, 1952, pp 127-311.

40. Leith GS, Ginther OJ: Characterisation of intrauterine mobility of the early equine conceptus. *Theriogenology* 22:401-408, 1984.

41. England G: Real-time ultrasonography for the diagnosis and management of equine pregnancy. *InPractice* 16:84-92, 1994.

42. Bergfelt DR, Adams GP, Pierson RA: Pregnancy. In Rantanen N, McKinnon AO, eds: *Equine Diagnostic Ultrasonography*. Baltimore: Williams & Wilkins, 1998, pp 125-140,.

43. Bain AM: The manual diagnosis of pregnancy in the Thoroughbred mare. *N Z Vet J* 15:227-230, 1967.

44. Ginther OJ: Mobility of the early equine conceptus. *Theriogenology* 19:603-611, 1983.

45. Ginther OJ: Fixation and orientation of the early equine conceptus. *Theriogenology* 19:613-623, 1983.

46. Chu JWK, Sharom FJ, Oriol JG, et al: Biochemical changes in the equine capsule following prostaglandin-induced pregnancy failure. *Mol Reprod Develop* 46:286-295, 1997.

47. Allen WR: Fetomaternal interactions and influences during equine pregnancy. *Reproduction* 121:513-527, 2001.

48. Short RV: Implantation and the maternal recognition of pregnancy. In Wolstenholme GEW, O'Connor M, eds: Ciba Foundation Symposium on Foetal Autonomy. London: J and A Churchill, 1969, pp 2-26.

49. Goff AK, Pontbriand D, Sirois J: Oxytocin stimulation of plasma 15-keto-13,14-dihydro prostaglandin $F_{2\alpha}$ during the oestrous cycle and early pregnancy in the mare. *J Reprod Fertil Suppl* 35:253-260, 1987.

50. Starbuck GR, Stout TAE, Lamming GE, et al: Endometrial oxytocin receptor and uterine prostaglandin secretion in mares during the oestrous cycle and early pregnancy. *J Reprod Fertil* 113:173-179, 1998.

51. Vanderwall DK, Silvia WJ, Fitzgerald BP: Concentrations of oxytocin in the intercavernous sinus of mares during luteolysis: temporal relationship with concentrations of 13,14-dihydro-15-keto-prostaglandin $F_{2\alpha}$. *J Reprod Fertil* 112:337-346, 1998.

52. Behrendt-Adam CY, Adams MH, Simpson KS, et al: Oxytocin-neurophysin I mRNA abundance in equine uterine endometrium. *Dom Anim Endocrinol* 16:183-192, 1999.

53. Stout TAE, Lamming GE, Allen WR: The uterus as a source of oxytocin in the cycling mare. *J Reprod Fertil Suppl* 56:281-287, 2000.

54. Watson ED, Buckingham J, Björkstén T, et al: Immunolocalization of oxytocin and neurophysin in the mare uterus. *J Reprod Fertil Suppl* 56:289-296, 2000.

55. Stout TAE, Lamming GE, Allen WR: Oxytocin administration prolongs luteal function in cyclic mares. *J Reprod Fertil* 116:315-320, 1999.

56. Hershman L, Douglas RH: The critical period for the maternal recognition of pregnancy in pony mares. *J Reprod Fertil Suppl* 27:395-401, 1979.

57. Sharp DC, McDowell KJ, Weithenauer J, et al: The continuum of events leading to maternal recognition of pregnancy in mares. *J Reprod Fertil Suppl* 37:101-107, 1989.

58. McDowell KJ, Sharp DC, Peck LS, et al: Effect of restricted conceptus mobility on maternal recognition of pregnancy in mares. *Equine Vet J Suppl* 3:23-24, 1985.

59. Brook D, Frankel K: Electrocoagulative removal of endometrial cysts in the mare. *Eq Vet Sci* 7:77-81, 1987.

60. Spencer TE, Burghardt RC, Johnson GA, et al: Conceptus signals for establishment and maintenance of pregnancy. *Anim Reprod Sci* 82-83:537-550, 2004.

61. Weithenauer J, Sharp DC, McDowell KJ, et al: Characterisation of the equine conceptus prostaglandin inhibitory product (Abstract). *Biol Reprod* 36(Suppl 1):329, 1987.

62. Ababneh MM, Troedsson MHT, Michelson JR, et al: Partial characterization of an equine conceptus prostaglandin inhibitory factor. *J Reprod Fertil Suppl* 56:607-613, 2000.

63. Stout TAE, Allen WR: Prostaglandin E₂ and F₂α production by equine conceptuses and concentrations in conceptus fluids and uterine flushings recovered from early pregnant and dioestrous mares. *Reproduction* 123:261-268, 2002.

64. Walters KW, Roser JF, Anderson GB: Maternal-conceptus signalling during early pregnancy in mares: oestrogen and insulin-like growth factor I. *Reproduction* 121:331-338, 2001.

65. Heap RB, Hamon MH, Allen WR: Oestrogen production by the preimplantation donkey conceptus compared with that of the horse and the effect of between-species embryo transfer. *J Reprod Fertil* 93:141-147, 1991.

66. Zavy MT, Mayer R, Vernon MW, et al: An investigation of the uterine luminal environment of non-pregnant and pregnant pony mares. *J Reprod Fertil Suppl* 27:403-411, 1979.

67. Silva LA, Gastal EL, Beg MA, et al: Changes in vascular perfusion of the endometrium in association with changes in location of the embryonic vesicle in mares. *Biol Reprod* 72:755-761, 2005.

68. Zavy MT, Sharp DC, Bazer FW, et al: Identification of stage-specific hormonally induced polypeptides in the uterine protein secretions of the mare during the oestrous cycle and pregnancy. *J Reprod Fertil* 64:199-207, 1982.

69. Palmer E, Driancourt MA: Use of ultrasonic echography in equine gynaecology. *Theriogenology* 13:203-216, 1980.

70. Simpson DJ, Greenwood RES, Ricketts SW, et al: Use of ultrasound echography for early diagnosis of single and twin pregnancy in the mare. *J Reprod Fertil Suppl* 32:431-439, 1982.

71. Jeffcott LB, Whitwell K: Twinning as a cause of foetal and neonatal loss in the Thoroughbred mare. *J Comp Pathol* 83:91-106, 1973.

72. Pascoe D, Pascoe R, Hughes J, et al: Comparison of two techniques and three hormone therapies for management of twin conceptuses by manual embryonic reduction. *J Reprod Fertil Suppl* 35:701-702, 1987.

73. Greenwood RES: The occurrence and successful veterinary management of twinning in the Thoroughbred mare. *Pferdeheilkunde* 15:603-607, 1999.

74. Morris LH, Allen WR: Reproductive efficiency of intensively managed Thoroughbred mares in Newmarket. *Equine Vet J* 34:51-60, 2002.

75. Ginther OJ: Intrauterine movement of the early conceptus in barren and post partum mares. *Theriogenology* 21:633-644, 1984.

76. McKinnon AO, Rantanen N: Twins. In Rantanen N, McKinnon AO, eds: *Equine Diagnostic Ultrasonography.* Baltimore Williams & Wilkins, 1998, pp 141-155.

77. van Niekerk CJ, Allen WR: Early embryonic development in the horse. *J Reprod Fertil Suppl* 23:495-498, 1975.

78. van Niekerk CH: The early diagnosis of pregnancy, the development of the foetal membranes and nidation in the mare. *J S Afr Vet Med Assoc* 36:483-488, 1965.

79. Allen WR, Hamilton DW, Moor RM: The origin of the equine endometrial cups. II. Invasion of the endometrium by trophoblast. *Anat Rec* 177:475-501, 1973.

80. Hamilton DW, Allen WR, Moore RM: The origin of the equine endometrial cups III. Light and electron microscopic study of fully developed endometrial cups. *Anat Rec* 117:503-518, 1973.

81. Urwin VE, Allen WR: Pituitary and chorionic gonadotrophin control of ovarian function during early pregnancy in equids. *J Reprod Fertil Suppl* 32:371-382, 1982.

82. Holtan DW, Squires EL, Lapin DR, et al: Effect of ovariectomy on pregnancy in mares. *J Reprod Fertil Suppl* 32:457-463, 1982.

83. Allen WR: The influence of fetal genotype upon endometrial cup development and PMSG and progesterone production in equids. *J Reprod Fertil Suppl* 23:405-413, 1975.

84. Mitchell D: Early fetal death and a serum gonadotrophin test for pregnancy in the mare. *Can Vet J* 12:42-44, 1971.

85. Henderson K, Stevens S, Bailey C, et al: Comparison of the merits of measuring equine chorionic gonadotrophin (eCG) and blood and faecal concentrations of oestrone sulphate for determining the pregnancy status of miniature horses. *Reprod Fertil Dev* 10:441-444, 1998.

86. Allen WR, Skidmore JA, Stewart F, et al: Effects of fetal genotype and uterine environment on placental development in equids. *J Reprod Fertil* 97:55-60, 1993.

87. Allen WR, Kydd JH, Boyle MS, et al: Extra-specific donkey-in-horse pregnancy as a model of early fetal death. *J Reprod Fertil Suppl* 35:197-209, 1987.

88. Rathwell AC, Asbury AC, Hansen PJ, et al: Reproductive function of mares given daily injections of prostaglandin F₂α at day 42 of pregnancy. *Theriogenology* 27:621-630, 1987.

89. Steiner J, Antczak DF, Wolfsdorf K, et al: Persistent endometrial cups. *Anim Reprod Sci* 94:274-275, 2006.

90. Samuel C, Allen WR, Steven DH: Studies on the equine placenta. I. Development of the microcotyledons. *J Reprod Fertil* 41:441-445, 1974.

91. Newcombe JR: Embryonic loss and abnormalities of early pregnancy. *Eq Vet Educ* 12:88-101, 2000.

92. Meadows SMJ, Binns MM, Newcombe JR, et al: Identical triplets in a Thoroughbred mare. *Eq Vet J* 27:394-397, 1995.

93. Ginther OJ: Twin embryos in the mare: I. From ovulation to fixation. *Eq Vet J* 21:161-170, 1989.

94. Ginther OJ: Twin embryos in the mare: II. Post fixation embryo reduction. *Eq Vet J* 21:171-174, 1989.

95. Ginther OJ: The nature of embryo reductions in mares with twin conceptuses: deprivation hypothesis. *Am J Vet Res* 50:45-53, 1989.

96. Ginther OJ, Griffin P: Natural outcome and ultrasonic identification of equine fetal twins. *Theriogenology* 41:1193-1199, 1994.

97. MacPherson ML, Reimer JM: Twin reduction in the mare: current options. *Anim Reprod Sci* 60-61:233-244, 2000.

98. Bowman T: Ultrasonic diagnosis and management of early twins in the mare. Proc Ann Conv Amer Assoc Equine Prac. Nashville: 1987, pp 35–43.

99. Roberts C: Termination of twin gestation by blastocyst crush in the broodmare. *J Reprod Fertil Suppl* 32:447-449, 1982.

100. Mari G, Iacono E, Merlo B, et al: Reduction of twin pregnancy in the mare by transvaginal ultrasound-guided aspiration. *Reprod Dom Anim* 39:434-437, 2004.

101. Allen WR, Brown L, Wright M, et al: Reproductive efficiency of flatrace and national hunt Thoroughbred mares and stallions in England. *Eq Vet J* 39:438-445, 2007.

102. Hemberg E, Lundeheim N, Einarsson S: Reproductive performance of Thoroughbred mares in Sweden. *Reprod Dom Anim* 39:81-85, 2004.

103. Allen WR: Luteal deficiency and embryo mortality in the mare. *Reprod Dom Anim* 36:121-131, 2001.

104. Ball BA: Embryonic loss in mares: Incidence, possible causes and diagnostic considerations. *Vet Clin North Am Eq Pract* 4:263-290, 1988.

105. Vanderwall D, Squires EL, Brinsko SP, et al: Diagnosis and management of abnormal embryonic development characterized by formation of an embryonic vesicle without an embryo in mares. *J Am Vet Med Assoc* 217:58-63, 2000.

106. King WA: Chromosome abnormalities and pregnancy failure in domestic animals. In McFeely RA, ed: *Domestic Animal Cytogenetics.* San Diego: Academic Press, 1990, pp 229–250.

107. Munne S, Alikani M, Tomkin G, et al: Embryo morphology, developmental rates, and maternal age are correlated with chromosome abnormalities. *Fertil Steril* 64:382-391, 1995.

108. Rambags BPB, van Boxtel DCJ, Tharasanit T, et al: Maturation in vitro leads to mitochondrial degeneration in oocytes recovered from aged but not young mares. *Anim Reprod Sci* 94:359-361, 2006.

109. Woods J, Bergfelt DR, Ginther OJ: Effects of time of insemination relative to ovulation on pregnancy rate and embryonic-loss rate in mares. *Eq Vet J* 22:410-415, 1990.

110. Kenney RM, Kent MG, Garcia MC: The use of DNA index and karyotype analyses as adjuncts to the estimation of fertility in stallions. *J Reprod Fertil Suppl* 44:69-75, 1991.

111. Love CC, Kenney RM: The relationship of increased susceptibility of sperm DNA to denaturation and fertility in the stallion. *Theriogenology* 50:955-972, 1998.

112. Ibrahim ME, Pedersen H: Acridine orange fluorescence as male fertility test. *Arch Androl* 20:125-129, 1988.

113. Bruyas JF, Bézard J, Lagneaux D, et al: Quantitative analysis of morphological modifications of day 6.5 horse embryos after cryopreservation: differential effects on inner cell mass and trophoblast cells. *J Reprod Fertil* 99:15-23, 1993.

114. Troedsson MHT: Uterine clearance and resistance to persistent endometritis in the mare. *Theriogenology* 52:461-471, 1999.

115. Adams GP, Kastelic JP, Bergfelt DR, et al: Effect of uterine inflammation and ultrasonically-detected uterine pathology on fertility in the mare. *J Reprod Fertil Suppl* 35:445-454, 1987.

116. Villahoz MD, Squires EL, Voss JL, et al: Some observations on early embryonic death in mares. *Theriogenology* 23:915-923, 1985.

117. Merkt H: Gunzel A-R: A survey of early pregnancy loss in West German Thoroughbred mares. *Eq Vet J* 11:256-258, 1979.

118. Bergfelt DR, Woods JA, Ginther OJ: Role of the embryonic vesicle and progesterone in embryonic loss in mares. *J Reprod Fertil* 95:339-347, 1992.

119. Newcombe JR: Observations on early pregnancy diagnosis and early embryonic loss in the mare. *Irish Vet J* 50:534-536, 1997.

120. Irvine CH, Sutton P, Turner JE, et al: Changes in plasma progesterone concentrations from days 17 to 42 of gestation in mares maintaining or losing pregnancy. *Eq Vet J* 22:104-106, 1990.

121. Stout TAE, Tremoleda JL, Knaap J, et al: Does compromised luteal function contribute to failure to establish pregnancy after non-surgical embryo transfer? In Alvarenga M, Wade JF: Havemeyer Foundation Monograph Series 14: Proceedings of the 6th Int. Symp. Equine Embryo Transfer, Newmarket: R&W Communications, 2005, pp 8-9.

122. Daels PF, Stabenfeldt GH, Hughes JP, et al: Effects of flunixin meglumine on endotoxin-induced prostaglandin F2 alpha secretion during early pregnancy in mares. *Am J Vet Res* 52:276-281, 1991.

123 Stout TAE, Tremoleda JL, Knaap J, et al: Mid-diestrus GnRH-analogue administration does not suppress the luteolytic mechanism in mares. *Theriogenology* 58:567-570, 2002.

124. Stout TAE, Allen WR: Oestrogens and pregnancy maintenance in the mare: For or against? *Pferdeheilkunde* 17:579-582, 2001.

125 Allen WE: Pregnancy failure induced by human chorionic gonadotrophin in pony mares. *Vet Rec* 96:88-90, 1975.

126. Urwin VE: Gonadotrophic control of ovarian function in pregnant equids. PhD Thesis. University of Cambridge, UK: 1985.

127. Ricketts SW, Alonso S: The effect of age and parity on the development of equine chronic endometrial disease. *Eq Vet J* 23:189-192, 1991.

128. Kenney RM: Cyclic and pathologic changes of the mare endometrium as detected by biopsy, with a note on early embryonic death. *J Am Vet Med Assoc* 172:241-262, 1978.

129. van Niekerk CH, Morgenthal JC: Fetal loss and the effect of stress on plasma progestagen levels in pregnant Thoroughbred mares. *J Reprod Fertil Suppl* 32:453-457, 1982.

130. Baucus KL, Ralston SL, Nockels CF, et al: Effects of transportation on embryonic death in mares. *J Anim Sci* 68:345-351, 1990.

131. van Niekerk FE, van Niekerk CH: The effect of dietary protein on reproduction in the mare. VII. Embryonic development, early embryonic death, foetal losses and their relationship with serum progestagen. *J S Afr Vet Assoc* 69:150-155, 1998.

132. McKinnon AO, Lescun TB, Walker JH, et al: The inability of some synthetic progestagens to maintain pregnancy in the mare. *Eq Vet J* 32:83-85, 2000.

133. Kastelic JP, Adams GR, Ginther OJ: Role of progesterone in mobility, fixation, orientation, and survival of the equine embryonic vesicle. *Theriogenology* 27:655-663, 1987.

134. Watson ED, Nikolakopoulos E, Lawler DF: Survival and normal development of an embryo after prostaglandin treatment. *Eq Vet Educ* 9:283-285, 1997.

135. Pycock JF, Newcombe JR: The effect of the gonadotrophin-releasing hormone analog, buserelin, administered in diestrus on pregnancy rates and pregnancy failure in mares. *Theriogenology* 46:1097-1101, 1996.

136. Newcombe JR, Martinez TA, Peters AR: The effect of the gonadotropin-releasing hormone analog, buserelin, on pregnancy rates in horse and pony mares. *Theriogenology* 55:1619-1631, 2001.

137. Kanitz W, Schneider F, Hoppen HO, et al: Pregnancy rates, LH and progesterone concentrations in mares treated with a GnRH agonist. *Anim Reprod Sci* 97:55-62, 2007.

138. Mann GE, Lamming GE, Fray MD: Plasma oestradiol and progesterone during early pregnancy in the cow and the effects of treatment with buserelin. *Anim Reprod Sci* 37:121-131, 1995.

FETAL MONITORING IN BROODMARES

KIM A. SPRAYBERRY

Monitoring of uteroplacental function and fetal well-being in broodmares is typically requested by owners when mares are in later stages of gestation, but it may begin anytime after pregnancy has been diagnosed. The type of monitoring undertaken varies with stage of pregnancy and client wishes, and the frequency and intensity with which mares should be monitored depend on the age, fertility, reproductive history, and present health of the mare. Although the most common causes of reproductive loss in mares can vary from region to region in the United States or among regions of the world, the overall causes of pregnancy loss can be broadly regarded as falling into infective or noninfective categories. Under these classifications, the frequency with which a given diagnosis for pregnancy loss is cited in one study may differ slightly from its reported frequency in another study, but the same conditions tend to comprise the top handful of causes in most studies. In a 1993 retrospective study[1] of broodmares in Kentucky, the most common infectious condition leading to reproductive loss (defined as abortion, stillbirth, and foal death within 24 hours of birth) was placentitis. In a similar study in which aborted fetuses, stillborn foals, and placentas from premature foals from 1988 and 1989 were analyzed,[2] placentitis and dystocia or birth asphyxia were the most common causes of reproductive loss, but noninfectious causes of reproductive loss exceeded the infectious causes by an approximate ratio of 2:1. In that study,[2] placental disorders were slightly more common than nonplacental disorders, and umbilical cord torsion was cited as an important cause of abortion. In a 2003 retrospective study[3] of abortion and neonatal death in horses in the United Kingdom, umbilical cord problems were the most frequent etiology, but placentitis was also an important cause of reproductive loss.

The most common noninfectious cause of abortion is placental insufficiency, which is most often a result of competition between twin conceptuses for available endometrial surface area or degenerative changes in the endometrium caused by age, parity, or past disease. Extensive microcotyledonary interdigitation and high cotyledonary surface density on the chorioallantoic surface, together with a functional and healthy endometrium with which to interact, are necessary for normal fetal development; conditions that influence either the maternal or fetal aspect of placentation directly influence fetal size and health.[4-8]

Widespread use of ultrasound in broodmare practice has led to improvement in practitioners' capabilities for early detection and reduction of twin pregnancies, leaving placentitis as the most common cause of pregnancy loss in some practices. In the author's practice, this effect is offset by the practice of breeding valuable broodmares into advanced age. Mares do not undergo cyclic endometrial shedding like primates, and increasing age and number of foals produced are associated with degeneration

and dysfunction of endometrial glands, degeneration and occlusion of endometrial vasculature, fibrosis in the endometrial stroma, myometrial atony, and development of endometrial cysts—changes collectively referred to as endometrosis.[7] As a result, pregnancy loss from uteroplacental insufficiency persists despite the low prevalence of undetected twin pregnancies. Once diagnosed, placental changes can be monitored with ultrasonographic imaging, and this information, combined with that obtained from endocrine assays and fetal biophysical profiling to monitor fetal responses, yields the most comprehensive body of information available to the practitioner at present. The commercial value of breeding horses or simply the costs a client may have expended in getting a mare bred and confirmed in foal, whatever her value, are such that attempting to preserve the pregnancy and treat a compromised fetus *in utero* is a feasible decision in many instances.

Mares with a high-risk pregnancy warrant fetal monitoring. Conditions considered to constitute a high-risk pregnancy include a history of abortion, prolonged pregnancy, dystocia, or other gestational problems; past delivery of a compromised foal; suboptimal endometrial function; prepartum uterine artery rupture and hemorrhage; recent episode of surgery or other physiologic stressor; present systemic illness; or inappropriately early signs of impending parturition, such as premature mammary development and lactation. In mares with any of these conditions or clinical signs, fetal monitoring is useful for evaluating uteroplacental appearance and fetal responses to the condition. Multiple methods of monitoring are available to the practitioner (Box 20-1). The most applicable methods for most practitioners are routine clinicopathologic testing, ultrasound imaging, and determination of serum hormone and fetal protein concentrations; this chapter focuses on discussion of these modalities.

PHYSICAL EXAMINATION AND ROUTINE CLINICOPATHOLOGIC TESTING

Physical examination of the pregnant mare is always important and should include a speculum examination if vaginal discharge has been observed. However, many conditions that result in fetal compromise do not cause illness in the dam, and mares may appear healthy and remain unaffected in the face of fetal compromise. Normal results of routine laboratory tests, such as a CBC, serum biochemical profile, and cytology and bacterial culture (of mammary secretions or vaginal exudate), do not rule out illness in the fetus. At the same time, illness in the mare that does result in abnormal values on clinicopathologic testing can certainly affect the fetus. Abnormal findings in maternal blood work may be considered a risk factor for fetal compromise and constitute justification of fetal assessment if they are anything more than very transient and mild. A fetus in a mare with leukopenia as a result of gastrointestinal disease or other inflammatory condition is at risk of compromise; at the same time, the fetus in a mare with placentitis may be substantially compromised despite the fact that the maternal peripheral cell count and fibrinogen concentration are within reference range.

DETERMINATION OF SERUM HORMONE CONCENTRATIONS

In addition to routine laboratory tests, serum hormone concentrations may also be assayed. Hormone assays are less-sensitive indicators of fetal viability than sonographic examination, because concentrations of hormones produced by the fetus or by the placenta do not always accurately predict fetal demise or decrease promptly after death of the conceptus or fetus.[9] Moreover, single-point concentrations are not altogether helpful, because hour-to-hour variation in concentrations is normal. If serum or plasma hormone concentrations are the sole basis on which fetal viability is to be determined, serial blood sampling and detection of trends or changes in mean concentrations is optimal. Once-monthly blood sampling for progesterone concentration was not useful in predicting abortion in one study of 33 pregnant mares.[10]

Progesterone and Progestagens

Progesterone concentration in pregnant mares remains high (>4 ng/ml) during the first half of gestation, in part because of synthesis by the primary corpus luteum (CL) associated with the ovulation that resulted in pregnancy. At approximately 55 to 60 days, progesterone from this source is supplemented by progesterone synthesized by accessory or secondary corpora lutea, which produce progesterone in response to pituitary follicle-stimulating hormone (FSH) and equine chorionic gonadotropin (eCG) secreted by the endometrial cup cells. Thus, progesterone from ovarian sources (primary and secondary CLs) maintains the pregnant state until mid-gestation, when placental synthesis of progestagens takes over this role.

The endometrial cups arise from the invasive trophoblast layer and invade the endometrium starting at days 35 to 40. The invasive nature of the endometrial cups is associated with their abbreviated lifespan, compared with that of the noninvasive trophoblast layer, which develops into the allantochorion. Exposure of the invasive trophoblastic tissue to the endometrium incites immune attack by maternal CD4+ and CD8+ lymphocytes against paternal cell antigens on the cup cells[11] and leads to regression in the cups' size by day 70 and discontinuation of function by days 120 to 150. As the endometrial cups and secondary corpora lutea regress, native progesterone concentrations in maternal serum decrease, reaching nadir levels at 240 to 300 days. Concentrations remain low throughout most of the remainder of gestation before increasing again during the last month.[12]

As measured concentrations of progesterone are decreasing at approximately 150 days of gestation, those of total progestagens are increasing, in part because the progesterone elaborated by fetal and maternal adrenal glands during this time undergoes metabolism by the placenta to other metabolites.[13,14] During the second half of gestation, these metabolites predominate in the mare's serum, and progesterone per se remains low, a fact that is unique to the mare among common domestic animals. The 5α dihydroprogesterone (5αDHP) metabolite of progesterone likely subserves the actions of progesterone in maintaining myometrial quiescence during the middle and last part of gestation. Progesterone and total progestagen concentrations both increase during the last month before parturition and the rate of increase becomes more rapid during the last week prior to parturition, with normal total progestagen concentrations of <10 ng/ml increasing to ≥20 µg/ml.[9] Concentrations then decrease precipitously in the hours to 1 to 2 days before parturition. Decreasing or low progestagen concentrations in the last month of gestation have been associated with abortion in mares with serious medical or surgical conditions, especially when fetal hypoxia is a consequence.[9] High progestagen concentrations (>10 ng/ml) detected in the middle and later stages of gestation may be an indicator of fetal stress or placentitis, reflecting an increased rate of hypothalamus-pituitary-adrenal (HPA) axis activity and fetal maturation.[15,16]

Because of these physiological patterns of change in progesterone and progestagen concentrations during gestation, single-point measurements of either hormone are not necessarily helpful, and serial sampling for determination of trends or mean concentrations during a given interval is recommended.[17] Practitioners must be familiar with what hormones a given endocrine assay is measuring; some tests are highly specific for progesterone (e.g., radioimmunoassay and ELISA), whereas others (competitive protein binding) reflect total progestagen concentration, and this information is crucial to interpretation of results.

Estrogens

Estrogen concentrations measured in maternal blood after day 40 of gestation chiefly reflect placental synthesis from circulating dehydroepiandrosterone, an androgen precursor produced by the transiently hypertrophic fetal gonads. At day 280 of gestation, fetal gonads decrease production of dehydroepiandrosterone, and estrogen concentrations in maternal blood decrease.

The mare is unique among domestic animals in maintaining high estrogen concentrations and low progesterone concentrations during most of gestation (although total progestagen concentrations are not low).

Estrone sulfate is a product of the conceptus and is useful for assessment of fetal well-being after day 40 to 45,[18,19] but plasma estrone sulfate concentrations may remain in reference range even after the fetus has died or been aborted in late-gestation mares.[9,20] Therefore, assay of estrone sulfate concentration for predicting abortion or determining fetal health in mares in advanced pregnancy may be less reliable. Although high estrone sulfate concentrations do not guarantee fetal viability, low concentrations are a reliable indicator of fetal demise. Determination of estrogens in pregnant mares thus may yield supporting or helpful information, but normal concentrations are not definitive proof of fetal viability. Commercial laboratories offering equine reproductive endocrine testing include BET Reproductive Laboratories (1501 Bull Lea Road, Suite 102, Lexington, KY 40511-3036) and Antech Diagnostics (1-800-872-1001 [East] or 1-800-745-4725 [West]).

Ultrasonographic Imaging

Visual assessment constitutes an important part of the examination of any patient, and ultrasonographic imaging enables sensitive and early visual detection of many changes in compromised fetuses or the intrauterine environment. Imaging studies of the fetus and uteroplacental unit are an important component of fetal monitoring, because fetal and placental structures can be performed visually and noninvasively on a real-time basis. Ultrasonography can be highly informative regarding the growth and well-being of equine fetuses, because measurements and dimensions of fetal structures can be compared against standardized growth curves. There are positive linear associations between gestational age and certain biophysical variables, although the variability in these associations increases with gestational age.[21] Imaging of the fetus and uteroplacenta facilitates early detection of disease and initiation of treatment (while the foal is in utero), which in turn enhance the likelihood of survival and chance for a favorable outcome for compromised fetuses.

Fetal ultrasonography is performed transabdominally and transrectally. After approximately 90 days, the fetus resides in the abdomen, and transabdominal imaging is the most informative. Transrectal ultrasound remains the most useful throughout pregnancy for early detection of uteroplacental thickening and placental separation in the caudal portion of the chorioallantois, the area most commonly affected with placentitis from ascending infection.[22,23]

Mare Preparation

For transabdominal scanning, images of the highest quality and precision are obtained when hair on the ventral abdomen is clipped with a no. 40 blade and coupling gel is applied to clean, dry skin. In the author's practice, ultrasound examinations are often performed during winter when it is inappropriate to remove large regions of the haircoat. In this scenario, mud and matted hair are removed by bathing if necessary but hair is not typically clipped or is clipped only partially. Liberal application of rubbing alcohol in the direction of hair growth usually facilitates adequate contact between skin and transducer to obtain a diagnostic imaging study. In the early stages of gestation (60 to 90 days), the fetus occupies the caudal portion of the abdomen, just cranial to the mammary gland, where the haircoat is naturally sparse. Later in gestation, much of the ventral aspect of the abdomen, from mammary gland to xiphoid, will be occupied by the fetus and fetal fluids.

Sedation should be avoided if fetal activity is being assessed, because fetal activity and cardiac rhythm will be altered and may remain altered for longer than the period of sedation lasts in the mare after administration of xylazine hydrochloride.[24] Because of their association with fetal oxygen supply and health, overall activity level, frequency of gross and fine motor activity, and cardiac rate and responsiveness to musculoskeletal activity are important features of ultrasonographic examination. Warming the rubbing alcohol before application facilitates acceptance of the procedure in most mares, and most do not require restraint for transabdominal ultrasonography. Ultrasound coupling gel is irritating to skin, especially after clipping, and should be removed after the examination. Sedation of mares may be necessary for safe transrectal imaging to determine uteroplacental thickness and fluid appearance at the cervical star and caudal portion of the uterus.

Transducers

Transabdominal fetal assessment necessitates imaging at 20- to 30-cm depths in light horse mares, and maximum information can be obtained with a macroconvex or sector array transducer operating at 2.5 to 5.0 MHz. For assessing the uteroplacental unit, scanning at frequencies of 3.5 to 7.5 MHz is optimal. Linear-array probes can be used to image portions of the uteroplacental area and fetal heart in some mares and have the advantage of a larger contact footprint and yielding high-resolution images. Although they are not suitable for thorough fetal assessment, use of a linear transrectal probe may nevertheless yield valuable information, such as uteroplacental thickness in the fetal horn and evidence of cardiac motility, depending on transducer wavelength and the mare's body wall thickness.

Transrectal imaging with a linear array probe operating at a frequency of 5.0 to 7.5 MHz is the best means of detecting changes in the chorioallantois in the caudal portion of the uterine body and fluids in the region of the cervical star.[22] Transrectal imaging should be used in examination of mares with suspected placentitis, since the ascending route of infection from the caudal portion of the reproductive tract is most common and changes at the cervical star can be seen earliest with transrectal imaging,[10] although the interval between time of entry of infection across the cervix to appearance of uteroplacental thickening or placental separation can vary.[25]

Imaging the Fetus

The fetus can typically be found immediately cranial to the mammary gland by approximately 60 days of gestation and lies in contact with the ventral abdominal wall after 90 days.[26,27] The area in which to examine the fetus extends cranially from the pre-mammary region to the xiphoid area as pregnancy advances.[27] The mare's abdomen is examined in quadrants until the fetal presentation can be confirmed. The pregnant horn, presentation, and number of fetuses present should be recorded. The non-pregnant horn is recognizable by the tubular cross-section and chorioallantoic infolding in the absence of overlying fetal structures. Detection of twins can be done by mapping the location of two hearts or two vertebral columns, but this process is not always straightforward. By the ninth month of gestation, the fetal presentation is fixed and imaging should confirm the fetus to be lying in anterior presentation either on its back (fetal vertebral column along dam's ventral midline) or partially on its side (i.e., anterior presentation and dorsopubic position). Ultrasonographic detection of the fetus in anything other than anterior presentation after 9 months should prompt concern for dystocia at parturition.

Fetal parameters are assessed to give the examiner an estimate of fetal size, which is an index of uteroplacental sufficiency, and to reveal signs of stress or fading, which are indicators of fetal hypoxia or asphyxia. Because the size of the equine fetus prevents simple measurement of length, size is estimated on the basis of measurements of smaller structures that can be correlated to overall fetal body size. This information is useful for the practitioner because abnormally small size indicates placental insufficiency and intrauterine growth retardation, whereas detection of abnormally large size can be used to prepare for a delivery that may be complicated by dystocia. Parameters assessed for judging fetal size include maximum thoracic width, aortic diameter during systole, femoral length, parietal width, and orbital dimensions. The latter two variables are usually assessed transrectally. Fetal variables that indicate whether oxygenation is adequate are heart rate, cardiac rhythm, and variability in rate related to episodes of musculoskeletal activity; breathing movements; overall activity level, nature of movements, and muscle tone; and appearance and volume of both compartments of fetal fluids. Uteroplacental variables evaluated are thickness and integrity of contact between uterus and chorioallantois. Reference ranges have been established and described in detail for the dimensions and appearance of these uteroplacental and fetal structures in late gestation.[22,27-31]

The complexity of fetal activity increases as gestation proceeds, with movements becoming more neurologically complex and thus more sensitive to the effects of asphyxia and hypoxia with gestational age. Equine fetuses appear to be more active than human fetuses, and in late gestation, a mean of 20 complex movements per hour has been reported as consistent with a healthy fetus.[32] Impairment in oxygen supply results in progressive loss of fetal activity, beginning with the more complex movements and progressing to decreases in simpler motions. Loss of variability in heart rate, breathing movements, and overall musculoskeletal activity and fetal tone are lost in that order under conditions of hypoxia in human fetuses.[26,33] Equine fetuses have been reported to have dormant periods lasting for 10 minutes or less, although quiescent periods may last for as long as 30 to 60 minutes. Most of the time, the activity of healthy equine fetuses is such that motion is observed frequently and sometimes complicates obtaining measurements during much of the ultrasound examination. In one study,[28] a mean of 10 episodes of cardiac acceleration was observed during 10-minute observation periods, although not all fetal activity elicited a cardiac acceleration. Absence of tone or movements or the appearance of flaccidity should prompt reexamination; periods of quiescence, inactivity, and absence of movements may be seen if the fetus is sleeping, but these findings may also be indications of severe fetal asphyxia and compromise.

Heart rate and rhythm and overall fetal activity should be recorded several times during the 20 to 30 minutes that are required to perform a complete fetal examination and biophysical profiling. Imaging in M mode is useful for ascertaining the cardiac rhythm once a suitable lateral view of the thorax has been found in B mode. Many ultrasound units are equipped with software for calculating heart rate when cursors are placed at identical sites in consecutive cardiac cycles. Reference ranges for fetal heart rate have been published; in brief, heart rate in healthy equine fetuses decreases over gestation, possibly as a result of increasing parasympathetic tone,[34] from a range of 61 to 85 bpm in fetuses < 330 days to a range of 52 to 81 bpm in fetuses > 329 days.[30,35] In the last weeks of gestation, baseline heart rate should be in the range of 60 to 75 bpm, with low values in the range of 40 to 75 bpm and high values in the range of 80 to 120 bpm.[36] The fetal heart should beat in normal sinus rhythm, with episodes of acceleration associated with fetal movement. Variation in heart rate in response to activity is an indicator of normal functioning of the sympathetic and parasympathetic divisions of the fetal nervous system and integration between central and peripheral nervous activity; disappearance of variability and of periods of heart rate acceleration suggests fetal hypoxia and is an unfavorable finding. Transient accelerations in heart rate of 25 to 40 bpm above baseline should be seen during or shortly after an episode of fetal activity.[27] Gross muscle activity and corresponding accelerations in heart rate increase with gestational age to an average frequency of approximately one episode per minute in healthy late-gestation fetuses and are a favorable finding.[27,28] The effects of sedation of the mare with xylazine and detomidine include depression of fetal heart rate and activity,[24,37] and although treatment of the mare for pain (as with colic) with these agents does not appear to impair fetal health, the effects on cardiac function and fetal activity make sedation of the mare inappropriate for accurate fetal monitoring. Persistent bradycardia is an ominous finding that signals a response to fetal hypoxia, possibly via a vagal response to low oxygen concentration, whereas persistent tachycardia in the absence of muscle activity signals fetal stress.[26] Both findings may be stages in a continuum of changes in fetal response to transient or chronic hypoxia and are unfavorable. Fetal heart rate can be assessed and monitored via fetal electrocardiography,[24,27,34] Doppler ultrasonography through the transabdominal window,[27] and via real-time transrectal or transabdominal ultrasonography.[29]

Breathing motions are an important feature of fetal health and, like other muscular activity, imply that neuromuscular function is normal and oxygenation is adequate. Imaging the subtle costal movement that signifies breathing in healthy fetuses can be challenging; these movements should be quantified during 20- to 30-second trains of consecutively observed breathing cycles, but this necessitates that the fetus remain relatively still, and confirmation of fetal thoracic excursions can be difficult to impossible during periods of fetal activity. The absence of breathing motions in a late-gestation fetus, like other musculoskeletal activity, denotes fetal depression in response to hypoxia.

Allantoic and amniotic fluid volumes should be measured at the point of deepest volume. The amniotic fluid volume is typically small, compared with allantoic fluid volume, and is usually best measured from pockets of fluid imaged at the junction of the fetal neck, shoulder, and thorax.[35] Normal values for maximum amniotic fluid depth are 0.8 to 14.9 cm; for maximum allantoic fluid depth, they are 4.7 to 22.1 cm.[35] The volume of fetal fluids represents the balance between fluid formation and excretion and serves as an index of fetal oxygenation, because both formation of the fluid in the fetal lungs and kidneys and removal by fetal swallowing and excretion are dependent on fetal oxygen sufficiency. Abnormally low volumes of fetal fluids suggest chronic fetal hypoxia and a resultant decrease in renal blood flow and diuresis,[37] although intrauterine rupture of placental membranes has also been reported as a cause of low fetal fluid volume.[31] Amniotic fluid is typically more echogenic than allantoic fluid, but a change in particle density in the amniotic fluid from one examination to the next may be a more important finding than the level of density seen at any single timepoint.[26] An abrupt increase in density of free-floating particulate density in the fetal fluids can represent fetal diarrhea (a stress response to acute hypoxia), hemorrhage (as with placental separation), or infection (as with placentitis). Fetal limb movement causes swirling of fetal fluids, and the density of free-floating particles may appear to be greater when observed in association with fetal movement.

Imaging the Uterus and Placenta

Parameters that pertain to the uteroplacental unit are the combined thickness of the uterus and placenta (CTUP) and the integrity of adherence between chorion allantois and endometrium. The thickness of the uterus and placenta (i.e., uteroplacental unit) This part of the examination is facilitated by use of a shorter-frequency ultrasound transducer (e.g., 5.0-10.0 mHZ) is measured as a unit because it is usually not possible (or necessary) to determine the demarcation between a cohesive placenta and endometrium and evaluate the structures separately unless a high-resolution transducer is used. Transabdominal measurement of uteroplacental width should be taken from segments of the chorioallantois lining the gravid horn where a pocket of allantoic fluid buoys the fetus from compressing the placenta.[35] Transrectal measurements of the CTUP are made in the caudal portion of the uterine body on the ventral aspect of the chorioallantois as it courses cranially from the cervical star. Uteroplacental width should be 7 to 13 mm when viewed transabdominally. Thickening of the CTUP is associated with placental edema, detachment, or inflammatory infiltration (placentitis). Detachment of the placenta is a serious indicator of compromise. Areas of separation are manifested as pockets of anechoic fluid between placenta and uterus and should not be confused with endometrial blood vessels. A so-called ribbon candy appearance of chorioallantoic infolding may be seen where it has separated from the uterus in severe instances. Separation of chorioallantois from endometrium causes loss of microcotyledon activity, leading to a decrease in oxygen and nutrient supply. Depending on the extent and severity of placental detachment, the hypoxic insult may be acute or chronic and ongoing; detection of multiple areas of edema, separation, or detachment should prompt sequential monitoring to evaluate the fetal response to the adverse conditions. Also, if areas of placental separation progress, the owner or farm manager should be informed of the possibility of premature placental separation during parturition and a red-bag delivery. Although placental separation is occasionally severe and progressive and early termination of pregnancy may be indicated, an anecdotal maxim holds that each additional day of gestation can be prolonged means one less day in the intensive care ward. Prolonging gestation also allows for continued maturation of the fetal HPA axis, readying the fetus for birth and permitting continued ossification of cuboidal bones. Conditions such as placentitis and placental separation or edema can lead to fetal demise because the decreased perfusion impairs delivery of glucose and other nutrients and removal of waste gases in addition to reducing oxygen supply. Skill in performing this type of ultrasonography requires repetition and practice; in many if not most instances, variation in the values of these variables assessed in profiling will only be associated with normal variation in a given fetus and variation in imaging techniques between examinations or among examiners.[36] Abnormal findings during ultrasonographic imaging should be confirmed by repeat examination. In a healthy fetus, it may be impossible to observe consecutive 20- or 30-second trains of breathing motions without interruption by gross or fine musculoskeletal movements as manifestations of fetal activity and thus complete the profile. The activity level of equine fetuses tends to increase with gestational age.[26]

Biophysical Profiling

Biophysical profiling refers to assessment of a limited group of variables, among all those that could be measured, that has proven to be best associated with outcome. Indices used in biophysical profiling of human fetuses are gross body movements, tone (manifested by fine motor movements), breathing movements, a heart rate that varies appropriately with periods of motor activity, and depth of amniotic fluid pockets.[38] Use of biophysical profiling to ascertain fetal well-being in equine fetuses is imprecise, compared with its application in human obstetrics.[38,39] It has been postulated that this is likely because, even when both transrectal and transabdominal imaging are performed, only part of the uteroplacental unit can be imaged in mares. In addition, the variables measured in human fetuses are used because they have known high correlation with fetal hypoxia, but the most sensitive variables for indicating fetal hypoxia in horses may not be the same as those in humans, may vary with gestational age, and have yet to be elucidated definitively.[36]

In mares, most biophysical profiling is undertaken to aid in preserving the pregnancy and monitoring fetal well-being, but other reasons for performing biophysical monitoring include selecting a twin for fetal reduction when twin pregnancy is diagnosed in later stages of pregnancy, deciding on the nature and timing of intervention for mares with hydrops conditions, providing information necessary for binding fetal insurance coverage, and making a decision to induce parturition for fetuses residing in a hostile uterine environment.

An early biophysical profile developed for use in mares included evaluation of fetal size, heart rate, movement, placental thickness, qualitative allantoic fluid appearance, and allantoic fluid volume estimation.[28] If values for all six variables fell into reference range, the profile was considered to be negative for fetal abnormalities, but abnormal values for a single parameter yielded a positive profile, indicative of fetal abnormalities. In the study[28] that led to that biophysical profile, seven of nine mares with a negative (satisfactory) profile delivered a normal foal and seven of eight mares with a positive (unsatisfactory) profile delivered an abnormal foal, but the mares used as controls were not closely matched with case mares with regard to gestational stage. Another biophysical profile reported in 1996 was developed on the basis of data from 30 mares with complicated pregnancies.[31] Variables evaluated in that study were fetal heart rate, activity, aortic diameter, maximum fetal fluid depths, and uteroplacental thickness and contact. Variables with values in normal range are assigned 2 points, and those with abnormal values are assigned a score of 0. If the overall score is 10 or less, the foal is likely to be compromised at birth. This yields information regarding intrapartum or post-partum problems that should be anticipated, and allows for arrangements to be made for transporting the mare to a hospital for foaling and neonatal intensive care (Table 20-1).

Table 20-1 | **Normal Values for Fetal and Maternal Variables in Mares During Late Gestation**

VARIABLE	MEAN ± SD*	RANGE
FETAL HEART RATE (HR)		
Low HR < 330 days (beats/min)	70.1 ± 6.8	61 – 85
Low HR > 329 days (beats/min)	66.4 ± 8.7	52 – 81
High HR (beats/min)	92.9 ± 11	56 – 118
Range in HR (beats/min)	16.7 ± 10	1 – 40
Mean HR (beats/min)	74.6 ± 7.4	53.8 – 87.8
AORTIC DIAMETER		
Ascending aorta (mm)	22.8 ± 2.2	18 – 27
THORACIC WIDTH		
At diaphragm (cm)	18.4 ± 1.2	16.2 – 21.3
Fetal breathing		
Presence and rhythm	Present and rhythmic	
FETAL ACTIVITY		
Scale of 0 to 3[†]	1.6 ± 0.6	1 – 3
FETAL TONE		
Presence	Present	
FETAL FLUID VOLUMES		
Allantoic fluid		
Maximum depth (cm)	13.4 ± 4.4	5.5 – 22.7
Quality (0 to 3) [‡]	1.41 ± 0.7	0 – 3
Amniotic fluid		
Maximum depth (cm)	7.9 ± 3.5	2 – 14.3
Quality (0 to 3) [‡]	1.6 ± 0.6	1 – 3
UTEROPLACENTAL THICKNESS		
Maximum thickness (mm)	11.5 ± 2.4	6 – 16
Minimum thickness (mm)	7.1 ± 1.6	4 – 11
UTEROPLACENTAL CONTACT		
Vessels	Small uterine and placental vessels detected	
Continuity	Rare small areas of discontinuity	

*Standard deviation.

[†]Scale for grading fetal activity: 0, no movement; 1, small degree of activity during imaging period (fetus active ≤ 33% of the time); 2, medium degree of activity (fetus active between 33% and 66% of the time); 3, highly active (fetus active > 66% of the time).

[‡]Scale for grading character of fetal fluids: 0, no particulate matter seen; 1, small amount of echogenic debris seen; 2, moderate amount of echogenic debris seen; 3, very echogenic fluid with numerous particles seen.

Performing both endocrine assays and ultrasonographic imaging yields the most comprehensive body of information regarding fetal health and is more sensitive for detection of abnormalities than performing either modality alone. Serum concentrations of progestagens and estrogenic compounds are imprecise indicators of fetal well-being, and use of endocrine assays alone cannot prove that the fetus is healthy, even if alive, because the changes in hormone concentrations are often too precipitous to be useful as predictors.[9,26] On the other hand, visual assessment of the fetus alone, by means of ultrasonography, may likewise render incomplete information; fetal responses to adverse conditions may go unrecognized because they are subtle, the range of normal values for a given parameter can be variable, normal findings on one occasion do not guarantee that fetal health will remain unchanged until parturition, or because of factors related to the examiner's skill. For these reasons, a combination of fetal or uteroplacental factors and endocrine testing has been advocated. In one study, transrectal imaging alone used with determination of progestagen profiles led to diagnosis of a compromised fetus in 20 of 22 mares with experimentally induced ascending placentitis.[25]

Placentitis

Given the prevalence of placentitis and the fact that many cases are amenable to treatment, this condition warrants detailed description. Histologically, placentitis is characterized by infiltration of inflammatory cells into the villous and subvillous layers of the chorioallantois.[8] The pathological changes seen with placentitis in the acute stages involve infiltration of the villous tips, whereas chronic changes involve inflammatory cell infiltrates in the subvillous tissue, necrosis of villous tips, and microabscess formation. The most common pathogens isolated from placental infections at a livestock diagnostic center in central Kentucky in 1988 and 1989 were *Streptococcus zooepidemicus*, *Leptospira* spp., *Escherichia coli*, a nocardioform actinomycete bacterium, fungi, *Pseudomonas aeruginosa*, *Streptococcus equisimilis*, *Enterobacter agglomerans*,

Klebsiella pneumoniae, and α-hemolytic streptococcal species.[40] The cardinal clinical signs of placentitis are premature udder development and lactation, with vaginal discharge in some, but not all, mares. Speculum examination of pregnant mares with purulent vaginal discharge usually reveals the exudate to originate from the cervix. Most placental infections are ascending in etiology. Bacteria that invade via this route first cause inflammation of the placenta in the area of the cervical star, and this may be followed by extension of infection along the umbilical cord to the amniotic fluid, where bacteria are aspirated or swallowed by the fetus.[41] The caudal portion of the chorioallantois can be sensitively evaluated sonographically. Thickening of the ventral arm of the chorioallantois as it extends cranially from the cervix is typically observed and may be accompanied by accumulation of exudate between the chorioallantois and uterus. This portion of the chorioallantois is the most consistent for measurements of the combined thickness of the uteroplacenta to be obtained, and reference range values have been established according to stage of gestation.[10,22] In brief, the uteroplacental thickness in this segment of chorioallantois should be <8 mm from 271 to 300 days, <10 mm from 301 to 330 days, and <12 mm from 331 days to term. The uterus and placenta are measured together as the combined thickness because they cannot typically be distinguished sonographically unless placental separation is observed.

The second most common route of infection in mares with placentitis is hematogenous delivery of pathogens to the uterus and placenta. Vaginal exudate may or may not be seen with this type of placentitis, and transabdominal imaging may reveal multifocal segments of placental thickening, separation, or both. A third scenario in which bacteria enter the uterus at the time of breeding and grow slowly enough that clinical signs are not seen until later in gestation is thought to be the possible etiology of so-called nocardioform placentitis, which is caused by infection with *Crossiella equi*; this route of infection and sequence of events has not been proven, but the distribution of lesions typical with this form of placentitis suggests that the infection is delivered via neither the ascending nor hematogenous routes. Mares with this form of placentitis develop the classic signs of placentitis but typically do not have vaginal discharge. Nocardioform placentitis is associated with excessive uteroplacental thickness and accumulation of exudate in the ventral segments of uterus, at the junction of horns and body. Large volumes of exudate may be appreciable sonographically that correspond with the sticky, mucoid (vs. suppurative), brown exudate seen grossly in that area of the placenta. Placentitis caused by *C. equi* has long been a disease thought to chiefly affect mares in north-central Kentucky, but infection has been reported in Europe and was recently reported in a mare that resided in Florida.[42]

Once disease of the uteroplacental unit or fetal compromise has been detected, the goals of management are to contain infection, modulate inflammation, promote myometrial quiescence, and maintain perfusion for gas exchange and nutrient flow. Equine fetuses that develop in an inflammatory or septic uterine environment undergo early maturation of the HPA axis, which accelerates readiness for birth and enhances adaptation to post-partum life. Affected fetuses are thus often candidates for medical treatment, which should be initiated while the foal is still *in utero* and continued after birth on the basis of clinicopathologic assessment and monitoring.

Whatever the etiology or route of infection, diagnosis of placentitis should prompt treatment with broad-spectrum anti-microbials (after bacterial and fungal culture and susceptibility testing; culture for suspected nocardioform pathogens must be specifically requested, and results take longer) and anti-inflammatory drugs such as flunixin meglumine, ketoprofen, or phenylbutazone. Many practitioners initiate antimicrobial treatment with a combination of penicillin or other β-lactam drug and gentamicin, administered intravenously (except for procaine penicillin G) or intramuscularly. Parenteral treatment with this regimen is often given for 5 to7 days, followed by a change to orally administered trimethoprim-sulfa. Oral treatment should probably be continued until foaling, although the same principles that apply to any horse receiving antimicrobials with regard to colonic disturbance must be kept in mind. Treatment with supplemental progesterone or a synthetic progestagen (altrenogest; 0.088 mg/kg [0.04 mg/lb], PO, q 24 hours) is usually recommended, and some clinicians also prescribe other tocolytics, such as clenbuterol (0.8 µg/kg [0.36 µg/lb], PO, q 12 hours; for Ventipulmin, administer 0.5 ml/100 lb). Mares with placentitis appear to have altered uterine motility,[43,44] but intravenously administered clenbuterol did not delay parturition in one study involving mares with normal pregnancies.[45] Tocolytic drugs may nonetheless help maintain myometrial quiescence in the face of placental inflammation and accelerated activation of the HPA axis in a stressed fetus. Pentoxifylline (7.5 mg/kg, PO, q 12 hours), a methylxanthine drug, has also been recommended because of its actions in increasing erythrocyte deformability (and hence promoting perfusion through capillaries and its immune-modulating properties).

A positive response to treatment can be seen as a decrease in mammary engorgement and milk dripping as well as decrease or resolution of vulvar discharge. Treatment is continued until the foal is born, even if the clinical signs of vaginal discharge and precocious mammary development resolve. Clients should be warned that the likelihood of fetal sepsis is high, and the foal should undergo complete examination with blood work at birth even if the initial clinical appearance is good. Clients may elect to board the mare where attendance of the birth by trained personnel can be arranged and where prompt referral can be made to a hospital with neonatal intensive care services.

Fetal monitoring enables assessment of the severity of compromise, the fetal response to treatment, and, in some instances, may help determine that the foal's chances of survival are better outside the uterus and that the pregnancy should be terminated, by Caesarean section or induced parturition. A truism that finds ready application in all aspects of fetal monitoring is that negative findings are sensitive for indicating fetal compromise, whereas normal values for biophysical variables or maternal serum hormone concentrations do not necessarily rule out fetal illness. Nonetheless, fetal monitoring provides a substantial service to the client and greatly enhances the level of care veterinarians can provide to the horses entrusted to their care. The most comprehensive body of information that can be compiled regarding the health of a fetus under evaluation is likely best obtained by combining endocrine testing and ultrasonographic imaging.

REFERENCES

1. Giles RC, Donahue JM, Hong CB, et al: Causes of abortion, stillbirth, and perinatal death in horses: 3,527 cases (1986-1991). *J Am Vet Med Assoc* 203:1170-1175, 1993.
2. Hong CB, Donahue JM, Giles RC Jr, et al: Equine abortion and stillbirth in central Kentucky during 1988 and 1989 foaling seasons. *J Vet Diagn Invest* 5:560-566, 1993.

3. Smith KC, Blunden AS, Whitwell KE, et al: A survey of equine abortion, stillbirth, and neonatal death in the UK from 1988 to 1997. *Equine Vet J* 35:496-501, 2003.
4. Steven DH, Samuel CA: Anatomy of the placental barrier in the mare. *J Reprod Fert* 23(suppl):579-582, 1975.
5. Wilsher S, Allen WR: The effects of maternal age and parity on placental and fetal development in the mare. *Equine Vet J* 35:476-483, 2003.
6. Abd-Elnaeim MM, Leiser R, Wilsher S, et al: Structure and haemovascular aspects of placental growth throughout gestation in young and aged mares. *Placenta* 27:1103-1113, 2006.
7. Allen WR, Stewart F: Equine placentation. *Reprod Fertil Dev* 13:623-634, 2001.
8. Cottrill CM, Jeffers-Lo J, Ousey JC, et al: The placenta as a determinant of fetal well-being in normal and abnormal equine pregnancies. *J Reprod Fertil Suppl* 44:591-601, 1991.
9. Santschi EM, LeBlanc MM, Rossdale PD: Preliminary investigation of progestagen and oestrone sulphate concentrations in the serum of late-term pregnant mares during severe medical and surgical stress. *Eq Vet J Suppl* 5:62, 1988 (abstract).
10. Troedsson MHT, Renaudin CD, Zent WW, et al: Transrectal ultrasonography of the placenta in normal mares and in mares with pending abortion: a field study. Proc 43rd Annu Meeting American Association of Equine Practitioners. 1997, pp 256-258.
11. Flaminio MJ, Antczak DF: Inhibition of lymphocyte proliferation and activation: a mechanism used by equine invasive trophoblast to escape the maternal immune response. *Placenta* 26:148-159, 2005.
12. Holtan DW, Nett TM, Estergreen VL: Plasma progestagens in pregnant mares. *J Reprod Fertil Suppl* 23:419-424, 1975.
13. Schutzer WE, Holtan DW: Steroid transformations in pregnant mares: metabolism of exogenous progestins and unusual metabolic activity in vivo and in vitro. *Steroids* 61:94-99, 1996.
14. Ousey JC, Forhead AJ, Rossdale PD, et al: Ontogeny of uteroplacental progestagen production in pregnant mares during the second half of gestation. *Biol Reprod* 69:540-548, 2003.
15. Rossdale PD, Ousey JC, Cottrill CM, et al: Effects of placental pathology on maternal plasma progestagen and mammary secretion calcium concentration and on neonatal adrenocortical function in the horse. *J Reprod Fertil Suppl* 44:579-590, 1991.
16. Lester G: Maturity of the neonatal foal. *Vet Clin North Am Pract Eq Pract* 21:333-355, 2005.
17. Troedsson MHT: Placentitis. In Robinson NER, ed: *Current Therapy in Equine Medicine V*. St Louis: WB Saunders, 2003, pp 297-300.
18. Kasman LH, Hughes JP, Stabenfeldt GH, et al: Estrone sulfate concentrations as an indicator of fetal demise in horses. *Am J Vet Res* 49:184-187, 1988.
19. Hyland JH, Langsford DA: Changes in urinary and plasma oestrone sulphate concentrations after induction of foetal death in mares at 45 days of gestation. *Aust Vet J* 67:349-351, 1990.
20. Santschi EM, LeBlanc MM, Rossdale PD: Preliminary investigation of progestagen and oestrone sulphate concentrations in the serum of late pregnant mares during severe medical and surgical stress. *Equine Vet J Suppl* 5:62, 1988.
21. Renaudin CD, Gillis CL, Tarantal AF, et al: Evaluation of equine fetal growth from day 100 of gestation to parturition by ultrasonography. *J Reprod Fertil Suppl* 56:651-660, 2000.
22. Renaudin CD, Troedsson MHT, Gillis CL, et al: Ultrasonographic evaluation of the equine placenta by transrectal and transabdominal approach in the normal pregnant mare. *Theriogenology* 47:559-573, 1997.
23. Renaudin CD, Troedsson MHT, Schrenzel MD: Transrectal ultrasonographic diagnosis of ascending placentitis in the mare: a report of two cases. *Equine Vet Ed* 11:69-74, 1991.
24. Schott HC II: Assessment of fetal well-being. In McKinnon AO, Voss JL, eds: *Equine Reproduction*. Philadelphia: Lea & Febiger, 1993, pp 964-975.
25. Morris S, Kelleman AA, Stawicki RJ, et al: Transrectal ultrasonography and plasma progestin profiles identifies feto-placental compromise in mares with experimentally induced placentitis. *Theriogenology* 67:681-691, 2007.
26. Vaala WE, Sertich PL: Management strategies for mares at risk for periparturient complications. *Vet Clin North Am Eq Pract* 10:237-265, 1994.
27. Adams-Brendemuehl CS: Fetal assessment. In Koterba AM, Drummond WH, Kosch PC, eds: *Equine Clinical Neonatology*. Philadelphia: Lea & Febiger, 1990, pp 16-33.
28. Adams-Brendemuehl CS, Pipers FS: Antepartum evaluations of the equine fetus. *J Reprod Fert Supp* 35:565-573, 1987.
29. Pipers FM, Adams-Brendemuehl CS: Techniques and application of transabdominal ultrasonography in the pregnant mare. *J Am Vet Med Assoc* 185:766-771, 1984.
30. Reef VB, Vaala WE, Worth LT, et al: Transabdominal ultrasonographic evaluation of the fetus and intrauterine environment in healthy mares during late gestation. *Vet Radiol Ultrasound* 36:533-541, 1995.
31. Reef VB, Vaala WE, Worth LT, et al: Ultrasonographic assessment of fetal well-being during late gestation: development of an equine biophysical profile. *Eq Vet J* 28:200-208, 1996.
32. Fraser AF, Hastie H, Callicott RB, et al: An exploratory ultrasonic study on quantitative foetal kinesis in the horse. *Appl Anim Ethol* 1:395-404, 1975.
33. Vintzileos AM, Fleming AD, Scorza WE, et al: Relationship between fetal biophysical activities and umbilical cord blood gas values. *Am J Obstet Gynecol* 165:707-713, 1991.
34. Matsui K, Sugano S, Masayuma I, et al: Alterations in the heart rate of Thoroughbred horse, pony, and Holstein cow through pre- and postnatal stages. *Jpn J Vet Sci (Nippon Juigaku Zasshi)* 46:505-509, 1984.
35. Reef VB: Fetal ultrasonography. In Reef VB, ed: *Equine Diagnostic Ultrasound*. Philadelphia: WB Saunders, 1998, pp 425-445.
36. Palmer J: Fetal monitoring. In *Proceedings*. Equine Symp Ann Conf Soc Therio and Am Coll Therio. 2000, pp 39-43.
37. Luukkanen L, Katila T, Koskinen E: Some effects of multiple administrations of detomidine during the last trimester of equine pregnancy. *Eq Vet J* 29:400-403, 1997.
38. Manning FA, Harman CR, Morrison I, et al: Fetal assessment based on fetal biophysical profile scoring IV. An analysis of perinatal morbidity and mortality. *Am J Obstet Gynecol* 162:703-709, 1991.
39. Manning FA, Harman CR, Menticoglou S, et al: Assessment of fetal well-being with ultrasound. *Obstet Gynecol Clin North Am* 18:891-905, 1991.
40. Hong CB, Donahue JM, Giles RC Jr, et al: Etiology and pathology of equine placentitis. *J Vet Diagn Invest* 5:56-63, 1993.
41. Calderwood Mays MB, LeBlanc MM, Paccamonti D: Route of fetal infection in a model of ascending placentitis (abstract). *Theriogenology* 58:791-792, 2002.
42. Christensen BW, Roberts JF, Malgorzata AP, et al: Nocardioform placentitis with isolation of *Amycolatopsis* spp in a Florida-bred mare. *J Am Vet Med Assoc* 228:1234-1239, 2006.
43. McGlothlin JA, Lester GD, Hansen PJ, et al: Alteration in uterine contractility in mares with experimentally induced placentitis. *Reproduction* 127:57-66, 2004.
44. Hendry JM, Lester GD, Hansen PJ, et al: Patterns of uterine myoelectrical activity in reproductively normal mares in late gestation and in mares with experimentally induced ascending placentitis. *Theriogenology* 58:853-855, 2002.
45. Palmer E, Chavatte-Palmer P, Duchamp G, et al: Lack of effect of clenbuterol for delaying parturition in late pregnant mares. *Theriogenology* 58:797-799, 2002.

Infectious Problems in the Last Trimester of Pregnancy

Sara K. Lyle

Infectious processes affecting the fetus or placenta during the last trimester can lead to abortion, stillbirth, or poor neonatal outcome depending on the causative agent and the time of infection in relation to the ontogeny of the fetus. Viral, bacterial, fungal, and protozoal agents are capable of causing abortion.

VIRAL AGENTS

Equine Herpesvirus-1 (Equine Rhinopneumonitis)

Equine herpesviruses (EHVs) are ubiquitous alpha viruses that cause respiratory tract disease, abortions, neurological disease, neonatal foal death, and chorioretinopathy. EHV-1 and EHV-4 are the two most studied and clinically significant herpesviruses of horses and are closely related but genetically and antigenically distinct.[1] EHV-1 is the predominant type responsible for abortion (usually after the fifth month of gestation), although sporadic abortions have been associated with more virulent strains of EHV-4.[2,3] The increased abortigenic nature of EHV-1 is related to its tissue tropism for endothelial cells in addition to respiratory epithelial cells, neuronal cells, and lymphoid cells.[2] In contrast, most strains of EHV-4 possess tropism only for epithelial cells and neuronal cells (trigeminal ganglion), limiting their ability to produce a viremia or disease in sites other than that of the respiratory tract (e.g., uterus or spinal cord).[2] Strains of EHV-1 can vary considerably in their pathogenicity, and therefore in their abortigenic potential. EHV-1 and EHV-4 replicate in the upper respiratory tract epithelium following inhalation of aerosolized, infective nasal secretions or by direct contact (inhalation or ingestion) with infected fomites. Infected fetuses, fetal membranes, and fetal fluids are other sources of EHV-1. Following exposure, EHV-1 can enter into either lytic or latent cycles of infection. Lytic cycles of infection involve virus replication, leading to nasal shedding, abortion, or ophthalmic or neurological sequelae. Latent infection cycles result when viral DNA is translocated to the nucleus, but transcription and translation of the viral genome are blocked with the exception of the latency associated transcript (LAT) of EHV-1 in the trigeminal ganglion[4] and CD8+ leukocytes.[5] Establishment of latently infected individuals is a significant feature of the epidemiology of herpesvirus infection, establishing a potential reservoir for EHV within a herd. Viremia following initial exposure or reactivation of latently infected individuals allows translocation of the virus to the placental endothelial cells, with vasculitis being most pronounced during months 5–9 of gestation compared with month 3 of gestation.[6] With profound endometrial vasculitis, abortion can occur without fetal infection,[7] and in a survey of field cases of abortion, six of nine abortions caused by EHV-1 were "atypical" with no fetal infection.[8] Experimentally the time from exposure

to abortion ranges from 9 to 29 days[7]; however, information on the frequency of reactivation of latently infected mares following stresses (e.g., transport, herd movements, weaning, corticosteroids) and the interval to abortion is unavailable.

Abortion caused by EHV-1 is typically sporadic and occurs during the last trimester, with little or no premonitory signs. Respiratory signs are usually not a feature, either in the aborting mare or within a band of mares. Fetuses are typically delivered dead with an intact amnion, or occasionally within an intact chorioallantois. Subsequent fertility following abortion is dependent on the mare's inherent fertility, and abortion caused by EHV in the following year is rare. Neonatal EHV foal disease is the rare result of either fetal infection near term gestation or infection immediately after birth. Foals are either ill at birth, or develop severe respiratory distress within the first few days of life, with high morbidity and mortality rates.[9]

Histopathologic examination of the aborted fetus and placenta is the most common method for diagnosing abortion caused by herpesvirus. Eosinophilic intranuclear inclusion bodies in airway epithelial and hepatic cells from fetuses, and vasculitis of the placenta are characteristic findings in hematoxylin and eosin–stained specimens. Other confirmatory tests included immunohistochemistry demonstrating the expression of viral antigens in infected epithelial and endothelial cells in fixed specimens, and *in situ* hybridization techniques demonstrating the presence of viral DNA. Serology can provide surveillance information on a herd; however, unless longitudinal sampling is possible, serology does not provide confirmatory evidence of herpesvirus as the causative agent of abortion. Complement fixation (CF) tests measure IgM antibodies, which begin to rise within several days of infection. A single high CF titer would provide strong supportive evidence of a recent EHV infection; demonstration of rising CF titers in paired samples is considered diagnostic. Virus neutralization (VN) tests measure predominantly IgG antibodies, which have a later and more persistent rise following infection than do IgM antibodies. Neither CF nor VN can differentiate between EHV-1 and EHV-4; only type-specific ELISAs are able to do so. Previous vaccination further confounds the usefulness of serology in diagnosing herpesvirus abortions. Surveys of broodmares and foals have shown that the seroprevalence of EHV-4 is greater than 99% in foals and mares,[10] whereas that of EHV-1 in mares varies from 26.2%[10] to >50% at the time of foaling.[11,12] With the exception of PCR tests on peripheral blood leukocytes, most latently infected animals are negative with current diagnostic tests, making it extremely difficult to diagnose latent infection. Reactivation of latent infections does lead to positive serology.

For four decades, vaccination has been used to control EHV-1 respiratory infection and abortion. Several of the available vaccines are labeled to provide protection against abortion, and vaccination during the fifth, seventh, and ninth month is recommended. Evidence that vaccination protects against abortion is somewhat conflicting, with field studies reporting a decrease in the incidence of abortion,[13] while in an experimental challenge study the same vaccine (Pnemobort K) failed to prevent abortion or reduce viremia.[14] Management probably plays a more significant role in reducing the incidence of abortion. Recommendations include hygiene, segregation of the farm population by age, isolation of pregnant mares by similar stage of gestation, attempt to reduce stresses to mares in the last half of gestation, and quarantine of new horses onto the farm.

Equine Arteritis Virus

Equine viral arteritis (EVA) is caused by equine arteritis virus (EAV), a single-stranded, enveloped RNA arterivirus in the family Arteriviridae. It can cause influenza-like illness in adult horses, abortion, and severe respiratory disease in young foals. Edema of limbs, scrotum, mammary glands, and the periorbital region are also described; however, the disease is commonly subclinical in healthy adults.[15] The most important routes of transmission are through aerosolized infective respiratory tract secretions from acutely infected horses and venereally from infective semen (see Chapter 10), but vertical *in utero* transmission and horizontal transmission via infective fomites has also been reported.[15] Following infection of mares, geldings, and prepubertal colts, transient shedding from the respiratory tract occurred for 7–14 days and was not detectable in bodily fluids by 28 days after challenge.[16] Persistent infection and shedding in stallions occurs 30%–60% of the time[17,18] and duration of shedding can range from weeks to years.[15] Abortions have been reported to range from 3 to 10 months of gestation, and rates vary considerably from <10% to as much as 60% in field situations, suggesting that there is variation in the abortigenic potential of different strains of EAV.[15] Diagnosis in cases of acute EAV infection is by a greater than four-fold increase in titer in acute and convalescent samples (21-28–day interval). Most fetuses and placentas do not have gross or microscopic lesions, but interlobular pulmonary edema as well as vascular changes in placenta, brain, liver, and spleen have been reported.[19] Virus isolation, RT-PCR, immunohistochemistry, and fetal serology are used to diagnosis abortion caused by EAV. There is only one approved modified live vaccine (Arvac, Fort Dodge Animal Health, Fort Dodge, IA) in the United States and Canada and is safe and effective in stallions and non-pregnant mares. Animals should be kept isolated for 28 days following vaccination.

BACTERIAL AND FUNGAL AGENTS

Placentitis

Placentitis has been reported to be responsible for 9.8,[20] 19.4,[21] 24.7,[22] and 33.5%[23] of abortions, stillbirths, and perinatal losses in horses. Fifty-three percent of these losses were due to bacterial infection; *Streptococcus equi* subsp. *zooepidemicus* (*S. zooepidemicus*) was isolated in 28% of these cases.[22] Other bacteria frequently identified were *Escherichia coli, Leptospira* spp. (see below), *Crossiella equi* (Fig. 21-1), *Pseudomonas* spp., *S. equisimilis, Enterobacter* spp., *Klebsiella* spp., α-hemolytic streptococci, *Staphylococcus* spp., and *Actinobacillus* spp.[22] The discrepancy in

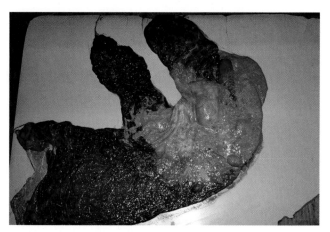

Figure 21-1. Placentitis due to *Crossiella equi*. Note that the affected portion of chorionic surface emanates from the ventral base of one uterine horn and there is copious mucoid exudate adherent to the surface of the chorion. (Courtesy Dr. Neil Williams, Livestock Disease Diagnostic Center, University of Kentucky, Lexington, KY.)

the reported incidences of placentitis lies in a considerably higher occurrence of umbilical cord problems (38.8%) in one of the survey populations,[20] compared with 4.5%[23] and 3.4%[22] in the other populations. The localization of placentitis to the cervical star was present in 95% of cases, supporting the argument that ascension of aerobic bacteria through the vagina and cervix is the most frequent route of infection.[24] Clinically, mares may have a vaginal discharge, show udder development, prenatally lactate, and deliver a premature or dead foal. The notable exception to the pattern of ascending infection through the cervix is nocardioform placentitis caused by actinomycetes. The majority of isolates have been *C. equi*,[25] although other species have been identified, including *Amycolatopsis* spp., *Streptomyces* spp., and *Cellulosimicrobium cellulans*. Most reported cases have been from Kentucky, but nocardioform placentitis has also been reported in South Africa, Florida, and Italy.[26-28] Inflammation of the chorion extends out from the cranial ventral uterine body, usually at the base of the uterine horn, with an adherent tan to brown mucoid exudate.[29] Mares occasionally have precocious udder development, but vaginal discharge is usually not observed. The majority of abortions occur during the ninth and tenth months of gestation. Interestingly, other non-nocardioform bacteria have been isolated from lesions that are grossly indistinguishable from nocardioform placentitis,[30] so perhaps the gross appearance of this form of placentitis is unique to its distribution pattern rather than to the causative agent. Nocardioform bacteria have been postulated to be introduced at insemination, then, either because of dormancy or an extremely slow-growing nature, fail to induce a placentitis until late gestation. Attempts to reproduce the disease by inoculation at breeding were not successful (Williams NM, personal communication, 2007).

Sporadic reports of fungi producing abortion include *Aspergillus fumigatus* and *Mucor* spp.,[31] *Allescheria boydii,*[32] *Histoplasma capsulatum,*[33] *Cryptococcus neoformans,*[34] and *Candida albicans.*[21] *Aspergillus* spp. are the most common isolates.[21,31] The incidence of fungal placentitis is considerably lower than that of bacterial placentitis, although grossly the lesions of the chorioallantois are indistinguishable from those produced by bacterial species. Inflammation of the chorioallantois near the cervical star and fetal emaciation as a result of *in utero* growth retardation are common features. Granulomatous pulmonary infiltrates are fairly common, but dermatitis is rare.

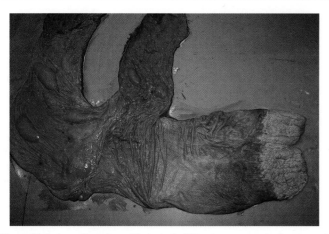

Figure 21-2. Ascending placentitis typical of *Streptococcus equi* subsp. *zooepidemicus* infection. (Courtesy Dr. Neil Williams, Livestock Disease Diagnostic Center, University of Kentucky, Lexington, KY.)

A model of the pathophysiology of ascending placentitis caused by *S. zooepidemicus* has been described,[35] wherein transcervically inoculated bacteria cross the chorioallantois, colonize the allantoic cavity, gain access to the amniotic cavity via the umbilical cord, and establish a fetal infection by either inhalation or swallowing of bacteria-laden amniotic fluid (Fig. 21-2). The resulting infection and inflammatory cascade is thought to produce observed increases in duration and intensity of uterine contractions,[36] elevated allantoic $PF_{2\alpha}$ and PGE_2,[35] increased expression of the proinflammatory cytokines interleukin-6 and interleukin-8,[37] and altered progestin profiles,[38] leading to preterm delivery of the fetal foal. Whereas the majority (14 of 16) of fetuses were delivered dead or non-viable, the remaining two foals were delivered premature (day 311 and 313), yet viable. These results suggest that acute infection is more likely to result in non-viable offspring, whereas infection of a more chronic nature may be more likely to result in precocious development *in utero*. Activation of the fetal hypothalamic-pituitary-adrenal axis (HPA), as determined by elevated amniotic cortisol and androgens, has been observed in human infants with infection-induced preterm delivery.[39] Studies examining the effect of maternally or intrafetally administered ACTH demonstrated that the equine fetal adrenal gland is relatively insensitive to precocious maturation until very late in gestation.[40-42] The fetal adrenal begins to respond to exogenous ACTH by day 304, but induced deliveries following ACTH administration at this stage of gestation were associated with poor neonatal outcomes. Pregnancies allowed to continue to spontaneous delivery had improved neonatal outcomes, and gestational length was shortened compared with controls.[41] Fetuses less than 295 days were unable to release cortisol in response to ACTH,[42] but whether *in utero* infection in the mare can accelerate the age of adrenal responsiveness is unknown. Recently, a novel minimally invasive technique for laparoscopic catheterization of the allantoic compartment of the mare was described that would allow for the determination of allantoic progestagen and cortisol concentrations and ultimately assessment of fetal HPA activation in response to transcervical inoculation of the chorioallantois.[43] Clearly there is need for further research in the area of equine fetal maturation in response to *in utero* inflammation and infection.

Mares exhibiting clinical symptoms of placentitis (vaginal discharge or premature udder development) are best monitored with transrectal and transabdominal ultrasonography (see Chapter 20). Ultrasonography is the preferred method of diagnosing placentitis and of monitoring the progression of fetal viability and placental changes. An increase in the combined thickness of the uterus and placenta (CTUP), especially with concomitant accumulation of echogenic fluid between the endometrial and chorionic surfaces (see Fig. 21-2), is characteristic of placentitis. A 5.0- to 7.5-MHz probe is positioned just cranial to the junction of the cervix and the uterine body. Small lateral movements are made until a vessel on the ventral border of the uterus is located. Several measurements are taken from the border of this vessel and the uterine wall and the allantoic surface and averaged. If serial monitoring is anticipated, it is beneficial to consistently measure the CTUP at the same distance from the cervix during each examination. Normal CTUP measurements have been established[44]; finding increases in the CTUP of >8 mm during the ninth month, >10 mm during the tenth month, and >12 mm after day 330 signals that placental failure and abortion may occur.[45] Certain circumstances can lead to CTUP values being greater than is considered normal in the absence of placentitis. Episodes of high fetal and uterine activity, especially when the fetus becomes positioned in the caudal uterine body, can produce CTUP values that are above the normal range for that stage of gestation. Apposition of the amnion with the allantois produces a slight increase in the CTUP. Edema of the chorioallantois at term is normal and simply indicates impending parturition. This change is also seen with experimentally induced placentitis in the 24 hours preceding abortion (Lyle SK, unpublished observations, 2006). Transabdominal ultrasonography is useful for assessing fetal heart rate (FHR), fetal activity, fetal position, character and depth of fetal fluids, as well as in cases of placentitis not due to ascension through cervix (e.g., nocardioform placentitis or hematogenous infection). Baseline FHRs in the last weeks of pregnancy are 60–75 bpm, with a range of 40–250 bpm. Low or high FHRs are cause for alarm if they are persistent with no accelerations or decelerations.[46]

Although amniocentesis is commonly used by physicians to diagnose chorioamnionitis in women and assess fetal maturity, allantocentesis is rarely used in cases of suspected placentitis in the mare either to document infection in the fetal fluid compartments or to ascertain readiness for birth. Lecithin:sphingomyelin ratio (L:S) and lamellar body count in amniotic fluid have been used in human medicine to predict the presence of phosphatidylglycerol, a marker for fetal lung maturity.[47] The L:S and lamellar body count in amniotic fluid in healthy equine term neonates have been measured[48]; however, neither the L:S nor the percentage phosphatidylglycerol were found to provide useful antepartum predictors of fetal maturity from day 292 to term.[49] Continued research is needed to identify reliable indicators of equine fetal maturity. In cases of hydrops, allantocentesis and amniocentesis have been used to determine whether hydrops amnion or hydrops allantois is present.[50] Although partial drainage of the allantoic compartment in mares with hydrops allantois has been used to maintain pregnancy, the risk of fetal infection is considered high.[51] Until markers for fetal maturity and for infection are identified, the use of allantocentesis in the diagnosis and management of placentitis should be undertaken with caution.

Empirical treatment for bacterial placentitis includes progestins to maintain uterine quiescence, broad-spectrum antibiotics to eliminate bacterial infection, immunomodulatory agents to reduce a proinflammatory cascade, and anti-inflammatory agents to prevent prostaglandin synthesis. Although these agents should address the basic problems of infection-induced prosta-glandin synthesis that leads to uterine contractions and fetal ex-pulsion, the efficacy of these regimens in the mare can be poor,[45] most likely because the attending veterinarian is unaware of when infection began, leading to a delay in initiating treatment. Non-human primate models of intra-amniotic group B strepto-coccal infection demonstrate that a combined therapeutic agent approach is associated with a significant delay in the onset of labor. Although maternally administered ampicillin effectively eliminated fetal infection, it was ineffective at preventing in-creases in IL-1, TNF-α, PGE_2, and $PGF_{2\alpha}$, and labor occurred sooner than in animals receiving ampicillin, dexamethasone, and indomethacin.[52] Allantoic fluid samples collected by an *in vitro* microdialysis system have been used to evaluate the ability of potassium penicillin G (22,000 IU/kg q 6 hours), gentamicin (6.6 mg/kg q 24 hours), trimethoprim-sulfamethoxazole (30 mg/kg q 12 hours), flunixin meglumine (1 mg/kg q 12 hours), and pent-oxifylline (8.5 mg/kg q 12 hours) to cross the placenta in normal pregnant pony mares. All of the antibiotics reached peak con-centrations greater than the MIC for targeted pathogenic species (*S. zooepidemicus* for penicillin, or *E. coli* or *Klebsiella* spp. for gentamicin); however, the length of time that allantoic concen-trations were above the MIC was only 3.25 hours for penicil-lin G and 4.75 hours for gentamicin.[53] Flunixin meglumine was undetectable in the allantoic fluid.[53] There was no difference in allantoic concentrations of trimethoprim sulfamethoxazole and pentoxifylline in control and experimentally infected mares.[54] Supplementation of the progestin 17α-hydroxyprogesterone was shown to reduce the incidence of spontaneous preterm delivery in women from 54.9% in the placebo group to 36.3% in the treatment group and improved postnatal outcome,[55] although this population did not include women with infective preterm delivery. The proposed mechanism of action was an inhibition of gap junction formation leading to myometrial relaxation.[56] Similarly, altrenogest (Regumate, 44 mg/day) protected 100% of mares (gestation days 93-153) treated with cloprostenol from aborting whereas only 63% of progesterone-treated (300 mg/day IM) maintained pregnancy. Based on these findings, altrenogest at a dose of 0.088 mg/kg once daily is recommended to maintain myometrial quiescence in cases of suspected or confirmed pla-centitis. Recently a long-acting progesterone formulation was found to be equally effective to altrenogest in maintaining preg-nancy following prostaglandin-induced luteolysis in mares be-tween 18 and 45 days of gestation.[57] Further studies are needed to assess the efficacy of long-acting progesterone in maintaining myometrial relaxation in cases of placentitis.

Leptospirosis

Leptospirosis is caused by motile gram-negative spirochetes, which are distributed worldwide and are probably infective to all mammalian species, including man. The taxonomy of *Lep-tospira* is complicated. Prior to 1987 only two species were identified: *L. biflexa* and *L. interrogans*, the former containing saprophytic (non-pathogenic) strains and the latter containing strains pathogenic for animals and man. Techniques such as DNA hybridization and restriction endonuclease analysis have more recently been used to determine that currently there are 18 species, 300 serovars in 30 named serogroups, and 14 unnamed serogroups.[29,58] The serovar designation is most commonly used for reporting field isolates and for describing the epide-miology of a suspected outbreak. The concept of maintenance

vs. accidental or incidental host is important to consider when determining the significance of a specific serovar's titer within an individual or herd. Maintenance hosts are mammalian spe-cies that have a commensal relationship with a pathogenic lepto-spire, producing little or no disease. Leptospires replicate within the host and produce prolonged (lifelong) urinary shedding, thereby maintaining an environmental population for infection of other maintenance hosts. Horses are proposed to be the main-tenance host for serovar Bratislava.[59] In contrast, accidental or incidental hosts are affected with disease (e.g., abortion) when infected with serovars from other species. Following infection, shedding is limited in duration once the animal is removed from the source of infection. The most common non-host–adapted se-rovars causing equine abortion in North America are kennewicki (also referred to as serovar Pomona-type kennewicki), grip-potyphosa, and hardjo; their respective maintenance hosts are skunks, raccoons, and cattle. Once infected, the horse can serve as a source of infection for other horses with non-host–adapted serovars for up to 14 weeks,[29] although direct horse-to-horse transmission is rare based on the finding that 86.7% of farms with mares aborting because of leptospirosis had only a single case per year.[60]

A generalized model of the pathogenesis of leptospirosis in animals has been described.[59] Following infection through the mucous membranes (conjunctiva, nasopharynx, genital tract) and a several-day incubation period, a subclinical bacteremic phase occurs that lasts for 2–7 days. Leptospires localize in renal tubules and in the male and female genital tract. Circulating anti-bodies appear 11–14 days after infection. Similarities of clinical disease in horses with other animals include bacteriemia, local-ization and persistence in the kidney, abortion, and excretion in uterine discharges. However, there are interesting differences in clinical findings from horses compared with other domestic animals, including no localization to the mammary gland with agalactia, no reported mare infertility, and no localization and persistence in the stallion. Abortions occur most frequently after the sixth month of gestation and are generally not accompanied by any premonitory signs. Placentas are edematous, with areas of necrosis and mucoid exudate; occasionally nodular, cystic al-lantoic masses are seen. The fetal liver is enlarged and pale to yellow, and the kidney is edematous with pale white streaks in the cortex and medulla.[61] Microscopic changes are seen most commonly in the placenta, liver, and kidney, and spirochetes can be found in the chorioallantoic stroma and villi and the renal tubules by Warthin-Starry staining (silver staining).[61,62]

Diagnosis is based on serology using the microscopic agglu-tination test (MAT) on sera from aborting dam and fetal fluids, or the demonstration of leptospires from the placenta or fetus by the fluorescent antibody test (FAT), silver staining, or dark-field microscopy. In studies from central Kentucky, MAT results from fetal fluids were both sensitive (81%) and highly specific (100%) in diagnosing abortion resulting from leptospirosis.[60] However, investigations from Ireland did not find MATs of fetal fluids to be a reliable means of confirming abortion caused by leptospirosis or in identifying the causative serovar.[63,64] The reasons for this difference are unclear. Although demonstration of an increase in a mare's MAT titer to a specific serovar following abortion should suggest the causative agent, this is not always the case. Mares frequently possess high titers to several serovars, compli-cating identification of the causative serovar.[60,65] Therefore, it is extremely important to pursue diagnostics on placental and fetal tissues and fluids when at all possible. The FAT on placental or fetal tissue is the preferred method for diagnosing leptospiral abortion. Results of FAT on fetal kidney yielded the highest sensitivity (98%) and specificity (100%), whereas placental tissue had a sensitivity of 87%.[60] Although culturing the organism is definitive for fetal infection, it is impractical and lengthy (results can take up to 6 months), and in one study only 53% of fetal kidney samples with a positive FAT yielded positive cultures.[60] Urine from mares having aborted or from infected neonates can be submitted for FAT, dark-field examination, or culture, provided this is done before antimicrobial therapy. The laboratory should be contacted before submission for recommendations on transport medium and sample handling.

Since abortion is frequently the first clinical sign of leptospiral infection, antibiotic therapy is not commonly used, and limited data are available on the efficacy of various antibiotics in horses. The most commonly recommended antibiotics are penicillin (10,000–15,000 IU/kg IM q 12 hours), oxytetracycline (5–10 mg/kg), and streptomycin (10 mg/kg IM q 12 hours).[66] Although antibiotic therapy has been proposed as a method of reducing or shortening the duration of shedding following abortion, there is little evidence that this is the case. Similarly, treatment of late gestation mares identified with rising titers resulted in delivery of clinical normal foals,[67] but without controls, it is unclear whether this was due to antibiotic therapy.

Following the diagnosis of a leptospiral abortion, several management considerations are recommended. In the face of a potential outbreak, serologic survey of the herd using the MAT to identify potential individuals at risk for impending abortion with acute exposure can be undertaken. Isolation of mares with high titers (>1:6400) to either serovars identified as abortifacient in that herd, or potentially abortifacient for that geographic locale would seem a logical step to reduce environmental contamination. However, since the majority of farms (87%) with leptospiral abortions experience only a single abortion in a given year, this may not significantly alter the pattern of abortion. Currently there is no approved vaccine against leptospirosis in horses, and although anecdotal reports of using leptospiral bacterins exist, there are no controlled data to support their efficacy. Preventing access to stagnant water and not spreading feed on the ground are two extremely important management practices that will reduce exposure to leptospires.

PARASITIC AGENTS

There have been sporadic reports in the literature of protozoal abortions resulting from *Trypanosoma evansi*, *Trypanosoma equiperdum*, *Babesia* spp., and *Neospora* spp., although the pathogenesis of abortion is largely unknown. In France, mares having recently aborted had higher titers to *Neospora caninum* than in other randomly chosen horses. *N. caninum* DNA was present in fetal brains (3 of 91), fetal hearts (2 of 77), and placenta (1 of 1). In cases where both maternal serum and fetal tissue was available, no *N. caninum* DNA was present,[68] making an association between *N. caninum* and reproductive loss open to consideration.

CONCLUSION

A wide variety of infectious agents are capable of causing abortion, some of which are contagious (EHV-1 and EAV), whereas others (placentitis) do not pose a threat to the remaining herd. General recommendations to reduce the incidence of abortion would include vaccinating mares for EHV-1, segregating pregnant mares from the remainder of the farm, isolating new arrivals for a minimum of 28 days before introduction to the herd, restricting access to stagnant water, practicing strict hygiene to avoid infective fomites, and avoiding stresses to late gestation mares. Every effort should be made to investigate the cause of each abortion in order to make appropriate recommendations to the farm owner and to avoid having a single abortion become a potential outbreak.

REFERENCES

1. Studdert MJ, Simpson T, Roizman B: Differentiation of respiratory and abortigenic isolates of equine herpesvirus 1 by restriction endonucleases. *Science* 214(4520):562-564, 1981.
2. Tearle JP, Smith KC, Platt AJ, et al: In vitro characterisation of high and low virulence isolates of equine herpesvirus-1 and -4. *Res Vet Sci* 75(1):83-86, 2003.
3. Gerst S, Borchers K, Gower SM, Smith KC: Detection of EHV-1 and EHV-4 in placental sections of naturally occurring EHV-1- and EHV-4-related abortions in the UK: Use of the placenta in diagnosis. *Eq Vet J* 35(5):430-433, 2003.
4. Baxi MK, Efstathiou S, Lawrence G, et al: The detection of latency-associated transcripts of equine herpesvirus 1 in ganglionic neurons. *J Gen Virol* 76(12):3113-3118, 1995.
5. Chesters PM, Allsop R, Purewal A, Edington N: Detection of latency-associated transcripts of equid herpesvirus 1 in equine leukocytes but not in trigeminal ganglia. *J Virol* 71(5):3437-3443, 1997.
6. Smith KC, Mumford JA, Lakhani K: A comparison of equid herpesvirus-1 (EHV-1) vascular lesions in the early versus late pregnant equine uterus. *J Comp Pathol* 114(3):231-247, 1996.
7. Smith KC, Whitwell KE, Binns MM, et al: Abortion of virologically negative foetuses following experimental challenge of pregnant pony mares with equid herpesvirus 1. *Eq Vet J* 24(4):256-259, 1992.
8. Smith KC, Whitwell KE, Blunden AS, et al: Equine herpesvirus-1 abortion: atypical cases with lesions largely or wholly restricted to the placenta. *Eq Vet J* 36(1):79-82, 2004.
9. Murray MJ, del Piero F, Jeffrey SC, et al: Neonatal equine herpesvirus type 1 infection on a Thoroughbred breeding farm. *J Vet Intern Med* 12(1):36-41, 1998.
10. Gilkerson JR, Whalley JM, Drummer HE, et al: Epidemiology of EHV-1 and EHV-4 in the mare and foal populations on a Hunter Valley stud farm: are mares the source of EHV-1 for unweaned foals? *Vet Microbiol* 68(1-2):27-34, 1999.
11. Brown JA, Mapes S, Ball BA, et al: Prevalence of equine herpesvirus-1 infection among Thoroughbreds residing on a farm on which the virus was endemic. *J Am Vet Med Assoc* 231(4):577-580, 2007.
12. Brown JA: Unpublished observations, 2007.
13. Bryans JT, Allen GP: Application of a chemically inactivated, adjuvanted vaccine to control abortigenic infection of mares by equine herpesvirus I. *Dev Biol Stand* 52:493-498, 1982.
14. Burrows R, Goodridge D, Denyer MS: Trials of an inactivated equid herpesvirus 1 vaccine: challenge with a subtype 1 virus. *Vet Rec* 114(15):369-374, 1984.
15. Timoney PJ, McCollum WH: Equine viral arteritis. *Vet Clin North Am Eq Pract* 9(2):295-309, 1993.
16. Fukunaga Y, Imagawa H, Tabuchhi E, et al: Clinical and virological findings on experimental equine viral arteritis in horses. *Bull Equine Res Inst Japan* 18:110-118, 1981.
17. Timoney PJ, McCollum WH: Equine viral arteritis: Current clinical and economic significance. In Proc 36th Annu Conv AAEP. Lexington, KY: 1990, pp 403-409.
18. Timoney PJ, McCollum WH, Murphy TW, et al: The carrier state in equine arteritis virus infection in the stallion with specific emphasis on the venereal mode of virus transmission. *J Reprod Fertil Suppl* 35:95-102, 1987.
19. Johnson B, Baldwin C, Timoney P, Ely R: Arteritis in equine fetuses aborted due to equine viral arteritis. *Vet Pathol* 28(3):248-250, 1991.
20. Smith KC, Blunden AS, Whitwell KE, et al: A survey of equine abortion, stillbirth and neonatal death in the UK from 1988 to 1997. *Eq Vet J* 35(5):496-501, 2003.

21. Hong CB, Donahue JM, Giles RC Jr, et al: Etiology and pathology of equine placentitis. *J Vet Diagn Invest* 5(1):56-63, 1993.
22. Giles RC, Donahue JM, Hong CB, et al: Causes of abortion, stillbirth, and perinatal death in horses: 3,527 cases (1986-1991). *J Am Vet Med Assoc* 203(8):1170-1175, 1993.
23. Hong CB, Donahue JM, Giles RC Jr, et al: Equine abortion and stillbirth in central Kentucky during 1988 and 1989 foaling seasons. *J Vet Diagn Invest* 5(4):560-566, 1993.
24. Whitwell KE: Infective placentitis in the mare. In Powell DG, ed: *Equine Infectious Diseases,* vol V. Lexington, KY: University Press of Kentucky, 1988, pp 172-180.
25. Donahue JM, Williams NM, Sells SF, Labeda DP: *Crossiella equi* sp. nov., isolated from equine placentas. *Int J Syst Evol Microbiol* 52(Pt 6):2169-2173, 2002.
26. Volkmann DH, Williams JH, Henton JH, et al: The first reported case of equine nocardioform placentitis in South Africa. *J S Afr Vet Assoc* 72(4):235-238, 2001.
27. Christensen BW, Roberts JF, Pozor MA, et al: Nocardioform placentitis with isolation of *Amycolatopsis* spp in a Florida-bred mare. *J Am Vet Med Assoc* 228(8):1234-1239, 2006.
28. Cattoli G, Vascellari M, Corro M, et al: First case of equine nocardioform placentitis caused by *Crossiella equi* in Europe. *Vet Rec* 154(23):730-731, 2004.
29. Donahue JM, Williams NM: Emergent causes of placentitis and abortion. *Vet Clin North Am Equine Pract* 16(3):443-456, viii, 2000.
30. Williams NM: Equine placental pathology: The common and the not so common. In *Uterine Infection in Mares & Women: A Comparative Study,* vol 2. Hilton Head, SC: Havemeyer Foundation, 2005.
31. Mahaffey LW, Adam NM: Abortions associated with mycotic lesions of the placenta in mares. *J Am Vet Med Assoc* 144:24-32, 1964.
32. Mahaffey LW, Rossdale PD: An abortion due to *Allescheria boydii* and general observations concerning mycotic abortions of mares. *Vet Rec* 77:541-545, 1965.
33. Rezabek GB, Donahue JM, Giles RC, et al: Histoplasmosis in horses. *J Comp Pathol* 109(1):47-55, 1993.
34. Petrites-Murphy MB, Robbins LA, Donahue JM, Smith B: Equine cryptococcal endometritis and placentitis with neonatal cryptococcal pneumonia. *J Vet Diagn Invest* 8(3):383-386, 1996.
35. LeBlanc MM, Brauer K, Paccamonti DL, et al: Premature delivery in ascending placentitis is associated with increased expression of placental cytokines and allantoic fluid prostaglandins E2 and F2alpha. *Theriogenology* 58:841-844, 2002.
36. McGlothlin JA, Lester GD, Hansen PJ, et al: Alteration in uterine contractility in mares with experimentally induced placentitis. *Reproduction* 127(1):57-66, 2004.
37. LeBlanc MM, Giguere S, Brauer K, et al: Premature delivery in ascending placentitis is associated with increased expression of placental cytokines and allantoic fluid prostaglandins E2 and F2alpha. *Theriogenology* 58:841-844, 2002.
38. Morris S, Kelleman AA, Stawicki RJ, et al: Transrectal ultrasonography and plasma progestin profiles identifies feto-placental compromise in mares with experimentally induced placentitis. *Theriogenology* 67(4):681-691, 2007.
39. Gravett M, Hitti J, Hess D, Eschenbach D: Intrauterine infection and preterm delivery: Evidence for activation of the fetal hypothalamic-pituitary-adrenal axis. *Am J Obstet Gynecol* 182(6):1404-1413, 2000.
40. Silver M, Fowden AL: Prepartum adrenocortical maturation in the fetal foal: responses to ACTH. *J Endocrinol* 142(3):417-425, 1994.
41. Ousey JC, Rossdale PD, Dudan FE, Fowden AL: The effects of intrafetal ACTH administration on the outcome of pregnancy in the mare. *Reprod Fertil Dev* 10(4):359-367, 1998.
42. Ousey JC, Rossdale PD, Palmer L, et al: Effects of maternally administered depot ACTH(1-24) on fetal maturation and the timing of parturition in the mare. *Eq Vet J* 32(6):489-496, 2000.
43. Lyle SK, Paccamonti DL, Hubert JD, et al: Laparoscopic placement of an indwelling catheter in the mare: Biochemical, cytologic, histologic, and microbiologic findings. *Anim Reprod Sci* 94:428-431, 2006.
44. Renaudin CD, Troedsson M, Gillis CL: Transrectal ultrasonographic evaluation of the normal equine placenta. *Eq Vet Educ* 11(2):75-76, 1999.
45. Renaudin CD, Liu IKM, Troedsson MHT, et al: Transrectal ultrasonographic diagnosis of ascending placentitis in the mare: a report of two cases. *Eq Vet Educ* 11(2):69-74, 1999.
46. Palmer JE: Fetal monitoring. In Society for Theriogenology Annual Conference. San Antonio, TX: 2000, pp 39-43.
47. Poggi SH, Spong CY, Pezzullo JC, et al: Lecithin/sphingomyelin ratio and lamellar body count. What values predict the presence of phosphatidylglycerol? *J Reprod Med* 48(5):330-334, 2003.
48. Castagnetti C, Mariella J, Serrazanetti GP, et al: Evaluation of lung maturity by amniotic fluid analysis in equine neonate. *Theriogenology* 67(9):1455-1462, 2007.
49. Williams MA, Schmidt AR, Carleton CL, et al: Amniotic fluid analysis for ante-partum foetal assessment in the horse. *Eq Vet J* 24(3):236-238, 1992.
50. Christensen BW, Troedsson MH, Murchie TA, et al: Management of hydrops amnion in a mare resulting in birth of a live foal. *J Am Vet Med Assoc* 228(8):1228-1233, 2006.
51. Bain FT, Wolfsdorf KE: Placental hydrops. In Robinson NE, ed: *Current Therapy in Equine Medicine,* vol 5. St Louis: Saunders, 2003, pp 301-302.
52. Gravett MG, Adams KM, Sadowsky DW, et al: Immunomodulators plus antibiotics delay preterm delivery after experimental intraamniotic infection in a nonhuman primate model. *Am J Obstet Gynecol* 197(5):518.e1-518.e8, 2007.
53. Murchie TA, Macpherson ML, LeBlanc MM, et al: A microdialysis model to detect drugs in the allantoic fluid of pregnant pony mares. In Proc 49th Annu Conv American Association of Equine Practitioners. New Orleans: 2003, pp 118-121.
54. Rebello S, Macpherson M, Murchie T, et al: The detection of placental drug transfer in equine allantoic fluid — Abstracts. *Theriogenology* 64(3):776-777, 2005.
55. Meis PJ, Klebanoff M, Thom E, et al: Prevention of recurrent preterm delivery by 17 alpha-hydroxyprogesterone caproate. *N Engl J Med* 348(24):2379-2385, 2003.
56. Garfield RE, Kannan MS, Daniel EE: Gap junction formation in myometrium: control by estrogens, progesterone, and prostaglandins. *Am J Physiol* 238(3):C81-89, 1980.
57. Vanderwall DK, Marquardt JL, Woods GL: Use of a compounded long-acting progesterone formulation for equine pregnancy maintenance. *J Eq Vet Sci* 27(2):62-66, 2007.
58. Human Leptospirosis: Guidance for Diagnosis, Surveillance, and Control. World Health Organization, 2003.
59. Ellis WA: Equine leptospirosis. In Eq Infect Dis VIII: Proc Eighth Inter Conf. Newmarket: R&W Publications Limited, 1999, pp 155-158.
60. Donahue JM, Smith BJ, Poonacha KB, et al: Prevalence and serovars of *Leptospira* involved in equine abortions in central Kentucky during the 1991-1993 foaling seasons. *J Vet Diagn Invest* 7(1):87-91, 1995.
61. Poonacha KB, Donahue JM, Giles RC, et al: Leptospirosis in equine fetuses, stillborn foals, and placentas. *Vet Pathol* 30(4):362-369, 1993.
62. Hodgin EC, Miller DA, Lozano F: *Leptospira* abortion in horses. *J Vet Diagn Invest* 1(4):283-287, 1989.
63. Ellis WA, O'Brien JJ: Leptospirosis in horses. In Powell DG, ed: *Equine Infectious Diseases.* Lexington, KY: University Press of Kentucky, 1988, pp 168-171.
64. Ellis WA, Bryson DG, O'Brien JJ, Neill SD: Leptospiral infection in aborted equine foetuses. *Eq Vet J* 15(4):321-324, 1983.
65. Williams DM, Smith BJ, Donahue JM, Poonacha KB: Serological and microbiological findings on 3 farms with equine leptospiral abortions. *Eq Vet J* 26(2):105-108, 1994.
66. Bernard WV: Leptospirosis. *Vet Clin North Am Eq Pract* 9(2):435-444, 1993.
67. Bernard WV, Bolin C, Riddle T, et al: Leptospiral abortion and leptospiruria in horses from the same farm. *J Am Vet Med Assoc* 202(8):1285-1286, 1993.
68. Pitel PH, Romand S, Pronost S, et al: Investigation of *Neospora* sp. antibodies in aborted mares from Normandy, France. *Vet Parasitol* 118(1-2):1-6, 2003.

PARTURITION AND EVALUATION OF THE PLACENTA

DALE PACCAMONTI

Various aspects of late gestation in the mare make horses unique among the domestic species. Gestation length is extremely variable, with the range for normal gestation length in horses encompassing a 6-week period and a reported range of delivery of normal healthy foals of 305–405 days. In no other species is the concept of "readiness for birth," as suggested by Rossdale and colleagues,[1,2] so apparent. Fetal maturation is important in timing the onset of parturition in most species, but variability is expressed in days, not weeks.

HORMONAL CHANGES

Increasing estrogens and declining progestogens at the end of gestation are characteristic of many domestic species. In horses, however, estrogens decline and progestogens rise in the last weeks of gestation, followed by a rapid decline in progestogens in the last days before delivery. Abnormal progestogen concentrations may signal placental disease (see Chapters 20 and 21). A precocious rise in progestogens is often observed with placentitis. Ousey et al.[3] reported that increased progestogens were found in mares with placentitis compared with mares with normal pregnancies, indicating increased fetal production or increased utero-placental metabolism in response to the chronic stress. Leblanc et al.[4] and Stawicki et al.[5] reported similar findings in a model of experimental placentitis. Conversely, an early decline in progestogens is usually associated with acute stress and abortion.[4]

As with many other species, fetal adrenocortical hormones increase near term, but in the horse, this change occurs only within a few days of parturition. The rise in fetal cortisol is associated with a number of changes associated with fetal maturation and readiness for birth, such as an increase in thyroid hormone, an increase in the neutrophil:lymphocyte ratio, and maturation of the fetal lung and gut. Foals delivered pre-term with precocious changes in progestogens often have concurrent precocious adrenocortical activity and have improved chances of survival.

MILK ELECTROLYTES

It is clear that a metric for fetal maturation is needed to be able to predict when parturition will occur or when intervention can be done safely. Peaker et al.[6] measured components of mammary secretions pre-partum and found that calcium rose to >10 mmol/L 1–6 days before foaling. This was followed by reports supporting the finding of a rapid pre-partum rise in calcium in mammary secretions.[7,8] Interestingly, a similar abrupt rise in calcium occurs in allantoic fluid shortly before parturition.[9] Not only does milk calcium rise rapidly, but the relative concentrations of sodium and potassium invert, with potassium concentrations becoming greater than sodium in the last few days of gestation.

Based on these characteristic changes, mammary secretions were deemed to be a very good way to assess fetal maturity or "readiness for birth."[7,8] Foals born from mares induced to foal when calcium was <10 mmol/L had a poorer chance for survival compared with foals induced when calcium was >10 mmol/L.[7,8]

Water hardness kits are useful for determining the concentration of calcium in mammary secretions.[10-12] However, the use of water hardness test kits is not without potential problems. Many kits test for divalent cations, which includes magnesium as well as calcium. Magnesium begins to increase earlier than calcium, and the rise is more gradual. Because of this slower, earlier rise in magnesium, water hardness tests that do not differentiate between magnesium and calcium complicate interpretation of results. Furthermore, the peak concentration of magnesium is reached earlier than is calcium, and magnesium often declines at parturition.[12,13] For these reasons, if a test is used to decide when to induce parturition, it is critical that the test measure only calcium. If the intent is merely to determine the likelihood of the mare foaling on a particular night, the type of test is not as important; however, those that test for only calcium will have a better predictive value.

Another potential confounding factor in the interpretation of milk calcium test results is that in the presence of placentitis or with twin pregnancy, there is often a premature rise in calcium. Elevated milk calcium before 310 days has been suggested to be an indication of an abnormal pregnancy.[14] Obtaining additional information by determining the concentration of sodium and potassium, in addition to calcium, is recommended if possible. If calcium is greater than 400 ppm, yet sodium remains greater than potassium, parturition should not be induced because a high probability of placentitis or undiagnosed twins exists.

Given that 10 mmol/L (400 ppm) calcium in mammary secretions has been well established as being a good indicator of fetal readiness for birth,[6-8,13] test results should be interpreted while keeping this standard in mind. Some manuscripts have referred to 200- or 250-ppm calcium carbonate as benchmarks for readiness for birth.[15,16] However, these values carry potential danger if used for induction of parturition. Calcium in milk is not in the form of calcium carbonate. Results from tests that measure calcium carbonate in a solution should be converted to calcium for correct interpretation. To convert ppm calcium carbonate to ppm calcium, results should be divided by 2.5 because the molecular weight of calcium carbonate is 100 and the molecular weight of calcium is 40 (100/2.5 = 40); ppm is derived by multiplying mmol × molecular weight). Therefore, 200- and 250-ppm calcium carbonate are equivalent to only 80- and 100-ppm calcium, respectively, or 2- and 2.5-mmol calcium carbonate or calcium (mmol are not dependent on molecular weight).

Mare mammary secretions usually need to be diluted before a water hardness test can be used to measure calcium. Therefore, if 1 ml of milk is diluted with 4 ml of distilled water, the test result should be multiplied by 5. As an example, a common test in the United States (Titrets, Chemetrics, Calverton, VA) is designed to measure calcium carbonate in water. If a dilution is made using 1 ml milk and 4 ml water, the test result should then be doubled to give ppm calcium.

Here is an example calculation:

$$\text{(Test result} \times 5) \text{ to correct for dilution effect}$$
$$\text{(Test result} / 2.5) \text{ to convert calcium carbonate to calcium}$$
$$\text{(Test result} \times 5 / 2.5 = \text{test result} \times 2)$$

In the manuscript using 200 ppm calcium carbonate (uncorrected results), as a predictor of foaling,[16] if the value is corrected for dilution and converted to calcium, the benchmark used is actually 560 ppm calcium, equivalent to 14 mmol/L; this is in agreement with the earlier reports.[7,8,12]

When used for estimating the likelihood of a mare foaling on a given night, milk calcium tests are more reliable for judging when a mare is not likely to foal than for predicting when she is likely to foal.[12] Of course, one reason for this is a mare's apparent ability to control when she goes into labor. It is a common observation that mares can seemingly withhold the onset of labor until surrounding conditions are suitable.[17] It is not unheard of for a mare with a milk calcium >10 mmol/L that is moved to a new environment where there is a lot of activity to not foal for days.

Another factor to consider in the interpretation of milk calcium tests is the rate of change. In general, the more rapid the rise, the more imminent is foaling. For example, a mare that has had calcium levels of 200, 195, 225, 225, 250, 250, and 500 ppm over the last week is more likely to foal that night than a mare that has had calcium levels of 200, 225, 250, 300, 325, 375, and 450 ppm. Calcium levels can also change rapidly during the day. A mare may have a milk calcium of only 300 ppm in the morning and over 700 by evening. Therefore, obtaining a milk sample for testing should be done either twice daily or late in the day.

INDUCTION OF PARTURITION

Pregnant mares with potential problems require close supervision for a successful foaling outcome. Mares with a ruptured prepubic tendon or a pelvic fracture may need assistance during delivery. Likewise, mares carrying suspected twins, or those with a history of previous dystocia, premature placental separation, or neonatal isoerythrolysis are further examples of situations in which it is prudent to have veterinary assistance available at the time of foaling. Because the length of gestation and timing of parturition are notoriously unpredictable in mares, it is difficult to ensure prompt veterinary care at the time of delivery. Induction of parturition is a means by which veterinary assistance can be guaranteed to be available at the time of delivery. In the past, induction of parturition gained a bad reputation in equine stud farm medicine because an accurate method to assess fetal maturity was not available; consequently, induction of parturition often resulted in the birth of premature foals that had a poor chance of survival.

Induction of parturition based on gestation length alone or even with the additional criteria of udder development and relaxation of the ligaments and cervix resulted in the delivery of premature foals that needed intensive care to survive and frequently died in spite of the care. With the knowledge of the changes in mammary secretion electrolytes, however, induction can now be performed safely.

The criteria to be met before induction include a minimum of 330 days gestation, colostrum in the udder, relaxation of the pelvic ligaments and cervix, and, most importantly, changes in the mammary secretions of >400 ppm (10 mmol) calcium and inversion of the Na:K ratio (K should be >Na in mammary secretions).

Because induction of parturition in mares is usually practiced when a high probability of complications or problems exists, extra precautions before beginning the procedure are warranted. Placing an intravenous catheter for the administration of oxytocin may seem unnecessary in most cases, but should complications arise that require intravenous administration of anesthetic agents or other drugs, it will prove fortunate. Similarly, preparation should be made in advance for any complications that may arise. Items such as obstetrical equipment and lubricant and supplies for neonatal care should be readied before beginning the induction procedure.

Oxytocin is the drug of choice for induction of parturition. Many dosages and routes of administration of oxytocin have been suggested for induction of parturition in mares.[18-20] Although many are effective, the guiding principle should be to mimic the natural process. The dose used is related to the intensity of parturition and the time to delivery. Therefore, a single low dose of oxytocin is preferred.[18,20] The smoothest induction is with a low dose (5–10 IU bolus IV or 10 IU in 200 ml over 15 minutes). Low doses, provided that the fetus has been determined to be "ready for birth," are sufficient to stimulate the cascade of events leading to parturition. Higher doses cause a more violent and rapid delivery. Explosive delivery is more likely to be associated with injury to the foal, such as fractured ribs, or to the mare, such as cervical trauma resulting in subsequent infertility.

A single dose of 10 IU oxytocin IV will usually result in the initiation of Stage II of parturition within 30 minutes of administration. Repeat administration is rarely necessary. Provided the criteria for readiness for birth have been met, complications are not expected. The incidence of retained placenta after induction of parturition is not increased and foal viability is normal.

Although some prostaglandin analogues are apparently safe and efficacious, they are not available in the United States. The natural $PGF_{2\alpha}$ has been associated with an increased incidence of premature placental separation and dystocia. Corticosteroids given repeatedly in high doses appear to induce precocious maturation and will shorten gestation length but are ineffective for inducing parturition within a matter of hours. Mares treated with 100 mg dexamethasone for 4 consecutive days beginning on Day 315 or 321 of gestation foaled at approximately 322 or 328 days of gestation, respectively,[21] Although foals appeared mature, they were smaller and quality of the available colostrum was poorer.[22]

CHARACTERISTICS OF PARTURITION IN MARES

Parturition is normally a very rapid process, often being completed in <20 minutes. Signs of impending parturition in the mare include udder development, observed 3–6 weeks before foaling; "waxing," or the presence of a very thick drop of sticky colostrum at the teat end, observed 1–72 hours before parturition; slight relaxation of the sacrosciatic ligaments, although this is not as evident as in cows, especially in the heavily muscled breeds like Quarterhorses; and the vulva becoming edematous and lengthening. Some mares may leak colostrum for days, to the extent that insufficient good quality colostrum is available when the foal is born.

Stage 1, the preparatory stage, is characterized by restlessness, walking, frequent urination, and sweating. The mare appears anxious while looking at her abdomen, getting up and laying down, and rolling. Most mares will rise at least once after laying down, but repeatedly getting up and down may signal a problem. The foal has an active role in its final positioning, going from a dorsopubic to a dorsosacral position. The duration of Stage 1 is usually about an hour or slightly longer, with a range of 10 minutes to 5.5 hours. Stage 1 ends with the rupture of the chorioallantois, normally at the cervical star. Rupture of the chorioallantois can be recognized by the passage of allantoic fluid, a brownish yellow, somewhat opaque-appearing fluid.

Stage 2 follows and consists of 15–30 minutes of very forceful expulsive efforts. The foal is presented in the intact amnion, a whitish membrane, which is usually seen at the vulva within 10 minutes of the rupture of the chorioallantois. A forefoot is first to appear, followed by a second forefoot approximately 6 inches behind it and then the muzzle. Delivery of the foal should progress rapidly. The long umbilical cord remains intact until the mare rises. It was once thought that significant blood flow, up to 1 L, occurred through the cord after birth, and attendees were cautioned about breaking the cord too soon. However, more recent studies have shown that there is no significant blood flow in the cord after birth and there is no difference in the PCV between foals in which the cord is broken soon after birth and those in which the cord is left intact. After delivery, the foal's navel should be disinfected with 0.5% chlorhexidine.[23] A 7% iodine (tincture of iodine) solution is associated with an increased incidence of patent urachus, and other problems because it is too harsh. Neither a 1% povidone-iodine nor 2% iodine solution were found to disinfect the umbilical stump adequately.[23]

Premature separation of the chorioallantois (or *red bag* in lay terms) is an obstetrical emergency. This can be recognized by the appearance of a red, velvety membrane at the vulva before delivery of the foal (Fig. 22-1). The chorioallantois must be ruptured immediately and delivery assisted because the foal will rapidly become hypoxic and anoxic. Clients should be made aware of this condition because if they do not take immediate action and instead await the arrival of a veterinarian, the foal will die of anoxia. Premature placental separation is associated with placentitis (the placenta is too thick to rupture at the cervical star area), fescue toxicity, twinning, inappropriate induction methods, and unknown causes. In many cases, the mare does not strain as in normal delivery and the premature separation and failure to rupture interferes with delivery. A more detailed description of placentitis is addressed in Chapters 20 and 21.

Dystocia, which means an abnormal birth, is not common in mares, but when it does occur, it can have serious consequences. Death of the foal and/or traumatic injury to the mare with a serious impact on future reproductive performance, or even death, may ensue. Prompt assessment of the cause of dystocia is important, as is relatively rapid decision-making as to the course of action. Dystocia is not usually due to feto-maternal disproportion in size, but rather to abnormalities of fetal posture, caused by the long limbs and neck of the foal, or congenital deformities such as wry neck, contracted tendons, or ankylosis of joints. Maternal causes, such as a tight vaginal-vestibular sphincter, a small vulva, or Caslick's that was not opened may also be involved. Because time is of the essence in management of dystocia, guidelines on when to intervene are important. The amnion should protrude from the vulva within 5 minutes after rupture of the chorioallantois (Fig. 22-2). As previously mentioned, appearance of the chorion at the vulva is an obstetrical emergency. After 10 minutes of strenuous labor and no sign of the fetus, a vaginal examination should be performed to determine the presentation, position, and posture of the foal. If both forefeet and the muzzle are in the canal, the mare should be allowed to continue. If strenuous contractions continue for another 10 minutes without significant progress, delivery should be assisted. Normally, the foal is an active participant in parturition. A weak or dead foal fails to assist in the process of parturition.

EVALUATION OF THE PLACENTA

Stage 3, delivery of the fetal membranes, usually occurs in <3 hours after parturition. Evaluation of the membranes should be a routine procedure after delivery. The membranes should be examined to be sure they have been passed in entirety. Retained

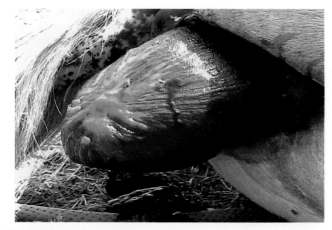

Figure 22-1. Premature separation of the placenta ("red bag"). The intact chorion is protruding from the vulva.

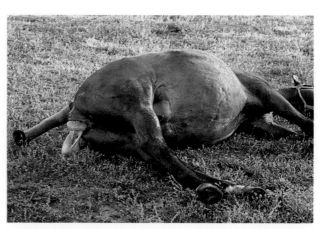

Figure 22-2. Normal parturition; the chorion has ruptured, and the amnion is protruding from the vulva.

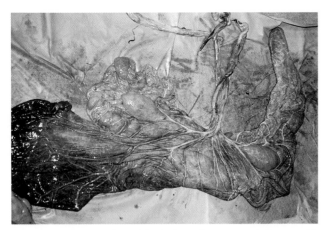

Figure 22-3. Allantoic surface of the fetal membranes passed after parturition. Usually the allantoic surface (shown on the right side of the photo) is outermost after passage, whereas the chorionic side (shown on the left side of the photo) is attached to the uterus.

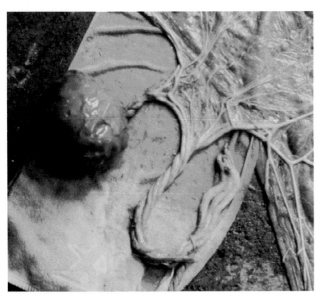

Figure 22-4. Amnion and umbilical cord with remnant of the yolk sac.

fetal membranes, most commonly in the nongravid horn, can have serious consequences such as metritis, endotoxemia, and laminitis if left unattended in a mare.

In addition, the membranes should be examined for any abnormalities (see Schlafer[24] for review). Normally, the fetal membranes are delivered inside out (i.e., with the allantoic surface outermost) (Fig. 22-3). First, the umbilical cord and amnion should be examined. The equine umbilical cord is quite long and tortuous and is normally twisted *in utero*. If umbilical torsion is suspected as the cause of stillbirth or abortion, the torsion must be accompanied by edema and congestion indicating impaired blood flow. A brownish, spherical hard object is occasionally observed (Fig. 22-5). Mistakenly referred to as an amorphous globosus or anomalous twin, this structure is actually the calcified remnant of the yolk sac. Meconium staining of the amnion is an indication of *in utero* fetal stress.

Next, the allantoic surface should be examined and then the placenta everted so the chorionic surface is now outermost. Typically, the fetal membranes are laid out in the shape of an F with the area of the uterine body corresponding to the vertical part of

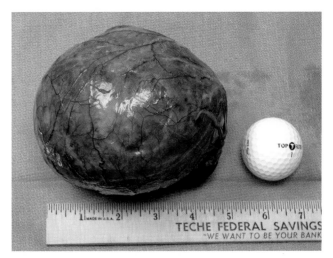

Figure 22-5. Calcified remnant of the yolk sac.

the F and the uterine horns to the horizontal arms (Fig. 22-3). Because normal chorionic epithelium develops when in apposition to normal endometrial epithelium, abnormalities observed in the chorion may be an indication of abnormal endometrium. The chorionic surface should be examined for areas of hypoplastic or aplastic villi. The chorion apposing the areas where the endometrial cups were located at the base of the gravid horn may be observed as areas lacking chorionic villi. Another area commonly lacking villi on the chorionic surface is the location of the umbilical attachment, usually at the base of the gravid horn, where the chorion may have been folded inward slightly, thus not in contact with the endometrium. In addition, the chorion in contact with the internal cervical os will lack villi, forming an area commonly referred to as the "cervical star" because of its stellate pattern. Areas of hypoplastic or aplastic villi may indicate endometrial pathology and warrant further investigation, especially in a mare that was difficult to get in foal or that had an abnormally long gestation.

The chorionic surface should be inspected closely for signs of placentitis, including discoloration, exudates, or abnormal thickening. If the placentitis is an ascending infection through the cervix, a thickened area extending from the cervical star will be evident. The affected portion of the placenta will be thickened and discolored, and the villi will be blunted. It may be covered with an exudate. Any abnormal areas may be a forewarning of septicemia of the foal. If indications of placentitis are detected at the time of delivery of the fetal membranes, treatment of the foal can be initiated immediately, before the foal begins to show signs of clinical illness. The initiation of early treatment may make the difference in success or failure of treatment. A more detailed description of the newborn is found in Chapter 23.

REFERENCES

1. Rossdale PD, Silver M: The concept of readiness for birth. *J Reprod Fertil Suppl* 32:507, 1982.
2. Rossdale PD, Ousey JC, Chavatte P: Readiness for birth: an endocrinological duet between fetal foal and mare. *Eq Vet J Suppl* 24:96, 1997.
3. Ousey JC, Houghton E, Grainger L, et al: Progestagen profiles during the last trimester of gestation in Thoroughbred mares with normal or compromised pregnancies. *Theriogenology* 63:1844, 2005.
4. LeBlanc MM, Macpherson M, Sheerin P: Ascending placentitis: What we know about pathophysiology, diagnosis, and treatment. *Proc Am Assoc Eq Pract* 50:127, 2004.

5. Stawicki RJ, Ruebel H, Hansen PJ, et al: Endocrinological findings in an experimental model of ascending placentitis in the mare. *Theriogenology* 58:849, 2002.
6. Peaker M, Rossdale PD, Forsyth IA, Falk M: Changes in mammary development and the composition of secretion during late pregnancy in the mare. *J Reprod Fertil Suppl* 27:555, 1979.
7. Ousey JC, Dudan F, Rossdale PD: Preliminary studies of mammary secretions in the mare to assess foetal readiness for birth. *Eq Vet J* 16:259, 1984.
8. Leadon DP, Jeffcott LB, Rossdale PD: Mammary secretions in normal spontaneous and induced premature parturition in the mare. *Eq Vet J* 16:256, 1984.
9. Paccamonti D, Swiderski C, Marx B, et al: Electrolytes and biochemical enzymes in amniotic and allantoic fluid of the equine fetus during late gestation. *Biol Reprod Mono* 1:39, 1995.
10. Camillo F, Cela M, Romagnoli S, et al: Day-time management of the foaling mare: Use of a rapid mammary Ca++ determination followed by a low dose of oxytocin. *Proc Intl Cong Anim Reprod* 2:883, 1992.
11. Cash RSG, Ousey JC, Rossdale PD: Rapid strip test method to assist management of foaling mares. *Eq Vet J* 17:61, 1985.
12. Ousey JC, Delclaux M, Rossdale PD: Evaluation of three strip tests for measuring electrolytes in mares' pre-partum mammary secretions and for predicting parturition. *Eq Vet J* 21:196, 1989.
13. Rook JS, Braselton WE, Nachreiner RF, et al: Multielement assay of mammary secretions and sera from periparturient mares by inductively-coupled argon plasma emission-spectroscopy. *Am J Vet Res* 58:376, 1997.
14. Rossdale PD, Ousey JC, Cottrill CM, et al: Effects of placental pathology on maternal plasma progestagen and mammary secretion calcium concentrations and on neonatal adrenocortical function in the horse. *J Reprod Fertil Suppl* 44:579, 1991.
15. Ley WB, Hoffman JL, Meacham TN, et al: Daytime management of the mare. 1: Pre-foaling mammary secretions testing. *J Eq Vet Sci* 9:88, 1989.
16. Ley WB, Bowen JM, Purswell BJ, et al: The sensitivity, specificity and predictive value of measuring calcium-carbonate in mares prepartum mammary secretions. *Theriogenology* 40:189, 1993.
17. Newcombe JR, Nout YS: Apparent effect of management on the hour of parturition in mares. *Vet Rec* 142:221, 1998.
18. Camillo F, Marmorini P, Romagnoli S, et al: Clinical studies on daily low dose oxytocin in mares at term. *Eq Vet J* 32:307, 2000.
19. Macpherson ML, Chaffin MK, Carroll GL, et al: 3 Methods of oxytocin-induced parturition and their effects on foals. *J Am Vet Med Assoc* 210:799, 1997.
20. Paccamonti DL: Elective termination of pregnancy in mares. *J Am Vet Med Assoc* 198:683, 1991.
21. Alm C, Sullivan JJ, First NL: Induction of premature parturition by parenteral administration of dexamethasone in the mare. *J Am Vet Med Assoc* 165:721, 1974.
22. Ousey JC, Kolling M, Allen WR: The effects of maternal dexamethasone treatment on gestation length and foal maturation in Thoroughbred mares. *Anim Reprod Sci* 94:436, 2006.
23. Lavan RP, Madigan JE, Walker R, Muller N: Effects of disinfectant treatments on the bacterial flora of the umbilicus of neonatal foals. *Biol Reprod Mono* 1:77, 1995.
24. Schlafer DH: Postmortem examination of the equine placenta, fetus and neonate: methods and interpretation of findings. *Proc Am Assoc Eq Pract* 50:144, 2004.

THE NEWBORN FOAL

Chapter 23

Deborah A. Parsons

The goal of any breeding program is a healthy, vibrant foal. After all the care taken to get the mare in foal and to maintain the pregnancy, proper attention to the management and care of the neonatal foal is imperative for a successful outcome. The majority of foalings are not attended by a veterinarian; this makes the experience and knowledge of caretakers (owner, groom, etc.) crucial to success. The more experienced the caretaker, the more likely he or she will be able to recognize problems early and will be better equipped to handle problems that occur. It will be the caretaker's responsibility to determine when help and intervention are needed. Every normal foal should have a veterinary examination within the first 12–24 hours post-partum. In order to recognize abnormalities, it is important to know the normal condition and behavior of the neonatal foal.

A normal healthy full-term foal should be energetic and the following events should occur post-partum (Box 23-1). Foals are usually able to obtain sternal recumbency within about 5 minutes of birth. They should have a strong suckle reflex within 20 minutes and stand within an hour (range:15–165 minutes). They usually start to make attempts to stand within 15–30 minutes, but occasionally a normal foal may take as long as 2 hours to successfully get and stay standing and nurse. The first few attempts to stand may be uncoordinated and aimless, but they should figure it out with minimal assistance. The longer it takes, the greater the chance there is a problem with the foal and veterinary assistance will be required. If the foal has not suckled within 4 hours, it should be considered abnormal. Anything that varies from these guidelines should be considered abnormal and veterinary care should be sought prior to the routine veterinary check. The chance of a positive outcome increases the sooner veterinary intervention is made.

RISK ASSESSMENT

The use of risk categories can improve the outcome of serious complications in neonatal foals by allowing for early monitoring, assessment, and intervention. These categories can be used to guide management practices and determine the amount of intervention needed and the need for the presence of a veterinarian at the time of parturition. The three-category system (low, moderate, and high risk) has been used successfully.[1-3] A two-category system has also been suggested that eliminates the moderate category and therefore allows more foals to be classified as high risk and receive more attention.[4] In determining the risk category of the foal, several factors are assessed, including the mare's reproductive history, maternal conditions during the pregnancy, ease of birth, management and environmental factors, and the foal's condition (Table 23-1). The risk category of the foal can be changed at any stage such that a foal that was considered "low risk" pre-partum suddenly becomes a "high risk" foal if a dystocia is encountered, or the foal is found to have an abnormality on assessment.

If the foal has only one factor in the high-risk group, it is classified as "moderate risk." Foals classified as a "high-risk" pre-partum can be decreased to moderate if the parturition is normal and the foal appears clinically normal. Increased observation is still warranted and many recommend placing these foals on broad-spectrum antibiotics with a good gram-negative spectrum (e.g., ceftiofur) for the first 48–72 hours of life.[1] Serial blood work should be performed in these foals over the first week of life. This would include testing for passive transfer of immunoglobulins (IgG), a complete blood count, and biochemistry profile. The foals should be monitored closely for energy, suckling, and weight gain. "Low-risk" foals are those with no identifiable abnormalities in any category and are basically normal foals in all regards.

Maternal factors include a combination of historical data regarding reproductive history, such as uterine infection, previous foalings, and illness of the mare during the pregnancy. Maternal risk factors include any factor that may interfere with the development or nourishment of the foal *in utero* or that interferes with the mare's ability to supply an adequate amount of good quality colostrum.[1,5] Examples of such conditions would include prior foals with neonatal isoerythrolysis (NI), hypoxic ischemic encephalopathy, dysmaturity, congenital defects, or poor-performance of undetermined cause, prior dystocias, twin pregnancies, premature lactation, or illness in the mare, among other things. Placental abnormalities such as placentitis, edema, or other placental irregularities can be identified pre-partum via ultrasound examination or post-partum by examination of the placenta, and they will increase the risk for the foal. Foals that are determined pre-partum to be at a "high risk" may be foaled out at a center that provides close monitoring and immediate veterinary attention at the time of parturition.

Box 23-1 | Normal Post-Partum Foal Events

Sternal in 1–2 minutes
Standing within 15 minutes to 2 hours
Nursing 35 minutes to 4 hours
Consider the foal abnormal if it has not stood and suckled in 4 hours.

Even though a mare and her gestation had seemed normal, any problems with the parturition process affect the foal's risk category by potentially altering blood flow or causing direct trauma to the foal.[1,5] Some of the conditions affecting the foal may be very obvious, such as dystocia, whereas others may be more subtle or unobserved. Any foal resulting from an unobserved delivery should be treated as "high risk" until determined otherwise. The same holds true for premature deliveries, premature placental separation, cesarean sections, or induced parturitions.

If obvious abnormalities with the foal's appearance or behavior are observed, the appropriate measures should be taken. Some foal factors that will result in a "high-risk" classification include congenital abnormalities, meconium aspiration, prematurity/dysmaturity, and failure of passive transfer (FPT). The environment that the foal is born into is also important in the risk of disease. If the environmental conditions are less than optimal, in terms of hygiene, climate, pathogen exposure, or the lack of observation, then the foal should be considered at higher risk of illness, especially sepsis.

INITIAL FOAL ASSESSMENT

All those attending foalings should be instructed on how to perform an immediate post-partum evaluation of the foal using the APGAR scoring system described in Table 23-2, or some modification thereof, to assist with recognition of early signs

Table 23-1 | **Risk Assessment**

MARE FACTORS	PLACENTAL FACTORS	PARTURITION FACTORS	FOAL FACTORS	MANAGEMENT FACTORS
Prior foals with neonatal isoerythrolysis, hypoxic ischemic encephalopathy, dysmaturity, congenital defects	Placentitis	Dystocia	Congenital abnormalities	Dirty foaling stall
Previous dystocia	Placental edema	Prematurity	Meconium staining	Cold, wet conditions
Vaginal discharge	Placental infarction	Prolonged gestation	Prematurity/dysmaturity	In foaling unit
Poor body condition		Premature placental separation	Small for gestational age	Suckling from a dirty mare
Poor pelvic or perineal conformation		Induced parturition	Twins	Infectious disease on farm
Twin pregnancy		Early cord rupture	Orphan foal	Excessive intervention in foaling
Prolonged pregnancy		Cesarean section	Trauma	Unobserved foaling
Premature lactation and loss of colostrum			Delayed ingestion of colostrum	Transport of mare to facility <4 weeks pre-partum
Agalactia			Failure of passive transfer	
Long transport within 1 month of parturition			Abnormal behavior post-partum	
Pyrexia			Not standing and suckling >4 hours	
Illness or injury				
Surgery or anesthesia				
Uterine torsion				
Hydrops				
Cesarean section				

Table 23-2 | **APGAR Scoring System**

PARAMETER	0 POINTS	1 POINT	2 POINTS
Appearance	Grey/blue mucous membranes	Pale pink mucous membranes	Pink mucous membranes
Pulse	Absent	<60, irregular	>60, regular
Grimace			
Nasal stimulation	No response	Grimace	Strong grimace, sneeze
Ear tickle	No response	Head/neck motion	Ear movement, head shaking
Thoracolumbar stimulation	No response	Head/neck motion	Attempt to stand with head, neck & limb motion
Attitude (muscle tone)	Limp, lateral recumbency	Semi-sternal, some limb flexion	Sternal
Respiration	Absent	<30, irregular	>30, regular, able to whinny

of problems and to determine the need for additional assistance and intervention.[3] This scoring is easy to perform even by inexperienced staff and should be obtained within the first 10–15 minutes post-partum. Each parameter is scored from 0 to 2. An optimal total score is 10, with normal foals usually scoring 9 or 10. Foals that score between 6 and 8 are usually considered to have mild asphyxia and may improve with stimulation by rubbing the core and limb manipulation. Assisting the foal into sternal recumbency may also be of benefit. Foals that score between 3 and 5 usually require oxygen therapy and cardiovascular support in addition to stimulation and placement in sternal recumbency. Preparations for intervention with respiratory and cardiovascular resuscitation should also be made. Aggressive therapy is usually required for foals that score <3, since full resuscitation is usually required.[3]

Foals that are considered "high risk" or that have questionable APGAR scores should be evaluated regularly over the first hour. If the foal is considered normal in all accounts and the foal has stood and suckled in the normal amount of time, they can be left undisturbed. Even though a foal has a normal APGAR score, this does not preclude a thorough veterinary examination within the first day of life (preferably 12–18 hours of age).

Vital Parameters

There are many immediate post-partum changes that will affect the foal's physical examination findings (Table 23-3). Most of these changes are due to accommodation of the cardiovascular and respiratory systems to life outside of the uterus. The pulse (HR) should be 40–80 bpm soon after birth and then increase to >100 bpm within the first hour of life. This increase usually coincides with the foal attempting to stand. It should take its first breath rather quickly after delivery, usually within the first 30 seconds. There may be an initial series of gasps that quickly change to a more normal breathing pattern. The respiratory rate (RR) should be >30 breaths/min and shallow just after birth. A slow RR is of more concern than a more rapid rate and may indicate the need for intervention and possible resuscitation.

Foals should also be monitored for urine production. Colts usually first urinate within the first 5–6 hours whereas fillies can take as long as 10–11 hours. If they are suckling normally, they will then void diluted urine frequently. Not considered by the APGAR scoring system, but still quite relevant to the health of the foal, is the rectal temperature. The most likely detrimental situation with a neonatal foal is hypothermia (<37°C). This may occur due to ambient temperature or circulatory deficiencies in the foal. Therefore, a climate-controlled environment is important and attempts should be made to warm these foals. Hyperthermia may occur due to sepsis but is also commonly associated

with a high ambient temperature or as a result of the energy expended while attempting to stand. Should there be any alterations in the normal temperature, the foals should be considered at greater risk and monitored appropriately.

Prematurity/Dysmaturity

An assessment of the foal's readiness for birth is also important in its initial assessment. Caretakers should be familiar with the signs of prematurity/dysmaturity as described in Box 23-2 in order to address the problems and potential complications that these foals may encounter. Prematurity should be assessed in each foal with a combination of the clinical appearance of the foal and the length of gestation. The presence of such signs warrants that the foal be treated as a "high-risk" foal and should be examined by a veterinarian before the routinely scheduled examination. Problems with premature/dysmature foals may include a variety of respiratory, metabolic, and infectious diseases.

The definition of prematurity is any foal that is born <320 days of gestation and appears clinically immature. The gestational length should really be only one of several criteria used to define a premature foal. As well as having its limits in identifying prematurity, gestational age is a poor indication of a foal's readiness for birth. A dysmature foal is generally considered to be a foal that is normal in terms of gestational age but immature in terms of size and physical appearance. The term *immaturity* is used to describe clinical signs despite the gestational age, whether it be premature or of the correct gestational age. These foals are not entirely ready for birth and may have difficulty maintaining homeostasis.

Foals with a body size that is too small for their gestational age have usually experienced some type of chronic derangement during gestation that interrupts the normal growth patterns *in utero,* resulting in intrauterine growth retardation. Such derangements would include *in utero* infections, twins, malnutrition, placentitis, severe uterine fibrosis, or other maternal illnesses. Symmetrical retardation results in all body parts proportionately decreased in size. This is thought to be due to diseases that inhibit mitosis, such as viral infections and prolonged compromise in the nutrient supply. Asymmetrical retardation is characterized by visceral and fat wasting with a relative preservation of fetal length and head circumference. This is most commonly due to uteroplacental vascular insufficiency late in gestation, sparing brain growth. Some of these small-for-gestational-age foals may actually exhibit more readiness for birth because of maturation of the adrenal glands with the chronic stress that results in normal cortisol levels and lung maturation at birth.

Premature/dysmature foals are usually smaller than would be expected and general weakness causes abnormally long times to

Table 23-3 | Neonatal Vital Parameters

	IMMEDIATELY POST-PARTUM	SEVERAL HOURS POST-PARTUM	FIRST WEEK POST-PARTUM
Temperature (°F)	99–102		
Heart rate	40–80	120–150	80–100
Respiratory rate	60–80	20–40	20–40
Urination	Colts: 5–6 hr Fillies: 10–11 hr		

Box 23-2 | Signs of Prematurity/Dysmaturity

Gestational age <320 days	Joint laxity
Low birth weight	Reduced body temperature
Soft lips	Respiratory distress syndrome
Incomplete ossification	Short, silky hair coat
Decreased suckle reflex	Bulging eyes
Abnormal behavior	Floppy ears
General weakness	Flexor tendon laxity
Domed forehead	Intolerance to oral feeding
Deep red tongue	

stand and suckle, if they ever do get up. A combination of factors might contribute to their weakness (e.g., immature musculoskeletal system, hypoglycemia). They usually also have a decreased suckle reflex, which further increases the chances of FPT. Care must be taken with feeding immature foals, especially when they are being fed by feeding tube, since they tend to be more intolerant to enteral feeding. The cause of this is not completely understood but may be due to immaturity of the enterocytes leading to maldigestion and malabsorption. This may affect the foal's ability to obtain adequate passive transfer, even if an adequate amount of good-quality colostrum has been fed by a nasogastric tube.

Immaturity in the musculoskeletal system includes joint laxity, flexor tendon laxity, and incomplete ossification of the cuboidal bones of the carpus and tarsus. Immature foals have a characteristic short, silky hair coat (Fig. 23-1). The hair matures from cranial to caudal and therefore the hair over the back and rear quarters will be the most immature. They can have a domed forehead, bulging eyes, soft lips, a deep red tongue, and floppy ears (Fig. 23-2). Immature foals will frequently have altered thermoregulation, so extra nursing care is required to prevent hypothermia (Fig. 23-3).

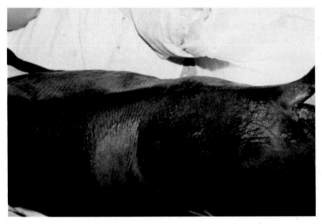

Figure 23-1. Short, silky hair coat of premature foal. (Courtesy Dr. Keith Chaffin)

POST-PARTUM CARE

Resuscitation

Any facility that is foaling a considerable number of mares should be equipped and have staff available that is trained in foal resuscitation. This is especially important if "high-risk" pregnancies are foaling in the facility. A veterinarian should be present for the delivery of "high-risk" foals and should be prepared to perform resuscitation as needed. Of course any facility that is considering delivering foals by cesarean section should be fully prepared for resuscitation and care of a severely compromised foal. Cesarean sections hold many potential complications for both the mare and the foal. The foal is subjected to the depressive effects of the anesthetics used in addition to a high incidence of hypoxia. They will not have many of the natural events of a normal delivery that assist in the transition from intrauterine to extra-uterine life. The action of compressing the foal through the pelvic canal expresses some of the amniotic fluid out of the lungs. The umbilical cord will be clamped, which brings about the concerns over the loss of blood and the increased risk of umbilical infection and patent urachus.

There are many causes of asphyxia in the foal, including maternal issues (e.g., systemic disease, hypotension, general anesthesia), placental abnormalities (e.g., placentitis, placental insufficiency), or fetal diseases (e.g., immaturity, infection, cardiac disease, umbilical cord compression). In addition, the delivery itself may be associated with asphyxia caused by dystocia, premature placental separation, or inappropriate positioning of the mare for delivery. When confronted with a lack of oxygen, the foal can start to breath *in utero,* which will result in complications such as meconium aspiration and reversion back to the fetal circulation. This will result in apnea when the foal is born. Resuscitation is required for any foals that are apneic or experiencing very low RRs (<10 breaths/min) or are gasping. Resuscitation is also in order should the pulse be absent or the foal flaccid and non-responsive. A prepared kit should be easily accessible that contains all that is required to allow for resuscitation (Box 23-3).

The approach to resuscitation should include a thorough assessment of the foal, followed by clearing of the airways. If the foal has just been delivered, the amniotic membranes must be removed from the nostrils. Any secretions in the airways should

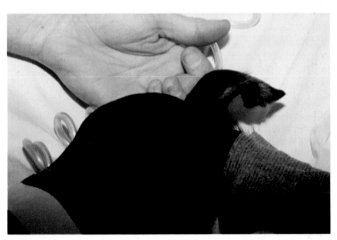

Figure 23-2. Floppy ears of premature foal. (Courtesy Dr. Keith Chaffin)

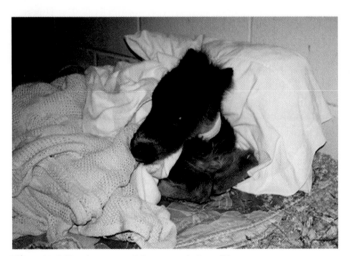

Figure 23-3. Nursing care and thermoregulation of the neonate.

be removed by positioning the head down, gentle pressure on the chest, and suctioning of the fluid from the nasal passages and pharynx. Attempts should be made to stimulate the foal to breathe by rubbing the foal briskly with towels, tickling the nasal mucosa or ear canal, flexing the limbs, or gently compressing the chest wall. The controversial use of doxapram (0.5 mg/kg IV) may be attempted. If a veterinarian or trained staff is present, the foal should be intubated (7-9–mm nasotracheal tube). Alternatively, a mask can be used to administer oxygen and breaths safely. Positive-pressure ventilation can be administered with the use of several devices. Care must be taken when using an Ambubag since a full compression is about 1 L, which would be too much for most foals. With 100% oxygen attached to the system, the inspired air has about 21% oxygen. Another easy-to-use device that can be used with or without oxygen is the C.D. Foal Resuscitator (Fig. 23-4). This unit contains two plastic cylinders that draw air through the induction valves and then expel it to the foal via a face mask. It has a bi-directional mask that allows the foal to exhale without removing the mask. It also has an adapter so that it can be used to aspirate fluid from the airways before resuscitation. If no units are available, positive-pressure ventilation can also be achieved by mouth-to-tube/nostril. If a demand valve is used in a clinic setting, care must be taken not to apply too much pressure. A breath should be administered just long enough to see the chest start to rise before being released immediately.

In addition to addressing respiration, resuscitation should also involve improvement of the foal's circulation. External chest

---

Box 23-3 | Foal Resuscitation Kit

Oxygen
Face mask for oxygen administration
Ambu resuscitator or C.D. Foal Resuscitator
Endotracheal tubes (7 and 9 mm); include 30-ml syringe for the cuff
Tracheostomy tube; surgical instruments for performing tracheostomy
Oxygen tubing
Intravenous catheters
Disinfecting scrub
Resuscitation drugs: epinephrine, doxapram, atropine, dobutamine, lidocaine, dexamethasone, furosemide, sodium bicarbonate, mannitol, lactated Ringer's solution with 5% dextrose, dextran 70, hypertonic saline
Needles and syringes

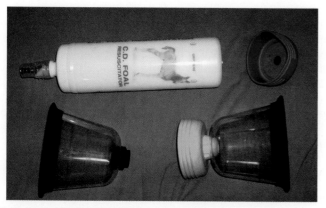

Figure 23-4. C.D. Foal Resuscitator. (Courtesy Dr. Sylvia Hall-Andrews.)

---

compressions should be administered 60–120 times each minute. The pulse and color of the mucous membranes should be re-evaluated frequently. If there is no improvement, intravenous fluids should be administered (lactated Ringer's solution with 5% dextrose, 7.5% hypertonic saline, Dextran, etc.). If this also fails to correct the situation, the administration of vasoconstrictors should be considered, along with the application of abdominal counter pressure or intermittent abdominal compressions.

Umbilical Care

The umbilicus usually ruptures within 6–8 minutes of birth about 3–5 cm from the body wall. Concern over premature rupture of the chord and the loss of blood were not clinically significant.[6] Using umbilical clamps can increase the chances of urachal and umbilical infections. The stump should be treated as soon as possible after the chord has ruptured. The use of chlorhexidine (0.5%) solution is preferred and appears to be superior to 2% iodine or povidone-iodine in decreasing the incidence of umbilical infection.[1,7] The stump should be treated every 6 hours for the first 24 hours and then continued based on need (e.g., recumbent foals may require prolonged treatment). The use of 7% iodine is discouraged since it is too caustic and can cause necrosis of the surrounding skin predisposing the foal to infections and patent urachus. The powdered preparations do not likely penetrate into pits in the skin and are not as effective as a solution. Therefore, dipping the stump into the solution is preferable. Solutions should not be used on multiple foals; each foal should have its own dip. To make the chlorhexidine solution add 1 part 2% chlorhexidine solution to 3 parts sterile water. This solution will not dry up the stump as quick as the iodine solutions. If more desiccation is desired, a small amount of alcohol can be added to the mixture (about 10% of the total volume).

Prophylactic Enemas

Meconium is the first feces that the foal must pass and is usually dark, firm, and pellet like. It can also appear as tarry, soft, sticky feces that can vary from dark brown to green. It is made up of digested amniotic fluid, mucus, epithelial cells, and bile. Should it be passed *in utero,* it is an indicator of fetal stress and the risk of pneumonia resulting from meconium aspiration is great and these foals should be treated as "high-risk" foals. All the meconium should normally be passed within 24 hours post-partum. The majority of foals pass it within 4 hours. Once the yellow milk feces are passed, the meconium can be deemed completely eliminated from the intestinal tract. Meconium impactions are the most common cause of colic in neonatal foals, and colts have a higher incidence than fillies, especially when considering impactions in the pelvic inlet.[1] Foals that have had prolonged gestations tend to have a higher incidence of meconium impactions.

Colostrum stimulates gastrointestinal motility and has some laxative properties. The act of suckling itself also stimulates gastrointestinal motility. Prophylactic enemas can be given to the foal soon after birth. The most frequently used are 100–120 ml of phosphate-buffered solution (Fleet) or mild soapy water. It is important for the caretaker to know how to administer the enema and how much and how frequently it may be given to avoid negative potential side effects. A precautionary measure is to leave instructions for the caretakers to administer the enema only once; if the foal fails to pass all the meconium or is showing signs of colic or straining, veterinary assistance should be sought. Veterinarians should use a soft tube when administering enemas while being careful not to irritate or rupture the rectum. Repeated enemas can cause mucosal irritation and may result in hemorrhage and edema that will then result in more straining and possibly further exacerbating the impaction. This makes it difficult to determine if the initial straining caused by the impaction has resolved. Persistent impactions can be treated with a retention enema with acetylcysteine diluted in water.

Colostrum Intake

Foals are born agammaglobulinemic and immunologically naïve but are immunocompetent.[8] Therefore, they rely on the immunity imparted by the colostrum to fight infection for the first 4–9 weeks of life. The foal's IgG concentration is a major factor in preventing infection in the neonates and therefore much attention is paid to ensure that the foal receives and absorbs adequate amounts.[9-11] When a foal fails to absorb sufficient maternal antibodies, it results in FPT. The commonly accepted value for FPT is any serum concentration that is below 400 mg/dL, while concentrations between 400 and 800 mg/dl are considered partial FPT.[12,13] Foals with FPT have an increased risk of morbidity and mortality because of septicemia, and early intervention and treatment with antibody supplementation helps to improve the outcome.[11,14]

Any foal that fails to suckle colostrum within the first 4 hours should be considered abnormal, and immediate intervention is recommended to get the colostrum into the foal (tube/bowl/bottle). Each foal should suckle at least 1 L of good-quality colostrum to provide adequate protection. Intervention is also in order should the colostrum itself not appear normal in character or quantity. Therefore, checking the colostrum and double-checking the foal's IgG absorption are imperative. Normal colostrum is creamy yellow and sticky. The quality of the colostrum depends on the IgG content. Generally an IgG concentration in the colostrum >70 g/L is considered adequate. This concentration of IgG is associated with a specific gravity >1.060 on a colostrometer or refractometer.[15] On a refractometer for measuring sugar concentrations, it should be at least 20%.[16] Special attention should be paid to the colostrum of maiden or older mares, mares with a history of poor colostrum production in the past, premature deliveries, or if the mare has been leaking colostrum before foaling. The easiest, although not very accurate, way to assess the colostrum is with its physical appearance. If it is white or dilute, it is definitely not adequate.

Simple, quick, commercial kits are available that allow the caretaker to identify poor-quality colostrum prior to the foal suckling. A semiquantitative glutaraldehyde precipitation (Gamma-Check-C, Veterinary Immunogenics Ltd., Cumbria, UK) test is one such test. Colostrum samples that clot within 3 minutes contain more than 60 g/L of immunoglobulins; if the sample clots in 3–10 minutes, it has ≥40 g/L of immunoglobulins. If the sample takes more than 10 minutes to clot or does not clot at all, an alternative source should definitely be sought for the foal. Another simple test that requires 20 minutes and can be done stall side is the Colostrum Equine IgG Midland Quick Test Kit (Midland BioProducts Corp, Boone, IA). This test uses 50 g/L of IgG as adequate colostral IgG concentration. Other tests are available that take longer for results and require a laboratory, like the single radial immuno-diffusion test (RID). These tests are very accurate but are better suited to test colostrum that is destined for a frozen colostrum bank as opposed to testing colostrum that is to be consumed by a newborn foal. When storing

colostrum for a colostrum bank, it may be stored in a normal domestic freezer. Although the nutritional components and some other immune proteins may be lost with this freezing, the colostrum should retain its IgG concentration for 12 months. The use of a −70°C freezer should result in the preservation of almost all the colostral components permanently.

Prophylactic Antibiotics

The use of prophylactic antibiotics should be restricted to cases where there is a clear indication, such as a "high-risk" foal or a history of disease on the farm. The antibiotics should be chosen based on targeted bacteria and the site of action. The potential side effects of the drug should also be considered. A single dose of long-acting penicillin is still extensively used, but the rationale for its use is questionable, especially since the majority of neonatal pathogens are gram-negative bacteria that are not usually sensitive to penicillin. Also, the practice of a single dose of the antibiotic brings into question the development of resistant pathogens on the farm.

ROUTINE VETERINARY EXAMINATION

Routine veterinary physical examinations are important to identify "high-risk" foals, formulate a list of differential diagnoses, direct ancillary tests, arrive at a presumptive diagnosis, and formulate a plan for initial therapy. Repeated veterinary examinations on subsequent days would be ideal and are commonly undertaken on large breeding farms. A foal's condition can change rapidly; it can appear normal during the veterinary examination and then within a few hours be severely compromised. Therefore, frequent examinations by the caretakers are recommended. When only a single veterinary examination is scheduled, it is usually performed between 12 and 18 hours of life to allow for assessment of colostral absorption at the same time. Assessing and addressing emergencies will take priority in the examination. In emergency situations, the major focus of the examination should involve evaluation of the respiratory and cardiovascular systems. Otherwise, a full detailed veterinary examination should be performed on all foals, even if they appear normal to the caretakers. Sick foals should have a sepsis score performed. This is a scoring system designed by Brewer and Koterba[10] to predict infection based on certain aspects of history, clinical pathology, and clinical examination. Points are assigned to the neutrophil count, the band neutrophil count, the presence of Döhle bodies, toxic granulation or vacuolization in neutrophils, and the fibrinogen concentration.[10] Other laboratory data that are scored include the presence of hypoglycemia, the IgG concentration, arterial oxygenation, and the presence of metabolic acidosis.[10] The clinical examination focuses on the presence of petechiation or scleral injection that is not a result of trauma, fever, hypotonia, coma, depression, or seizures as well as the presence of uveitis, diarrhea, respiratory distress, swollen joints, and open wounds.[10] Historical data of concern include placentitis, the presence of vaginal discharge, and dystocia.[10] The identification of prematurity on this scoring system is based on days of gestation alone.[10]

Every veterinary examination should start with observation of the foal's behavior from afar, assessment of the environment, and a critical history related to the mare, the gestation, the delivery, and the post-partum events, including the quality and quantity of colostrum consumed. The examination of the foal

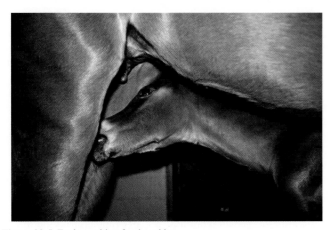

Figure 23-5. Foal searching for the udder.

is incomplete without the examination of the mare and the placenta. Critical assessment of the foal's behavior can be useful to identify problems, or merely to identify that there is something not quite normal with the foal and therefore closer attention and more frequent examinations are warranted. This can include both the way the foal responds to the mare as well as how it interacts with its environment. The behavior of the mare can also be of importance, especially when rejection is a possibility or she is too anxious to allow the foal to suckle adequately. The frequency, efficiency, and vigor at which the foal suckles are also of importance (Fig. 23-5). The mare's udder can be a good gauge as to how much the foal is suckling, whether the mare is producing an adequate amount of milk, and whether intervention and supplementation are required. The mare should be examined for excessive milk/colostrum dried on her hind limbs, which may indicate premature loss of the colostrum. After suckling, the foal should be assessed for milk in the nostrils. This can usually be done after the clinical examination is complete, since after the stress of the examination, the foal will usually head straight to the udder and suckle upon release. Milk on the foal's face and head can indicate that the foal has at least been searching for the udder in the right place, but it can also indicate more significant problems such as early signs of colic where the foal will stand under the udder and even mouth the udder without truly suckling. This will cause the mare to release milk on the foal. This is sometimes the first sign of a problem related to the gastrointestinal tract in the foal. The foal should be observed for lethargy, one of the first signs of illness.

Generally the same principles apply in performing a physical examination on a foal as with an adult, with a few additions. The initial examination should start with an assessment of the general appearance of the foal, including discoloration of the hair (meconium staining), mentation, and physical appearance (e.g., congenital defects). The vital parameters change over the first few hours of life and then stabilize. The rectal temperature is normally 37°–38.9°C (99°–102°F). The pulse quality should be strong and can be assessed by palpating the facial, brachial, or greater metatarsal arteries. At this time the temperature of the distal limbs can also be assessed. The mucous membranes of a normal neonatal foal should be moist and pink with a capillary refill time of <2 seconds. With early sepsis, these can become hyperemic and be accompanied by scleral injection and red coronary bands. Should they become icteric, especially in a foal that has suckled colostrum, this can be one of the first indicators of NI. It may also indicate hepatic problems, or hemolysis.

Petechiae of the oral or nasal mucous membranes or inside of the pinna of the ears is another sign of sepsis. Severe hypoxia can result in the membranes becoming cyanotic. This color can also be seen with circulatory collapse (hypotensive, endotoxemic, or hypovolemic shock).

Examination of the neonatal gastrointestinal tract includes assessment of the abdominal size, auscultation, and palpation of the inguinal rings and umbilical area. Examination of the quantity and quality of fecal production is important. The inability to palpate meconium per rectum and the owner's report of meconium passage does not rule out an impaction orad to the pelvic rim. The passage of yellow-brown feces is indicative of successful elimination of the meconium. Abdominal distention can result from gas or fluid accumulation in bowel or the accumulation of urine, blood, or excessive peritoneal fluid free in the abdominal cavity. Ballottement of the abdomen can sometimes distinguish free peritoneal fluid from fluid within the viscus. Bruxism, ptyalism, and rolling in dorsal recumbency are common signs of gastric ulceration in foals.

Immunoglobulin Determination

Determination of the foal's IgG concentration at 8–12 hours of age has benefits and should be incorporated into any routine foal examination. Early identification of FPT allows for the administration of an alternative source of IgGs orally. The absorption can be reassessed in 5–6 hours. If testing is postponed until peak absorption at about 18 hours of age, the practitioner is restricted to the use of intravenous plasma since there is minimal oral absorption of IgG at this time. The financial benefits of waiting may be offset by the cost of the plasma administration. The prevalence of FPT in foals is reported to be between 3% and 20%, and early identification of these cases can ensure timely intervention and minimize morbidity, mortality, and financial loss.[11,14,17,18] Those foals identified as having partial FPT may not require intervention if the foal is healthy and on a well-managed farm with no known illness, since there is no greater morbidity or mortality than foals with values >800 mg/dl.[19] However, this concentration of IgG may not be adequate for foals that are sick or compromised in any fashion.[20-23]

There are many tests available to determine a foal's serum IgG concentration. The test chosen should be reliable and easy to perform and have results available in a short period.[24] The gold standard has remained the single radial-immunodiffusion (SRID) which is the most accurate test available at this time.[25] The home/practice prepared SRID kits must be calibrated (Equine IgG RID, Veterinary Medical Research and Development, Pullman, WA) but gives useful accurate quantitative results. They are expensive and require more technical skill to perform, and there is usually a 24-hour delay in receiving the results. In order to decrease the amount of time that the foal is left susceptible to infection, the use of a quick stall side test is preferable, such as zinc sulfate, sodium sulfite, glutaraldehyde precipitation, latex agglutination, CITE, or SNAP test. The zinc sulfate turbidity test is a simple test in the field that is quick, accurate, and cheap. The need for serum instead of plasma may prolong the testing time in the field. The tests tend to be less accurate at IgG concentrations <400 mg/dl.[26,27] In addition, hemolysis of the sample may result in falsely elevated results.[28] The sodium sulfite turbidity test results are too unpredictable for use. The glutaraldehyde precipitation test is marred by a poor specificity for IgG concentrations <800 mg/dl and hemolysis may result in false-positive results, and it will detect other serum proteins in addition to IgGs.[13,28]

One of the most commonly used tests in the field is an enzyme-linked immunoassay that comes as a convenient on-site test (SNAP Foal IgG Test Kit, IDEXX Laboratories, Westbrook, ME). This test measures the foal's IgG concentration with a species-specific anti-IgG antibody.[12,13,29,30] This semiquantitative test is easy to perform and inexpensive. and the results are available within 10 minutes. This makes it a very good screening test for FPT. The SNAP test is impaired by a low specificity, a poor positive predictive value compared with SRID, and its use of heat- and contamination-sensitive reagents.[13,30,31] It has a different sensitivity and specificity depending on the concentration of IgG in the sample. When testing a sample with ≤400 mg/dl of IgG, the sensitivity is 90% and the specificity is only 79%, but with samples of ≤800 mg/dl, the sensitivity increases to 95% while the specificity decreases to 52%. The specificity of this test on samples with ≤800 mg/dl was found to be lower in foals with a sepsis score of ≥11 and bacteremia, whereas samples with ≤400 mg/dl were unaffected by the fibrinogen concentration, sepsis score, or bacteremia.[24] This will ensure that foals with an IgG concentration of ≤800 mg/dl are identified and treated, but some foals that do have adequate passive transfer will be identified with FPT and may be treated unnecessarily. The detrimental effects of plasma administration are minimal other than cost, since adverse reactions are rare and usually minor in the foal, especially when using a commercial source of plasma.[29,32,33]

A recent report indicated that Fourier-transformed infrared spectroscopy (IR) had a diagnostic accuracy that was as good or better than the other tests but would prove to be more economical.[34] This test is performed by transmitting IR radiation through a sample and an IR spectrometer records the wavelength dependence of radiation absorption by the sample.[34] It can quantify the IgG concentration accurately with a specificity of 92.5%, similar to calorimetric assay, but it is superior to the published results for all other assays, especially the ELISA. The sensitivity is better than the ELISA and other turbimetric assays at 96.8% but is lower than the calorimetric assay and similar to glutaraldehyde coagulation and zinc sulfate assays.[34] The positive predictive value (88.1%) is high, allowing this test to reduce unnecessary treatments.[34] The negative predictive value is high like most tests at 98%.[34] Of course these values will vary with the prevalence of FPT in the population being tested. This test is not compromised by hemolysis or other chemicals that can interfere with other tests.[34] The results are available within minutes and no standards or reagents are required; therefore, the cost per test is low and performing repeated tests is inexpensive.[34] When this test becomes commercially available, it will have the additional advantage in that it can also provide results for total protein, albumin, cholesterol, glucose, and triglyceride.[34]

Use of Plasma

Any foal with FPT who is older than 18 hours of age, and colostrum is not available or not being absorbed appropriately by the foal, requires intravenous plasma administration. There are some local enteric benefits to the oral administration of colostrum even after the time for IgG absorption has passed.[35,36] In addition to the laxative properties, colostrum provides local immunity for enteric infections. Foals with complete FPT will most likely require at least 2 L of plasma to increase the IgG concentration to >800 mg/dl. A rule of thumb is that 1 L of good-quality plasma will increase a 50-kg foal's IgG concentration by 200 mg/dl. After the administration of plasma, the foal's IgG concentration should be re-evaluated in 6–12 hours. In ill or "high-risk" foals. it may be necessary to re-evaluate the IgG concentration repeatedly since there is the possibility of sequestration of the IgG, loss from clearance of complexes formed between the transfused IgG and existing foreign antigen, or increased demand and usage of the IgG if disease or infection is present.

When plasma is required, it can be obtained from the dam or another horse on the same farm or preferably commercial hyperimmune plasma can be given.[37] Examples of commercial plasma include Polymune (Veterinary Immunogenics, Templeton, CA), HiGamm (Equi Lake Immunogenics, Ontario, NY), or High-Glo (Mg Biologics, Ames, IA). The commercial products may appear more expensive, but they are less time consuming to use and more consistently of high quality and usually contain certain protective antibodies against gram-negative endotoxins, equine rotavirus, *Rhodococcus equi*, tetanus, and equine influenza. Many are also concentrated to allow maximum IgG delivery in a smaller volume of plasma. They are usually designated specific pathogen free and are tested to ensure that they do not contain A, Q, or C antibodies. The donors are "universal" donors; therefore, cross-matching is not required as it would be if a horse on the farm was going to be used as a donor. When the safety of commercial plasma is compared with harvested plasma and the time costs for performing the cross-match, blood collection, and plasma harvest, the cost of the commercial plasma is very reasonable. Apart from the cost, disadvantages of commercial plasma are that it is frozen and therefore complement and some other components of the plasma are denatured and there may be a lack of specific antibodies for the local pathogens. Plasma should be administered with careful attention to aseptic techniques. An intravenous jugular catheter is usually placed, although cephalic catheters can also be used. Either short- or long-term catheters may be chosen depending on the other requirements of the foal. If there are any signs of reaction during administration, such as agitation, increases in heart or respiratory rates or temperature, or hives, the rate of delivery should be decreased for 5–10 minutes. If the signs resolve, the rate can be increased again. If signs persist, the practitioner should discontinue and find an alternative source of plasma. Prednisolone or dexamethasone may be administered intravenously as needed for signs of plasma reaction. Severe reactions may require epinephrine; therefore, a crash kit should be available. Such reactions are very rare in the foal and are more likely to be encountered with the administration of whole blood than plasma.

Hematology and Biochemistry in Neonates

If there are any concerns with a foal, a complete blood count and biochemistry profile should be performed. Some perform such blood work routinely on any foals to provide early identification of any potentially ill foals. This would be ideal but is frequently not undertaken because of financial restraints placed on the veterinarian. Should there be any indications of early sepsis, either through clinical examination or based on abnormalities on routine blood work, a blood culture should be performed. The blood cultures are useful should the foal become ill and be non-responsive to the antibiotics selected; more importantly, they are a good monitor of the pathogens in circulation in that population. The sensitivity patterns of the common pathogens recovered may alter the antibiotic usage in subsequent foals.

Performing routine blood work on every foal allows for the detection of FPT, early septicemia, NI, and altered renal function (especially important before the administration of oxytetracycline for limb contracture), among other conditions. If finances are restricted, the immunoglobulin G (IgG) determination is the most important, followed by the complete blood count and fibrinogen. IgG determination is a must for any "high-risk" or sick foal.

Alterations occur within the first few weeks of life in several parameters commonly evaluated in foals. The packed cell volume (PCV) will increase shortly after birth and then declines for the first few weeks of life. This is a physiological anemia and not pathological. The total protein will be very low at birth and increases as the foal suckles and absorbs the immunoglobulins from the colostrum. Normal foals frequently have increased bilirubin and appear mildly icteric. This will be due to a physiological icterus with an increase in both the total and unconjugated bilirubin. This is thought to be due to an increased bilirubin load and immaturity of the hepatocytes. With severe icterus the conjugated bilirubin will be increased. This is seen with NI, septicemia, and hepatitis. The creatine kinase is frequently increased in newborns from unknown causes. Bone growth, intestinal pinocytosis, and hepatic maturation are thought to contribute to the increased alkaline phosphatase that is seen in foals for months post-partum. In addition, hepatocellular maturation during the first few weeks of life results in elevations in gamma glutamyl transferase, sorbitol dehydrogenase, and aspartate amino transferase. The serum creatinine measured in the early post-partum period is more of a reflection of placental function; for this reason creatinine is frequently elevated in the first 24–48 hours and decreases steadily if the foal's renal function is normal. Caution should be taken with any foal until the creatinine concentration is within normal limits.

Neonatal Isoerythrolysis

The one condition in which the foal should be prevented from consuming the mare's colostrum is the risk of NI. In this condition there is incompatibility between the foal's blood and the antibodies in the mare's colostrum (alloantibodies), resulting in rupture or lysis of the foal's red blood cells. Prevention of this condition is preferred over treatment. In these situations an alternative source of colostrum or plasma should be administered to ensure that the foal has adequate immunological protection without the risk of developing NI. Such actions should be taken if the mare has had previous foals with NI and she is re-bred without knowledge of compatibility between the mare and the stallion blood types. The ideal situation would be to blood-type all mares that are to be bred and all stallions to ensure compatibility. If just the mares are tested, those mares whose blood types are Aa and Qa negative are at an increased risk of producing a foal with NI. Breeding to stallions that are Aa and Qa negative will also decrease the possibility of NI, but the blood types for most stallions are not made available. Alternatively, the mares can be tested 2–3 weeks pre-partum for alloantibodies to determine the risk to the foal. It is important to wait until the end of pregnancy for this test, since testing earlier may produce negative results. Multiparous mares are more likely to produce a foal with NI, although primiparous mares can infrequently produce an NI foal; therefore, testing should be considered.

Foals that develop NI are usually born normal and can continue to appear normal for up to 7 days or they can succumb rapidly within the first 24–48 hours. The severity of the disease and the rate of deterioration of the foal are determined by the quantity and activity of the absorbed alloantibodies. The most reliable diagnostic test is the hemolytic cross-match using washed foal erythrocytes, mare serum, and an exogenous source of absorbed complement. Although this will give an accurate risk of the development of NI, it must be performed in a laboratory, with a significant delay in results; therefore, it is impractical in private field practice. A simple cross-match, or jaundiced foal agglutination test, can be done in the field with the foal's blood and either the colostrum or the mare's serum. A Coombs' test may be useful with these cases, although false negatives are common, and this would put the foals at risk if the colostrum is not withheld since it does not address hemolysins.

ORGAN SYSTEM EXAMINATION AND DISORDERS

Respiratory System

Evaluation of the respiratory system should begin prior to entering the stall, if possible, to avoid excitation and artificial increase in the rate. Respirations should be assessed for rate, effort, and character. Both high and low RRs are significant in the foal. An RR of 60–80 breaths per minute in the immediate post-partum period decreases to around 20–40 breaths per minute within an hour and remains there for the first few weeks of life. Although the respiratory pattern of standing foals is fairly regular, when sleeping it becomes irregular with fast, shallow breaths alternating with periods of apnea. Apnea or low RRs can be associated with primary respiratory disorders or with metabolic disturbances. Hypothermia can also lead to decreased respirations and apnea. Advanced prematurity and hypoxia-induced suppression of the respiratory center can result in a low RR and poor respiratory excursions. Cyanotic mucous membranes are not a sensitive indicator of lung function and oxygenation, since a Pao_2 of <40 mmHg is required before cyanosis is evident. Arterial blood gases or pulse oximetry (in well-perfused foals) are better at assessing oxygenation. Foals with immature lungs may appear normal for the first 24–48 hours before they develop respiratory distress caused by surfactant disorders. During initial lung auscultation, there are fine inspiratory rales associated with inflation of the fluid-filled alveoli. These sounds will change as more alveoli open and fetal fluid is absorbed across the airways. During the first few hours, the lung sounds are moist, and crackles can be heard in the normal dependent lungs when the foal is in lateral recumbency. Thoracic auscultation is not reliable for assessing the lower respiratory tract in neonatal foals since the changes are subtle, if not inappreciable, even with severe pulmonary disease, and they do not correlate well with the severity of pathology. More information can be gained by assessing the respiratory rate, effort, and pattern of respiration. Flared nostrils, increased abdominal effort, and rib retractions are better indicators of disease than auscultation. To further complicate the diagnosis, coughing and nasal discharge is rarely a component of pulmonary disease in the neonatal foal. The presence of nasal discharge, especially milk or what appears like meconium, is of vital importance. Thoracic radiographs and arterial blood gas analysis allows for the best assessment of respiratory function in these neonates, including immaturity. Ultrasonography can be useful when a diaphragmatic hernia, hemothorax, fractured ribs, or lung contusions are suspected.

In the early neonatal period, lung disease is usually the result of an infection acquired in utero or immediately post-partum either alone or combined with atelectasis caused by recumbency, immaturity, or surfactant dysfunction. Other conditions can lead to increased RRs and effort, including pain or stress. Careful palpation of the ribs, feeling for fractures with medial displacement of the distal fragment of the rib or crepitus, is essential. On auscultation a clicking sound during inspiration on the affected side and grunting on expiration may be heard. Foals with rib fractures usually prefer to lie on the normal side, provided the fractures are unilateral. Rib fractures can be a cause of sudden death in foals because of trauma to the myocardium, a ruptured diaphragm, or pneumothorax. These fractures are best treated conservatively.

If the tachypnea and tachycardia are more pronounced when the foal is standing, musculoskeletal structures should be assessed while looking for a source of pain. Fractures can occur during dystocias that require assistance. Accidental trauma can occur to the limbs by the mare, especially with maiden mares or when mares are showing signs of rejecting the foal. Intervention may eliminate this possibility.

Respiratory Distress Syndrome

The cause of respiratory distress syndrome in neonatal foals is an inadequate amount of mature surfactant in the lungs. Surfactant is a complex phospholipid produced by type II pneumocytes, and its function is to reduce the surface tension in the alveoli, thereby increasing the compliance in the lungs. The composition of the surfactant changes over the course of gestation and is not fully mature until term. A deficiency in mature surfactant results in an increased surface tension that in turn decreases the compliance of the lungs and increases the effort required to expand the lungs. This results in pulmonary collapse or atelectasis and ventilation/perfusion mismatch. The increased tension in the alveoli also reduces the hydrostatic pressure in the tissues around the capillaries in the lungs and draws fluid into the lungs, resulting in pulmonary edema. This deficiency may also result in direct lung injury resulting in epithelial disruption and leakage of protein into the alveolar spaces. All of this results in the impairment of effective gas exchange at the alveolar level. This is further complicated by recumbency, which leads to positional atelectasis and ventilation/perfusion mismatch. The inability to take deep breaths results in incomplete expansions of the lungs. These factors as well as the lack of evacuation of respiratory fluids all predispose the foal to pneumonia.

Congenital Malformations of the Head

Assessment of the upper respiratory tract for congenital defects should be done early in the examination. Malformations may involve the nares, nasal passages, pharynx, larynx, or trachea. These may include cleft palate, stenotic nares, choanal atresia, subepiglottic cyst, collapsing trachea, and guttural pouch tympany, to name a few. Identification of a cleft palate should be done prior to addressing any other abnormalities that might prove costly. The success rate of surgical correction of a cleft palate in the foal is quite low, but if it is identified early, the risk of aspiration pneumonia can be reduced by preventing the foal from suckling and instead feeding it through a feeding tube. The identification of a cleft palate may be quite simple with a good oral examination, but in some cases only the very distal portion of the soft palate is affected. These foals require endoscopy to confirm the diagnosis. Affected foals will usually regurgitate milk out of one or both nostrils after suckling. Other conditions with a similar presentation include hypoxic-ischemic syndrome, prematurity, weakness caused by sepsis or conditions such as the presence of subepiglottic cysts, white muscle disease, or pharyngeal weakness of unknown cause. With primary pharyngeal weakness, the dysphagia will usually resolve with age, but intervention must be made early to avoid aspiration of milk and subsequent associated illnesses.

Wry nose is lateral deviation of the nasal septum and the premaxilla. Surgical correction with extensive reconstruction is possible in some cases, although there is some question as to the heritability, which would then question the ethics of surgical correction. The immediate concern with these foals is whether they can latch on to the udder and suckle. Specific attention to passive transfer and ensuring that the foal is consuming enough milk is important. An alternative method of feeding, such as from a bowl or bucket, may be required.

The most common malocclusion seen in foals is brachygnathia (parrot mouth, overbite). Although this fault can lead to eating difficulties, it is usually not a significant issue for the survival of the foal. Surgical correction is discouraged because of the possible heritability of the condition. The opposite condition, prognathism, is commonly seen in conjunction with forelimb contracture and incomplete ossification of the cuboidal bones in Western Canada and the Pacific Northwest of the United States. This condition is due to congenital hypothyroidism. These foals may have other signs of dysmaturity despite a possible prolonged gestational length. They frequently appear with fine hair coats, lethargy, and FPT. The FPT can be attributed to difficulties standing and suckling combined with frequent agalactia. The malocclusion will usually correct itself with age. The tendon contracture should be addressed, as it would with any other foal with a similar presentation, including nursing care, bandaging/splints, casts if required, and possibly oxytetracycline therapy. It is also important to take radiographs of these foals to assess the maturation of the cuboidal bones.

Cardiovascular System

As previously discussed, the HR of the neonate varies with the age post-partum and stabilizes at 80–100 bpm in the first week of life. Tachycardia can be associated with pain, excitement, sepsis, hypocalcemia, or primary cardiac disease. A sinus arrhythmia and possibly ventricular premature complexes are not uncommon in the immediate post-partum period. These should disappear after a few hours. Because of the foal's thin chest wall, the heart sounds and murmurs are easily auscultated and the palpable apex beat is much more prominent. A left-sided murmur can usually be auscultated in the immediate post-partum period. This murmur is usually benign and associated with the ductus arteriosus (DA). Functional closure usually occurs within the first 24–72 hours post-partum, although it can be present longer without causing a problem. Premature foals and those with persistent pulmonary hypertension are more likely to develop a patent DA (PDA). The clinical signs noted will depend on the magnitude of the shunt through the PDA. A definitive diagnosis can be difficult since it is hard to visualize the DA ultrasonographically because of the location of the lungs. When a PDA becomes pathological, the foal may become hypoxic because the fetal circulation is maintained or the circulation has reverted back. In this situation, unoxygenated blood is delivered to the systemic circulation. When there is no reversion of the circulation, the long-term sequelae include stunted growth and exercise intolerance. With more severe cases that involve unoxygenated blood in the systemic circulation, the prognosis is poor. Surgical correction may be attempted, but the prognosis is guarded. Other persistent murmurs that can be identified in neonatal foals include ventricular septal defects and valvular deficits. These may also result in poor growth and exercise intolerance as long as there is no delivery of unoxygenated blood to the systemic circulation.

Vascular perfusion can be roughly assessed on physical examination by assessing the temperature of the distal extremities and the quality of the peripheral pulses. When assessing the distal extremities, the ambient temperature must be taken into account. Cardiovascular collapse and hypotension may be represented by a thready pulse. Hypotension is an indication of septic or hypovolemic shock, severe asphyxia, or advanced prematurity. Referral to an intensive care facility is in order for these foals to allow accurate assessment of the foal's blood pressure and to take the appropriate measures to resolve the problem.

Musculoskeletal System

The musculoskeletal system should be assessed for maturity, congenital anomalies, fractures, or angular limb deformities. Common traumatic injuries include fractured ribs, dislocated physis, soft tissue trauma leading to focal limb swelling, hematomas, and other limb fractures. All joint swellings in foals should be considered possibly septic until proven otherwise. Joints are considered septic if a white blood cell count of >10,000 cells/µl is found in the joint fluid, regardless of whether bacteria are cultured from the fluid.

All foals should be assessed during their fist veterinary examination for conformation. The foal should be assessed for signs of trauma during parturition. Exercise programs for each foal should take into account the musculoskeletal soundness of the foal. Regular assessment by the caregivers should include an assessment of the conformation of the foal, since circumstances can change rapidly and may need intervention and alteration of the exercise program. Unless problems are identified, the foal should first be seen by a farrier at about 1 month of age and then every 4–6 weeks unless problems develop.

Contracted Foal Syndrome

The most common musculoskeletal disorder seen in neonatal foals is contracture of one or more of the limbs. The contracture is usually bilateral and involves the joints of the fore limbs, although it can also involve the hind limbs or both fore and hind limbs. The fetlock is the most common joint affected. Radiographs of the affected area are recommended to ensure that there are not any underlying skeletal malformations. Mild cases can be treated with physical therapy and bandaging. The judicious use of non-steroidal anti-inflammatories (NSAIDs) is helpful to reduce the discomfort experienced by the foal and encourage the foal to bear full weight on the limb. The use of selective COX-2 NSAIDs, such as Veda Profen, may be preferential to decrease the potential negative side effects. More severely affected foals will benefit from heavy support bandages and splints in addition to the use of oxytetracycline (1–3 gm IV bolus in 250-500ml saline). This can be administered once every 24 hours for up to 3 days.[38] Care must be taken in foals that are also compromised and potentially dehydrated or already suffering from renal compromise. It is recommended to perform a biochemistry panel prior to the administration of multiple doses of oxytetracycline. Casts can also be used in severe cases, but have to be placed with care and changed frequently to avoid cast sores and subsequent potentially devastating consequences. These treatments are of course in addition to exercise restriction and the administration of NSAIDs. In severe cases where the foal is unable to stand without assistance, nursing care is very important and will be required around the clock to allow them to stand and suckle from the mare and keep them clean to avoid scalding and pressure sores. Referral to a neonatal intensive care facility should be considered, if possible, because of the intensive nursing care required and the high risk of secondary problems. Rupture of the extensor tendons is not uncommon and requires no specific therapy besides exercise restriction. In time most of these foals will move normally. Gastric ulcer prophylaxis is recommended in these foals.

Older foals with contracture should be thoroughly assessed for a source of lameness. These acquired contractures are usually the results of abnormal weight-bearing caused by pain. The contracture most often involves the coffin joint or the fetlock. Treatments include addressing the primary source of lameness, NSAIDs, corrective hoof trimming, and possible surgical intervention (e.g., check ligament desmotomy).

Tendon Laxity

Many foals are born with tendons that are too lax. Mild cases usually required restricted exercise on good footing and most will improve in the first 48–72 hours. When the laxity is more severe, heel extensions may be required to allow more correct weight-bearing and to take the pressure off the heels, which can become traumatized (Fig. 23-6). Glue-on shoes work well, but they must be removed in 10–14 days to prevent contracture of the hoof. A light wrap may be required to minimize the trauma to the soft tissues, but heavy bandaging should be avoided since it will further weaken the soft tissues. Exercise should be restricted to short periods several times a day.

Angular Limb Deformities

Angular limb deformities can be present either immediately after birth or acquired shortly after. These can be the result of soft tissue laxity, *in utero* malpositioning, or incomplete ossification

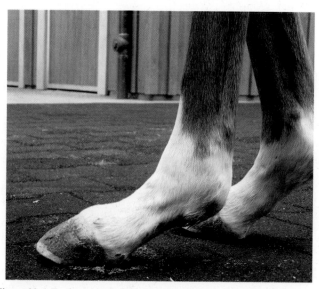

Figure 23-6. Tendon laxity in the hind limbs. (Courtesy Brian Leight.)

of the cuboidal bones. The most common angular deformity is mild carpal valgus, where the distal limb deviates laterally, resulting in a knock-kneed appearance. This is usually self correcting within the first few weeks but should be monitored closely. Exercise should be restricted to avoid irregular wear on the joints. Corrective hoof trimming should be attempted with many cases early in the condition. Should carpus valgus not resolve by 5 months of age, surgery should be considered. With fetlock varus, where the limb distal to the fetlock is deviated medially, the time period for surgical intervention is much shorter

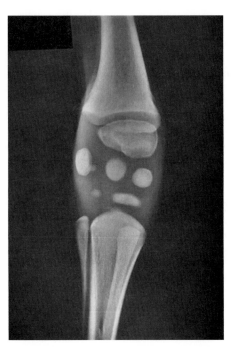

Figure 23-7. Incomplete ossification of the carpus. (Courtesy Dr. Keith Chaffin.)

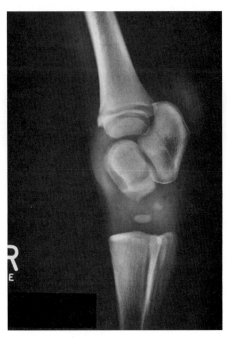

Figure 23-8. Incomplete ossification of the hock. (Courtesy Dr. Keith Chaffin.)

and should be undertaken if medical attempts at correction have not worked by 2 months of age.

Incomplete Ossification

Immaturity of the skeleton can result in laxity of the joints and is best assessed with radiographs. Both lateral and AP views of both the carpi and the tarsi are taken soon after birth to crudely estimate the development in other parts of the skeleton (Figs. 23-7 and 23-8). The templates for the carpal and tarsal bones and the epiphyses of the adjacent long bones usually ossify during the last 2 months of gestation. This process should have progressed to the periphery of the bones at the time of birth and should be complete by 1 month of age. Depending on the degree of ossification present, recommendations may vary from splints or casting to mere stall restriction on good footing while awaiting maturation. The progression of skeletal ossification in these foals should be assessed regularly with radiographs, and alterations to the exercise program and degree of support should follow.

NEUROLOGICAL AND OPHTHALMOLOGICAL SYSTEMS

Overt neurological signs can include depression, seizures, or abnormal behaviors. Foals with decreased oxygen delivery to the brain or hypoxic-ischemic encephalopathy will have clinical signs that depend on the severity of asphyxia and subsequent brain cell damage. Frequently these signs develop slowly over the first 24–48 hours post-partum. Full body seizures in the foal are not always present and can be manifested by facial grimacing, twitching, chewing, repetitive blinking, or most commonly increased head and neck rigidity. Other causes of neurological derangements include congenital malformations (hydrocephalus), viral and bacterial infections, trauma, metabolic abnormalities (hypoglycemia, hyperbilirubinemia), and epilepsy of unknown origin.

Although important, it is difficult to fully assess a neonatal foal's vision. The pupillary light response is present but slower than in adults and should normalize within the first week of life. The pupils are large but should be of equal size. They are more circular initially and then by 1 week of life they will have decreased in size and become more oval. The menace response in a neonate is usually not present for the first 2 weeks of life due to the ongoing development of the vision pathways through the cerebellum and cerebral cortex. Once developed, the loss of the menace response can be associated with cerebral edema because of birth asphyxia, septic optic neuritis, or other ocular deficits, which can include retinal detachment and optic nerve hypoplasia. Observations on how the foal reacts to its environment and to the mare can help with vision assessment. Fixed and dilated pupils are associated with severe mid-brain swelling. This can be due to head trauma or severe hypoxic-ischemic encephalopathy. Nystagmus or retinal hemorrhages may accompany alterations in the pupils and results in a high suspicion of brain swelling. Scleral hemorrhages are common and usually indicate a dystocia or cranial trauma during the birthing process. These can take several weeks to resolve, and no specific therapy is required.

Care should be taken to evaluate the foal for entropion, in which the eyelids roll in towards the cornea, especially if there are signs of prematurity/dysmaturity, disease, or dehydration. Entropion can be acquired or congenital. It is important to address entropion early since it can result in corneal edema or ulceration. Acquired entropion can be due to self-trauma, dehydration, or prematurity and lack of periorbital fat. Correction of mild cases can be done by manual eversion of the eyelids several times a day while protecting the cornea with frequent application of topical antibiotic ointments. If the condition is more severe, procaine penicillin G can be injected subcutaneously into the lower eyelids or sutures can be placed in the lower eyelids, taking care to ensure that the suture ends are not contacting the cornea. Foals with entropion should have their corneas evaluated frequently to ensure that ulcers are not missed. Frequent staining for corneal ulcers and the prophylactic use of artificial tears or antibiotic ointment are also in order for neonatal foals that are recumbent. These foals have reduced corneal sensitivity and decreased tear production, making them especially susceptible to corneal ulcers.

Hypopyon and uveitis, inflammation of the iris, ciliary body, and choroid can be associated with systemic bacterial infections or viral infections. The corneas should be clear, although mild corneal edema may be considered normal for a few hours after birth. The posterior and anterior Y-sutures are commonly seen on the lenses of neonatal foals. These should be differentiated from congenital cataracts. The normal lens may appear cloudy for the first few weeks. The pupillary membranes usually persist and are visible sometime until about 12 months of age and no treatment is required.

UROGENITAL SYSTEM

Examination of the urogenital system usually focuses on the external structures, including the umbilicus. If discolored urine is noted, additional investigation should be performed to determine if this is hematuria, hemoglobinuria, or myoglobinuria.

Umbilical Abnormalities

Swelling around the umbilical stump is not uncommon. It may be associated with hemorrhage from the umbilical structures, may be a result of hernia formation and trauma to the muscle layers, or inflammation resulting from reaction to the umbilical dip, which is more common when iodine solutions are used. It can also be associated with urine accumulation, either from a bladder or urethral rupture, and the associated inflammation. If the umbilicus is found to be moist after the first 24 hours or is inflamed, it should be examined for patent urachus or umbilical infection. The best way to evaluate an umbilicus is with ultrasonography. This allows examination of the internal umbilical remnants. The ultrasound examination can be done using a 5-7.5–MHz transducer. The vein and both umbilical arteries should measure <1.0 cm. The umbilical stump that contains the two arteries and the urachus should be <1.5 cm × 2.5 cm.[39] If there is any concern over the umbilical structures, broad-spectrum antibiotics should be administered to the foal. If there are gas echoes in the umbilical structures, this would indicate an anaerobic infection and the appropriate antibiotic should be added to the treatment protocol (e.g., metronidazole). Medical therapy should be attempted first in most cases of umbilical infections. If antibiotics are started early and the foal is treated aggressively, medical therapy is more likely to be successful. If medical treatment fails, or there is a large abscess, or the abscess is approaching the liver, then surgical removal of the umbilicus is in order in conjunction with aggressive antibiotic therapy.

Patent Urachus

Patent urachus is another common disorder of neonatal foals that can be congenital or acquired. The urachus, the canal that drains the urinary bladder through the umbilicus in the fetus, usually closes at birth or very soon after, atrophies, and scars to become the scar on the apex of the bladder. Patency becomes an issue since it is a source of irritation, and more importantly it is a route for infection. Congenital patent urachus can be the result of overdistention of the urachus *in utero* or during parturition. Acquired patent urachus is more common and it is often associated with infection. This occurs more frequently in foals that experience prolonged recumbency with urine scalding of the umbilical area. It also occurs more frequently in foals that have had umbilical irritation or ligation and in foals in which the umbilical cord has been cut. The use of an inappropriate concentration of iodine solutions or too frequent application of strong disinfectants can also be associated with an increased incidence of patent urachus since it leads to premature sloughing of the umbilical stump before the urachus has atrophied and scarred. Conditions that cause increased intra-abdominal pressure will also increase the risk of the development of patent urachus. Such conditions would include causes of tenesmus such as constipation, dysuria, cystitis, urachitis, urachal diverticulum, and uroperitoneum, or would result from bladder catheterization.

Evaluation of foals with a patent urachus with ultrasonography is recommended to assess the abdomen, bladder, and umbilical structures to ensure there is no underlying cause for the condition and to identify signs of infection. The treatment of patent urachus includes cautery with 2% iodine or silver nitrate or surgical removal of the umbilical remnants. Cautery may cause additional tenesmus that could exacerbate the situation. In addition to the treatment of the urachus itself, the primary cause should be addressed and antibiotic therapy should be initiated.

Uroperitoneum

Uroperitoneum involves the leakage of urine from any portion of the urinary tract into the abdomen. Leakage can also occur into the subcutaneous tissues and the retroperitoneal space. The most common source of urine leakage is from the bladder. Defects in the bladder wall can be congenital and occur during foaling or post-partum. Congenital ruptures are due to a failure of the muscular layer of the bladder to close. This is usually on the dorsal midline. Ruptures can occur during foaling and are a result of increased pressure placed on the caudal abdomen as the foal is passed through the pelvic inlet. Chances are increased if the foal has a full bladder at the time of parturition or dystocia is encountered. Again, these tears involve the dorsal wall, which is thought to be weaker. Colts are more prone to ruptured bladders than fillies, which may be due to the relatively smaller urethral size in the colts. Fillies appear to be more prone to ureteral anomalies or ruptures, which can lead to uroperitoneum, although these are rare. Rupture of the bladder can also occur post-partum because of urachal infections or as a result of trauma or excessive pressure placed on the caudal abdomen, as can occur with improper lifting of the foal. This is especially true for compromised foals that require intensive care management. Therefore, extra care should be taken when lifting and moving these foals.

With ruptured bladders, the rate at which the abdomen distends with urine depends on the size of the defect in the bladder wall and the amount of urine being produced by the foal. The production of a normal stream of urine does not rule out the possibility of a ruptured bladder. As the abdomen fills with fluid, it distends at the ventral aspect. This differentiates the abdominal distention from that caused by excessive gas in the intestines, which will produce more distention dorsally. In addition, a fluid wave can frequently be palpated in the foal's abdomen. Apart from abdominal distention, other clinical signs associated with ruptured bladders include mild colic, anorexia, straining to urinate, ventral or preputial edema, depression, and decreased suckling and activity. Straining to urinate is frequently mistaken for straining to defecate, and therefore assessment and treatment can be delayed if the caretakers are administering repeated enemas (Fig. 23-9). As the abdomen continues to distend, the foal will eventually develop respiratory difficulties. Colts will commonly fill their scrotums with urine and develop preputial swelling. A very large volume of fluid can collect in the abdomen before the foal exhibits clinical signs that alert caretakers to a problem that requires veterinary attention. This can take 1–3 days post-partum, especially if the foal is still urinating fairly normally. With very small defects, the foal may not be presented for examination for up to 5 days. Ultrasound examination can reveal variable amounts of free abdominal fluid depending on the stage at which the examination is performed. The intestines appear to be floating in fluid, but otherwise appear normal. The integrity of the walls of the bladder, urachus, or ureter may be altered.

Treatment of a ruptured bladder in most cases requires surgical repair. This can be undertaken only after the foal is metabolically stabilized. The electrolyte imbalances should be addressed immediately. The typical electrolyte profile for a foal with a ruptured bladder would include hyponatremia, hypochloremia, and hyperkalemia. Metabolic acidosis usually accompanies these abnormalities in the electrolytes. Bradycardia may develop because of these imbalances. Neurological signs can also develop, which can include seizures, hyperesthesia, dementia, or ataxia. In addition, these foals are frequently azotemic with a dramatic increase in the creatinine concentration. Of note is that this typical picture may not be apparent in sick neonatal foals that are receiving intravenous fluid therapy. Radiographs will show ventral opacity to the abdomen, indicating free abdominal fluid. With uroperitoneum the creatinine concentration in the abdominal fluid should be more than twice the concentration in the serum. This may not be present early in the condition.

The electrolytes and respiratory system are of immediate concern, since the hyperkalemia can lead to fatal arrhythmias. Treatments include intravenous saline and dextrose with or without sodium bicarbonate. If the foal is not ventilating adequately because of the pressure on the diaphragm, care must be taken when choosing to administer bicarbonate. General anesthesia should be avoided until the serum potassium concentration falls below 5.5 mEq/L. The abdomen should be drained, especially if there is compromise to respiratory excursions. This will also help to decrease the possibility of an abrupt drop in blood pressure in surgery once the abdomen is opened and the fluid is evacuated. In addition, a urinary catheter should be placed to prevent further urine accumulation in the abdomen while awaiting surgical correction. One should not forget the use of broad-spectrum antibiotics in these cases.

GASTROINTESTINAL SYSTEM

Abnormalities involving the gastrointestinal system can present early in the post-partum period. Any evidence of blood in the stool or melena should be a signal for immediate intervention and thorough assessment of the foal. The two most common causes of melena in a neonatal foal are clostridial enterocolitis and hypoxic-ischemic bowel injury. Aggressive intervention is recommended in both these conditions. Enlargement of the abdomen can signify several disorders, including uroperitoneum and small- or large-bowel distention. If the distention is accompanied by signs of colic, the foal should be assessed thoroughly for ileus, peritonitis, meconium impactions, or other intestinal obstructions. Ultrasonography is useful for differentiating these conditions and guiding appropriate therapy.

Congenital atresia coli, atresia recti, or ani should also be considered in foals where no feces have been seen. In overo Paint horses the lethal white syndrome should be considered, especially if the foal is all white. In this condition there is atrophy of the distal small intestine and colon because of myenteric agangliosis. They usually develop progressive colic signs over the first 24 hours of life. There is no cure at this time for this condition.

If a gastrointestinal problem is identified, further diagnostics should include ultrasonography, radiography with or without barium, and abdominocentesis. In foals with colic, vital parameters do not always distinguish between surgical and medical cases. Foals tend to be less tolerant of abdominal pain than adults, but if the pain is non-responsive to analgesics, surgical exploration may be required.

MISCELLANEOUS DISORDERS

Hernias

Umbilical, inguinal, and scrotal hernias can occur in the foal and should be assessed early and monitored closely. Most congenital hernias are small, usually <5–6 cm in diameter, and reducible. These usually resolve spontaneously, but should be monitored by the caretakers and manually reduced at regular intervals. Usually umbilical hernias will have healed by about 6 months of age; if not, surgical correction should be considered. Umbilical clamps must be used with caution, since serious side effects can occur. If the umbilical hernias are >10 cm in diameter, they

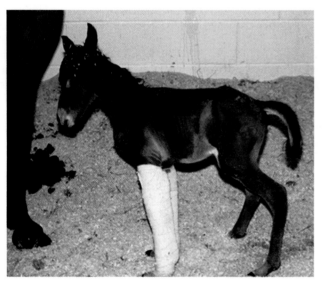

Figure 23-9. Foal straining to urinate.

usually require surgical correction. Fortunately these large hernias tend to be uncommon.

Inguinal hernias can contain omentum or bowel that has descended into the inguinal canal. If the contents descend past both the deep and superficial inguinal ring, they are considered scrotal hernia. Most are indirect hernias with the vaginal process or tunica vaginalis forming the hernial sac. A direct hernia would be one in which there is rupture of the tunica vaginalis. It is best to evaluate these hernias in lateral recumbency. Surgery should be considered if the hernia is not reducible. Also, should the hernia continue to enlarge or not resolve by 6 months of age, surgery should be considered.

IMMUNIZATION OF THE LATE-TERM MARE AND THE NEWBORN FOAL

Vaccinations to be administered to a foal will depend on the geographical location of the foal, the immunity of the mare, the farm history of disease, the plans for travel, and the risks involved with vaccination. Timing of vaccination is determined by the foal's ability to respond to the vaccine and on the mare's vaccination history. Vaccines are given to foals to protect them from diseases that they are at risk of acquiring during the foal and weanling stages, as well as those pathogens that will become a threat later in life. Diseases that should be considered for an immunization program include tetanus, influenza, herpesvirus 1 and 4, rotavirus, botulism, West Nile virus strangles, or encephalopathies such as eastern, western, and Venezuelan encephalomyelitis virus.

Management practices to reduce the exposure are equally as important as vaccinations and become even more important when considering those foal diseases that do not have good vaccines available (e.g., clostridial diarrhea, *R. equi*), Detailed vaccination recommendations for these diseases are further discussed in Chapter 25.

ANTHELMINTIC USE

Parasite control is important for the health and well-being of the foal and should be addressed early. Measures should be taken to reduce the parasite load on the fields that the foals will occupy even before the foal has arrived. Therefore, in addition to paying close attention to the deworming strategies used in the foals, the adult management is important as well. The lower the exposure to the foal, the better. This will require a combination of anthelmintic control and management strategies.

Deworming the mare with ivermectin at the time of parturition can delay the initial anthelmintic administration to the foal until 6–10 weeks of age, unless there is a recognized parasite problem on the farm. Alternatively, ivermectin can be given at 1 week of age. This is to target infection with *Strongyloides*. Moxidectin should not be used in foals <4 months of age. In the post-neonatal foal, the worms of greatest concern are the strongyles and the ascarids. Because of the development of ivermectin resistance in ascarids, the use of pyrantel pamoate in addition to ivermectin is recommended. Antiparasitic strategies are further addressed in Chapter 25.

ENVIRONMENT AND HYGIENE

As important as vaccinations, antibiotics, and passive transfer is the environment into which the foal is born. Weather conditions can vary during the foaling season, which will play a significant role in the risk assessment of the foal. This is especially true where the weather dictates that mares foaling early in the season are indoors. The use of designated foaling stalls have some advantages in that strict attention can be paid to ambient temperature, monitoring and intervention with foaling, and strict disinfection protocols, but they also lead to increased pathogen accumulation. Any stall that is to be used for foaling should be warm with clean bedding and it should not have been used for multiple horses without thorough disinfection in between. There is a trend for pathogens to accumulate within the environment as the foaling season progresses that puts foals born later in the season at greater risk. More rigorous disinfection should be performed as the season progresses. The mare herself poses a considerable risk to the foal for disease transmission. As the foal initially searches for the udder, it will mouth the mare all over. Therefore, cleaning the udder as well as the rest of her body, while concentrating on the hind limbs, will help to decrease the oral challenge with pathogens for the foal.

The risk of disease transmission lies not only with the physical environment of the foal, but any handlers, including veterinarians, also pose a risk. The use of gloves and designated clothing (e.g., gowns, coveralls) for each farm and each mare and foal pair is important to decrease the risk to the foal. If any disease is present on the premises, these precautions are a must and strict adherence to isolation of each foal is important. The use of designated boots and foot baths should also be part of the farm management. On the initial examination by the veterinarian, the environment should be assessed for cleanliness and suitability. In addition, animals that have contact with the foal, either directly or indirectly, should be assessed for disease. This will allow the veterinarian to take into account the risk to the foal when making decisions.

ORPHAN FOAL MANAGEMENT

The orphan foal requires different management considerations and special attention. Of course, all that applies to other foals also applies to the orphan. Depending on when the foal is orphaned, passive transfer may be of prime concern. After the provision of passive immunity, providing adequate nutrition to allow for good health and normal growth in the foal is imperative. The only way to provide a normal feeding schedule, as much as seven times per hour, is to provide a nurse mare. This is always the best option for the foal, since it provides companionship and education for the foal in addition to nutrition. It is possible to induce lactation in mares that have had at least one foal in previous years. The selection of a mare for induction of lactation should include a mare that has proven to be a good mother. There are several methods for inducing lactation, including the use of estradiol-benzoate, altrenogest, and sulpiride or domperidone, or alternatively dinoprost etradiole-benzoate altrenogest, and domperidone.[40]

If a nurse mare is not available, the foal can be trained to drink from a bucket. Feeding from a bowl or bucket is preferred to bottle feeding since it will reduce the bonding to humans and makes feeding easier after they are trained to drink. This will also decrease the chances of aspiration, which can occur when foals are fed via bottles. Several milk replacers are available that are specifically formulated for foals. These are recommended over goat milk or calf milk replacer. Milk replacers formulated for veal calves should be avoided since they are low in iron and can lead to anemia. Once a replacer is selected, changes should be avoided if possible, since this can lead to diarrhea or rejection of the milk by the foal.

Foals should generally be fed about 20%–30% of their body weight in milk each day (e.g., about 12 L for a 50-kg foal). The age of the foal at the time feeding is initiated will determine the amount of milk fed. The milk should be fed in several feedings. The normal foal will suckle up to seven times per hour, which is not feasible for an orphan foal; therefore, initially the foal should be fed every 2 hours for foals <5 days of age. This can gradually be increased with the goal being feeding every 6 hours by the time the foal is 10 days of age. If digestive problems such as colic or diarrhea develop, the quantity of milk fed should be decreased and the number of feedings increased. The foal's weight should be monitored and it should be gaining 1–2 kg per day.

Hay can start to be fed at about 10 days of age and grain can be introduced around 4–6 weeks of age. Milk-based pellets can be fed in addition to the milk, but these are poorly accepted by foals. In addition, foals should have fresh water available. Most orphan foals are ready to be weaned from milk at 3–4 months of age. Depression can be a significant issue with orphan foals. A companion in an adjacent stall or a goat may help to comfort the foal. The foal should be turned out in an individual paddock, since turning it out with other horses can result in injury to the foal.

REFERENCES

1. Madigan JE: *Manual of Equine Neonatal Medicine*, ed 3. Woodland, CA: Live Oak Publishing, 1997.
2. Koterba AM: Identification and early management of the high-risk neonatal foal: averting disasters. *Eq Vet Ed* 1:9-14, 1989.
3. Vaala WE, Sertich PL: Management strategies for mares at risk for periparturient complications. *Vet Clin North Am Eq Pract* 10:237-265, 1994.
4. Knottenbelt DC, Holdstock N, Madigan JE: Risk category of the foal. In *Equine Neonatology Medicine and Surgery*. Philadelphia, Saunders.
5. Vaala WE: Management of the high risk pregnancy; the peripartum period. Proc Amer College Vet Intern Med 7th ACVIM Forum. 1989, 417-420.
6. Doran RT, Threlfall WR, Kline R: Umbilical blood flow and effects of premature severance in the neonatal horse. Proceedings of the Society of Theriogenology 1985, pp 175–178.
7. Lavan RP, Madigan JE, Walker R, et al: Effects of disinfectant treatments on the bacterial flora of the umbilicus of neonatal foals. *Biol Reprod* 1:77-85, 1995.
8. McGuire TC, Crawford TB: Passive immunity in the foal: measurement of immunoglobulin classes and specific antibody. *Am J Vet Res* 34:1299-1303, 1973.
9. Cohen N: Causes of and farm management factors associated with disease and death in foals. *J Am Vet Med Assoc* 204:1644-1651, 1994.
10. Brewer BD, Koterba AM: Development of a scoring system for the early diagnosis of equine neonatal sepsis. *Eq Vet J* 20:18-22, 1988.
11. Robinson JA, Allen GK, Green EM, et al: A prospective study of septicemia in colostrum-deprived foals. *Eq Vet J* 25:214-219, 1993.
12. McClure JT, DeLuca JL, Miller J: Comparison of 5 screening tests for the detection of failure of passive transfer in foals. Proceedings of the 20th American College of Veterinary Internal Medicine Forum. 20:770, 2002.
13. McClure JT, Miller J, DeLuca JL: Comparison of two ELISA screening tests and a non-commercial glutaraldehyde screening test for the detection of failure of passive transfer in neonatal foals. *Proc Am Assoc Eq Pract* 49:301-305, 2003.
14. McGuire TC, Crawford TB, Hallowell AL, et al: Failure of colostral immunoglobulin transfer as an explanation for most infections and deaths of neonatal foals. *J Am Vet Med Assoc* 170:1302-1304, 1977.
15. Massey RE, LeBlanc MM, Klapstein EF: Colostrum feeding of foals and colostrum banking. *Proc Am Assoc Eq Pract* 37:1-8, 1991.
16. Cash RSG: Colostral quality determined by refractometry. *Eq Vet Educ* 11(1):36-38, 1999.
17. Morris DD, Meirs DA, Merryman GS: Passive transfer failure in horses: incidence and causative factors on a breeding farm. *Am J Vet Res* 46:2294-2299, 1985.
18. Kalinbacak A, Guzel M, Altintas I: Incidence of failure of immune passive transfer (FPT) in Thoroughbred foals—Interest of a rapid diagnosis for FPT. *Revue Méd Vét* 156:163-165, 2005.
19. Brewer B, Koterba A: Development of a scoring system for the early diagnosis of equine neonatal sepsis. *Eq Vet J* 20:18-22, 1988.
20. Wilkins PA, Dewan-Mix S: Efficacy of intravenous plasma to transfer passive immunity in clinically healthy and clinically ill equine neonates with failure of passive transfer. *Cornell Vet* 84:7-14, 1994.
21. McClure JT, Sellon DC, Hines MT: Immunologic disorders, equine immunodeficiency diseases. In Smith BP, ed: *Large Animal Internal Medicine*, ed 3. St Louis: Mosby, 2002.
22. Koterba AM, Brewer BD, Tarplee FA: Clinical and clinicopathological characteristics of the septicemic neonatal foal: review of 38 cases. *Eq Vet J* 16:376-382, 1984.
23. Clabough DL, Levine JF, Grant GL, et al: Factors associated with failure of passive transfer of colostral antibodies in standardbred foals. *J Vet Intern Med* 5:335-340, 1991.
24. Metzger N, Hinchcliff KW, Hardy J, et al: Usefulness of a commercial equine IgG test and serum protein concentration as indicators of failure of transfer of passive immunity in hospitalized foals. *J Vet Intern Med* 20:382-387, 2006.
25. Rumbaugh GE, Ardans AA, Ginno D, et al: Measurement of neonatal equine immunoglobulins for assessment of colostral immunoglobulin transfer: Comparison of single radioimmunodiffusion with zinc sulfate turbidity test, serum protein electrophoresis, refractory for total serum protein and sodium sulfate precipitation test. *J Am Vet Med Assoc* 172:321-325, 1978.
26. Buening GM, Perryman LE, McGuire TC: Practical methods of determining serum immunoglobulin M and immunoglobulin G concentrations in foals. *J Am Vet Med Assoc* 171:455-458, 1977.
27. LeBlanc MM: A modified zinc sulfate turbidity test for the detection of immune status in newly born foals. *J Eq Vet Sci* 10:36-40, 1990.
28. Clabough DL, Conboy HS, Roberts MC: Comparison of four screening techniques for the diagnosis of equine neonatal hypogammaglobulinemia. *J Am Vet Med Assoc* 194:1717-1720, 1989.
29. McClure JT, DeLuca JL, Lunn DP, et al: Evaluation of IgG concentration and IgG subisotypes in foals with complete or partial failure of passive transfer after administration of intravenous serum or plasma. *Eq Vet J* 33:681-686, 2001.
30. McClure JT, Davis R, Giguére S: Evaluation of five commercially available assays and measurement of serum total protein concentration via refractometry for the diagnosis of failure of passive transfer of immunity in foals. *J Am Vet Med Assoc* 227:1640-1645, 2005.
31. Davis DG, Schaefer DM, Hinchcliff KW, et al: Measurement of serum IgG in foals by radial immunodiffusion and automated turbidimetric immunoassay. *J Vet Intern Med* 19:93-96, 2005.
32. Pemberton DH, Thomas KW, Terry MJ: Hypogammaglobulinemia in foals: Prevalence on Victorian studs and simple methods for detection and correction in the field. *Aust Vet J* 56:469-473, 1980.
33. LeBlanc MM: Immunologic considerations. In Koterba AM, Drummond WN, Kosch PC, eds: *Equine Clinical Neonatology*. Philadelphia: Lea & Febiger, 1990.
34. Riley CB, McClure JT, Low-Ying S, et al: Use of Fourier-transform infrared spectroscopy for the diagnosis of failure of passive immunity and measurement of immunoglobulin concentrations in horses. *J Vet Intern Med* 21:828-834, 2007.
35. Rumbaigh GE, Ardans AA, Ginno D, et al: Identification and treatment of colostrum deficient foals. *J Am Vet Med Assoc* 174:273-275, 1979.
36. White S: The use of plasma in foals with failure of passive transfer and/or sepsis. *Proc Am Assoc Eq Pract* 43:215-218. 1989.
37. Stoneham SJ: Collection and administration of plasma to a newborn foal. *InPractice* 20:384-384, 1997.
38. Lokai MD, Meyer RJ: Preliminary observations on oxytetracycline treatment of congenital flexural deformities in foals. *Mod Vet Pract* 66:237-239, 1985.
39. Reef VB: *Equine Diagnostic Ultrasound*. Philadelphia: WB Saunders, 1998.
40. Daels PF, Bowers-Lepore J: How to induce lactation in a mare and make her adopt an orphan foal: What 5 years of experience have taught us. *Proc Am Assoc Eq Pract* 353:349-353, 2007.

BREEDING THE POST-PARTUM MARE

PHIL MATTHEWS AND JUAN C. SAMPER

It has been shown that in order to keep a 12-month inter-foaling interval, the average number of days from foaling to conception must be around 25 days. Therefore, mares must be bred at the earliest opportunity that will give them the best chance for conceiving and maintaining the pregnancy.

In order to determine this optimal time, it is important to know the physiology of the post-partum mare. On average, mares start their first post-partum heat around 6 or 7 days and ovulate on days 9–11. Therefore, mares that have foaled normally have been normal since foaling and are to be bred on foal heat should be examined by day 6, 7, or 8 post-partum. This allows for several goals to be achieved during this examination. The mare's reproductive health can be ascertained, where she is in her cycle can be determined, and plans can be made to obtain semen or book her to a stallion in time to be bred prior to ovulation. (The growth size of her ovulatory follicle will determine if sequential examinations are necessary prior to breeding this cycle.) This first foal heat examination should consist of a thorough visual examination of the external genitalia, vestibule, vagina, and cervix, as well as an assessment of the uterus, broad ligament, and ovaries by transrectal palpation and ultrasonography.

Mares that appear to have no foaling complications are still examined for tears and bruising of the vulva and vestibule as well as lacerations to the vagina and cervix. The more difficult the birth, the more likely these traumas are to occur; however, they can occur in any foaling mare and with an increased frequency in primiparous mares. Therefore, a careful vaginal speculum examination is necessary; if there is any doubt of cervical trauma on the part of the veterinarian, he or she should perform a digital examination on the cervix to determine the extent of the damage. Not only unexpected trauma may be discovered during this examination, but a not-yet-detected uterine discharge may be discovered during this foal heat examination. As mentioned, careful palpation and ultrasonographic evaluation is also necessary at this time to not only assess estral status, but to ascertain signs of internal trauma such as hematomas caused by uterine artery ruptures and bleeding in to the broad ligament.

However, this initial examination should take place prior to foal heat if the foaling was abnormal, the placenta was retained or was grossly abnormal, or the mare develops an abnormal uterine discharge. Obviously an abnormal birth or placenta will be realized at or soon after parturition, but a uterine discharge may not develop for several days. Therefore, it is incumbent upon the breeder to be looking for signs of discharge that sometimes can be obvious visually. However, there are those that are not, and monitoring the temperature daily on these post-partum mares can be valuable in detecting a uterine discharge in that most will develop a fever of varying degrees. Mares that are unable to go outside and exercise in the days after foaling will have a greater chance of developing a uterine discharge. When inclement weather or problems with the foal dictate that the mare stay in the barn, she is unable to exercise normally and is less likely to get up and down and roll as she would outside. These normal activities are part of the physical process of uterine clearance in the post-foaling uterus as it involutes. Administration of oxytocin may help avoid a uterine discharge by aiding with uterine clearance.

STRATEGIES FOR POST-PARTUM BREEDING

Foal Heat

Assessing the foal heat begins at day 6, 7, or 8, depending on how much notice is needed in getting on the stallion's breeding book or ordering cooled semen. As mentioned previously, the examination should consist of the visual assessment of the perineum, the speculum examination, and the transrectal palpation and ultrasound examination. As with any pre-breeding examination, the cervical relaxation, uterine edema, and follicle size are all monitored and their progression is used to predict ovulation or to time the administration of an ovulatory agent.

Foal heat is somewhat different from subsequent heats in this process because of the possibility of post-foaling trauma or uterine discharge. Prudently, evidence of trauma of any severity would mean not breeding this heat and giving the mare time to heal and recover from such. Uterine discharge would also mean "passing" this heat, but would also indicate treatment by uterine lavage, ecbolics, and possibly systemic antibiotics and anti-inflammatories in severe cases.

During the transrectal ultrasound examination of the foal heat mare, there is a slightly increased propensity to find more uterine fluid than in subsequent cycles. The fluid is often of a normal character (anechoic) but of more volume than expected. These mares may be candidates for "passing" as well, especially if the fluid does not resolve with administration of an ecbolic.

Some breeders will determine whether to breed on foal heat based on when ovulation is predicted to occur. There is certainly anecdotal evidence to support that mares that ovulate later in foal heat (after 10 days) have a higher conception rate than those ovulating early (before day 9). Studies have also shown that mares that are selectively bred on foal heat perform as well as mares that are bred in subsequent cycles. These studies also indicate that there is no significant difference in the fetal loss of mares bred on foal heat compared with mares bred later.[10,11]

Routine culturing of foal heat mares is not rewarding. Often the cultures will be positive for contaminants or mixed growth of potential pathogens. The examination itself is going to be more telling in determining whether or not this foal heat mare is suitable to breed.[7,8]

Although teasing of the post-partum mare can be helpful, it can be unreliable. Most mares have a protective instinct toward the newborn foal and the signs of estrus can be very subtle or non-existent even though the mare is cycling. This problem is even more accentuated in mares with their first foal at foot. Most mares tend to display better behavior with age or as the number of estrus cycles increases.

Recent data by Agricola et al.[1] from examining biopsies of mares 14 and 22 days post-partum revealed that on day 14, 100% of the mares had RBCs and siderophages in the endometrium. By day 22, these were only present on 40% and 70% of the mares, respectively. However, by Day 14, 40% of the post-partum mares had neutrophils and 70% had glandular dilatation. By day 22, no mares had dilated glands nor neutrophils. This clearly indicates that the clean-up process in the mares endometrium takes at least more than 14 days and would support the common belief that mares should not be bred prior to day 10.

DELAYING THE FOAL HEAT

Because mares tend to have a reduction in fertility when bred early after foaling, veterinarians and broodmare managers have tried to delay the onset of foal heat with the use of progesterone and estradiol to block follicular development. For this, mares are treated with 150 mg of progesterone and 10 mg of estradiol-17β for 3 or 4 days. The treatment must begin in the first 24 hours after foaling, or it will not work properly.[6,13] In the author's opinion, it should be started within the first 6 hours after foaling for the best results; if started later than 24 hours, the mare's natural drive to have a foal heat will override the treatment and she will ovulate in spite of the therapy. This will delay the mare's natural follicular development for as many days as the veterinarian treats her, and in this manner the management can be sure that the mare will ovulate 10 days or later post-partum. In several trials this therapy has worked very well.

SHORT CYCLE AFTER FOAL HEAT OVULATION

Since it has been shown that uterine involution is incomplete and inflammatory products are still in the uterus in most mares until day 14 post-partum, an alternative method for mare management is to short cycle the post-partum mare after her foal heat ovulation. This should allow these mares to be bred approximately 10 days before the natural subsequent cycle. This method is achieved by administering prostaglandin F2α to the mare on day 6 after ovulation. This management effort is best achieved if the mare's foal heat is monitored so that the day of ovulation can be determined. It is important to realize that the interval between prostaglandin treatment and ovulation may vary greatly depending on the presence of diestral follicles at the time of treatment. Mares should be examined at the time of treatment in order to assess the presence of diestral follicles; follicles >30 mm will tend to move much faster than smaller follicles. Mares with even larger follicles may come in to heat and ovulate so quickly that it is difficult to arrange for getting them bred. Therefore, by performing this transrectal ultrasound examination at the time of prostaglandin treatment, the breeding manager and veterinarian are provided with a good indication of how quickly the mare

will return to estrus and ovulate. This same examination can help avoid previously undetected ovulations that could have further delayed the return to estrus.

SECOND NATURAL OVULATION

Once the mare has had her first ovulation post-partum and if her reproductive tract is normal (including no bacterial contamination of the uterus), she should start to have regular 19-22–day interovulatory intervals. Veterinarians must realize the importance of the 8-10–day post-partum examination. This examination not only provides information on the degree of uterine involution, but will also help predict when the mare should come into heat and ovulate in her second natural estrus. Mares that have an early second post-partum ovulation should be considered abnormal and appropriate diagnostic techniques such as ultrasound, culture, and cytology should be pursued in order to determine the cause. On the other hand, mares that do not appear to have a foal heat ovulation must also be evaluated for bacterial contamination of the uterus or inadequate nutritional practices. It should be highlighted that lack of behavioral signs of estrus does not necessarily indicate a lack of cyclicity.

Other possible explanations for mares failing to cycle after foal heat are seasonal anestrus and lactational anestrus. Mares that foal early in the year may have a foal heat, but some may regress to a seasonal anestrus whereas others may not have an ovulation at all after foaling. When this occurs, it is unfortunate because the foaling advantage gained by this early foaling will now be lost for next year. As with seasonal anestrus with any mare, the only treatment is exposure to an extended photoperiod, which will take approximately 6–8 weeks to stimulate ovulation. This regression can be prevented by putting the pregnant mares under lights prior to foaling, mimicking the same schedule that is used with the barren mares.

Lactational anestrus is described as a failure to ovulate because of the physical activity of lactating and suckling a foal. Whether this in fact occurs or not is controversial.[2,3] Certainly poor body condition may contribute to poor reproductive performance, and some think that the mares that are being labeled as exhibiting lactational anestrus are actually being influenced by a combination of the effects of poor body condition, lactational demands, and season of the year.[4] It has been reported that weaning these mares will result in follicular activity and ovulation.

POST-FOALING THERAPIES

Mares with perineal conformation problems should have their vulva closed as soon as practical after foaling. How soon the mare's vulva is sutured will depend on how poor her conformation is. If the mare has been opened before foaling, she should be sutured as soon as possible. Caslick's operation can be performed immediately after foaling or even in the first few days; however, it is not recommended to put unnecessary stress in the mare that could increase the mare's blood pressure and precipitate other problems.

Management of mares during the post-partum period and immediately after breeding should be done aggressively, but the indiscriminate treatment of mares or blanket therapies on post-foaling mares is not recommended. Some clinicians believe in the routine treatment of mares with antibiotics or uterine lavage; however, these therapies should be performed based on clinical signs. Although it is important to remove fluid and debris from post-partum mares that have a problem, the procedure is not appropriate for every mare.[12] In a controlled study using 100 mares, 50% were flushed on day 4 post-partum and 50% served as controls; the most important factor affecting foal-heat conception was the foaling-to-ovulation interval whereas flushing appeared to have no effect.[5] Routine lavage should be performed in mares with heavy purulent vaginal discharges, febrile mares post-partum, and mares with retained placentas.

Reducing the foaling-to-breeding interval is important in the overall management of a commercial breeding operation. Proper assessment of the post-foaling mare should be carried out in any cases where the foaling was not routine or the mare has had a problem since foaling, such as a uterine discharge. A thorough examination should be made of the foal heat mare to assess her reproductive health, whether she is a good candidate to breed on foal heat or to document her ovulation for short cycling. When the clinician has decided to breed the mare, aggressive post-breeding examinations and therapies are perhaps the most cost-effective way to approach the breeding cycle by helping to ensure that pregnancy ensues from the breeding. Therapies such as uterine lavage and the use of ecbolic agents such as oxytocin, carbetocin, or cloprostenol should be considered, depending on fluid accumulation and the amount of inflammation after breeding.

REFERENCES

1. Agricola R, Pessa P, Barbosa M, et al: Microvascularization and proliferation of cell nuclear antigen expression in the post-partum endometrium in the mare. *Anim Reprod Sci* 94:417-419, 2006.
2. Loy RG: Characteristics of post-partum fertility in the mare. *Vet Clin North Am Large Anim Pract* 2:345-359, 1980.
3. Palmer E, Drincourt MA: Some interactions of season of foaling, fertile period and ovarian activity in the equine. *Livestock Prod Sci* 10:197, 1983.
4. Ginther OJ: *Reproductive Biology of the Mare*, ed 2. Cross Plains, WI: Equiservices 1992.
5. Blanchard TL, Varner DD, Brinsko SP, et al: Effects of postparturient uterine lavage on uterine involution in the mare. *Theriogenology* 32(4):527-535, 1989.
6. Bruemmer JE, Brady HA, Blanchard TL: Uterine involution, day and variance of first postpartum ovulation in mares treated with progesterone and estradiol-17beta for 1 or 2 days postpartum. *Theriogenology* 57(2):989-995, 2002.
7. Huhtinen M, Reilas T, Katila T: Recovery rate and quality of embryos from mares inseminated at the first post-partum oestrus. *Acta Vet Scand* 37(3):343-350, 1996.
8. Katila T, Koskinen E, Oijala M, Parviainen P: Evaluation of the post-partum mare in relation to foal heat breeding. II. Uterine swabbing and biopsies. *Zentralbl Veterinarmed A* 35(5):331-333, 1988.
9. Lowis TC, Hyland JH: Analysis of post-partum fertility in mares on a thoroughbred stud in southern Victoria. *Aust Vet J* 68(9):304-306, 1991.
10. McCue PM, Hughes JP: The effect of postpartum uterine lavage on foal heat pregnancy rate. *Theriogenology* 33(5):1121-1129, 1990.
11. McKinnon AO, Squires EL, Harrison LA, et al: Ultrasonographic studies on the reproductive tract of mares after parturition: effect of involution and uterine fluid on pregnancy rates in mares with normal and delayed first postpartum ovulatory cycles. *J Am Vet Med Assoc* 192(3):350-353, 1988.
12. McPhearson M, Blanchard TL: Breeding mares in foal heat. *Eq Vet Educ* 17:200-204, 2005.
13. Sexton PE, Bristol FM: Uterine involution in mares treated with progesterone and estradiol-17 beta. *J Am Vet Med Assoc* 186(3):252-256, 1985.

PREVENTIVE MEDICINE AND MANAGEMENT OF THE BROODMARE AND THE FOAL

NELSON I. PINTO

In the first weeks of life, the foal will be challenged by different pathogens such as infectious agents and parasites. Proper management of the broodmare in the last third of gestation is very important to improve the immunological response of the foal against those infectious agents and to decrease the exposure to some parasites.

VACCINATION

Several authors have reviewed vaccination protocols for broodmares and foals, providing important guidelines in different publications.[1-8] This chapter was written based on a review of these publications and several scientific studies.

Infectious agents are the most important cause of morbidity and mortality in human and veterinary medicine. In animal health they are responsible for significant economic losses represented in cost of treatment, delay in animal development, or animal losses.

Dr. Edward Jenner discovered the vaccine against smallpox in cows in 1798,[9] and since then vaccination or immunization became one of the biggest strategies to control and eradicate infectious diseases in human and animal populations. Depending on the situation, the objective of vaccination is to prevent, ameliorate, or treat infections. Vaccination programs have to be designed based on clinical and epidemiological observations and economic constraints in order to be rational and effective.

Epidemiology is one of the sciences that helps understand the relationship between the causal agent, the host, and the environment in the disease process. These three factors determine the presence and severity of the infectious disease. Epidemiological and clinical studies provide valuable data about infectious disease, such as mechanism of transmission, latent period, incubation period, route of contamination, geographic distribution of the disease, population susceptibility, and shedding patterns of the organism from infected individuals. The knowledge of these elements allows us to design better control programs and prevention against infectious diseases.

Other important variables in the design of a vaccination program are the immunological features of the available vaccines. Vaccine characteristics include its capacity to generate antibodies and/or cellular responses, the type of vaccine (live or killed), the type of antibodies produced, and longevity of the immunological response to that particular antigen. In addition, the risk for adverse reactions—and in the case of the broodmare and the neonate, information regarding immunoglobulin levels in the colostrum and the duration of maternal immunity in the neonate—should be taken into account. Another important aspect that needs to be taken into account is the possible interference of maternal immunity on the foal's ability to produce antibodies. Unfortunately, information about passive transfer of immunity and antibody production in the foal is available only for a limited amount of the commercial vaccines, which makes it difficult to design an ideal vaccination protocol for the broodmare and the newborn foal.

Immunology and Mechanism of Action

After the vaccine is administered, it induces an adaptive response of the immune system in the patient. This adaptive response is mediated either by antibodies or effector cells such as cytotoxic T lymphocytes (CTLs). The CTLs express a CD8 molecule and T-helper (TH) lymphocytes express a CD4 molecule. The TH lymphocytes can be TH-1 or TH-2; TH-1 induces cytotoxic and inflammatory responses, and TH-2 stimulates antibody response.

In order for the lymphocyte to respond, the antigen has to be presented either by infected cells or by specialized cells such as macrophages. Those antigens are presented through the major histocompatibility complex (MHC) molecules. The Type I molecules are present in all cells, and the Type II molecules are present in specialized antigen-presenting cells. The CD8 and CD4 molecules in the lymphocyte act as a receptor for the MHC molecules. As a result, cytotoxic lymphocytes (CD8+) respond only to antigens presented through MHC I molecules because of cellular infection and TH lymphocytes will respond to those antigens presented, through MHC II.[1,2]

Types of Vaccines

The type and extension of the immune response after the vaccine administration, as well as the frequency of dosage, are strongly related to the type of vaccine.

There are two different types of vaccines in equine medicine:
1. Killed vaccines: Inactivated pathogen and subunit vaccines are listed as killed vaccines. In the inactivated pathogen vaccines, the agent is treated with heat or chemicals to be inactivated, but their antigenicity is preserved. The subunit vaccines are made from extracted proteins from the pathogen.

These vaccines are biologically safe, but they need strong adjuvants to stimulate the immune system.

Killed vaccines are less likely to induce disease in immunocompromised individuals, but some of them can fail to induce protective cellular immune responses because they are unlikely to generate CTL response.[1] Also, their efficacy depends on the production of antibodies and the antibody longevity. With killed vaccines the patient requires more frequent boosters to keep the antibody level at protective levels. The presence of certain adjuvants in inactivated vaccines and the frequent dosing can increase the risk for adverse local and allergic reactions. Several types of vaccine adjuvants are used at present; the adjuvant enhances the immune response (humoral or cellular) against the antigen included in the vaccine, and they aim to induce less adverse reactions.[10,11]

2. Live vaccines: There are three different classes of live vaccines: (1) modified-live, (2) recombinant, and (3) chimera vaccines. In modified-live vaccines the agent is alive but attenuated; these vaccines induce both humoral and cellular immune responses. Recombinant vaccines use a vector or a carrier such as a bacterium or a virus (Canarypox) to express the antigen. In chimera vaccines, the pathogen and the vector belong to the same family. This type of vaccine has been used against viral infections such as West Nile virus. All types of live vaccines have good antigenicity, providing longer immunity, but sick or immunocompromised animals could develop the disease that they are being vaccinated against. In addition, live vaccines can reverse their pathogenicity. The use of live vaccines in pregnant mares is not recommended because they can induce some type of infection and/or abortion, and in the case of herpesvirus 1, the risk could be higher.[2,11]

IMMUNOLOGY OF THE FOAL

Understanding the immunological status of the neonate is very important in designing the vaccination protocol of both the pregnant mare and the foal. Proper vaccination of the mare facilitates the production of good-quality colostrum, which should have higher levels of antibodies against the more prevalent infectious agents for the foal in their particular geographical area.

The fetal immune system is able to respond and produce immunoglobulins against specific antigens at Day 200 of gestation, and at birth the equine neonate has a fully developed immune system with lymphocyte counts close to those reported in adult horses. However, the epitheliochorial placentation in the mare acts as a barrier between mare and fetus for maternal immunoglobulin transfer. For this reason foals have low levels of circulating immunoglobulins at birth, and therefore the presence of high levels of IgG in a newborn foal before nursing is indicative of *in utero* immunological stimulation.[7]

The main source of immunoglobulins for the newborn is colostrum, which the mare produces in the last 2–3 weeks of pregnancy. The levels of immunoglobulins in serum and colostrum in the mare do not show a direct relationship, suggesting that the production of some of the immunoglobulins occurs in the mammary gland.[12] Colostrum composition in addition to immunoglobulins includes cells such as lymphocytes, macrophages, neutrophils, and epithelial cells. In addition, colostrum has other components such as hormones, growth factors, and enzymes.[13-16]

After ingestion of colostrum, the IgG is absorbed in the small intestine by pinocytosis in a non-selective process. This capacity of absorption decreases rapidly with time; it is reduced by 22% at 3 hours and is <1% by 20 hours. This is the reason why providing colostrum to the newborn foal in the first hours of life is vital; otherwise the risk for failure of passive transfer and sepsis is higher.[17] Several factors can influence the level of IgG in the foal after colostrum ingestion, such as insufficient and/or late intake, lack of absorption, lack of production for the mare, and poor quality of the colostrum.

Several types of immunoglobulins are found in the colostrum with different concentrations and circulatory half-life in the foal. IgG is the highest in colostrum, followed by IgA and IgM. The IgG has three different types: IgGb, IgGa, and IgG(T), with IgGb being predominant in the colostrum. The half-life for IgGa in the foal is 18 days, 32 days for IgGb, and 21 days for IgG(T). IgG reaches the lowest concentration between 1 and 2 months of life. Other immunoglobulins such as IgA and IgM reach their lowest concentration in the foal by 3–4 weeks of age.[13,14] Starting around 3 months, lymphocyte (T and B) population duplicates, resulting in an increase of IgG and IgM levels.[16,18]

The ingestion of colostrum has been related to partial suppression of immune response in equine neonates; however, foals depend exclusively of this source of antibodies to be protected against the environmental pathogens. The timing on the foal vaccination is critical. Several studies have shown the relationship between vaccinations before 6 months of age and poor immunological responses to some vaccines, suggesting that some vaccines administered to foals before the levels of maternal antibodies are low can induce inadequate production of antibodies in the foal and can induce the failing of subsequent doses by inducing a possible immunotolerance to those particular vaccines.[19-23] With all of these facts in mind, it is plausible to vaccinate the foals after 4–6 months of life.[5]

VACCINATION IN THE BROODMARE AND THE FOAL

The goals in broodmare vaccination are (1) protecting the mare from infectious diseases that can affect her directly and/or induce abortion, and (2) protecting the foal by improving the quality of colostrum in the mare. On the other hand, vaccination in the foal aims to protect it after the maternal antibodies decrease. Based on these premises, several vaccines can be added to the core vaccines in the broodmare. Broodmares should be vaccinated in the last 4–8 weeks of pregnancy against those diseases that the foal is at high risk for in its first few months of life. Also, the foals have to be vaccinated against those organisms that affect them after the maternal immunity decreases.

As of July 2007, the U.S. Department of Agriculture–licensed biological products for use in equine include those to prevent infectious diseases such as tetanus, eastern equine encephalomyelitis (EEE), western equine encephalomyelitis (WEE), Venezuelan equine encephalomyelitis (VEE), West Nile virus (WNV), equine herpes virus type 1 (EHV-1), equine herpes virus type 4 (EHV-4), equine viral arteritis (EVA), equine influenza, strangles, rabies, Potomac horse fever (PHF), and botulism type B. Vaccines such as rotavirus and equine protozoal encephalomyelitis (EPM) are conditionally licensed.

Recent publications recommend core vaccines for horses. These vaccines are aimed at controlling diseases widely spread in the country and/or having high mortality and/or public health relevance. The core vaccines include tetanus, EEE, WEE, WNV, and more recently rabies. In the case of broodmares, EHV-1 is included in the core vaccination to prevent abortion. Other vaccines can be added based on the geographic area or if the individual will travel to areas endemic of a particular disease.[5,6,8]

Specific Vaccines

Equine Encephalitis (EEE, WEE, and VEE)

The viruses that cause equine encephalitis belong to the Togaviridae family, and although transmitted mainly by mosquitoes, birds and rodents are the reservoirs because of their ability to support high viremias. Their incubation period in the horse is 2–3 days, but can go up to 3 weeks. Initial clinical signs include fever, and with time neurological signs are present such as depression, ataxia, and paralysis consequence of brain stem, cortical, and spinal cord dysfunction. The clinical signs are progressive and the disease prolonged for 2–14 days. Clinical cases are more common during the summer and early fall. Prevention plans include mosquito control and frequent vaccinations in areas where the disease is endemic. Only inactivated vaccines are available in the United States: bivalent (EEE and WEE) or trivalent (WEE, EEV and EEE). EEV vaccine is not commonly used based on the lack of clinical cases for more than 20 years. Vaccination in the broodmare is recommended 4–6 weeks before foaling to induce good maternal immunity in the foals. Like other vaccines, maternal immunity against equine encephalitis has an inhibitory effect on the foal to produce its own antibodies, even after two vaccinations; for this reason, vaccination in foals from vaccinated mares should start between 4 to 6 months of age, with two doses 4–6 weeks apart, and a third dose at 10–12 months of age or before the start of the mosquito season. In endemic areas such as the southeastern United States, vaccination in foals from vaccinated mares starts at 2–3 months of age, with three doses 4 weeks apart, and the fourth dose at 10–12 months of age. In the case of foals from unvaccinated mares, vaccination starts at 3–4 months of age; they need two doses 4 weeks apart, and a third at 10–12 months or before the mosquito season starts.[5,8,24]

West Nile Virus (WNV)

First diagnosed in North America in 1999, WNV spread rapidly throughout the United States and Canada. This endemic condition and the severity of the disease made WNV vaccine a core vaccine. WNV, as other encephalitides viruses, is transmitted mainly by some species of mosquitoes. Birds are the main reservoir, where the virus replicates, and the virus is transmitted to the mosquito, which inoculates birds, humans, and horses, among other species.

The WNV vaccines available for horses have shown good efficacy, and they are (1) inactivated vaccine, (2) the live canarypox vector vaccine, and (3) the live flavivirus-chimera vaccine. The inactivated vaccine provides protection and adequate production of antibodies, reducing the viremia in horses. The canarypox vaccine provides early protection, with one dose and two doses 5 weeks apart administered and challenged after a mosquito infected challenge model.[25,26] It also provided coverage in an intrathecal infection model.[27] The flavivirus vaccine has proved to be safe at higher doses, and it induces early protection at 10 days after vaccination for up to a year.[28,29] In one study all three vaccines were compared in an intrathecal challenge model; all vaccinated horses survived, but the group with the chimera vaccine showed fewer clinical signs compared with the control group and the inactivated vaccine group.[30]

Vaccination against this disease is strongly recommended for every horse; broodmares need to be vaccinated 4 weeks before foaling to provide good maternal immunity to the foal.[3] At some point the safety of the WNV vaccines in pregnant mares was questioned, but no evidence of the relationship between malformed fetuses or stillbirths has been found using the inactivated vaccine.[31] Maternal immunity does not inhibit the foals' ability to produce antibodies, and foals can then be vaccinated as early as 4 months of age with good antibody production.[4,5] The most recent review recommends different vaccination protocols according to the type of vaccine (Tables 25-1 and 25-2).[8]

Rabies

The incidence of rabies in North America is low, but vaccination is recommended in areas where the disease is prevalent in wildlife. There are three different inactivated vaccines, and their use in broodmares is recommended 4–6 weeks before foaling. In foals from vaccinated mares, the vaccine should be administered twice with a 4-6–week interval, starting at 6 months of age, and a third dose should be administered between 10 and 12 months of age; in the case of foals from non-vaccinated mares, the initial vaccine starts at 3 months of age.[8] After a primary vaccination the antibodies reach the highest level at 28 days, and it is considered immunized at that time. Booster is required 1 month after the first dose and on a yearly basis thereafter.

Equine Herpes Virus 1 and 4

There are nine different equine herpes viruses, five of which infect the domestic horse (1-5), and two (6 and 9) are often associated with wild equid infection. Herpes virus can survive in the environment between 7 and 35 days but are susceptible to regular disinfectants and heat. Among the herpes viruses, the alpha herpes viruses (1 and 4) are most commonly associated with disease in horses. Those two viruses are highly contagious and can spread through nasal secretion, and the remnants of abortions are highly contaminated with infectious particles. The infection is transmitted by aerosol and/or ingestion. The EHV-1 affects the endothelium and produces viremia and neurological signs, and in pregnant mares it can infect the fetus and induce abortion. In contrast, EHV-4 is more associated with respiratory disease and does not have an affinity for the endothelium.

An important epidemiological characteristic of EHV is that some horses can be infected without clinical signs (latent infection). Those individuals became reservoirs of the virus and are responsible for the spread of disease.[32] The latently infected horse can develop a new episode of virus replication and shedding without clinical signs, especially after a stressful situation. As a consequence, new clinical cases will be seen on those farms. The latently infected individual with EHV-1 can also develop clinical signs such as neurological symptoms or abortion under stress situations.[33]

Inactivated vaccines with EHV-1 and EHV-4 are available. Pregnant mares should be vaccinated at 5, 7, and 9 months of pregnancy to reduce the incidence of abortion,[34] although some studies do not show significant differences between vaccinated and non-vaccinated mares.[2] Vaccination in weanlings with a combined EHV-1 and EHV-4 was protective with two doses 4 weeks apart and challenged 2 weeks after the last vaccination with EHV-4. Also, the vaccinated weanlings shed virus for less time and the clinical signs were milder compared with the control group.[34]

Table 25-1 | **Vaccinations in the Broodmare**[*]

DISEASE	BROODMARES PREVIOUSLY VACCINATED	BROODMARES NON-VACCINATED OR UNKNOWN VACCINATION HISTORY
Tetanus	Annual 4–6 weeks pre-partum	2-dose series (4–6 weeks apart). Revaccinate 4–6 weeks pre-partum.
EEE/WEE	Annual 4–6 weeks pre-partum	2-dose series (4 weeks apart). Revaccinate 4–6 weeks pre-partum.
WNV	Annual 4–6 weeks pre-partum	In areas of high risk: Inactivated vaccine: 2-dose series, 4–6 weeks apart. Revaccinate prior to the onset of the next vector season. Recombinant canary pox vaccine: 2-dose series, 4–6 weeks apart. Revaccinate prior to the onset of the next vector season. Flavivirus chimera vaccine: Single dose Another dose is recommended prior to the onset of the next vector season.
Rabies	Annual 4–6 weeks pre-partum or before breeding	Annual
Botulism	Annual 4–6 weeks pre-partum	3-dose series 8, 9, and 10 months gestation.
EHV	3-dose series with product labeled for protection against EHV abortion. Give at 5, 7, and 9 months of gestation.	Annually, but consider 6-month revaccination interval for: <ul><li>Horses <5 years of age</li><li>Horses on breeding farms or in contact with pregnant mares</li><li>Performance or show horses at high risk</li></ul>
EVA	Not recommended unless high risk. Vaccinate when mares are open.	Not recommended unless high risk.
Influenza	Previously vaccinated: Inactivated vaccine: Semi-annual with one dose administered 4–6 weeks pre-partum. Canarypox vector vaccine: Semi-annual with one dose administered 4–6 weeks prepartum	Inactivated vaccine: 3-dose series <ul><li>2nd dose 4–6 weeks after 1st dose</li><li>3rd dose 4–6 weeks pre-partum</li></ul> Canarypox vector vaccine: 2-dose series <ul><li>2nd dose 4–6 weeks after 1st dose but no later than 4 weeks pre-partum</li></ul>
Potomac horse fever (PHF)	Semi-annual, with one dose given 4–6 weeks prepartum	2-dose series <ul><li>1st dose 7–9 weeks pre-partum.</li><li>2nd dose 4–6 weeks pre-partum.</li></ul>
Rotavirus	3-dose series <ul><li>1st dose at 8 months gestation</li><li>2nd and 3rd doses at 4-week intervals thereafter.</li></ul>	3-dose series <ul><li>1st dose at 8 months gestation.</li><li>2nd and 3rd doses at 4-week intervals thereafter.</li></ul>
Strangles *Streptococcus equi*	Killed vaccine containing M protein): Semi-annual with one dose given 4–6 weeks pre-partum.	Killed vaccine containing M protein): 3-dose series <ul><li>2nd dose 2–4 weeks after 1st dose</li><li>3rd dose 4–6 weeks pre-partum</li></ul>

[*]Vaccinations for Adult Horses developed by the American Association of Equine Practitioners Infectious Disease Committee, 2008. Available at: http://www.aaep.org/images/files/Adultvaccinationtablerevised108.pdf.

The use of a modified-live EHV-1 vaccine has been proposed as an alternative to prevent abortion for some practitioners, and it is claimed that this vaccine provides cross protection against EHV-4. When it is used in pregnant mares at breeding time and 6–8 weeks before foaling, it results in improved colostrum quality against both pathogens and protecting the foal from respiratory disease produced by EHV-1 or EHV-4.[3]

There is evidence that foals from vaccinated mares have a reduced ability to produce antibodies after administration of inactivated vaccines (EHV-1, and EHV-1 and EHV-4) for up to 5 months of age,[4,35] but cellular immune response was evident against both viruses in foals vaccinated with a modified live EHV-1 vaccine.[36] The consequence of this maternal immunity interference suggests that vaccination in foals against herpes virus should start between 4 and 6 months of age. Two doses are indicated at 4- to 6-week intervals, and a third dose should be administered between 10 and 12 months of age. This vaccination protocol in foals is valid for inactivated and modified live herpes virus vaccines.[3,4,8]

Tetanus

Among the equine vaccines, tetanus is perhaps the most used. Tetanus is a sporadic non-contagious infectious disease. Because of its characteristics, it is difficult to perform extensive studies regarding vaccine efficacy. However, it has been reported that

Table 25-2 | **Clinical Pharmacologic Features and Spectra of Activity of Equine Anthelminthics**

CLASS	ANTHELMINTHIC	DOSE MG/KG	ADULT STRONGYLES	STRONGYLE MIGRATING LARVAE	SMALL STRONGYLE ADULTS	SMALL STRONGYLE INHIBITED LARVA (MUCOSA)	TAPEWORMS	ASCARIDS	BOOTS
Macrocyclic lactones	Ivermectin	0.2	++++	++++	++++			++++	++++
	Moxidectin	0.4	++++	++++	++++	++++		++++	
Benzimid-azoles	Fenbendazole	5–10	++++	++++	++++	++++		++++	
	Mebendazole	8.8	++++		++++				
	Oxibendazole	10–15	++++		++++				
	Oxfendazole	10	++++	+++	++++			++++	
	Thiabendazole	44	++++	++++	++++			++++	
Pyrimidines	Pyrantel pamoate	6.6	++++		++++		++++		
	Pyrantel embonate	19	++++		++++		++++		
	Pyrantel tartrate	2.6	++++	++++	++++		++++		
Heterocyclics	Piperazine	88	++		++++			++++	
Pryazinoiso-quinolines	Praziquantel	1.5	Unknown				++++		

Modified from Love S. Treatment and prevention of intestinal parasite-associated disease. *Vet Clin North Am Equine Pract* 19:791-806, 2003.
++, 50% efficacy; +++, 60%-75% efficacy; ++++, 90% efficacy.

the lack of vaccination is the most common risk factor for horses that acquire tetanus. A toxoid and an antitoxin are available for horses; the antitoxin induces passive immunity for a 3-week period.

Broodmares should be vaccinated with the toxoid and booster in the last 4–6 weeks of pregnancy to ensure good antibody levels in the colostrum. A common practice in newborns is the administration of tetanus antitoxin. This practice appears unnecessary if the mare had a proper vaccination plan during the pregnancy. In addition, administration of tetanus antitoxin increases the risk of inducing serum sickness in the foal.[7] Antibodies from maternal immunity are still present in foals up to 18 weeks of age. Foal immunization should start between 4 and 6 months of age with two doses 4 weeks apart and a third dose between 10 and 12 months of age.[5,8,37]

Strangles

This disease, caused by *Streptococcus equi* subsp *equi,* is more common in young horses, although older horses can acquire it if they are unprotected. Clinical signs of the disease are nasal discharge, fever, and abscessation of the retropharyngeal and/ or submandibular lymph nodes. The purulent material from affected horses is the main source of contamination to other horses directly or indirectly through fomites.

Licensed vaccines are the inactivated, adjuvanted cell wall SeM extracts and the attenuated live vaccine. Inactivated vaccines are effective in reducing the magnitude of clinical signs as well as in reducing the development of disease after challenging vaccinated individuals. Adverse effects include abscessation and inflammation at the injection site.[38,39] Vaccination of the broodmare induces the presence of IgG and IgA in colostrum, which is absorbed by the foal and ultimately distributed in the nasopharyngeal mucosa, protecting those foals until they are weaned.[40] A certain degree of inhibitory effect from the maternal immunity is seen with inactivated vaccines. The modified live vaccine is prescribed for intranasal use, and it improves the production of local immune response.[41,42]

Vaccination in the broodmare is recommended 4–6 weeks before foaling with the inactivated vaccine. Foals are more susceptible between 4 and 8 months of age and in endemic areas and should be vaccinated with the intranasal vaccine as earlier as 4 months of age with two doses 3–4 weeks apart, and a third dose administered 3 months later. Boosters are required every 6–12 months. The use of the inactivated vaccine in foals should start between 4 and 6 months of age, three doses at 3- to 6-week intervals, and then booster semi-annually until the high risk is present.[6,8]

Botulism

Clostridium botulinum is a gram-positive, spore-forming anaerobic rod that produces the toxin that causes botulism. The bacteria can produce eight different neurotoxins, all of which produce identical clinical signs, but it is relevant to know which one is involved when antitoxin is used in the treatment. The toxin produces flaccid paralysis and paresis impeding the release of acetylcholine in the neuromuscular junction. Horses are affected by the types A, B, C, and D. Clinical signs include difficulty swallowing or dysphagia, flaccid paralysis, lack of pupillary response, and other signs compatible with lack of muscle tone. The type B toxoid vaccine is the only product available in the United States.

Botulism occurs through three different mechanisms: (1) ingestion of the toxin, (2) ingestion of the spores and subsequent intestinal infection and toxin production (toxicoinfectious), or (3) wound contamination and infection. In foals it is the toxicoinfectious form of the disease and can affect them as young as 7 days of age, but more often between 1 and 3 months. The disease is present mainly in Kentucky and the mid-Atlantic sea border states.[3,6,43]

Horses in endemic areas should be vaccinated because botulism can be present at any age, but foals between 2 and 4 months are more susceptible. Vaccination of the broodmare at 8, 9, and 10 months of gestation is indicated to produce enough coverage for the foal until the third month of age.[3,44] If the broodmare was vaccinated in a previous pregnancy, a single dose 4–6 weeks before foaling is required.[8] Vaccination for foals from vaccinated mares in endemic areas should start between 2 and 3 months of age, three doses with a 4-week interval. Foals from unvaccinated mares should begin immunizations at 1–3 months of age. Where there is high risk or incidence of disease, all foals can start vaccination at 2 weeks of age.[8]

Rotavirus

Rotavirus is a double-stranded RNA virus, highly contagious and resistant to several disinfectants, and is considered the most important viral cause of diarrhea in foals. Transmission is through the fecal–oral route, with an incubation period of 1 day. In addition to vaccination, special management of bedding and instruments is vital to prevent spread the virus in the farm. Mares can be vaccinated, with an inactivated virus vaccine at 8, 9, and 10 months of every gestation to induce adequate production of antibodies in the colostrum, and the levels of IgG in the foal last for 90 days. The vaccine also decreases the incidence and severity of the clinical signs.[45]

Influenza EIV

The influenza A type A2 virus belongs to the Orthomyxoviridae family. Equine influenza is a highly contagious respiratory disease in immunologically naïve individuals. Clinical signs include fever, serous nasal discharge, cough, and in some cases lymphadenopathy. Secondary problems to an influenza infection include bacterial pneumonia, myositis, myocarditis, and limb edema. Mortality has been reported in foals.[46]

Prevention of the disease is achieved by vaccination. There are several products licensed in the United States, each of which contains one of the three different types of influenza antigen: killed virus, lived modified virus, and the live canarypox vector. The inactivated vaccine induces an adequate production of antibodies, which is correlated with the level of protection,[1,47-49] but the cellular response with those vaccines is not optimal.[1] There is evidence that the inactivated vaccines do not reduce the risk of disease in recently vaccinated horses[49]; however, the duration of clinical signs was reduced.[50] On the other hand, the live modified vaccine, which is administered intranasally, protects horses for 6 months with a single dose; vaccinated horses developed significantly less severe clinical signs and a shorter course than the control group. Also, the correlation between the antibody level with the level of protection was not found, suggesting mucosal and cellular imunity.[49,51] The canarypox vaccine is administered intramuscularly. In studies conducted by Edmund Toulemonde et al.[52] and Minke et al.,[53] it was observed that vaccinated horses, after viral challenge, develop mild signs of disease and complete suppression of viral excretion compared with the controls. Protection was seen up to 5 months after the second dose.

Maternal immunity with EIV has been extensively reported. Maternal antibodies are present at 5 months in the foal, and vaccination in those individuals is recommended to start at 6 months of age.[20-23] Control of this condition includes vaccination of the entire population of the farm, and if any horses are coming to the farm, vaccination should be enforced. If possible, new horses need to be vaccinated and isolated for 4 weeks after. The schedule of vaccination can change depending on the vaccine selected (see Tables 25-1 and 25-2).[8]

Equine Viral Arteritis (EVA)

The transmission of EVA occurs through aerosol and the reproductive route, which is the most common. The stallion can shed the virus from a few weeks to several years, and it is considered as the reservoir of disease. During artificial insemination the virus can be transmitted through fresh, cooled, or frozen semen. Clinical signs are variable between fever and nasal discharge, ocular discharge and peripheral edema in adult horses, abortion in pregnant mares, and interstitial pneumonia in foals. A detailed discussion on EVA is found in Chapter 10.

A live-modified vaccine is available in North America, which protects stallions against the carrier state and mares from abortion.[2] The vaccination in mares is performed before they are bred and the booster is administered between the foaling and the new breeding.[8] Although the use of the vaccine in pregnant mares is controversial, a recent study reported that vaccination of a limited number of mares in their last trimester of gestation had no adverse effects in the mare or in the foal after birth. The vaccine is not indicated for foals <6 weeks of age.[54] Vaccination protocol in colts who could become stallions should start at 6 months, when the maternal antibodies are not detectable (2–6 months of age).[55]

Potomac Horse Fever

Potomac horse fever is caused by the gram-negative coccus. *Neorickettsia risticii* The disease is commonly seen near water sources such as rivers as well as on irrigated pastures, and it occurs more often between May and November. The organism has been isolated from different trematodes, which are currently considered as the vector of the disease. The incubation period varies between 1 and 3 weeks. Clinical signs initially are depression, anorexia, and fever, followed by diarrhea (60% of the cases), peripheral edema, and in some cases toxemia and laminitis can develop as a complication. It is also documented that the disease and the experimental infection can produce abortion.[56,57]

Several inactivated vaccines are available. Vaccination is recommended only for horses that live in, or for those traveling to, endemic areas. Foals appear to be less susceptible than adult horses. Few scientific studies about the efficacy of this bacterin are available in the literature and the results are controversial. In one of those the vaccination was not associated with decrease in the incidence of disease nor the severity of the clinical signs, nor was the economic benefit seen.[58,59]

The presentation of the disease is seasonal with a higher incidence in the late summer and early fall. The use of the vaccine is recommended in broodmares 4–6 weeks before foaling; the maternal immunity is present in the foal for up to 3–5 months of age; foals can be first vaccinated at that time.[6,8]

PARASITE CONTROL

Appropriate control and treatment of the pregnant mare against gastrointestinal parasites are a critical determinant to prevent severe infestation in the newborn foal.

Management practices such as monitoring for anthelminthic resistance, adequate quarantine and anthelminthic therapy of incoming horses, not over-stocking the pasture, and appropriate use and rest of nursery fields can reduce the foal contamination with strongyles and ascarids.[60,61]

Depending on the age, the foal is susceptible to different parasites. In the first weeks of life they are more susceptible to parasites such as ascarids and strongyloides, which is the parasite that is transmitted through the milk, the skin, or in a pre-natal infestation through the placenta. Other parasites such as strongyles are rare in foals <4 months, and cyathostomes are more common in weanlings. Cestodes do not affect foals in the first year.[61]

In general, deworming treatments are mainly administered between 8 and 12 weeks apart using two or three classes of anthelminthics. This interval, which can be either insufficient or excessive, depends on the degree of pasture contamination. In some cases the owner decides which anthelminthic to use, based mainly on marketing and not on potential pharmacologic resistance.[62]

Table 25-2 summarizes the five classes of anthelminthics presently available:

1. Macrocyclic lactones (ivermectin and moxidectin): These drugs induce selective paralysis of the parasite by increasing permeability of chloride in their muscle. Moxidectin has a longer half-life in adipose tissue than ivermectin because of its liposolubility. This is the reason for adult horses in poor body condition and young foals to be more susceptible to toxicity with moxidectin.[63,64]
2. Benzimidazoles: Fenbendazole, oxibendazole, mebendazole, and oxfendazole are commonly used. They inhibit the formation of microtubules inducing intestinal cell disruption and inhibit egg production.
3. Pyrimidines: Three pyrantel salts are used in horses, producing spastic paralysis of the nematode by agonist action at nicotinic acetylcholine receptors on their muscle cells. They are also effective against cestodes (tape worms), at double of the dose.[65]
4. Heterocyclics: Piperazine produces spastic paralyses in the nematode, but its spectrum includes only adult ascarids and cyatostomes.
5. Pryazinoisoquinolines: Praziquantel is commonly combined with other anthelminthics due to its efficacy against cestodes. Praziquantel induces parasite muscular contraction and paralysis.

In terms of diagnosis, the fecal egg count is used to determine infestation and resistance. Arbitrarily, established egg cell counts >100 eggs per gram are indicative for treatment; other sources used 300 eggs per gram. Unfortunately, the level of correlation or sensitivity and specificity of the egg cell count is low to diagnose the severity of the infestation. Resistance is considered if after 14 days after treatment the egg cell count reduction is <85%. Lack of sensitivity and specificity are limitations on the fecal egg count.[60]

Some authors recommend treating the pregnant mare, based on parasite resistance, 1 month before foaling with a complete dose, and also 10 days before the due date. After foaling a larvacidal dose is suggested around Day 10. The foal should be treated around 6 weeks of age with benzimidazoles or pyrimidines (fenbendazole or pyrantel), then every 4 weeks, until the sixth month.[61]

REFERENCES

1. Lunn DP, Townsend HGG: Equine vaccination. *Vet Clin North Am Equine Pract* 16:199-226, 2000.
2. Barquero N, Gilkerson JR, Newton JR: Evidence-based immunization in horses. *Vet Clin North Am Equine Pract* 23:481-508, 2007.
3. Riddle WT: Preparation of the mare for normal parturition. Proc 49th Annu Conf Am Assoc Eq Pract 2003, pp 1-5.
4. Wilson WD: Vaccination programs for foals and weanlings. Proc 45th Annu Conf Am Assoc Eq Pract.1999, pp 254-263.
5. Wilson WD: Strategies for vaccinating mares, foals, and weanlings. Proc 51st Annu Conf Am Assoc Eq Pract. 2005, pp 421-438.
6. Wilson WD, Pusterla N: Immunoprophylaxis. In Sellon DC, Long MT: *Equine Infectious Diseases.* St Louis: Saunders, 2007, pp 556-577.
7. Lunn DP: Practical foal vaccination strategies. Proc 47th Annu Conf Am Assoc Eq Pract.1997, pp 57-60.
8. AAEP, Infectious disease committee: Guidelines for the vaccination of horses. 2008. Available at: http://www.aaep.org/vaccination_guidelines.htm. Accessed July 21, 2008.
9. Jenner E: *The Three Original Publications on Vaccination Against Smallpox,* Vol XXXVIII, Part 4. The Harvard Classics. New York: P.F. Collier & Son, 2001, pp 1909-1914. Available at: www.bartleby.com.
10. Spickler AR, Roth JA: Adjuvants in veterinary vaccines: modes of action and adverse effects. *J Vet Intern Med* 17:273-281, 2003.
11. Aguilar JC, Rodriguez EG: Vaccine adjuvants revisited. *Vaccine* 25:3752-3762, 2007.
12. Giguere S, Polkes AC: Immunologic disorders in neonatal foals. *Vet Clin North Am Eq Pract* 21:241-272, 2005.
13. Kohn CW, Knight D, Hueston W: Colostral and serum IgG, IgA, and IgM concentrations in Standardbred mares and their foals at parturition. *J Am Vet Med Assoc* 195:64-68, 1989.
14. Zou E, Brady HA, Hurley WL: Protective factors in mammary gland secretions during the periparturient period in the mare. *J Eq Vet Sci* 18:184-188, 1998.
15. Jeffcott LB: Studies on passive immunity in the foal II. The absorption of 125I-labelled PVP (polyvinyl pyrrolidone) by the neonatal intestine. *J Comp Pathol* 84:279-289, 1974.
16. Kelly GS: Bovine colostrums: a review of clinical uses. *Altern Med Rev* 8:378-394, 2003.
17. Holzangel DL, Hussey S, Mihaly JE, et al: Onset of immunoglobulin production in foals. *Eq Vet J* 35:620-622, 2003.
18. Flaminio MJ, Rush BR, Shuman W: Peripheral blood lymphocyte subpopulations and immunoglobulin concentrations in healthy foals and foals with *Rhodococcus equi* pneumonia. *J Vet Intern Med* 13:206-212, 1999.
19. Smith R III, Chaffin MK, Cohen ND, Martens RJ: Age-related changes in lymphocyte subsets of quarter horse foals. *Am J Vet Res* 63:531-537, 2002.
20. van Maanen C, Bruin G, de Boer-Luijtze E, et al: Interference of maternal antibodies with the immune response of foals after vaccination against equine influenza. *Vet Q* 14:13-17, 1992.
21. Wilson WD, Mihalyi JE, Hussey S, Lunn DP: Passive transfer of maternal immunoglobulin isotype antibodies against tetanus and influenza and their effect on the response of foals to vaccination. *Eq Vet J* 33:644-650, 2001.
22. van Oirschot JT, Bruin G, de Boer-Luytze E, Smolders G: Maternal antibodies against equine influenza virus in foals and their interference with vaccination. *Zentralbl Veterinarmed B* 38:391-396, 1991.
23. Conboy HS, Berry DB, Fallon EH, et al: Failure of foal seroconversion following equine influenza vaccination. *Proc 43th Conf Am Assoc Eq Pract* 43:22-23, 1997.
24. Ferguson JA, Reeves WC, Hardy JL: Studies on immunity to alphaviruses in foals. *Am J Vet Res* 40:5-10, 1979.
25. Siger L, Bowen RA, Karaca K, et al: Assessment of the efficacy of a single dose of a recombinant vaccine against West Nile virus in response to natural challenge with West Nile virus-infected mosquitoes in horses. *Am J Vet Res* 65:1459-1462, 2004.
26. Minke JM, Siger L, Karaca K, et al: Recombinant canarypoxvirus vaccine carrying the prM/E genes of West Nile virus protects horses against a West Nile virus-mosquito challenge. *Arch Virol Suppl* 18:221-230, 2004.
27. Siger L, Bowen R, Karaca K, et al: Evaluation of the efficacy provided by a recombinant canarypox-vectored equine West Nile virus vaccine against an experimental West Nile virus intrathecal challenge in horses. *Vet Ther* 7:249-256, 2006.
28. Long MT, Gibbs EP, Mellencamp MW, et al: Efficacy, duration, and onset of immunogenicity of a West Nile virus vaccine, live Flavivirus chimera, in horses with a clinical disease challenge model. *Eq Vet J* 39:491-497, 2007.
29. Long MT, Gibbs EP, Mellencamp MW, et al: Safety of an attenuated West Nile virus vaccine, live Flavivirus chimera in horses. *Eq Vet J* 39:486-490, 2007.
30. Seino KK, Long MT, Gibbs EP, et al: Comparative efficacies of three commercially available vaccines against West Nile Virus (WNV) in a short-duration challenge trial involving an equine WNV encephalitis model. *Clin Vac Immunol* 14:1465-1471, 2007.
31. Vest DJ, Cohen ND, Berezowski CJ, et al: Evaluation of administration of West Nile virus vaccine to pregnant broodmares. *J Am Vet Med Assoc* 225:1894-1897, 2004.
32. Allen GP: Epidemic disease caused by equine herpesvirus-1: recommendations for prevention and control. *Eq Vet Educ* 14:136-142, 2002.
33. Slater JD, Borchers K, Thackray AM, Field HJ: The trigeminal ganglion is a location for equine herpesvirus 1 latency and reactivation in the horse. *J Gen Virol* 75:2007-2016, 1994.

34. Heldens JG, Kersten AJ, Weststrate MW, et al: Duration of immunity induced by an adjuvanted and inactivated equine influenza, tetanus and equine herpesvirus 1 and 4 combination vaccine. *Vet Q* 23:210-217, 2001.

35. Burki F, Nowotny N, Rossmainth W, et al: Training of the immune system of foals against ERP virus infections by frequent vaccination with presently available commercial vaccines. *Dtsch Tierarztl Wochenschr* 96:162-165, 1989.

36. Ellis JA, Steeves E, Wright AK, et al: Cell-mediated cytolysis of equine herpesvirus-infected cells by leukocytes from young vaccinated horses. *Vet Immunol Immunopathol* 57:201-214, 1997.

37. Jansen BC, Knoetze PC: The immune response of horses to tetanus toxoid. *Onderstepoort J Vet Res* 46:211-216, 1979.

38. Hoffman AM, Staempfli HR, Prescott JF, et al: Field evaluation of a commercial M-protein vaccine against *Streptococcus equi* infection in foals. *Am J Vet Res* 52:589-592, 1991.

39. Bryant S, Brown KK, Lewis S et al: Protection against strangles with an enzymatic *Streptococcus equi* extract. *Vet Med* 80:58-70, 1985.

40. Sheoran AS, Timoney JF, Holmes MA et al: Immunoglobulin isotypes in sera and nasal mucosal secretions and their neonatal transfer and distribution in horses. *Am J Vet Res* 61:1099-1105, 2000.

41. Sheoran AS, Sponseller BT, Holmes MA et al: Serum and mucosal antibody isotype responses to M-like protein (SeM) of *Streptococcus equi* in convalescent and vaccinated horses. *Vet Immunol Immunopathol* 59:239-251, 1997.

42. Galan JE, Timoney JF: Mucosal nasopharyngeal immune responses of horses to protein antigens of *Streptococcus equi. Infect Immunol* 47:623-628, 1985.

43. Whitlock RH, Buckley C: *Botulism. Vet Clin North Am Equine Pract* 13:107-128, 1997.

44. Wilkins PA, Palmer JE: Botulism in foals less than 6 months of age: 30 cases (1989-2002). *J Vet Intern Med* 17:702-707, 2003.

45. Powell DG, Dwyer RM,Traug-Dargatz JL, et al: Field study of the safety, immunogenicity, and efficacy of an inactivated equine rotavirus vaccine. *J Am Vet Med Assoc* 211:193-198, 1997.

46. Peek SF, Landolt G, Karasin AI, et al: Acute respiratory distress syndrome and fatal interstitial pneumonia associated with equine influenza in a neonatal foal. *J Vet Intern Med* 18:132-134, 2004.

47. Morley PS, Townsend HG, Bogdan JR, Haines DM: Risk factors for disease associated with influenza virus infections during three epidemics in horses. *J Am Vet Med Assoc* 216:545-550, 2000.

48. Wood JM, Mumford J, Folkers C, et al: Studies with inactivated equine influenza vaccine. 1. Serological responses of ponies to graded doses of vaccine. *J Hyg (Lond)* 90:371-384, 1983.

49. Paillot R, Hannant D, Kydd JH, Daly JM: Vaccination against equine influenza: quid novi?. *Vaccine* 24:4047-4061, 2006.

50. Morley PS, Townsend HG, Bogdan JR, Haines DM: l: Efficacy of a commercial vaccine for preventing disease caused by influenza virus infection in horses. *J Am Vet Med Assoc* 215:61-66, 1999.

51. Townsend HGG, Penner SJ, Watts TC, et al: Efficacy of a cold-adapted, intranasal, equine influenza vaccine: challenge trials. *Eq Vet J* 33:637-643, 2001.

52. Toulemonde CE, Daly J, Sindle T, et al: Efficacy of a recombinant equine influenza vaccine against challenge with an American lineage H3N8 influenza virus responsible for the 2003 outbreak in the United Kingdom. *Vet Rec* 156:367-371, 2005.

53. Minke JM, Toulemonde CE, Coupier H, et al: Efficacy of a canary-pox-vectored recombinant vaccine expressing the hemagglutinin gene of equine influenza H3N8 virus in the protection of ponies from viral challenge. *Am J Vet Res* 68:213-219, 2007.

54. Moore BD, Balasuriya UB, Nurton JP et al: Differentiation of strains of equine arteritis virus of differing virulence to horses by growth in equine endothelial cells. *Am J Vet Res* 64:779-784, 2003.

55. Timoney PJ, McCollum WH: Equine viral arteritis. *Vet Clin North Am Eq Pract* 39:295-309, 1999.

56. Long MT, Goetz TE, Whiteley HE, et al: Identification of *Ehrlichia risticii* as the causative agent of two equine abortions following natural maternal infection. *J Vet Diagn Invest* 7:201-205, 1995.

57. Long MT, Goetz TE, Kakoma I, et al: Evaluation of fetal infection and abortion in pregnant ponies experimentally infected with *Ehrlichia risticii. Am J Vet Res* 56:1307, 1995.

58. Atwill ER, Mohammed HO: Evaluation of vaccination of horses as a strategy to control equine monocytic ehrlichiosis. *J Am Vet Med Assoc* 208:1290-1294, 1996.

59. Atwill ER, Mohammed HO: Benefit-cost analysis of vaccination of horses as a strategy to control equine monocytic ehrlichiosis. *J Am Vet Med Assoc* 208:1295-1299, 1996.

60. Coles CC, Jackson F, Pomroy WE et al: The detection of anthelmintic resistance in nematodes of veterinary importance. *Vet Parasitol* 136:167-185, 2006.

61. Knottenbelt D, Pascoe R: Routine stud management procedures. In Knottenbelt D, LeBlanc M, Lopate CH, Pascoe R: *Equine Stud Farm Medicine and Surgery.* St Louis: Saunders, 2003, pp 25-41.

62. Lloyd S, Smith J, Connan RM, et al: Parasite control methods used by horse owners: factors predisposing to the development of anthelmintic resistance in nematodes. *Vet Rec* 146:487-492, 2000.

63. Goehring LS: van Oldruitenborgh-Oosterbaan MM: Moxidectin poisoning in a foal? *Tijdschr Diergeneeskd* 124:412-414, 1999.

64. Johnson PJ, Mrad DR, Schwartz AJ, Kellam L: Presumed moxidectin toxicosis in three foals. *J Am Vet Med Assoc* 214:678-680, 1999.

65. Love S: Treatment and prevention of intestinal parasite-associated disease. *Vet Clin North Am Equine Pract* 193:791-806, 2003.

EVALUATION OF REPRODUCTIVE EFFICIENCY

CHARLES C. LOVE

Evaluation of the reproufffctive efficiency (RE) in the horse breeding industry is an important aspect of routine mare and stallion management. Although many breeding enterprises have systems that record day-to-day breeding activities, there are no accounting systems that monitor and summarize the day-to-day breeding activities so that management has current information regarding breeding success and failure. Since reproductive outcome directly affects financial outcome, however, reproductive outcome is often not determined until the breeding season is over; therefore, it is too late to implement changes in management strategy. In addition, clinicians should make evaluation of reproductive efficiency a routine aspect of the stallion breeding evaluation.

Historically, RE is restricted to the determination of seasonal pregnancy rate and cycle/pregnancy, two measures that reflect a stallion's *average* fertility, usually after the conclusion of the breeding season. However, limiting the evaluation of reproductive success to these two values alone assumes that the only source of reduced fertility is confined to the stallion while ignoring the effects of mare type and management. There are additional measures of RE that can pinpoint specific areas of reduced fertility in a breeding establishment that is often not related to a primary stallion limitation.

What is reproductive efficiency? For the purposes of this chapter RE is defined as the thorough evaluation of all available stallion, mare, and management information. Stallion factors include those endpoints associated with the breeding soundness evaluation such as semen quality, testes health, and the physical condition of the stallion. These factors have been previously described and outlined in the stallion manual published by The Society for Theriogenology.[1] Measurable mare factors include the reproductive status of the mare (i.e., maiden, barren, or foaling), mare age at the time of breeding, foaling date, and interestrous interval. Factors controlled by management include the size of a stallion's mare book, composition of the book (e.g., number of maiden, foaling, and barren mares), and intensity of mare management leading up to and through breeding (i.e., how is ovulation determined, how often are mares bred when in heat).

The goal of breeding record evaluation is to describe and define non-sperm factors and the role they play in understanding and diagnosing the primary cause(s) of reduced fertility in the stallion and mare. Although subjective, a working estimate is that sperm quality accounts for 20%–40% of the variability in the fertility of the average stallion. This assumes that the stallion does not have a dramatic sperm-limiting factor such as extremely poor semen quality or very low sperm numbers. This hypothesis suggests, therefore, that 60%–80% of a stallion's fertility can be explained by non-sperm factors, broadly categorized as management and mare factors.[2]

Historically, the overall (average) fertility of a stallion can be described by determining the *seasonal pregnancy rate* and *cycles per pregnancy.*[1]

Seasonal pregnancy rate (SPR) is represented as a percentage and is based on the number of mares diagnosed as pregnant at a particular point in time divided by the total number of mares that have been bred to that stallion up to that point in time. This value is usually determined following the breeding season, but it can be evaluated at any time during the season. SPR is an important economic endpoint but is not a sensitive indicator of a stallion's fertility because it does not reflect the total number of cycles that a mare is bred to achieve the pregnancy (i.e., efficiency). As an example, a stallion can achieve a relatively low pregnancy rate per cycle yet end the season with a seasonal pregnancy rate similar to a stallion achieving a relatively high pregnancy rate per cycle; the only difference is the stallion with a relatively low pregnancy rate per cycle must breed the mares in his book more times (i.e., less efficiently) during the season to reach the same seasonal pregnancy rate. Therefore, although SPR is important economically and is the one most familiar to the horse breeder, it is not a sensitive endpoint when trying to describe and identify the source of reduced fertility.

Several factors are important when determining SPR. The time of year (e.g., during the breeding season, shortly after the breeding season, or many months after the breeding season) when SPR is determined will influence the value. As the point in time approaches the next breeding season, the value will more closely approximate the *foaling rate.* How often a mare was bred during the season (the number of estrous cycles) will also affect SPR. The more opportunity a mare has to become pregnant, the more likely she is to get pregnant. Mares added to the book at the end of the season or mares removed from the book and passed to another stallion may be bred only once, thereby artificially inflating the mare book size and resulting in the appearance of a lower SPR. Therefore, when a stallion is presented with a low SPR, determination of adequate mare exposure is important. In addition, the inclusion or exclusion of mares that exhibit early embryonic death (EED) will also modulate SPR. Most embryonic loss is probably mare rather than stallion related. Therefore, to describe a stallion's inherent fertility, all diagnosed pregnancies (which indicate that the stallion was able to accomplish fertilization in those mares) should be included in calculating the SPR. Yet, including EED as a pregnancy when figuring seasonal pregnancy rate is of no economic relevance (i.e., no foal results and no stud fees will be transferred), and an inflated end of season economic picture will be assumed.

Cycles per pregnancy (pregnancy rate/cycle, or *C/P)* is a more sensitive indication of a stallion's fertility because it measures how *efficient* a stallion is in establishing pregnancies. This value is determined by counting *all* estrous cycles from *all* mares that a stallion has bred and dividing it by the total number of pregnancies. The *total number of cycles* can be determined by counting all dates bred excluding multiple matings in the same estrous period (i.e., doubles). The assumption is made that all mares were in normal estrus at the time of breeding and were bred near the time of ovulation. This assumption is not always correct, especially when artificial insemination (AI) is used, since mares can be bred regardless of whether they are in standing estrus.

SPR and C/P are the two most common endpoints initially determined when evaluating stallion fertility. They are, however, *seasonal averages* that measure overall fertility of not just the stallion, but the mares and management as well. It is possible, however, to be more specific when one is interested in identifying the specific source of a reduced SPR or elevated C/P. Although cutoff/threshold values are not always appropriate, a SPR of 80% and C/P of 2.0 can be used as working reference points, below and above which one might consider to investigate sources of reduced fertility.

There are several broad categories, as outlined in the following text, that record analysis should evaluate as well as the endpoints that can be used to evaluate those categories.

INFLUENCE OF MARE TYPE ON PREGNANCY OUTCOME

Mare type refers to the reproductive status of the mare coming into the breeding season and is commonly divided into maiden, barren, and foaling mares. These groupings are important because of differences in inherent fertility and opportunity to be bred.

Barren

This group contains non-pregnant mares coming into the breeding season of interest. Mares in this group will usually have lower fertility than the other groups. There are several reasons why a mare might be barren, including:

Not bred the previous season. This can occur because the owner simply decided not to breed the mare, or the mare may have foaled late in the previous season and did not have ample opportunity to become pregnant. Mares barren because of these reasons have normal fertility.

Subfertile. These mares have intrinsic fertility problems that contributed to failure to become pregnant the previous breeding season, and they are commonly older than the rest of the mare population. In most cases, the subfertile mares will account for the majority of the mares classified as barren.

Mares that have aborted. Mares that have aborted during the previous breeding season. Some managers and computer programs use the term *slipped* instead of the term *aborted*.

Foaling

These are mares that produced a foal in the current breeding season and will be rebred during the same season. One should expect high fertility in this group of mares, as they recently conceived and carried a foal to term. This group may exhibit reduced fertility if a predominant proportion of the mares foaled late in the breeding season, thus having only one estrous cycle available for breeding. Fertility in this group may also be reduced

if some event (injury/illness to the stallion) prematurely shortens the breeding season.

Maiden

These are mares that have never been bred. Mares in this group are generally young; however, occasional maiden mares are older because of owner election not to breed when young (usually because of a continuing performance career). Older maiden mares are generally less fertile than young maiden mares. Mares that are recently retired from performance careers may not be cycling regularly when they first become available for mating (typically in February) and thus may require more time and subsequently more breedings to become pregnant. However, since maiden mares are generally available for breeding early in the season, their chances of eventually becoming pregnant are high.

Evaluation of Mare Type

The number of each mare type and their percentage contribution to the book can be determined. In general, foaling mares account for 50%–60% of the book with barren (20%–30%) and maiden mares (10%–20%) accounting for the rest. In unusual cases these ratios are different and can affect SPR and C/P. These proportions are important because the foaling mares are the primary influence of fertility because of their large numbers, but this does not preclude a smaller number of very subfertile barren mares from having a prominent effect on fertility. Stallions that become less popular tend to attract barren mares of poorer reproductive quality; in which case the barren mares may contribute to a larger proportion of the stallion's book as well as require more cycles to become pregnant. This will reduce a stallion's overall SPR and C/P below that expected based on sperm quality alone.

MARE AGE

The age of the mare population to which a stallion is bred can be an important influence on a stallion's fertility. As mares age and approach 12–14 years of age, as a population, fertility declines. Some stallions may accumulate a larger group of mares that are older than that of the average stallion and will experience reduced fertility, usually because these mares tend to be barren. Therefore, identifying and recording mare age is an important determinant in evaluating fertility.

SEASONALITY OF PREGNANCY

The breeding season officially starts February 15 and extends to the end of June and early July and therefore includes both non-physiological (short day lengths) and physiological (longer day lengths) breeding seasons. The fertility of a stallion can vary considerably on a month-to-month basis based on a number of factors. Ideally, mares that are anticipated to be bred early in the breeding season have been exposed to long-day length conditions using artificial lighting to initiate normal cyclicity. Sometimes while mares may have been exposed to lighting, there may be an inadequate response, resulting in prolonged cycles or a transitional-like state. The determination of interestrous or interbreeding intervals can give the clinician a clue regarding whether mares are cycling normally early in the breeding season. Another cause of a reduction in fertility early in the breeding season is a large book of barren mares and/or maiden mares that are in poor reproductive shape. If the barren mare group is extremely poor, she will continue to be bred and remain open until the end of the season and therefore will result in poor fertility late in the breeding season as well. As a general rule, fertility from February through May should be similar when mares are cycling normally and there is no influence of mare type or breeding frequency on fertility. Fertility tends to decline in June and July because mares still being bred at this time are intrinsically less fertile or subfertile.

MATHEMATICS OF HORSE BREEDING

Although there are many factors involved in horse breeding, perhaps none is more simple yet critical than realizing that mares need adequate stallion exposure to for high fertility (i.e., a 100% pregnancy rate per cycle is not achievable, so mares not becoming pregnant on first service must be bred a sufficient number of times to afford a realistic opportunity to become pregnant during the season). To illustrate this principle, if a stallion achieves a 50% pregnancy rate per cycle, mares must on average be bred at least two estrous cycles to yield a 75% seasonal pregnancy rate. Yet, a 75% seasonal pregnancy rate would be considered to be low on well-managed breeding farms.

Opportunity To Become Pregnant

The ability of a mare to become pregnant is influenced, to a certain degree, simply by the number of estrous cycles that she is bred regardless of the intrinsic fertility of the stallion. A reproductively normal mare that is bred once to a stallion that has a 50% per cycle pregnancy rate has a 50% chance of getting pregnant; two cycles, a 75% chance; and three cycles, an 87.5% chance. Opportunity is less important when highly fertile stallions (i.e., high per cycle pregnancy rate) are bred because they require fewer cycles to render a mare pregnant, making opportunity more important as the fertility of a stallion decreases. However, when stallions of average (i.e., 50% per cycle pregnancy rate) or below fertility, or artificial breeding techniques such as cooled-shipped or frozen semen are used, then *opportunity* becomes a critical component of the fertility equation.

Measures of Opportunity

The *average day of first breeding* for each mare type—This is determined by averaging the first day (e.g., March 1, April 10) of breeding for all mares in each mare type. The intent of this value is to determine when mares in each group started to be bred in the breeding season. Maiden and barren mares have the potential to start February 15, since they enter the breeding season not pregnant. In contrast, foaling mares must wait until they foal before they can be rebred and therefore, as a group, will start the breeding season later. As a general rule the average day of first breeding for maiden and barren mares should be sometime in the first half of the month of March, whereas foaling mares tend to start in mid to late April, a month or more later than the maiden and barren mares.

Cycles/mare for each mare type—This endpoint determines the number of estrous cycles that each mare was bred. Maiden and foaling mares are bred approximately 1.3–1.6 cycles per mare, with barren mares approaching 2.0 cycles per mare. Maiden mares are low because they tend to be a highly fertile group and therefore get pregnant at an

efficient rate and simply do not need to be bred more; whereas foaling mares are lower than barren mares because they must foal before they can be bred. In the latter case, the foaling mares have a lack of opportunity in some cases because the end of the breeding season occurs before they can be bred again; in effect, they run out of time. In some cases this may result in a lower-than-anticipated SPR in foaling mares—not because the stallion is at fault, but because the mares were not bred enough. Interestingly, in some cases, barren mares will have a higher SPR than foaling mares—not because they are intrinsically more fertile, but because they were bred more.

Overbreeding

Stallions may possess highly fertile sperm characteristics (excellent sperm motility, high percent of morphologically normal sperm) but may be limited by the ability to deliver a threshold level of normal sperm at each breeding for the number of mares in their mare book, resulting in overbreeding. The effects of overbreeding are usually manifest as a reduction in the *efficiency* (cycles/pregnancy) by which a stallion renders his mares pregnant, which, if dramatic enough, will result in a reduction in seasonal pregnancy rate.

Daily Pregnancy Rate Based on the Number of Mares Bred per Day

When mares are bred using AI, the number of sperm inseminated varies from day to day because of variation in the amount of sperm ejaculated by the stallion as well as the variation in the number of mares bred on a daily basis. If a stallion is limited in the amount of sperm he can produce for the number of mares he must breed, it is likely that he will not deliver a threshold number of sperm to maximize fertility to all mares throughout the breeding season. This results in fertility fluctuations caused by variation in inseminated sperm numbers above and below the threshold for maximum fertility.[3]

Several approaches can be used when evaluating the effect of sperm numbers on fertility. One is to evaluate the number of mares bred per day. Theoretically, a stallion that breeds only one mare per day should deposit more sperm in the uterus than when he breeds two, three, or four mares per day. This value simply compares the overall pregnancy rate on days when one mare is bred vs. two vs. three vs. four, etc., and it determines whether pregnancy rate declines as more mares are bred per day. A second and more relevant approach is to determine the relationship between the insemination dose of sperm and pregnancy. If sperm level is a determining factor, then as sperm numbers increase, so should fertility. This can be plotted as shown in Fig. 26-1. In this example, when insemination dose is <400 million progressively motile sperm, the pregnancy rate is 50% (i.e. average fertility); when above that level, fertility rises to 65%.

In the Thoroughbred industry, because of the use of natural cover, insemination dose cannot be measured, but the *order* (cover number) in which a mare is bred during the day has the potential to affect fertility. Pregnancy rates of those mares that were the stallion's first cover of the day are compared with pregnancy rates from mares that were bred the second, third, and fourth covers of the day. If overbreeding occurs, and the number of sperm that a stallion delivers is below the optimal threshold, pregnancy rates will decline in the latter covers.

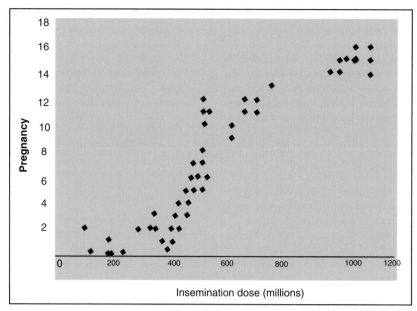

Figure 26-1. The relationship between pregnancy outcome and insemination dose (millions of progressively motile sperm). Through March 3, this stallion had bred 54 mares; SPR: 72%; C/P: 1.64 (61%). Mare fertility: foaling, 55%; maiden, 83%; barren, 60%.

Effect of Breeding Frequency

One factor that will modulate fertility during the breeding season is the frequency of stallion use. For a farm that is using natural cover, the *breeding frequency* represents the number of times a stallion is bred in a given period (i.e., the number of times bred in a day or week). On farms where artificial breeding is used, the *breeding frequency* represents the number of mares bred with an individual ejaculate. No stallion will have mares presented for breeding at even intervals throughout the breeding season. Therefore, pregnancy rates achieved by the stallion when used for different breeding frequencies can be used to evaluate whether overuse of the stallion has occurred (i.e., whether he has been bred too frequently for ejaculates to contain sufficient numbers of sperm to effect good fertility). Use of breeding frequencies to evaluate this phenomenon is presented in Figs. 26-1 to 26-3. These figures have been created using a custom-designed Excel spreadsheet and rely on the following parameters:

Number of mares bred in last week—Identifies the number of mares bred in the week previous to the day in question. This parameter is an evaluation of the long-term effect of frequent breedings, with the intent of determining whether there is a threshold breeding frequency above which fertility of the stallion declines.

Number of mares bred the previous day—Identifies the number of mares bred (either by natural or artificial breeding) on that day.

Pregnancy differential—For each date a mare is bred, a pregnancy score is given (+1 if pregnancy results, −1 if no pregnancy results). The scores are summed for the week previous to a particular date and graphically indicate the fertility of a stallion for the previous week.

Cumulative pregnancy value—This value represents the summed pregnancy scores (+1 or −1) for the entire breeding season leading up to the date of interest. The zero line represents a 50% pregnancy rate per cycle from the start of the breeding season to that point in time.

To illustrate the effects of breeding frequency, see Fig. 26-2. The arrow (March 7) represents the date for recording the following breeding frequency values: number of mares bred in last week = 10; number of mares bred previous day = 3; pregnancy differential = 3; and cumulative pregnancy value = 17. Interpretation of these data reveals that on March 7, there were 10 mares bred in the previous week, 3 more mares became pregnant than were non-pregnant (pregnancy differential), and for the breeding season on this date there are 17 more mares pregnant than non-pregnant.

NATURAL COVER VERSUS ARTIFICIAL INSEMINATION

Natural Cover

Historically, stallions were bred using either natural cover, in which the stallion actually breeds the mare, or AI. In either case the stallion was bred with fresh sperm or sperm that had not been altered by cooling, freezing, or long-term storage. In the last 15–20 years the increased use of shipped and frozen sperm has increased dramatically as breed registries have allowed its use. Coincidental with the marketing of these "semen technologies" has been an increase in the incidence of reduced fertility in some stallions that were "fertile" prior to the application of these techniques. Some of the advantages of natural cover/breeding over AI include the following:

1. In almost all cases mares are exposed to a greater than threshold level of normal sperm and are therefore ensured adequate sperm numbers deposited in their uterus.
2. Mares are in standing estrus. Almost by definition this must occur if the stallion is going to safely mount and be able to breed the mare. This ensures that no mares are bred that are not in heat or due to client pressure to breed them when they may not be ready.
3. Semen is not handled and therefore there is no possibility that otherwise good-quality sperm will be compromised by poor handling technique or be exposed to toxic substances.

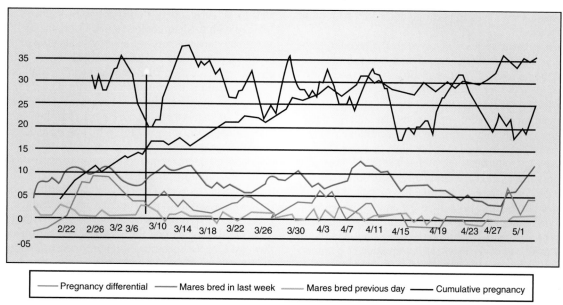

Figure 26-2. This figure graphically represents an example of a highly fertile Thoroughbred stallion bred by natural cover. Notice that the cumulative pregnancy value continues to climb regardless of preceding breeding frequencies. There is no indication that a threshold breeding frequency, above which fertility declines, has been reached. Although there are peaks and valleys in the pregnancy differential, they are probably related to non-stallion factors. This stallion would be expected to achieve a 90% seasonal pregnancy rate, requiring less than an average of 1.5 estrous cycles per pregnancy, in a book of 100 mares bred by natural service.

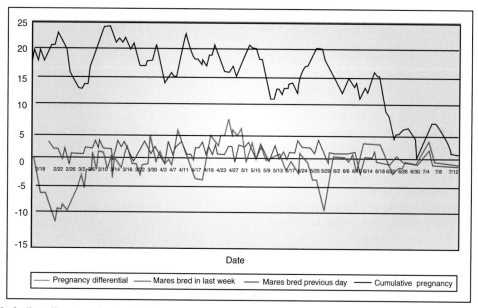

Figure 26-3. Example of a fertile stallion (mare book: 182; SPR: 84%; C/P: 1.97 [51%]), which is of lesser fertility than the stallion in Figure 26-1. This stallion has a period of reduced fertility early in the breeding season from February to April 21. This can be traced to the poor fertility of the barren mares (SPR: 77%; C/P: 2.63 [38%]). Once foaling mares predominate in April and May, fertility improves.

4. Intensively managed Thoroughbred mares are monitored such that ovulation is closely timed with breeding in an attempt to ensure that the mare is bred only once, close to ovulation, to minimize the number of times that a stallion will breed a mare during one estrous period. It is uncommon for an intensively managed Thoroughbred stallion to have more than 10% of estrous cycles in which mares will be bred more than once. Breeds in which AI is used will breed a mare more often when she is in estrus, because of the ease of doing so. Although AI allows the breeder to theoretically breed more mares with a single ejaculate, there are instances in which a popular stallion does not have sufficient sperm to accommodate all the mares that must be bred in a particular period. In most cases all mares will receive semen, but each inseminate will be a less-than-threshold level required for optimal fertility. The Thoroughbred industry appears to be able, in many cases, to breed similar numbers of mares and is able to do so by reducing the number of times the average

mare is bred during the estrous period compared with those breeds that use AI.

5. Fewer management systems involved in the breeding process. The widespread use of shipped and frozen semen has increased the number of individuals involved in the breeding of a mare and, therefore, fertility can be limited by the abilities of the weakest link. Prior to the use of shipped and frozen semen, most breeding operations had both the mares and stallion on the same farm under a common management or mares were shipped to the stallion. In either case the mares were bred with fresh sperm that was at the most only a few hours since ejaculation. Shipped and frozen semen has enabled more individuals to become involved in the breeding industry but has also resulted in the dilution of breeding expertise. In addition, the cooling and shipping or freezing of sperm has stretched the abilities of some stallion's sperm to remain at a level of fertility that accommodates commercial viability. Although these marginal stallions can be managed to be commercially fertile when fresh semen is used, their fertility may be dramatically reduced when the sperm is processed.

Artificial Insemination

Breeds that use AI have additional factors that influence overall fertility. For example, mares may be inseminated with *fresh semen* that is *inseminated immediately* after collection, with stallions and mares being managed on the same farm. Assuming good management, this method of artificial breeding is expected to result in the highest fertility. *Tailgate breeding* may also occur, in which case the mare is trailered to the farm, inseminated in the trailer, and immediately returned to the farm of origin. Since mares bred by tailgate breeding are under different management, pregnancy rates may be variable and sometimes lower than that achieved for mares managed at the farm where the stallion stands at stud. For mares bred with *transported cooled semen*, each mare is also under variable management. Additional factors that may adversely affect pregnancy rates when mares are bred with transported cooled semen are that insemination timing in relation to ovulation can be more variable, and some stallions do not achieve the same level of fertility with cooled semen as with fresh semen. Pregnancy rates achieved with *frozen semen* tend to be substantially lower for most stallions than they can achieve with fresh or cooled semen inseminations. Therefore, in addition to those factors outlined for evaluation of the Thoroughbred breeding operation, additional parameters must be considered when evaluating fertility achieved by a stallion used for AI.

Insemination dose tends to vary considerably in AI programs throughout the breeding season because of the variation in the number of mares bred on any particular day. Because of this phenomenon, the effect of insemination dose on fertility can be displayed graphically (see Fig. 26-1). Historically, the "threshold dose" of sperm required to "maximize fertility" is reported to be 500 million progressively motile sperm. In reality this threshold varies considerably with the stallion and may range from as low as 5 million if the deep-horn insemination technique is used to over a billion when stallions of lesser fertility are bred. This plotting technique allows the clinician to determine that threshold for the specific stallion of interest. The stallion in Fig. 26-1 had "good" fertility (50% per cycle) when bred with <400 million sperm, but "excellent" fertility (65% per cycle) when bred with >400 million sperm.

The evaluation of breeding records is an integral part of the stallion breeding soundness evaluation. Although there are reductions in fertility that are solely stallion related, reduced fertility is often multifactorial (i.e., mare, management, and stallion); therefore, diagnosis and appropriate treatment and management can be attained only if all factors that influence fertility are critically evaluated. In addition, breeding records should be evaluated routinely, regardless of the fertility level, to monitor and identify areas of the breeding process that are successful as well as those in need of improvement.

REFERENCES

1. Kenney RM, Hurtgen JP, Pierson H, et al: Manual for clinical fertility evaluation of the stallion. Hastings, NE: Society for Theriogenology, 1983.
2. Love CC: The role of breeding record evaluation in the evaluation of the stallion for breeding soundness. Proc Annu Conf Soc Theriogenology, Columbus, OH, 2003, pp 68-77.
3. Love CC: Evaluation of breeding records. In *Manual of Equine Reproduction*, ed 2, St Louis, 2003, Mosby.

Significance of the Equine Genome for the Horse Industry

Doug F. Antczak

Over the past dozen years a consortium of veterinary geneticists and clinicians have worked together to advance knowledge of the genome of the horse. Participants in the Horse Genome Project from 22 laboratories in 12 countries collaborated to produce the initial linkage, physical, and comparative equine gene maps. This international cooperation has been essential to the success of the project. In early 2006 these efforts were given an enormous boost when the U.S. National Human Genome Research Institute of the National Institutes of Health added the horse to the list of mammalian species to be sequenced. Now, just 2 years later, a whole genome sequence of the horse has been produced and is available to researchers and clinicians worldwide in public DNA databases. The explosion in information about the equine genome has already produced important new diagnostic tests for inherited diseases that can be used clinically to eliminate genetically determined conditions through selective breeding. The future will no doubt bring even more rapid advances in genetic-based technologies that will have the power to transform traditional horse-breeding practices. This will lead to more interactions between geneticists and horse breeders who have the shared goal of "improving the breed."

STATUS OF THE EQUINE GENOME AND GENOMIC RESOURCES

Characterization of the genome of the horse has progressed rapidly from a state <20 years ago, when only a handful of equine genes had been sequenced and mapped, to the situation today, where virtually the entire genome sequence is available online. The speed at which the equine genome has been characterized has produced some technologies and research tools that have become obsolete as quickly as they have been developed and defined. This makes it challenging to create a summary of the state-of-the-art technology that will have a long duration.

Like the various types of maps that are available for geographic information, different experimental approaches have yielded information that provides complementary views of the genomic landscape of the horse. Furthermore, increasing levels of resolution provide ever more detailed information. The *linkage maps* of the horse based on polymorphic microsatellites[1,2] remain useful tools for mapping traits to chromosomes or to sub-chromosomal levels. Fine mapping and gene identification requires additional or alternative methods. *Physical maps* of many horse chromosomes have been produced, most from the research group at Texas A&M University (reviewed in Chowdhary and Raudsepp[3]). These include highly detailed maps of the equine X and Y chromosomes.[4,5] *Comparative maps* made across genomes provide reference points and identify conserved chromosomal regions. So-called chromosome painting has been very informative in these studies. This technique uses fluorescently labeled gene probes from individual chromosomes or chromosome arms in hybridization experiments using chromosome smears from the same species used to generate the probes, or from different species. In the case of the horse, a high degree of conservation of gene content has been demonstrated between human and horse chromosomes.[6,7] This has been very useful in predicting gene content and even gene order on individual horse chromosomes.

The U.S. Government–sponsored whole genome sequencing of the horse can be justified on the basis of the comparative genomic information obtained that will help decipher the secrets of the human genome. However, the benefits to the horse may be even more important. The whole genome sequencing effort undertaken at MIT's Broad Institute produced a 6.8× coverage of the equine genome. On average, every section of DNA from the donor horse was sequenced 6.8 times. Some parts of the genome are more difficult to sequence than others, such as the genes of the immune system that are highly polymorphic, contain duplicated genes, and have many DNA repeat sequences. Overall, a 6.8× coverage of the equine genome means that about 85%–90% of the donor horse's DNA has been determined. This is still a very high level of coverage compared with most mammals that have been sequenced, with the exception of humans and mice. The raw sequence data must be assembled into the order found on the chromosomes, and annotated, so that the 20,000+ genes of the horse can be named using a nomenclature system that is consistent with that used in other mammals. The assembly and annotation processes are very large and complex tasks, and refinements will continue for several years to come. We know that the horse genome contains about 2.68 billion base pairs that are spread across 31 autosomes and the sex chromosomes. The overall polymorphism rate of 1/1500 base pairs in the equine genome has been estimated. Several relevant websites that contain information about the Horse Genome Project and the equine genome are listed in Box 27-1.

CHARACTERIZATION OF INHERITED DISEASES OF THE HORSE

Compared with humans, dogs, and cats, there have been relatively few inherited diseases identified in horses, and mutations are known for only eight (Table 27-1, reviewed in Finno et al.[8]). This makes the horse more like the other livestock species, where selection for production or performance traits seems to have had a beneficial effect on overall genetic makeup. However, among the few genetically determined equine diseases identified thus

Box 27-1 | **Websites Relevant to Horse Genetics**

Horse Genome Project (HGP) University of Kentucky	http://www.uky.edu/Ag/Horsemap/
Horse Genome Resources (NIH)	http://www.ncbi.nlm.nih.gov/genome/guide/horse/
Horse Genome Project (NIH)	http://www.ncbi.nlm.nih.gov/sites/entrez?db=genomeprj&cmd=Retrieve&dopt=Overview&list_uids=11760
Horse Genome Browser Gateway (University of California Santa Cruz)	http://genome.ucsc.edu/cgi-bin/hgGateway
Ensembl Horse Database	http://www.ensembl.org/Equus_caballus/index.html
Horse Genome Project (MIT Broad Institute)	http://www.broad.mit.edu/mammals/horse/
Horsemap Database (France)	http://locus.jouy.inra.fr/cgi-bin/lgbc/mapping/common/intro2.pl?BASE=horse
Horse Genome Project Bacterial Artificial Chromosome Resource (Hannover, Germany)	http://www.tiho-hannover.de/einricht/zucht/hgp/index.htm
Veterinary Genetics Laboratory—Horse Tests (University of California Davis)	http://www.vgl.ucdavis.edu/services/horse.php
VetGen Corp. (commercial genetic testing company)	http://www.vetgen.com/

Table 27-1 | **Inherited Diseases of the Horse with Known Genetic Mutations**

CONDITION	ABBREVIATION	AFFECTED BREED(S)	MODE OF INHERITANCE
Severe combined immunodeficiency disease[9]	SCID	Arabian	Autosomal recessive
Hyperkalemic periodic paralysis[10]	HYPP	Quarter Horses and QH crosses	Autosomal dominant
Overo lethal white syndrome[11,12]	OLWS	Primarily Paint horses	Autosomal recessive
Hereditary equine regional dermal asthenia[13]	HERDA	Quarter Horses and QH crosses	Autosomal recessive
Glycogen branching enzyme deficiency[14]	GBED	Quarter Horses, Paint horses	Autosomal recessive
Polysaccharide storage myopathy[15]	PSSM	Quarter Horses, Paint horses, Appaloosas, Warmbloods, and draft breeds	Autosomal dominant
Junctional epidermolysis bullosa[16]	JEB	Belgian, other draft breeds, American Saddlebred	Autosomal recessive
Malignant hyperthermia[17]	MH	Quarter Horses	Autosomal dominant

far are some that are of significance in the affected breeds and widely known among horsemen. These include severe combined immunodeficiency disease (SCID) in Arabians, hyperkalemic periodic paralysis (HYPP) of Quarter Horses, the lethal white syndrome of frame overo Paint horses, and hereditary equine regional dermal asthenia (HERDA) in Quarter Horses.

Although these inherited diseases in general do not have negative influences on fertility, they can affect breeding strategies. Breed organizations can require genetic testing and identification of heterozygous carriers for autosomal recessive conditions, and prospective buyers can request the results of genetic tests for specific diseases before purchasing a horse. At least two laboratories offer commercial genetic testing for a limited number of inherited equine diseases (see Table 27-1). For autosomal recessive conditions, one breeding strategy is to avoid carrier-to-carrier matings. This will eliminate affected animals from the population, but it will not eliminate the deleterious mutation from the breed. A more stringent approach would be to ban from breeding affected animals carrying autosomal dominant traits or carriers of autosomal recessive traits. Both of these strategies limit the possible mating pairs within the breeding population and, therefore, require greater care and skill in reproductive management. Horses have

been selected for speed, size, coat color, and athletic ability, but seldom has fertility been a major consideration.

CHROMOSOMAL ABNORMALITIES AND INFERTILITY

Beginning in the 1970s, cytogeneticists began to describe equine chromosome abnormalities that were often associated with infertility. These included XY and XX sex reversal, X chromosome monosomy, Y chromosome disomy, and sex chromosome mosaicism. Improved chromosome banding techniques later led to the identification of autosomal deletions, autosomal trisomy, and most recently, autosomal translocations (reviewed in Lear and Bailey[18]). The molecular resources and tools of the Horse Genome Project have added to the traditional techniques based upon banding patterns. In particular, the chromosome painting technique described previously and the use of bacterial artificial chromosome (BAC) probes in fluorescent *in situ* hybridization have greatly increased the sensitivity and specificity of investigations of autosomal translocations.[19,20] Breakpoints identified using molecular approaches were at the fusion boundary of human chromosomes 10 and 15 on horse chromosome 1 and at human chromosome 3p and 3q on horse chromosome 16.[20] Thus, these breakpoints used in the evolution of the equids may be fragile sites and more likely to lead to further rearrangements. Importantly, autosomal translocations can result in reduced fertility, with some meiotic segregations leading to normal zygotes, and others resulting in embryonic lethals.[20] This possibility should alert equine reproductive specialists to consider chromosomal abnormalities in their differential diagnoses in horses with reduced fertility.

PROSPECTS FOR THE FUTURE

A number of equine diseases suspected of having a simple genetic basis remain to be solved. These include lavender foal syndrome, Fell Pony immunodeficiency, cerebellar abiotrophy, recurrent exertional rhabdomyolysis, and degenerative suspensory ligament desmitis. It is also likely that additional conditions caused by single-gene mutations will be identified as awareness of the importance of genetic determinants of disease increases among equine practitioners. Great challenges are still before us in the area of complex diseases and traits that result from gene–environment or gene–gene interactions. For example, recurrent airway obstruction (heaves), insect bite hypersensitivity, and the skin tumor sarcoid, are known to have both genetic and environmental components.[21-23] A whole genome scan using microsatellites has identified a quantitative trait locus on horse chromosome 4 that contributes to osteochondritis dissecans in fetlock joints.[24] Conformation and performance are multigenic traits that are also strongly influenced by environment. The genes influencing many complex diseases often result in increased risk for an individual in developing the condition. However, because there is often an associated environmental trigger, not all susceptible individuals develop disease. This makes the development of control strategies for complex diseases based on selective breeding very complicated.

Addressing these challenges will require application of the new molecular tools of the Horse Genome Project. Single nucleotide polymorphism (SNP) DNA arrays (commonly referred to as SNP Chips) permit evaluation of genetic variation across the entire genome in single tests, and furthermore facilitate dissection and identification of different forms of complex diseases.[25] A 60,000 equine SNP chip has been produced in early 2008 and is now undergoing evaluation before release to the equine research community.

Expression microarrays allow evaluation of gene expression from thousands of genes in isolated cells or tissues. Thus far the only reports of horse-specific microarrays have used an expression array containing about 3000 gene probes.[26] However, newer iterations of the equine expression array containing many more genes are in various stages of development and testing, and it is likely that expression arrays containing all of the 20,000+ horse genes will be available commercially by 2009. These expression arrays should find wide application in many areas of equine medicine and surgery. For example, they can be used to identify changes in gene expression in equine joint disease that may lead to improved therapeutics.

The Horse Genome Project has spawned the development of important new tools for the veterinary geneticist, and benefits have already begun to accrue to the equine industry from genetic studies of the horse. The elimination of specific undesirable traits from horse breeds using selection based on molecular biology is taking place now. Advances in DNA sequencing speed and increased cost-effectiveness of testing hold the promise for new applications that could address more challenging goals. Will horsemen be able to harness the information in the genome to breed sounder, more durable horses? In today's world of rapidly advancing technology, the possibilities seem limited only by our imagination.

REFERENCES

1. Guérin G, Bailey E, Bernoco D, et al: Report of the International Equine Gene Mapping Workshop: Male Linkage Map. *Anim Genet* 30:341, 1999.
2. Swinburne J, Gerstenberg C, Breen M, et al: First comprehensive low-density horse linkage map based on two 3-generation, full-sibling, cross-bred horse reference families. *Genomics* 66:123, 2000.
3. Chowdhary BP, Raudsepp T: The horse genome derby: racing from map to whole genome sequence. *Chromosome Res* 16:109, 2008.
4. Raudsepp T, Lee EJ, Kata SR, et al: Exceptional conservation of horse-human gene order on X chromosome revealed by high-resolution radiation hybrid mapping. *Proc Natl Acad Sci U S A* 101:2386, 2004.
5. Raudsepp T, Santani A, Wallner B, et al: A detailed physical map of the horse Y chromosome. *Proc Natl Acad Sci U S A* 101:9321, 2004.
6. Raudsepp T, Frönicke L, Scherthan H, et al: Zoo-FISH delineates conserved chromosomal segments in horse and man. *Chromosome Res* 4:218, 1996.
7. Yang F, Fu B, O'Brien PC, et al: Refined genome-wide comparative map of the domestic horse, donkey and human based on cross-species chromosome painting: insight into the occasional fertility of mules. *Chromosome Res* 12:65, 2004.
8. Finno CJ, Spier SJ, Valberg SJ: Equine diseases caused by known genetic mutations. *Vet J* May 8 [Epub ahead of print], 2008.
9. Wiler R, Leber R, Moore BB, et al: Equine severe combined immunodeficiency: A defect in V(D)J recombination and DNA-dependent protein kinase activity. *Proc Nat Acad Sci USA* 92:11485, 1995.
10. Rudolph A, Spier SJ, Byrns G, et al: Periodic paralysis in Quarter Horses: a sodium channel mutation disseminated by selective breeding. *Nat Genet* 2:144, 1992.
11. Metallinos DL, Bowling AT, Rine J: A missense mutation in the endothelin-B receptor gene is associated with lethal white foal syndrome: an equine version of Hirschsprung disease. *Mamm Genome* 9:426, 1998.
12. Santschi EM, Purdy AK, Valberg SJ, et al: Endothelin receptor B polymorphism associated with lethal white foal syndrome in horses. *Mamm Genome* 9:306, 1998.
13. Tryon RC, White SD, Bannasch DL: Homozygosity mapping approach identifies a missense mutation in equine cyclophilin B (PPIB) associated with HERDA in the American Quarter Horse. *Genomics* 90:93, 2007.
14. Ward TL, Valberg SJ, Adelson DL, et al: Glycogen branching enzyme (GBE1) mutation causing equine glycogen storage disease IV. *Mamm Genome* 15:570, 2004.
15. McCue ME, Valberg SJ, Miller MB, et al: Glycogen synthase (GYS1) mutation causes a novel skeletal muscle glycogenosis. *Genomics* 91:458, 2008.
16. Spirito F, Charlesworth A, Linder K, et al: Animal models for skin blistering conditions: absence of laminin 5 causes hereditary junctional mechanobullous disease in the Belgian horse. *J Invest Dermatol* 119:684, 2002.
17. Aleman M, Riehl J, Aldridge BM, et al: Association of a mutation in the ryanodine receptor 1 gene with equine malignant hyperthermia. *Muscle Nerve* 30:356, 2004.
18. Lear TL, Bailey E: Equine clinical cytogenetics: the past and future. *Cytogenet Genome Res* 120:42, 2008.
19. Lear TL, Layton G: Use of zoo-FISH to characterise a reciprocal translocation in a Thoroughbred mare: t(1;16)(q16;q21.3). *Equine Vet J* 34:207, 2002.
20. Lear TL, Lundquist J, Zent WW, et al: Three autosomal chromosome translocations associated with repeated early embryonic loss (REEL) in the domestic horse *(Equus caballus)*. *Cytogenet Genome Res* 120:117, 2008.
21. Marti E, Gerber H, Essich G, et al: On the genetic basis of equine allergic diseases. I. Chronic hypersensitivity bronchitis. *Eq Vet J* 23:457, 1991.

22. Marti E, Gerber H, Lazary, S: On the genetic basis of equine allergic diseases. II. Insect bite dermal hypersensitivity. *Eq Vet J* 24:113, 1992.

23. Lazary S, Gerber H, Glatt, PA, et al: Equine leucocyte antigens in sarcoid affected horses. *Eq Vet J* 17:283, 1985.

24. Wittwer C, Dierks C, Hamann H, et al: Associations between candidate gene markers at a quantitative trait locus on equine chromosome 4 responsible for osteochondrosis dissecans in fetlock joints of South German Coldblood horses. *J Hered* 99:125, 2008.

25. Antoniou AC, Spurdle AB, Sinilnikova OM, et al: Common breast cancer-predisposition alleles are associated with breast cancer risk in BRCA1 and BRCA2 mutation carriers. *Am J Hum Genet* 82:937, 2008.

26. Gu W, Bertone AL: Generation and performance of an equine-specific large-scale gene expression microarray. *Am J Vet Res* 65:1664, 2004.

Page numbers followed by f indicate figures; t, tables; b, boxes.